Atlas of Heart Anatomy and Development

Florin Mihail Filipoiu

Atlas of Heart Anatomy and Development

Springer

Florin Mihail Filipoiu, PhD, MD
Anatomy Department
University of Medicine and Pharmacy
Carol Davila
Bucharest
Romania

Previously published in Romanian by Editura Prior & Books as *Cordul: Anatomie, repere embriologice si notiuni de infrastructura a miocardului - Atlas explicitat si comentat* by Florin Mihail Filipoiu, [2012], ISBN 978-6-0692-5063-1

ISBN 978-1-4471-7246-8 ISBN 978-1-4471-5382-5 (eBook)
DOI 10.1007/978-1-4471-5382-5
Springer London Heidelberg New York Dordrecht

Printed on acid-free paper

Springer is part of Springer Science+Business Media (www.springer.com)

Preface

To write a book utilizing the extraordinary sources of information, which so many people have access to, seems to have over-simplified our field. Perhaps, this is the way it should be. However, it is my sincere belief that when one purchases a book, one must choose wisely as it will influence their future. The method of how a book is written will influence your professional development.

Beyond the abundance of information lies the writer's style, belief and respect for the subject and his peers. Basic information can be useful; however when combined with love, experience and "savoire faire", it actually shapes the readers.

The development of this book took over 8 years. During this time, several times per week, side-by-side with my assistants and a few enthusiastic students, we would spend hours in the dissection laboratory. In the beginning, I did not wear glasses – however during this time, my prescription doubled. My assistants went from being single to having children of their own who now attend school. It took us over a year to realize what we did not know and subsequently rediscovered structure by structure.

I discovered the phenomenal history of how anatomical structures were initially described. I read about anatomists who are no longer even mentioned; however their contribution to our profession has been so powerful that they deserve to be recognized with statues. I have compared opposite theories about the same structure and have supported those scientists that were ignored by the contemporaries of their time. After a few years of this research, I was able to develop a macro view. Ontogenesis and the cardiac anatomy were intertwined and supplemented admirably. After a while, we began to view information based on its clinical utility. Subsequently, we commenced to form our own opinions which developed into theory.

I reached a profound moment when I was able to describe the myocardial architecture, through the prism of biological utility and clinical function. It was like winning the World Cup – only for me, it happened to be while I was alone, in front of my computer, late at night. The hardest part was assembling my thoughts and ultimately my conclusions in a final product. The difficulty of the editing process, however, was mitigated by virtue of the people that I worked with. Along with my team-mates, I actually learned a new skill. I sincerely thank them for their support and dedication. Towards the end, honestly, I even asked myself if all this time and effort was worth it. I discovered that it was actually hard to be sincere with myself. I immediately decided that I had to be sincere with you, my readers.

To write a book that has taken such a long time to put together and that required significant resources and energy is something that is very difficult to recommend embarking upon. However, to experience the creation of intellectual capacity and the unparalleled feeling of elation is something that is reserved for the souls of aristocrats. In the end, it is all a matter of self-reflection.

This book is dedicated to my children, Zoran and Serena, my niece Sabina and my parents. A special thank you to my wife, Mirela, who has taught me the extraordinary lessons of will power, ideals and priorities.

Bucharest, Romania

Florin Mihail Filipoiu, PhD, MD

Contents

The General Development Period

1

1.1 The General Development Period [1, 2]

During this period, the developing heart goes through several developing phases; they shall be named according to each dominant stage.

1.1.1 The Germ Disk Stage

In the 18th and 19th day, the developing embryo is found in the trilaminar germ disk stage, with the following composing part:

- The ectodermal tissue that exhibits the primitive streak on its dorsal surface (a central sulcus lying longitudinally) along side which the right to left symmetry is orientated.
- the mesodermal tissue
- the endodermal tissue

The trilaminar germ disk is flanked by the amniotic cavity and the yolk sac.

1.1.2 The Formation of the Endocardial Tubes

(A) *The differentiation of the cardiogenic area* (the cardiogenic mesoderm) is created as a meshing of the mesoderm into the cephalic end of the germ disk with the mesoderm located above the *prechordal plate* (the future *oropharyngeal membrane*)

(B) *The formation of the two tubes* takes place as follows:

- The cardiogenic mesoderm wraps around the upper end of the neural plate – as a right and left cardiogenic mesodermal plane (the primary cardiogenic fields) [3]. A transversal section performed here shows that groups of cardiogenic angioblastic cells are found along each side of the lateral mesoderm of the germ disk. These two cellular groups form two full cords which immediately tunnel creating the right and left endocardial tubes.

In the germ disk there are multiple movements of the various cellular groups. The developing embryo undergoes folding movements in a transversal and longitudinal direction while other cells undergo the so called process of descensus.

The embryonic movements are not self initiated but they result from the cellular multiplication, differentiation and variable growth rates of the neighboring regions.

1.1.3 The Primitive Heart Tube Formation

This formation process occurs on the 22nd day, by the median merging of the two tubes and the transversal folding of the embryonic disk.

As the embryonic transversal folding occurs, the two endocardial tubes move closer. A fusing process follows that creates the primitive heart tube found in the ventral mesentery of the primitive gut.

This tube has a dorsal connection with the anterior portion of the primitive gut and is attached to the walls of the future pericardial cavity by groups of cells that form the dorsal mesocardium, the ventral mesocardium (this structure quickly disappears), the arterial and venous mesocardium (Fig. 1.1).

The endocardium develops from the primitive cardiac tube. The adjacent mesoderm called the mioepicardic plate, gives rise to the developing myocardium and epicardium. Between the endocardium and the plate there is a new structure called the cardiac jelly which is invaded by endocardiac cells and leads to the formation of the cardioglia (Figs. 1.2 and 1.3).

The cardiac jelly contains about 50 proteins, such as: collagen, fibronectin, fibrillin, fibulin and growth factors [4].

F.M. Filipoiu, *Atlas of Heart Anatomy and Development*,
DOI 10.1007/978-1-4471-5382-5_1, © Springer-Verlag London 2014

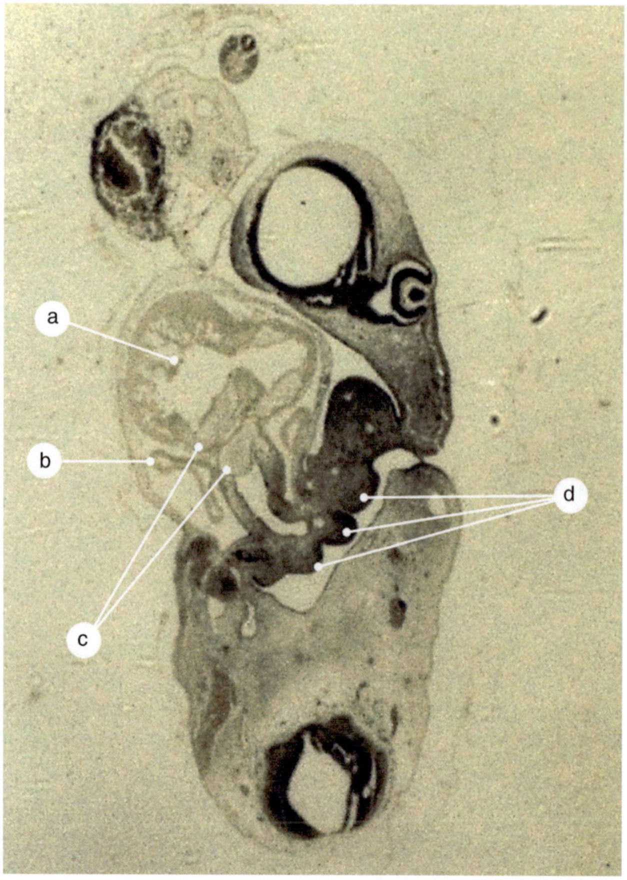

Fig. 1.1 Arterial mesocardium represented by the truncus arteriosus and branchial arches region junction. *a* Primitive ventricle, *b* right atrium, *c* endocardial crests in the truncus arteriosus, *d* branchial arches region

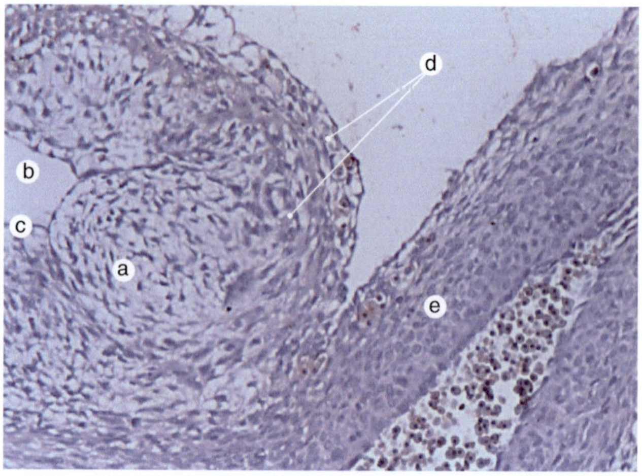

Fig. 1.2 Myoepicardial plate and cardioglia. *a* Cardioglia, *b* ventricle, *c* endocardium, *d* myoepicardial plate, *e* truncus arteriosus

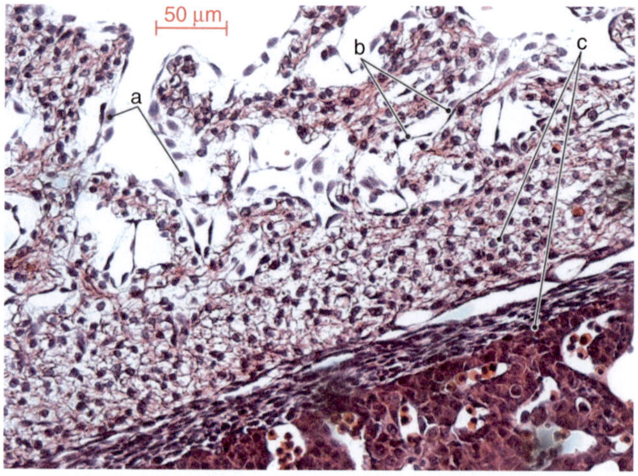

Fig. 1.3 Myoepicardial plate and endocardium. *a* Blood cells in the ventricular cavity organized by the contact with the endocardium, *b* endocardium, *c* myoepicardial plate

1.1.4 The Formation of the Cardiac Prominence

The cardiac prominence becomes structured in the following way: the transversal folding movement occurs simultaneously with the longitudinal folding of the germ disk. The primitive cardiac tube location lies on the ventral side of the embryonic body, inferior to the stomodeum in the future cervical region. The cells proliferate and differentiate, creating the endocardial prominence. This prominence lies superiorly to the transverse septum and the vitelline sac. A more correct terminology is the hepatocardiac prominence (Fig. 1.4)

Between the heart and hepatic primordium lies the transverse septum, a large area of "embryologic unrest" which influences the hepatic and cardiac development.

Throughout the development stage, the heart undergoes a process of *descensus*. More precisely, the heart descends from the cervical to the thoracic area, above the diaphragm (already differentiated from the septum transversum). This process is not considered a cardiac descending as much as a growth at different speeds of the neighboring regions (*pseudodescensus*). On the 23rd day the first inefficient (arrhythmic) contractions occur with progression to the 28th day when they become rhythmic and efficient.

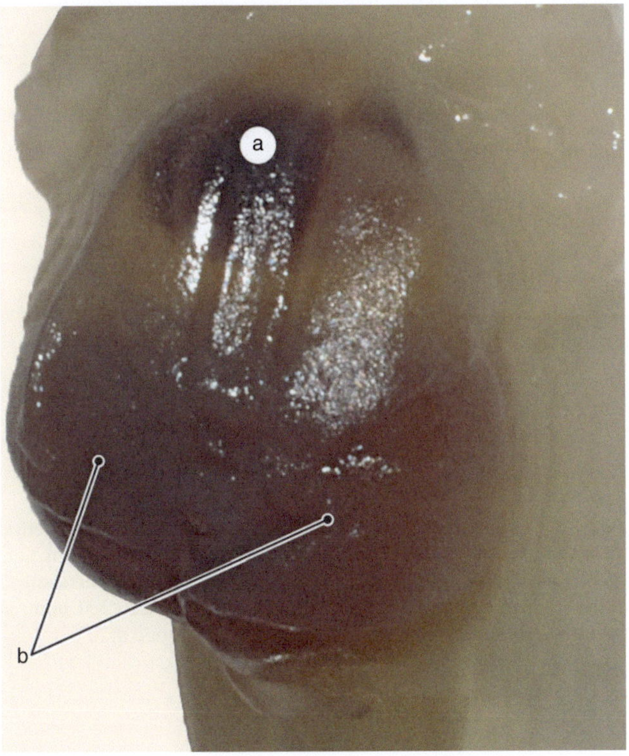

Fig. 1.4 Hepatocardiac bulge. *a* Cardiac bulge, *b* hepatic bulge

1.1.5 The Stage of Linear Cardiac Tube

As a result of the different types of movements and due to the disappearance of the ventral mesocardium, the cardiac tube remains fixed at the extremities, superior through the arterial mesocardium and inferior through the venous mesocardium (including the sinus venosus). The sinus is fixed to the transverse septum. Actually the horns of the sinus arise from the transverse septum and connect above it. The mesocardial sinus covers the space between the two horns and continues posteriorly with the dorsal mesocardium, tying the atrium and sinus venosus to the primitive gut (Figs. 1.5 and 1.6).

Immediately superior to the sinus venosus, the walls of the primitive atrium reflect posteriorly, between the leaflets of the dorsal mesocardium, creating the atrio (myocardial)-mesodermal junction. The junction is therefore created between the cardiac mesoderm and the mesoderm lying anterior to the primitive gut [5] (Fig. 1.7)

This junction is a true *mesodermal pedicle* of the primitive atrium, covered on its exterior by the dorsal mesocardium.

The dorsal mesocardium disappears posteriorly from the cardiac tube. Its inferior segment remains and covers the mesodermal pedicle. A thin band of embryonic tissue called the mesocardial taenia (Fig. 1.8) will point for a short duration to the insertion of the mesocardium on the cardiac tube.

The myocardial-mesodermal junction has a central depression called the *pulmonary facet*, where the primitive pulmonary vein will attach to the primitive atrial wall.

The mesodermal pedicle is the location where the extracardiac mesoderm can migrate into the myocardial mass (Fig. 1.9).

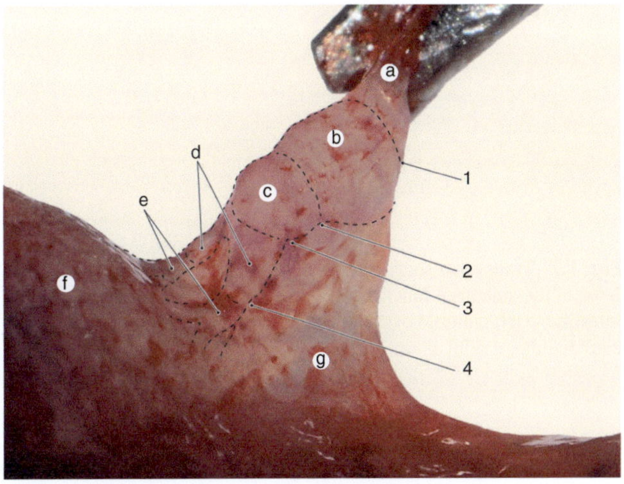

Fig. 1.5 Primitive cardiac tube with dorsal mesocardium – lateral view. *a* Dorsal aortae, *b* aortic bulb, *c* primitive bulb, *d* primitive ventricle, *e* primitive atrium, *f* septum transversum, *g* dorsal mesocardium undergoing reduction, *1* bulbo-aortic sulcus, *2* interbulbar sulcus, *3* bulboventricular sulcus, *4* atrioventricular sulcus

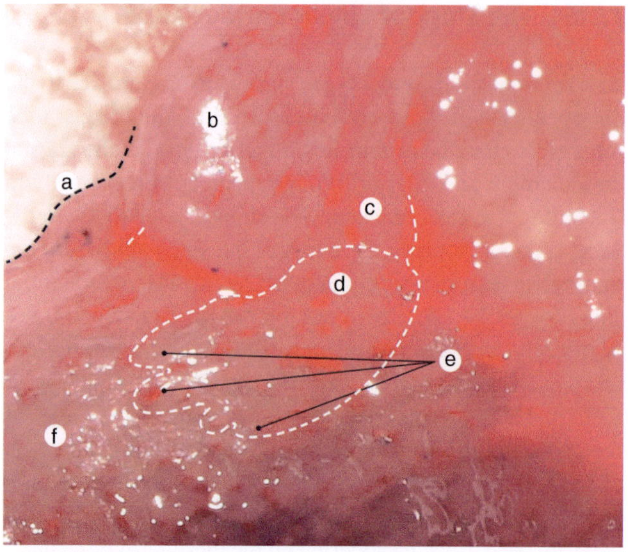

Fig. 1.6 Septum transversum with sinus horns, detail. Left anterolateral view. *a* Right primitive ventricle, *b* primitive bulbus, *c* left primitive ventricle, *d* left primitive atrium, *e* sinus tributaries, *f* septum transversum

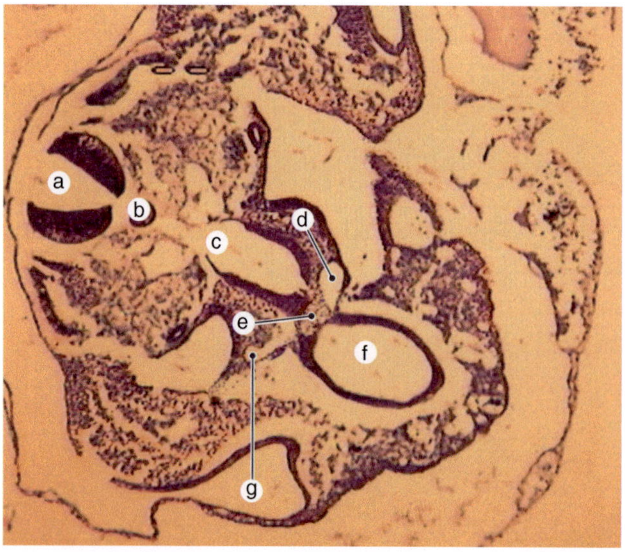

Fig. 1.7 Transverse section through the primitive cardiac tube at the level of the sinoatrial junction. *a* Neural tube, *b* notochord, *c* primitive intestine, *d* left sinusal horn, *e* dorsal mesocardium taenia, *f* endocardial cardiac tube, *g* right sinusal horn

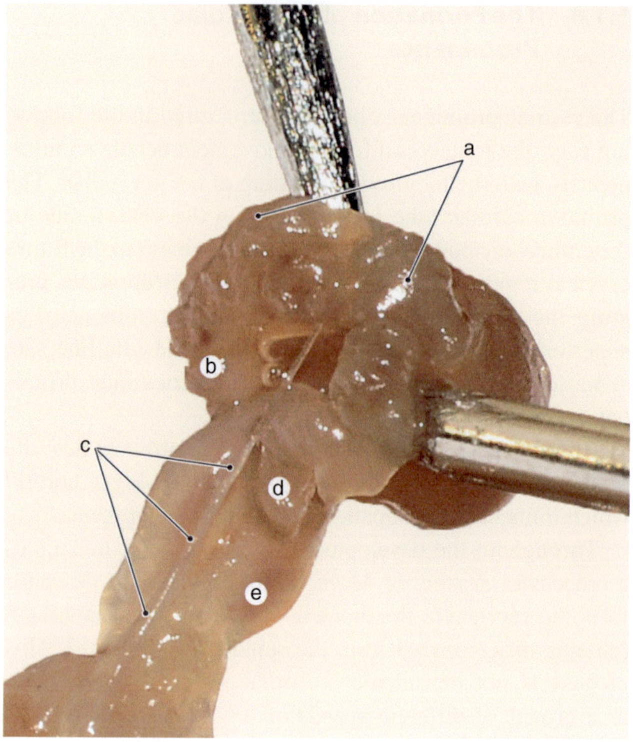

Fig. 1.8 Taenia mesocardica. *a* Primitive atrium, *b* right auricle, *c* taenia mesocardica, *d* left auricle, *e* reversed arterial pedicle

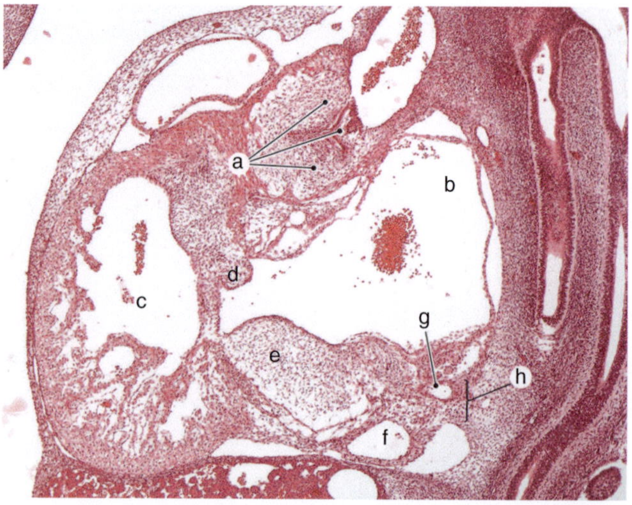

Fig. 1.9 Migration of extracadiac dorsal mesoderm into the inferior endocardial cushion and formation of the pulmonary vein. *a* Formation of the aortic valves, *b* left atrium, *c* left ventricle, *d* superior endocardial cushion, *e* inferior endocardial cushion, *f* sinus venosus left horn, *g* primitive pulmonary vein, *h* extracardiac dorsal mesoderm

This migration is known in literature as the "*dorsal extracardiac mesoderm protrusion in the atrial wall*". The mesodermal myocardial junction takes the shape of a horseshoe around the pulmonary facet with the inferior concavity towards the atrial wall. As a result along both sides of the mesodermal pedicle, the atrial cavity is populated by two cellular masses conventionally called the *right and left pulmonary edges* (Fig. 2.11).

These edges are located postero-superiorly to the atrial opening of the primitive pulmonary vein [6].

The migration (protrusion) of the dorsal extracardiac mesoderm towards the atrial wall is an important step in the progression of atrial septation and development. The alteration of the mesodermal protrusion is followed by defects in atrial septation and even in deficits of the intermediate septum formation.

- Lying in the developing cardiac wall are different types of extracardiac cells:
- Neural crest cells can migrate to the heart through brachial arches, the arterial pedicle or through the dorsal mesocardium;
- cells developed from the dorsal mesenchyme;
- epicardial cells;
- angioblast cells.

The primitive cardiac tube has a relatively straight shape, with a superior part that continues with the two *dorsal aortae* and an inferior part called the *sinus venosus*. The sinus has two extensions called the left and right horns which end in three pairs of veins: the vitelline, umbilical and common cardinal veins.

During this phase, the cardiac tube is composed of many segments (dilated areas) [7]: the aortic bulb (sac), the bulbus cordis (its distal part will arise into the truncus arteriosus), primitive ventricle, primitive atrium and sinus venosus (Fig. 1.10).

From the moment the cardiac tube is formed, nature takes its course of admirably solving a very difficult problem: how to effectively create an entry and exit point from a relatively straight cardiac tube, to create a four chamber organ with six large entry vessels and two exit vessels… This highly successful story is not completely known or understood today, we are still at an initial phase of studying the major development phases. The key to these mechanisms is in a biochemical, molecular and genetic realm.

After the formation process, the looping stage occurs, followed by the torsion and differentiation of the cardiac tube- a process that has two stages. Please note the cardiac folding is not a simple occurrence, but a complex repositioning and a dimensional modification of the cardiac tube segments. Further, the changes occur at different speeds and rhythms corresponding to the various regions.

There is a permanent constant process of cellular differentiation and proliferation, as well as structural alterations resulting from the apoptosis process.

The simple cardiac tube looping produces identical changes on both sides of the looped tube. On the internal aspect, the looping could even lead to lumen stenosis, a process that obviously does not occur.

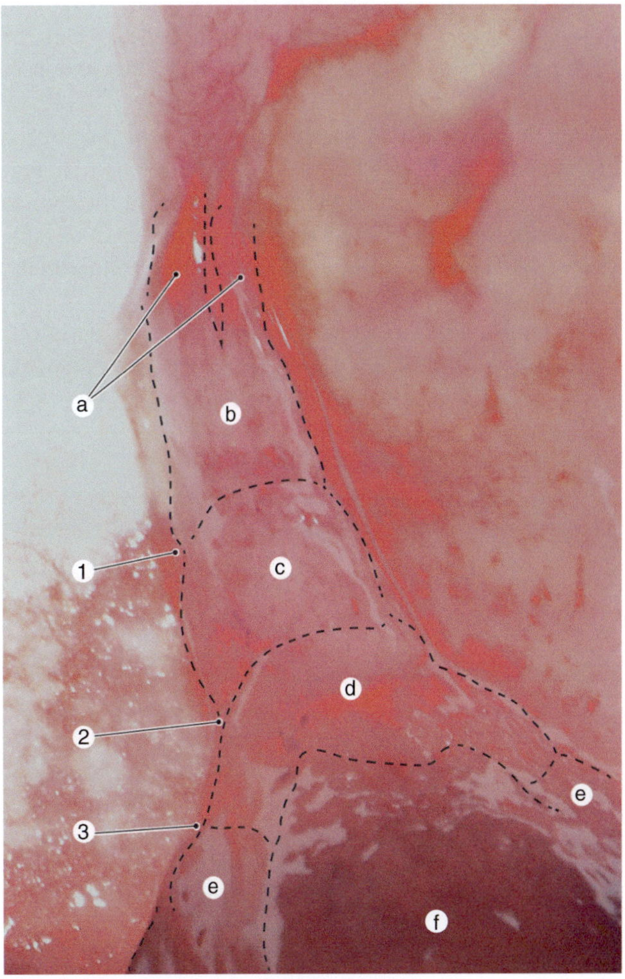

Fig. 1.10 Straight primitive cardiac tube. *a* Dorsal aortae, *b* aortic bulbus, *c* primitive bulbus, *d* primitive ventricle, *e* primitive atria continuing the future sinusal horns, *f* septum transversum, *1* interbulbar sulcus, *2* bulboventricular sulcus, *3* atrioventricular sulcus

1.1.6 The Cardiac Loop Stage (The "U" Shaped Heart)

The transformation process from a rectangular tube into a looped tube occurs such that the entrance of the cardiac tube remains posteriorly and superiorly oriented. The middle ventricular region forms the inferior concavity and the rear aspect of the cardiac tube arrives by the entrance part, anteriorly located and slightly to the right.

More precisely, the conotruncal junction (to be described below) will be found anterior to the atrioventricular junction (Fig. 1.11a, b)

Between the cavities narrow sulci appear, called atrioventricular sulcus (future atrioventricular junction), bulboventricular sulcus (future interventricular sulcus) and the conoventricular sulcus (located between the future trabecular aspect of the right ventricle and conus) (Fig. 1.11a, b).

During this stage, the cardiac tube's growth is marked by the important dilatation (ballooning) of the ventricular segment. As a result, the general arrangement of the cardiac tube appears with a single loop (the concave part towards the right superior aspect), making its shape similar to the letter "U" (Figs. 1.12, 1.13 and 1.14)

The ballooning process has a major contribution to the development of the future sternocostal and diaphragmatic aspects of the heart and also towards the future right ventricle.

The outer areas of these regions grow at a higher rate, in comparison to the atrioventricular canal. The size differences lead to understanding the septation process.

The sinus venosus will be fixed in a postero- inferior position to the level of septum transversus (Fig. 1.15). The left sided tributaries decrease in size, as a result the right atrium's development predominates.

The looping of the primitive cardiac tube and the formation of the "U" shaped heart align the direction of the primitive atrium towards the left side. This creates a developmental asymmetry of the two atria.

The atrioventricular canal is found on the left side of the middle line, along the future left atrium, while the sinoatrial junction is found to the right of the middle line, on the posterior wall of the future right atrium. The primitive atrium extends as a transversal tube between these two structures [8].

The blood initially flows through the cardiac tube in this order: sinus venosus- right atrium- left atrium- atrioventricular canal- presumptive left ventricle- presumptive right ventricle- truncus arteriosus.

The heart loop is composed of an internal concave and an external convex side. The ventricular development begins by the intense ballooning of the ventricular region along the convex side. On the internal side, which is slower in development, the bulboventricular sulcus starts to form and distally nearby the conoventricular sulcus also becomes visible. The two sulci superimpose forming the conoventricular fold (Fig. 1.11b).

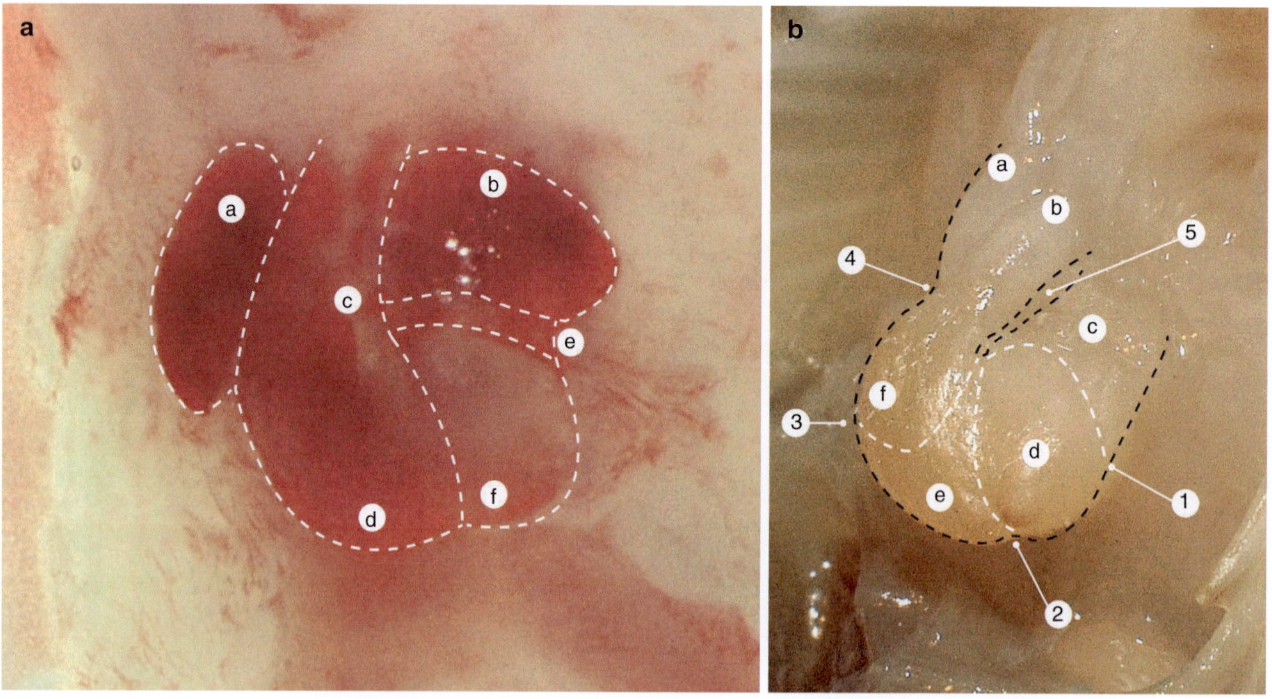

Fig. 1.11 (**a**) Conotruncal junction overlaying the atrioventricular sulcus. *a* Right auricle, *b* left auricle, *c* conotruncal junction, *d* right ventricle, *e* atrioventricular sulcus, *f* left ventricle. (**b**) Highlighting of the conoventricular fold. *a* Aorta, *b* pulmonary trunk, *c* atrioventricular junction, *d* future left ventricle, *e* future trabeculated part of the right ventricle, *f* conus region, *1* Atrioventricular limit, *2* bulboventricular sulcus, *3* conoventricular limit, *4* sinotubular junction, *5* conoventricular fold

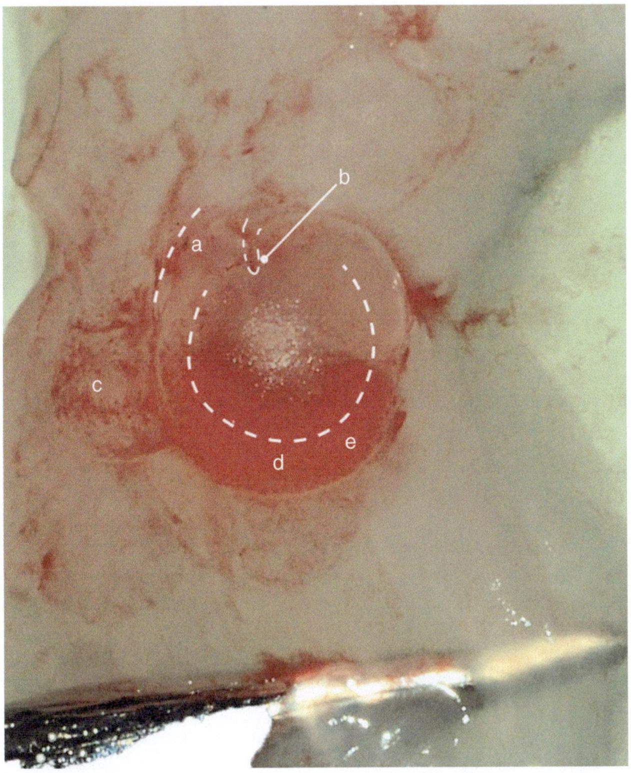

Fig. 1.12 "U"-shaped heart. *a* Truncus arteriosus, *b* bulboventricular fold, *c* right auricle, *d* future right ventricle, *e* future left ventricle

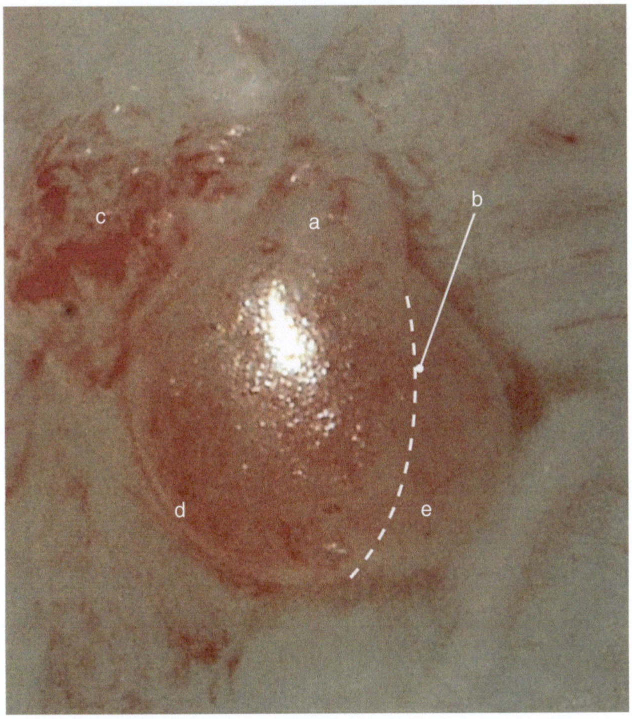

Fig. 1.13 "U"-shaped heart. *a* Truncus arteriosus, *b* bulboventricular sulcus, *c* right auricle, *d* right ventricle, *e* left ventricle

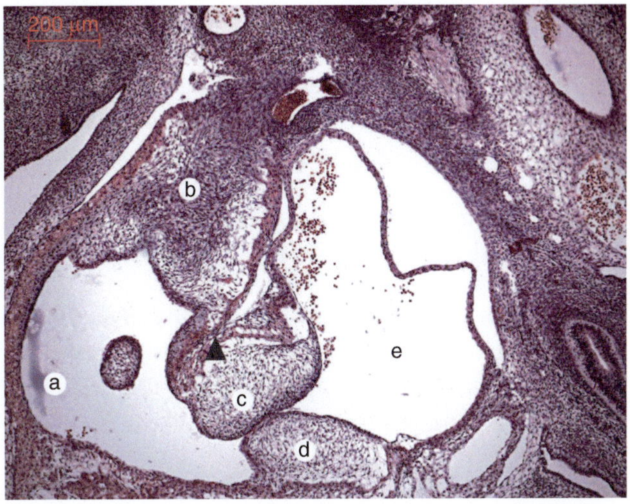

Fig. 1.14 "U"-shaped heart. Endocardial cushions at the level of the atrioventricular junction and truncus arteriosus. The *arrowhead* indicates the conoventricular fold. *a* Primitive ventricle, *b* spiral septum in the truncus arteriosus lumen rezulting from the fusion of the endocardial crests, *c* superior endocardial cushion, *d* inferior endocardial cushion, *e* primitive atrium

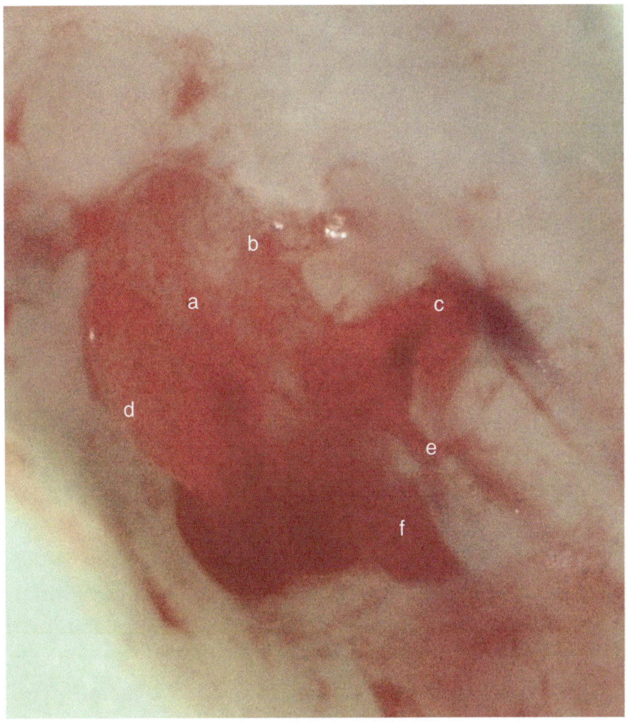

Fig. 1.15 Reversed "U"-shaped heart. Diaphragmatic surface. Sinusal horns and primitive pulmonary vein. *a* Interventricular sulcus, *b* left ventricle, *c* sinus venosus left horn, *d* right ventricle, *e* primitive pulmonary vein, *f* sinus venosus right horn

1.1.7 The "Cor Sigmoideum" Stage

During this phase, the cardiac tube continues to develop in length, as the extremities remain fixed, it curves and becomes similar to the letter "S". This is the following structural arrangement:

- sinus venosus lies posterior and inferior
- primitive atrium is situated in the middle but above the sinus
- the bulboventricular loop lies inferior and anterior.

The sinus venosus, the primitive atrium and its mesocardial pedicle (in which the primitive pulmonary vein will form) but also the primitive ventricle, form the inflow pole of the cardiac tube.

The bulbus cordis together with the truncus arteriosus and aortic sac will form the outflow pole of the cardiac tube.

The primitive ventricle will create the largest portion of the left ventricle. The bulbus cordis will form the trabeculated part of the right ventricle, the subostial portion of the large arteries (the cones or roots of the large arteries) and the truncus arteriosus. The latter will create the intrapericardial part of the aortic and pulmonary trunk [9].

The final looping process:

- The outflow pole lies anterior to the atrioventricular canal and primitive atrium.
- The left ventricle is ballooned and well structured, while the right ventricular conus still has a tubular shape, attached to the anterolateral side of the left ventricle (Fig. 1.16). The difference in the developmental rate between the two ventricles is very evident here. The anterior interventricular sulcus and the left ventricular apex are well defined in the seventh to eighth week. On the diaphragmatic surface the posterior interventricular sulcus is barely visible (Fig. 1.17) This difference in cardiac evolution, suggests that this so called looping process does not occur on the diaphragmatic side with the same intensity as on the sternocostal side, therefore this process is not about the entire diameter of the cardiac tube (pseudolooping process).

The bulboventricular sulcus situated on the underdeveloped internal edge will remain deep within the conoventricular fold. Only on this edge the conoventricular sulcus will superimpose with the bulboventricular sulcus. As a result, the direction of the bulbar segment will reach the atrioventricular canal and the incoming blood will flow to the bulbar region without passing through the future left ventricle (Figs. 1.14 and 1.18)

At the end of this stage, the arterial blood reaches both ventricles simultaneously not successively, the left ventricle followed by the right [10].

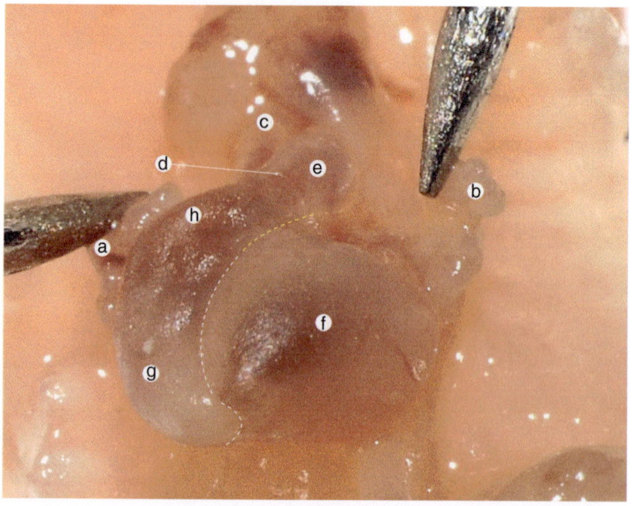

Fig. 1.16 Cor sigmoideum. Sternocostal surface. *a* Right auricle, *b* left auricle, *c* aorta, *d* Limits of conus muscularization, *e* subpulmonary infundibulum, *f* left ventricle, *g* future trabeculated part of the right ventricle, *h* conus side of the right ventricle. The *white dotted line* corresponds to the bulboventricular sulcus and the *yellow dotted line* indicates the fusion area between conus and primitive ventricle

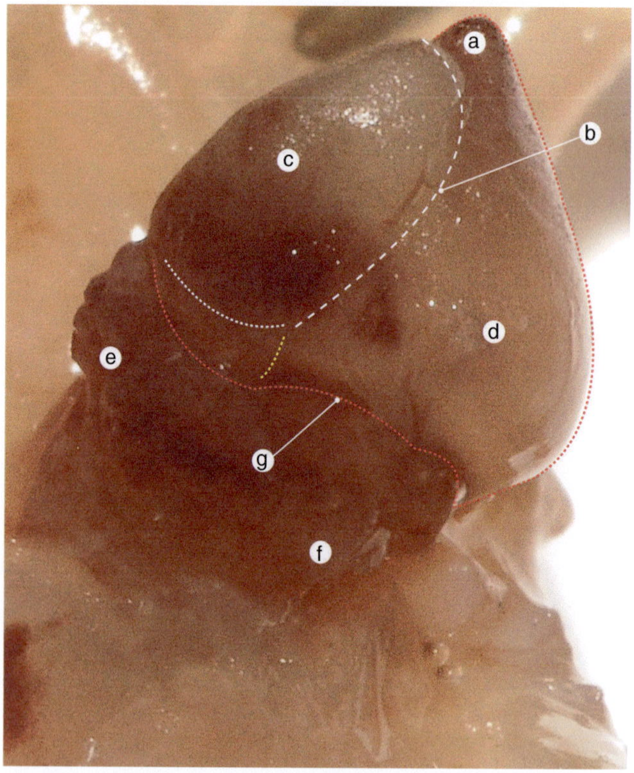

Fig. 1.17 Cor sigmoideum-diaphragmatic surface. The *red dotted line* circumscribes the primitive ventricular territory. The *yellow line* represents the imaginary continuation of the posterior interventricular sulcus towards the atrioventricular junction. The *white dotted line* limits with the *red line* the region of the atrioventricular junction. *a* Apex, *b* posterior interventricular sulcus, *c* right ventricle, *d* left ventricle, *e* right atrium, *f* left atrium, *g* atrioventricular junction

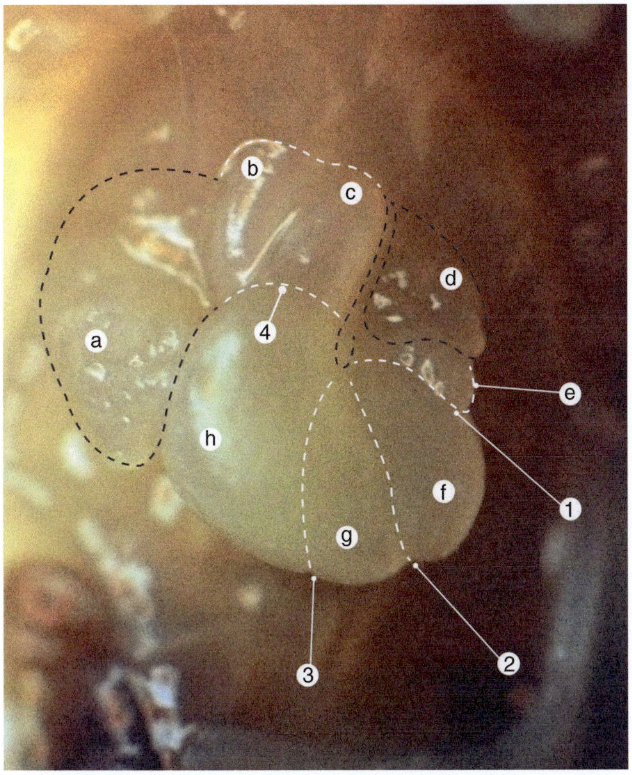

Fig. 1.18 Evolution of the intersegmental sulci. *a* Right atrium, *b* aorta, *c* pulmonary trunk, *d* left atrium, *e* atrioventricular junction, *f* future left ventricle, *g* future trabeculated part of the right ventricle, *h* conus region, *1* Atrioventricular junction, *2* bulboventricular sulcus, *3* conoventricular sulcus, *4* sinotubular junction

References

1. Moore K. The developing human clinically oriented embryology. Philadelphia: Elsevier; 2007.
2. Schoenwolf GC, Bleyl SB, Brauer PR, Francis-West PH. Larsen's human embryology, 4th ed. New York, Edinburgh: Churchill Livingstone; 2009.
3. Abu–Issa R, Kirby ML. Patterning of the heart field in the chick. Dev Biol. 2008;319(2):223–33.
4. Eisenberg LM, Markwald RR. Molecular regulation of atrioventricular valvuloseptal morphogenesis. Circ Res. 1995;77(1):1–6.
5. Webb S, Brown NA, Anderson RH. Formation of the atrioventricular septal structures in the normal mouse. Circ Res. 1997;82:645–56.
6. Webb S, Brown NA, Wessels A, Anderson RH. Development of the murine pulmonary vein and its relationship to the embryonic venous sinus. Anat Rec. 1998;250:325–34.
7. Sadler TW. Langman's Embriologie medicala. 10th ed. Bucuresti: Editura medicala Callisto; 2008. p. 380.
8. Christoffels VM, Habets PE, Franco D, Campione M, de Jong F, Lamers WH, Bao ZZ, Palmer S, Biben C, Harvey RP, Moorman AF. Chamber formation and morphogenesis in the developing mammalian heart. Dev Biol. 2000;223(2):266–78.
9. Anderson RH, Becker AE. The development of the heart. Cardiac anatomy. London: Gower Medical Publishing; 1980.
10. Rodeck CH, Whittle MJ. Fetal medicine: basic science and clinical practice. London/New York: Churchill Livingstone Elsevier; 2009.

2 The Specific Development Period

2.1 The Formation and Septation of Atria

Atria develop mostly from the primitive atrium. Initially there is a unique cavity, which has membranous walls (the endocardial tube). During development, these membranous walls will gain muscle fibers.

The muscle fiber invasion of the atrial wall is discussed later in this chapter.

The inner surface of atria varies during development. The definitive atrial wall contains neighboring structures, therefore we can consider that the atrial wall has an ontogenetic, morphologic and physiologic heterogeneity.

In the adult atrium the auricles develop from the primitive atrium and the definitive atria will integrate parts of the atrioventricular canal (which will later form the vestibular areas), as well as parts from the sinus venosus (which will later form sinus venarum and the dorsosinusal space) and the primitive pulmonary vein (which will form the atrial wall between the ostias of the pulmonary veins).

The dorsal extracardiac mesoderm migrates within the interatrial septum. At the base of this septum, the atrial wall derives from extensions of the endocardial cushions.

Muscle fiber development within the interatrial septum may take place in different ways: through the evolution of adult myocytes from myoblasts, the transformations of the mesenchyme towards the myocyte cell line or the transformation of extracardial mesoderm into myocytes.

Simultaneous development of cardiac myocytes and cardiac vasculature suggests an epicardial involvement in myocyte development (see proepicardial development).

Atrial septation takes place in days 27–36 in the embryos which evolve 4–17 mm. Atrial septation is part of a general and simultaneous process of primitive heart septation. Due to didactic considerations we decided to try to create a schematization according to the dominance and territories of each stage.

2.1.1 The Formation of Septum Intermedium

On the right and left walls of the atrioventricular canal, through cardioglial accumulation, two endocardial prominences develop. After the cardiac tube rotation they take their final position, becoming sagittal – and will be named the superior and inferior endocardial cushions.

Despite their name, the endocardial cushions are genetically lateralized structures.

These cushions will fuse and form the septum intermedium (Figs. 2.1, 2.2, 2.3, 2.4 and 1.14). Both cushions have atrial and ventricular elongations.

The formation of septum intermedium finalizes in weeks 6–7 with the help of the mesoderm (probably extracardial mesoderm) which migrates at this level through the septum primum (Fig. 2.4).

The septum intermedium separates right and left atrioventricular orifices. These orifices are initially narrow with the aspect of "gullets" (Figs. 2.5, 2.6 and 2.7).

Cells derived from the endocardium classically form the mesenchyme of the endocardial cushions. However, in these cushions also arrive cells derived from the epicardium [1].

F.M. Filipoiu, *Atlas of Heart Anatomy and Development*,
DOI 10.1007/978-1-4471-5382-5_2, © Springer-Verlag London 2014

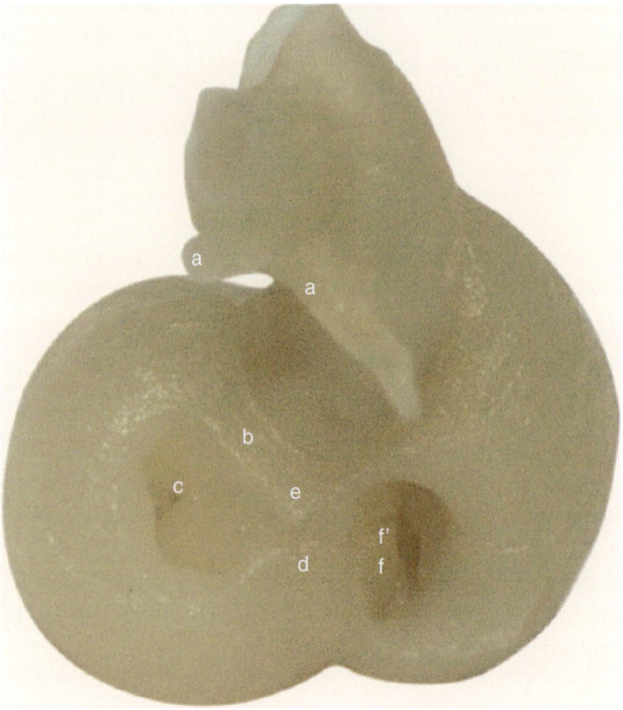

Fig. 2.1 Around 7 weeks old heart, after the removal of the atria. Posterior view. Endocardial cushions are merging. Their extensions are delaminating, leading to cusps formation. The protrusion of the aorta in the superior endocardial cushion separates its mesenchyme into two extensions: a *left one*, which becomes the mitral-aortic continuity and a *right one*, which becomes the membranous septum. *a* Pulmonary arteries, *b* the future mitral-aortic continuity, *c* endocardial cushions forming the anterior cusp, *d* inferior endocardial cushion, *e* superior endocardial cushion, *f*, *f'* endocardial cushions engaged in forming the septal cusp

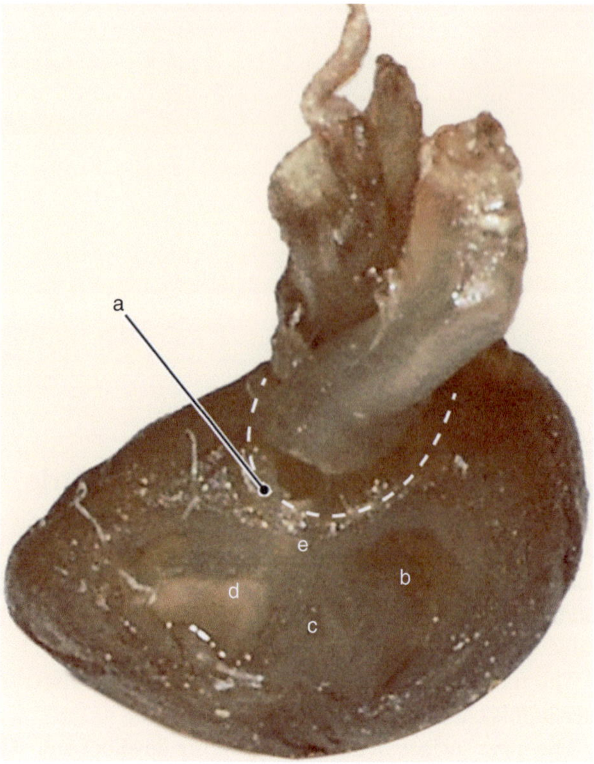

Fig. 2.2 Around 7 weeks old heart. After atrial removal, the aorta is also removed at the level of the conotruncal junction. The merging between the wall of the aorta and the septum intermedium is visible. *a* Aortic protrusion in the superior endocardial cushion, *b* septal cusp, *c* inferior endocardial cushion, *d* anterior mitral cusp, *e* superior endocardial cusp

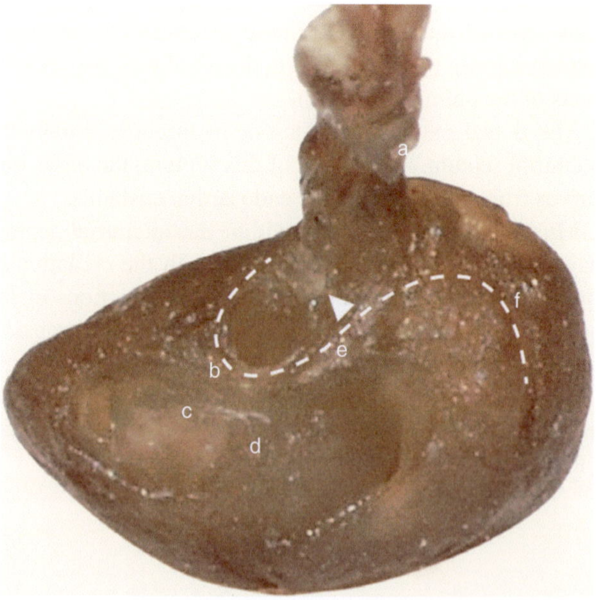

Fig. 2.3 The aortic protrusion separates the superior endocardial cushion into a left extension, which will generate the mitral-aortic continuity and a right one, which will generate the membranous atrioventricular septum. Conal septum superior part (*arrowhead*) separates the aorta from the pulmonary trunk, subvalvulary. *a* Pulmonary artery, *b* the left extension of the superior endocardial cushion, *c* anterior mitral cusp, *d* inferior endocardial cushion, *e* the right extension of the superior endocardial cushion, *f* superior bulboventricular sulcus

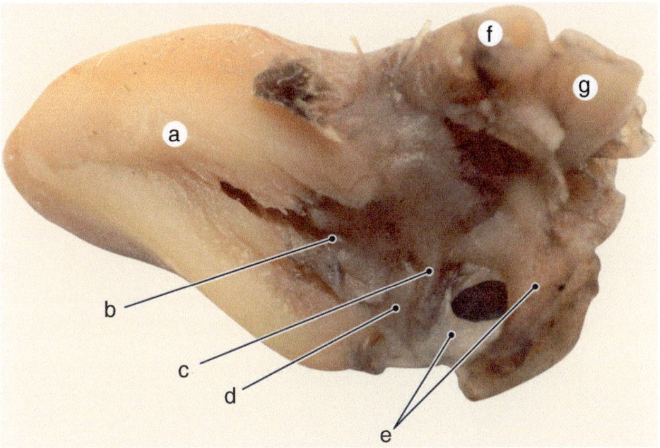

Fig. 2.4 A 12 week old heart. Sagittal section, left to the interatrial septum. The way that different structures fuse at the base of the septum is visible. *a* Left ventricle, *b* anterior mitral cusp, *c* superior endocardial cushion extension, *d* inferior endocardial cushion extension, *e* fascicular and membranous part of the septum primum, *f* pulmonary trunk, *g* aorta

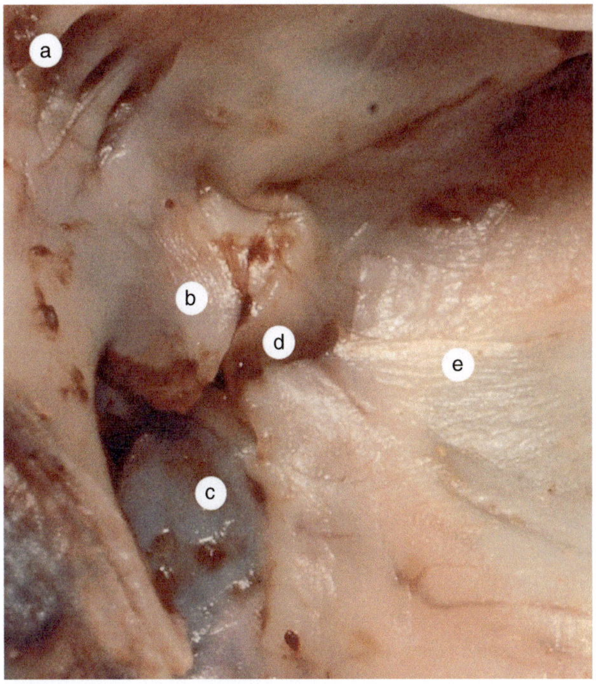

Fig. 2.6 A 12 weeks old heart. The left side of the interatrial septum base. A defect in the merging of the endocardial cushions indicates that the structures participate in the forming of the septum intermedium. *a* Left atrium, *b* the surface of the superior endocardial cushion, *c* anterior mitral cusp, *d* the surface of the inferior endocardial cushion, *e* the inferior limb of the septum primum

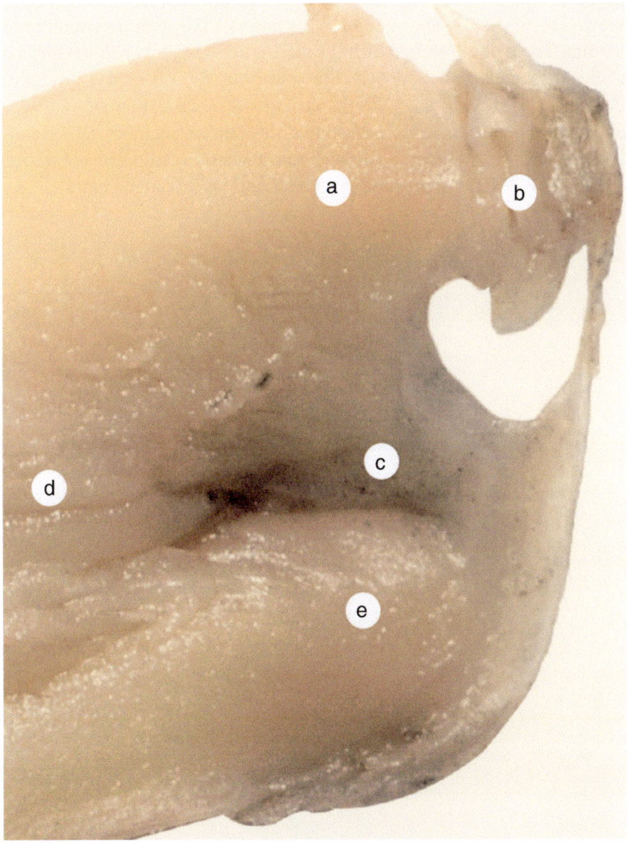

Fig. 2.5 Sagittal section at the right of the previous. The continuity of the interventricular septum, with the endocardial cushions about to merge, is visible. Septum primum material takes part in the fusion of the endocardial cushions in an obvious manner. *a* Inferior endocardial cushion, *b* coronary sinus, *c* septum primum completes the fusion of the two cushions, *d* interventricular septum, *e* superior edocardial cushion

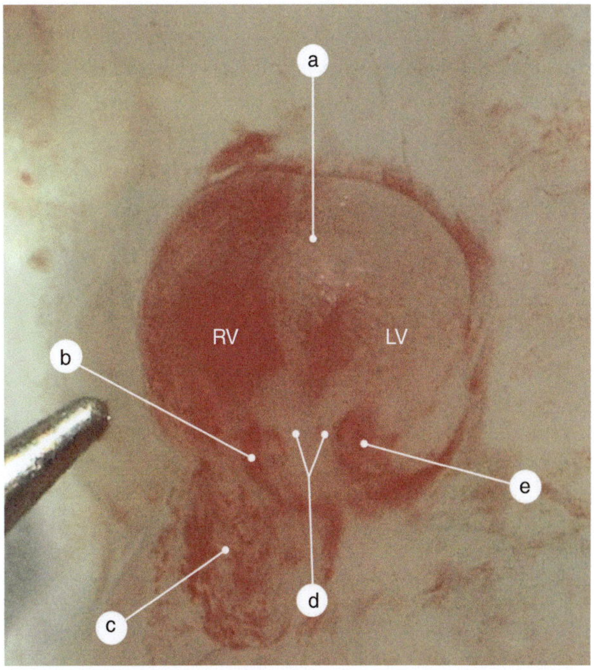

Fig. 2.7 Rat's heart, 10 days old. The tip of the needle indicates the real size. The heart is reversed. Through the endocardial transparency the septum primum and its two extensions are visible. The right extension merges with the interventricular septum. The atrioventicular ducts are permeable and full with blood. *a* Interventicular septum, *b* right atrioventricular duct, *c* right auricle, *d* the extension of the septum intermedium which continues the inferior endocardial cushion, *e* left atrioventricular duct, *RV* right ventricle, *LV* left ventricle

2.1.2 The Formation of Septum Primum

A hemodynamic problem has to be solved through atrial septation: how can an orifice temporarily allow blood to flow from the right atrium to the left atrium until birth and this flow stop after birth?

A series of partially unknown events solve this problem, events which we will further describe in detail in the following lines.

An endocardial fold named septum primum develops on the wall of the primitive atrium, opposite to the septum intermedium (posterior-superior wall). This septum primum develops downwards in a falciform pattern. Between septum primum and septum intermedium an orifice is defined – foramen primum. Septum primum continues to develop and fuses with septum intermedium and therefore foramen primum disappears. During this last event another orifice develops in the superior part of septum primum – foramen secundum.

This is the classical succinct way to present the development of septum primum and foramen secundum.

We consider that an alternate theory may be helpful for cardiologists, and we decided to state and describe it.

Septum primum develops on the atrial wall opposite to septum intermedium (postero-superior atrial wall) like an arch-like fascicular mesenchymal mass (a mesenchymal fasciculum which continues the endocardial cushions) which tends to unite both endocardial cushions (Figs. 2.8, 2.9, 2.10, 2.11 and 2.12).

There is the possibility that this endocardial fold derives from cells from the fusion line of both endocardial tubes. This fusion line is represented by the mesocardic taenia (Fig. 1.8) and corresponds to the base of septum primum.

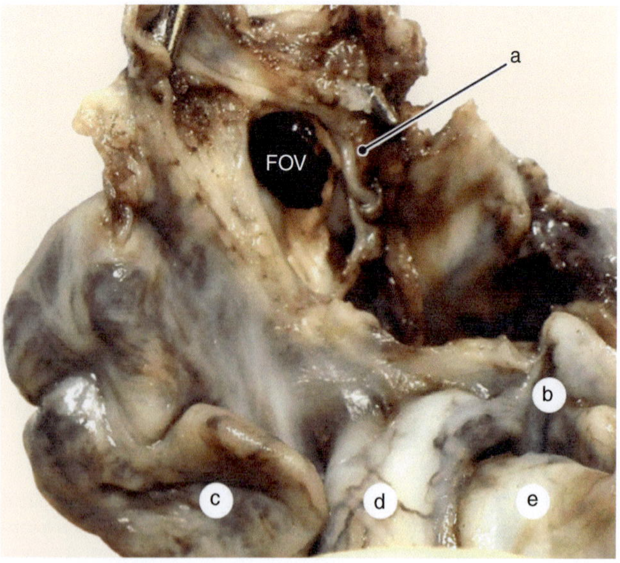

Fig. 2.8 A 12 weeks old heart. The left side of the interatrial septum. The left atrium is removed. The septum primum fascicular part resembles a fold in the atrial celling. *a* Fascicular part of the septum primum, *b* left auricle, *c* right auricle, *d* aorta, *e* pulmonary artery, *FOV* fossa ovalis

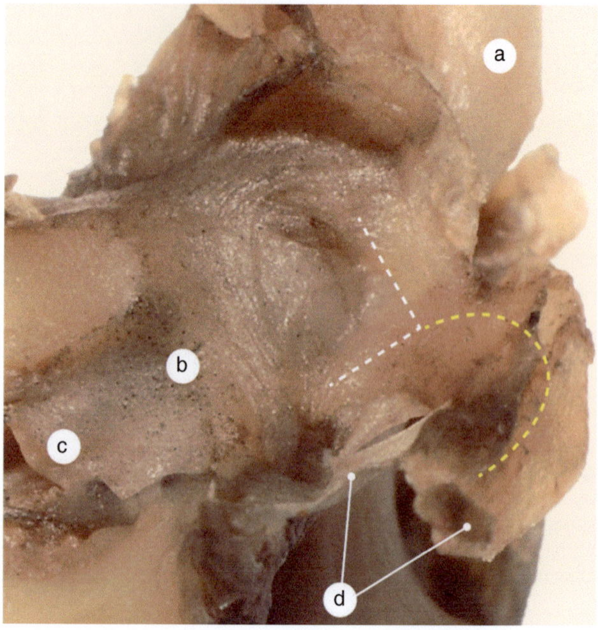

Fig. 2.9 A 12 weeks old heart. Left atrium opened, left and posterior view. The fascicular and membranous parts of the septum primum are visible. The origin fascicle of the superior endocardial cushion surface dissociates and participates in the mitral-aortic continuity structure. Between the arms of the "V", the atrial wall remains membranous for an extended period. Even in adulthood this certain segment can be easily damaged by traction. *a* Aorta, *b* mitral-aortic continuity, *c* anterior mitral cusp, *d* septum primum fascicular and membranous parts

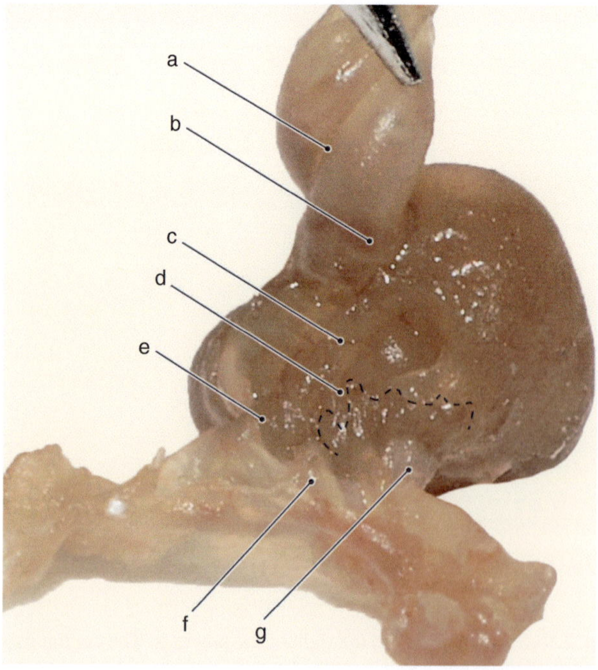

Fig. 2.10 Approximately 7 weeks old heart. Atria have been previously sectioned at the base and than reversed. The septum primum is visible junctioning with the inferior endocardial cushion. Sinus septi bulges in the right valve of the sinus venosus. The left pulmonary margin flanks the septum primum base. *a* Spiral septum, *b* aorta with forming valves, *c* superior endocardial cushion, *d* sinus septi, *e* left pulmonary margin, *f* septum primum, *g* right valve. The *dotted line* shows the inferior contour of the right valve

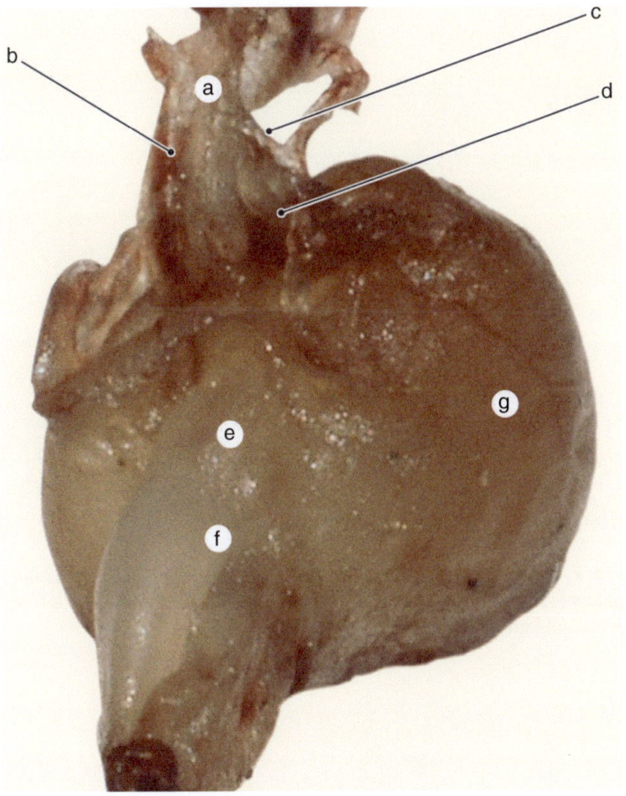

Fig. 2.11 Approximately 7 weeks old heart. The arterial pedicle is drawn anteriorly. Only the junction between the septum primum and the inferior endocardial cushion remained from the anterior wall. In this area, septum primum is flanked by the two pulmonary ridges (margins). Left to the septum primum, the pulmonary fosset is visible- the place where the primitive pulmonary vein opens. *a* septum primum, *b* right pulmonary margin, *c* left pulmonary margin, *d* pulmonary vein fosset, *e* aorta with forming valves, *f* spiral septum, *g* left ventricle

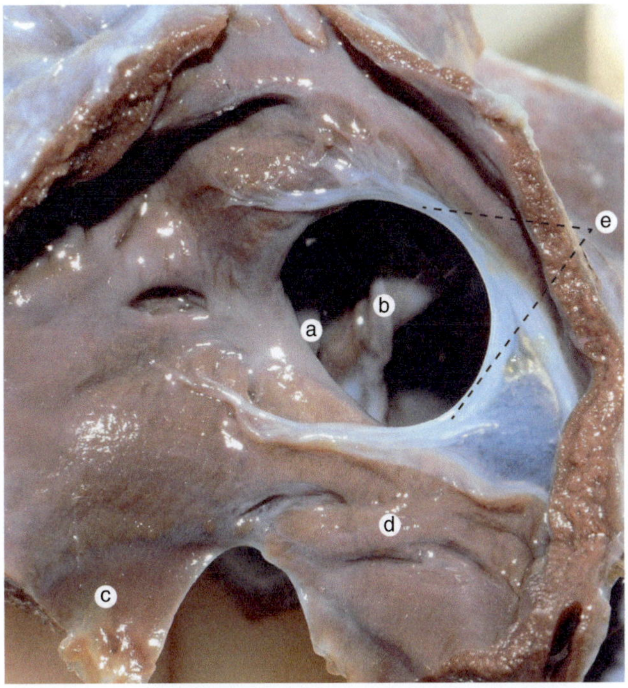

Fig. 2.12 Three and a half months old heart. Septum primum viewed from the left atrium. Large interatrial communication, a true "foramen ovale". The migrating mesenchyme is visible in the thickness of the mitral cups. *a* Septum secundum, *b* foramen ovale, *c* anterior mitral cusp, *d* inferior endocardial cushion extension, *e* septum primum with superior and inferior limbs

We should try to understand cardiac septation like a complex and almost simultaneous process which occurs in the atria and ventricles. There are two falciform septums (interatrial and interventricular) which evolve towards each other and will fuse at the level of the fused endocardial cushions. A third septum, the spiral septum, which divides the emerging pole of the ventricle, also fuses with the interventricular septum and septum intermedium, finalizing the septation.

Anteriorly, the septum primum commences from the union of two mesenchymal fascicles, which continue the superior endocardial cushion. The anterior extremity of this septum consequently has the shape of a reversed "V" (Figs. 2.9, 2.18 and 2.22).

Posteriorly, septum primum does not directly reach the inferior endocardial cushion but ends just above it, more precisely, above the pulmonary vein fossa.

The posterior extremity of the septum has a complex aspect. This extremity is flanked laterally by two prominences named the left and right pulmonary ridges (Figs. 2.10 and 2.11) thus named because of their boundary with the pulmonary vein fossa.

The right pulmonary ridge is considered to be Hiss' spina vestibuli. At its level protrudes into the atrium wall the dorsal extracardiac mesenchyme.

The left pulmonary ridge evolves towards musculization and attenuates at some point due to the evolution of the pulmonary vein towards the left atrium. This ridge also participates in the consolidation of the septum primum base.

The inferior margin of the septum primum contains, throughout its evolution, a sheath of mesodermal cells, endocardially migrated here through the spina vestibuli.

If we closely observe the aspect of the septum primum we can notice the following elements:

- a fixed part, basal part – derived from the mesenchyme, continuing the superior endocardial cushion located on the atrial roof. This part quickly suffers a muscular transformation.
- a relatively mobile part – the membranous part, with an endocardial fold aspect. Like any other fold it has two sheaths, which cover like a mantle the fascicular part. In our opinion, only this part develops inferiorly and to the left in order to fuse with both endocardial cushions which are on the verge of fusioning (the space between both sheaths represents

A possible way for the extracardiac mesenchyme, which has protruded the septum primum via spina vestibuli, to participate in the endocardial cushions fusion) (Figs. 2.12, 2.13, 2.14, 2.15 and 2.16).

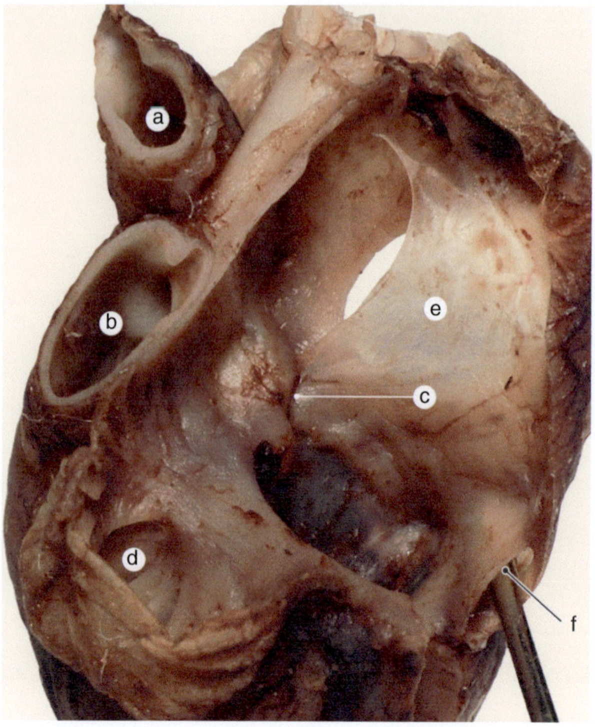

Fig. 2.13 A 4 months old heart. A defect in the merging of the two endocardial cushions material can be seen. Hence delineation of the areas depending on the two cushions and their area of fusion is possible. *a* Aorta, *b* pulmonary artery, *c* a merging vice of the endocardial cushions, *d* left auricle, *e* septum primum with superior and inferior limbs, *f* coronary venous sinus

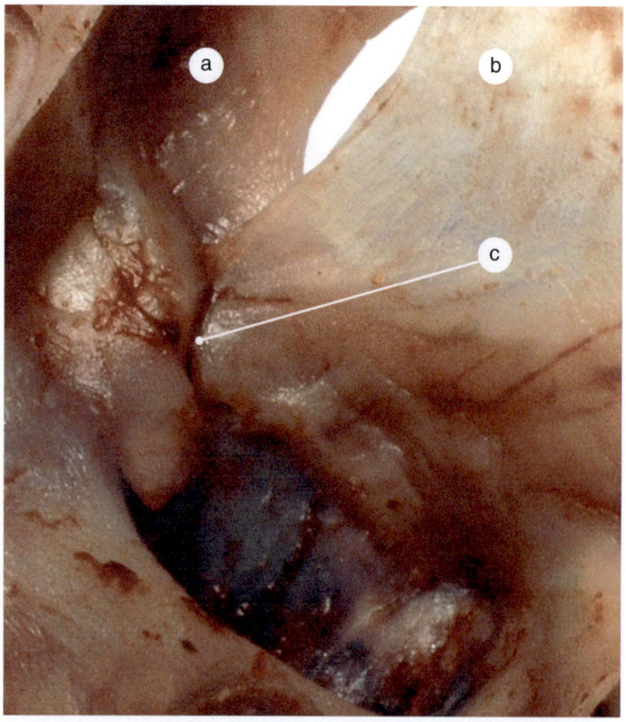

Fig. 2.14 Detail of the previous image. Septum primum can be clearly seen participating in the merging of the two cushions. *a* Septum secundum, *b* septum primum, *c* merging defect

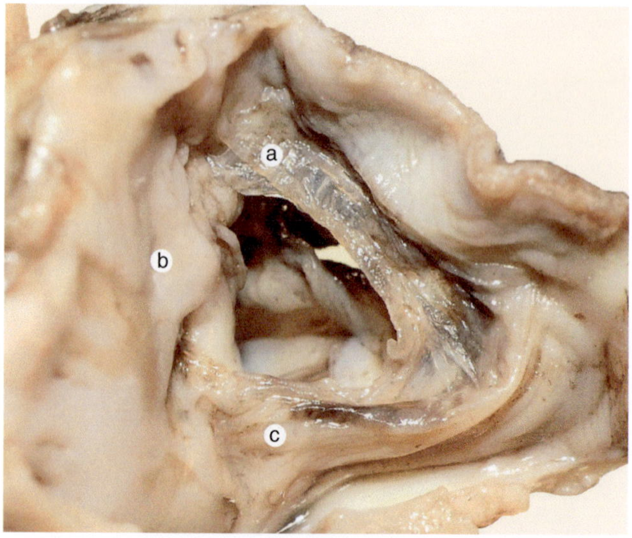

Fig. 2.15 A 3 months old heart. Inferior limb of the septum primum enters the area of merging of the endocardial cushions. *a* Superior limb, *b* merging area, *c* inferior limb

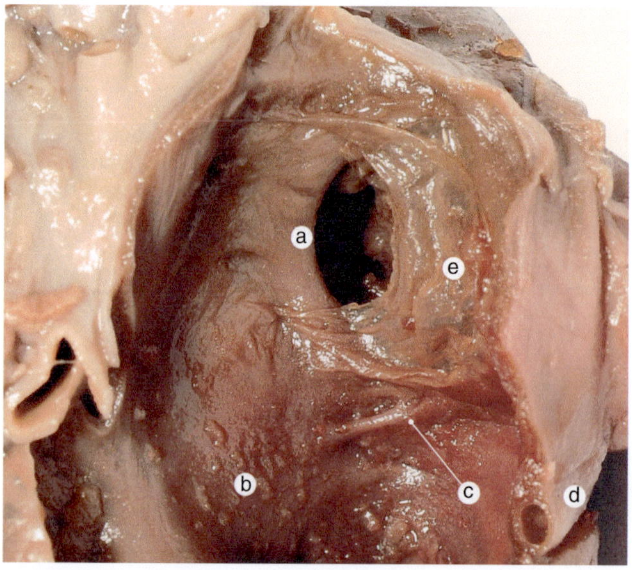

Fig. 2.16 A 4 months old heart. The left side of the interatrial septum. The inferior cushion extension strengthens the intermediate septum and forming of the anterior mitral cusp. *a* Septum secundum, *b* anterior mitral cusp, *c* inferior cushion extension, *d* venous sinus, *e* septum primum

Following the fusion of the three structures (two endocardial cushions and the membranous part of septum primum) and the participation of the extracardiac dorsal mesenchyme, the foramen primum closes (Fig. 2.5).

This evolution might explain why the pathology of septum primum is associated with septum intermedium pathology.

The membranous part of septum primum later suffers a variable fibrous transformation (after the third month) and a much later muscular transformation (just before parturition).

Septum primum evolves like a falciform separating wall. It's free margin, which is placed anteriorly and concave, will finally become falx septi – the valve of the fossa ovalis. This margin has a superior and an inferior limb (Figs. 2.12, 2.13, 2.14, 2.15, 2.16 and 2.17).

The base of septum primum (the part adherent to the wall) develops anteriorly, and passes along with the inferior limb over the endocardial cushions' fusion line at the level of septum intermedium (Fig. 2.18). In this the way the extracardiac mesenchyme, migrated between the two sheaths of the septum, may participate in the endocardial cushions' fusion and in the finalization of the septum intermedium. Through the same pathway the extracardiac mesenchyme might reach the anterior mitral cusp (Figs. 2.12 and 2.14).

As we have shown, the membranous part of septum primum has a free margin (anterior – superior) which does not participate in the cushions' fusion. It has a falciform shape and is shifted towards the left. Between it's concavity, the anterior atrial wall and septum secundum, it remains throughout fetal development a hemodynamically efficient orifice which allows blood-flow from the right atrium to the left atrium (see preceding fig.). This margin is called falx septi.

The membranous part of the septum primum will finally form the floor of the fossa ovalis. The membranous aspect disappears due to a variable evolution, either through fibrous transformation or muscular transformation.

The space between falx septi and the anterior atrial wall ensures an efficient interatrial communication and is frequently mistaken with foramen secundum. This space, however, is the equivalent of the oval foramen (an ambiguous term to be explained in the following lines).

We consider that the evolution of foramen secundum is not fully clarified in specialty literature.

If foramen secundum would be a compulsory step during atrial septation, it would mean that it appears as a fusion of small orifices which occur in the posterior-superior part of septum primum (according to literature). These small orifices would fuse, resulting a single hemodynamically efficient orifice – foramen secundum. All these events should take place along with the closing of foramen primum – a risky period for the survival of the embryo (if these stages are not well-synchronized there is the risk of right-left atrial blood-flow blockage). Later, through apoptotic processes, the septum primum, which lies anterior to foramen secundum, should disappear and the margin of foramen secundum would become falx septi.

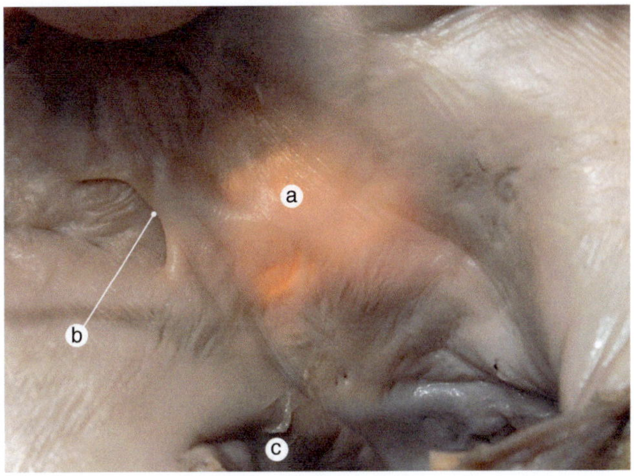

Fig. 2.17 Adult heart. Interatrial septum viewed from the left atrium. Transillumination. The valve of fossa ovale – falx septi- has merged with the septum secundum, closing the interatrial communication. Fossa ovale does not overlap the merging area. *a* Fossa ovale visible by means of transillumination, *b* Falx septi, *c* mitral orifice

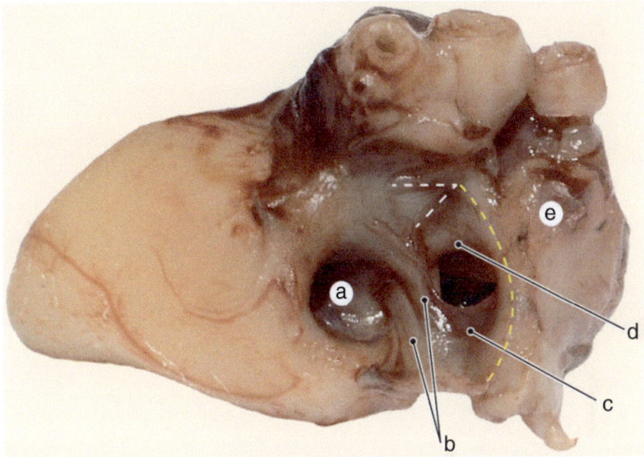

Fig. 2.18 A 3 months old heart. Left side of the interatrial septum. The extensions of the endocardial cushions are very well represented. *a* Anterior mitral cusp, *b* endocardial cushions extensions, c septum primum, *d* septum secundum, *e* superior vena cava

Therefore, we consider that Odger's [2] statement that says "foramen secundum is rather a lack of development than an involution of an already formed septum" should be reconsidered. Furthermore, we consider that foramen secundum is "an incident" in the evolution of septum primum, which sometimes cannot be compensated and remains after birth as a foramen secundum septal defect (Figs. 2.19 and 2.20).

The occurrence of this "incident" is favored by the fact that septum primum does not directly fuse posteriorly with the inferior endocardial cushion due to the interposition of the pulmonary edges and the orifice of the primitive pulmonary

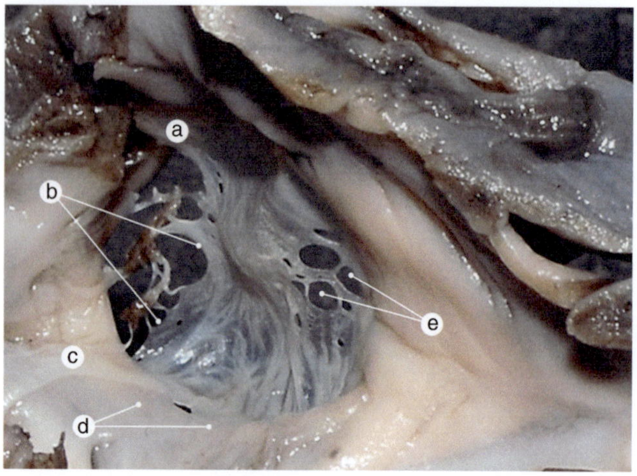

Fig. 2.19 A 7 months old heart. "Classic" ostium secundum in a complex malformation. View from the left atrium. *a* Superior limb, *b* Falx septi, *c* inferior limb of septum primum, *d* the area of the former ostium primum, *e* ostium secundum

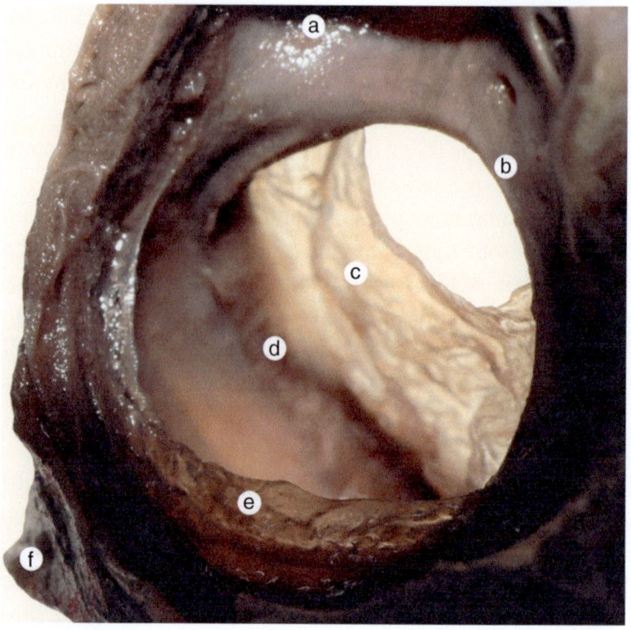

Fig. 2.21 View from the right atrium. The left valve of the sinus venous moulds the posterior edge of a very well defined septum secundum, and than merges with septum primum. The ensemble this way formed with the right valve generates an interatrial conduit. Septum secundum is a true "crista dividens" for the bloodstream (see also Fig. 2.34). *a* Superior vena cava, *b* septum secundum, *c* septum primum, *d* left valve, *e* right valve, *f* inferior vena cava

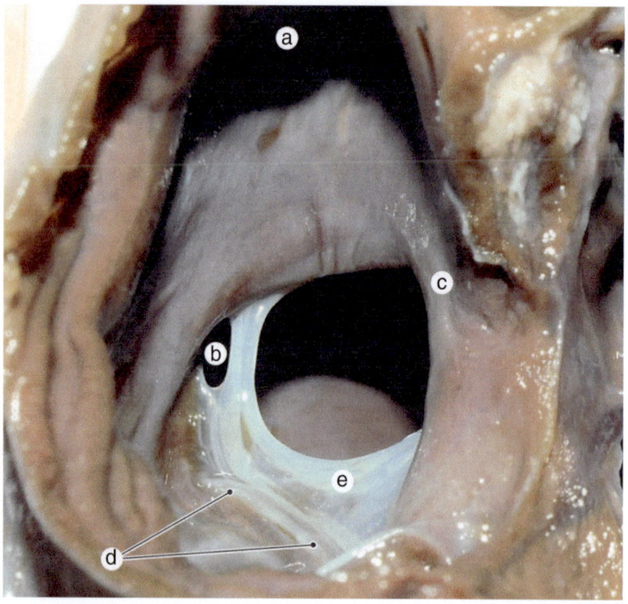

Fig. 2.20 View from the right atrium. A 5 months old heart. Uncompensated ostium secundum. Muscular septum secundum is very well defined. Between the left valve and septum primum is a fine layer of muscular tissue, perhaps from the protusion of the extracardiac mesenchyme (see also Fig. 2.32). *a* Superior vena cava, *b* ostium secundum, *c* primitive sinus left valve merged with septum primum, *d* septum secundum, *e* septum primum

vein. In this region, the finalizing of the inter-atrial septum is achieved mainly by overlapping of the left valve of the sinus venosus with the mesenchymal part of the spina vestibuli and the septum primum (Fig. 2.32).

As we underlined, there is a complex aspect of the junction between the septum primum and the inferior endocardial cushion. The superior part of the septum primum and the pulmonary edges limit superiorly the pulmonary vein fossa. Inferior to this fossa there lies the inferior endocardial cushion.

The fusion between the left valve of the sinus venosus and the right pulmonary edge (spina vestibuli) creates along with the septum primum the left wall of a conduit which allows blood to flow from the right atrium to the left atrium. The right wall of this conduit is represented by the right valve of the sinus venosus (Fig. 2.21).

In order to avoid any confusion this intraatrial conduit is different from the intraseptal conduit, which is going to be detailed in the following lines.

This ensemble creates pressure, which can determine the evolution of the primitive pulmonary vein towards the left atrium. The inclusion of the pulmonary vein within the left atrium wall is guided superiorly by a prominence.

It looks like an endocardial fold and is represented by a posterior elongation of the inferior endocardial cushion (Figs. 2.22 and 2.23). This elongation (septum intermedius) may participate in the fusion of the endocardial cushions. In the same time, this elongation serves as a pathway through which cells of the endocardial cushion participate in forming of the anterior mitral cusp (Fig. 2.24). The opposite edge of this elongation disappears in the posterior left atrial wall. In most cases this ridge involves therefore it strengthens the left side of septum primum's base. As we underlined before, we consider the elongation of the inferior endocardial cushion is involved in the directing of the incorporation of the pulmonary vein in the left atrial wall (see the following lines).

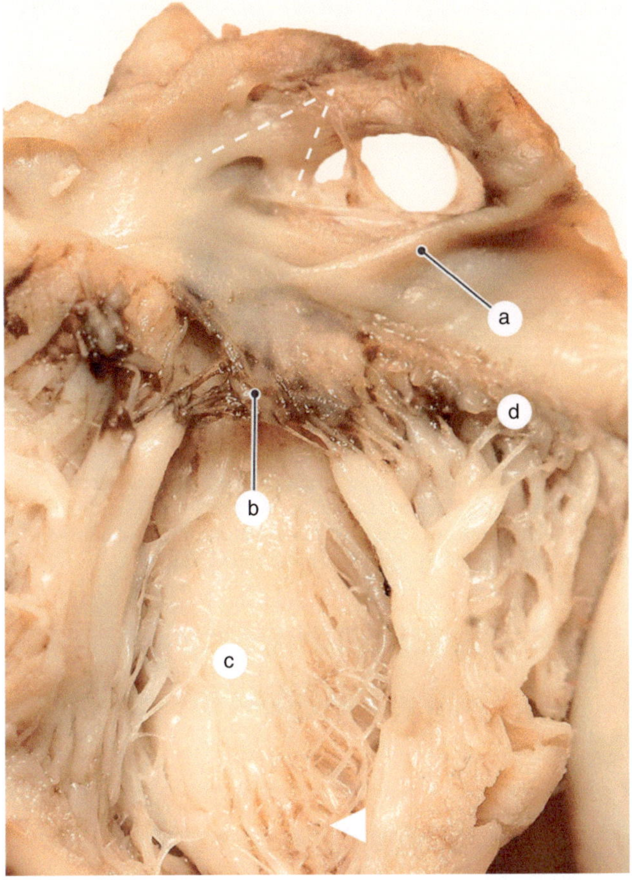

Fig. 2.22 Two and a half months old heart, opened on the obtuse edge. The left side of the septal structures. The form of a reversed "V" of the fascicular part of the septum primum is easily visible, as well as the extension of the inferior endocardial cushion, which forms the anterior mitral cusp. The *arrowhead* represents Purkinje network. *a* The extension of the inferior endocardial cushion, *b* the anterior mitral cusp, *c* left ventricle, *d* the posterior mitral cusp

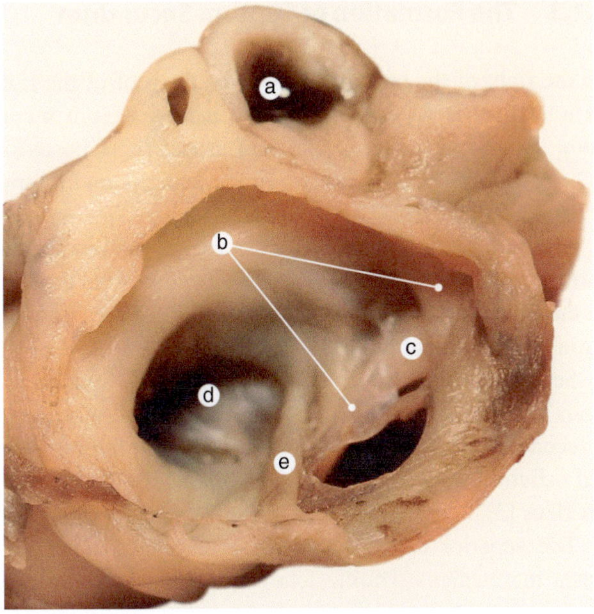

Fig. 2.23 View from the left atrium and posterior of the interatrial septum. Septum primum and septum secundum diverge towards anterior and converge toward posterior. This disposition lessens the interatrial communication. *a* Pulmonary artery, *b* septum primum, *c* septum secundum, *d* anterior mitral cusp, *e* extension of the inferior endocardial cushion

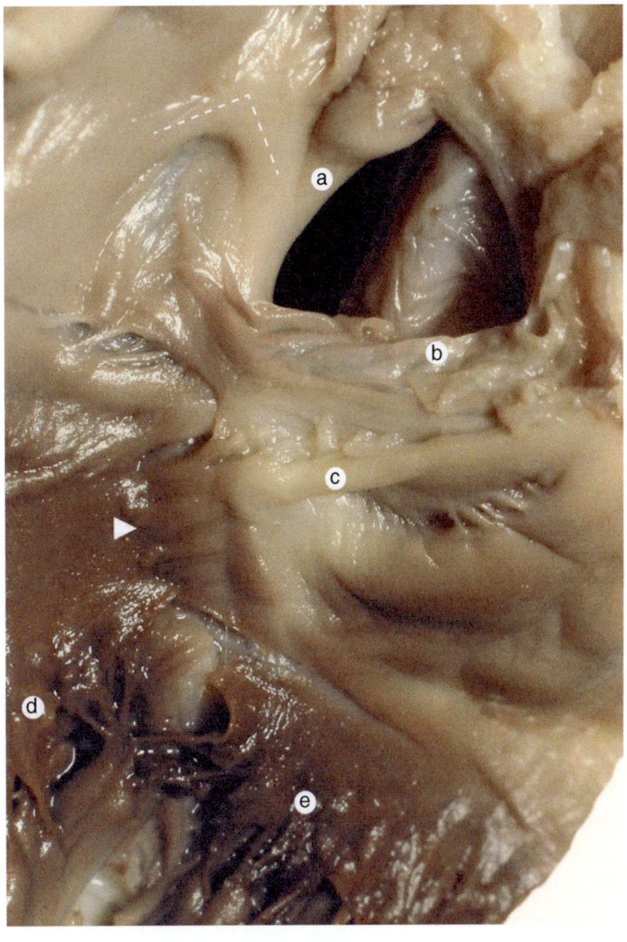

Fig. 2.24 The base of the interatrial septum seen from the left atrium. The septum primum origin in reversed "V", traces on the wall of the primitive atrium an unmusculed, membranous area, of the anterior atrial wall. It is now understood why this area of the atrial wall has a low level of resistance if tractioned. A migrating cellular population enters the mitral anterior cusp (*arrowhead*) trough the inferior endocardial cushion. *a* Septum secundum, *b* septum primum, c extension of the inferior endocardial cushion, *d* anterior mitral cusp, *e* posterior cusp

2.1.3 The Formation of Septum Secundum

To the right of the septum primum, on the roof of the right atrium, there is an endocardial fold named septum secundum. This septum has a falciform aspect (it is posterior-inferiorly concave) and has two limbs: superior and inferior (Figs. 2.25, 2.26, 2.27, 2.28 and 2.29).

In its anterior-superior part it's a proper septum and it's formed by an elongation of the superior endocardial cushion. In the following pictures we tried to underline the structural variability of this septum.

Septum secundum divides the blood flow within the sinus venosus in a main course towards the left atrium and a secondary course, which flows towards the future tricuspid ostium. Due to this fact this septum is also called crista dividens [3].

The superior edge of septum secundum is a veritable crista interveniens. During fetal development, at its level, there can sometimes be found a small prominence named *the intercaval tubercle of Lower* (Figs. 2.30 and 2.31). This structure guides the blood of the superior vena cava towards the tricuspid valve.

During evolution:

- reptiles have a heart with three chambers and a partially separated ventricle. There is no septum secundum.
- birds have a heart with four chambers. There is no septum secundum [4].
- Septum secundum occurs in mammals as an evolutional gain in the development of a four-chambered heart.

Septum secundum will become the most massive atrial septum and will form most of the interatrial septum, in the segment which lies superiorly and anteriorly to the fossa ovalis. Septum secundum (a muscular structure), on its' left side, is covered by the superior limb of septum primum (a membranous structure). Both structures will suffer a variable coalescence process that will lead to the closing of the interatrial conduit.

The occurrence of septum secundum is accompanied by a folding of the atrial wall on the opposite side, therefore septum secundum in the posterior-inferior part looks more like a fold of the atrial wall, to the right of septum primum. The free margin of this fold undergoes a coalescence and a fibromuscular transformation process. So, this margin has a special individual aspect.

Septum secundum is formed only after the left valve of sinus venosus fuses with septum primum. Due to the fact that posteriorly, septum secundum is formed like a fold in the atrial wall, it is considered that this fold rises the left valve while fusing with septum primum. Some authors consider that the left valve fuses with septum secundum (Fig. 2.32).

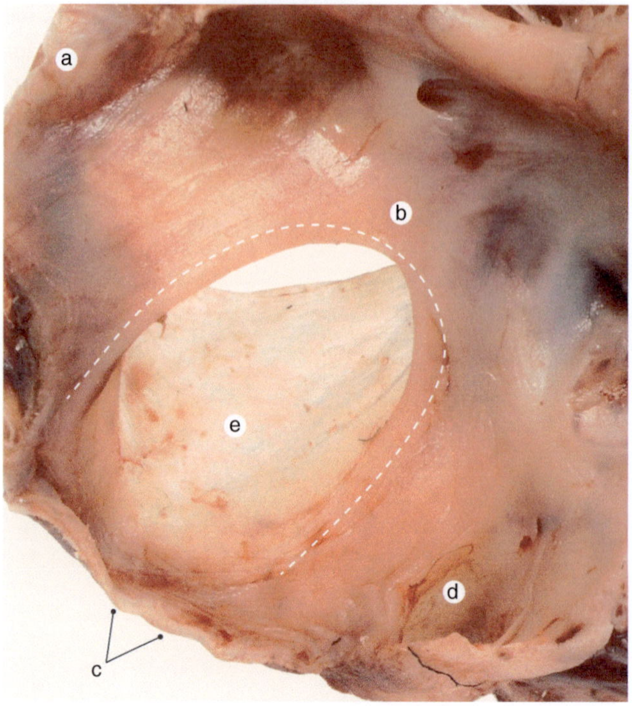

Fig. 2.25 View from the right atrium of the interatrial septum. A 5 months old heart. Septum secundum is well formed, resembling a "tight" fold. *a* Superior vena cava, *b* septum secundum, *c* inferior vena cava, *d* ostium of the coronary sinus, *e* septum primum

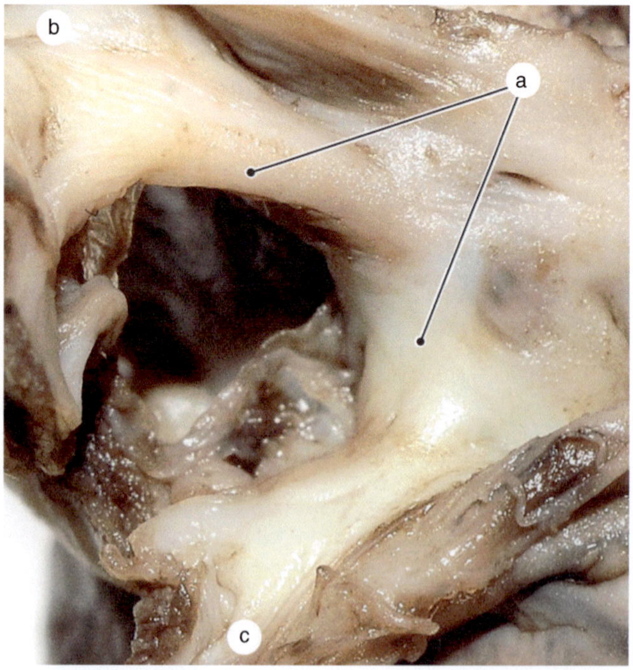

Fig. 2.26 A 3 months old heart. View from the right atrium. Septum secundum is well defined, resembling a "wide" fold. *a* Septum secundum, *b* superior vena cava, *c* inferior vena cava

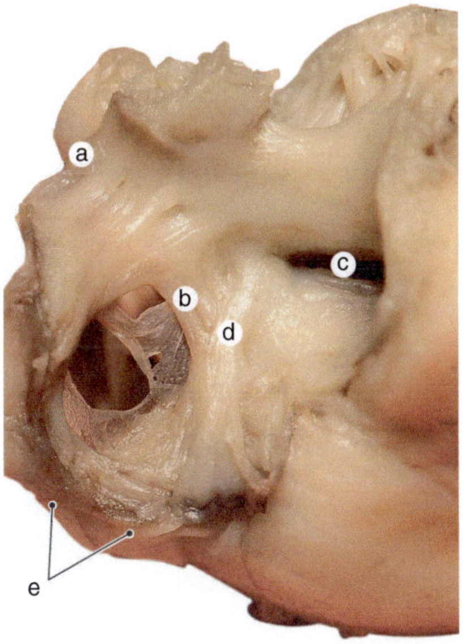

Fig. 2.27 Two months and a half old heart. View from the right atrium. Septum secundum towards the anterior has the obvious aspect of a muscular septum and not one of a fold on the wall. *a* Superior vena cava, *b* septum secundum, *c* tricuspid hole, *d* tendon of Todaro, e inferior vena cava

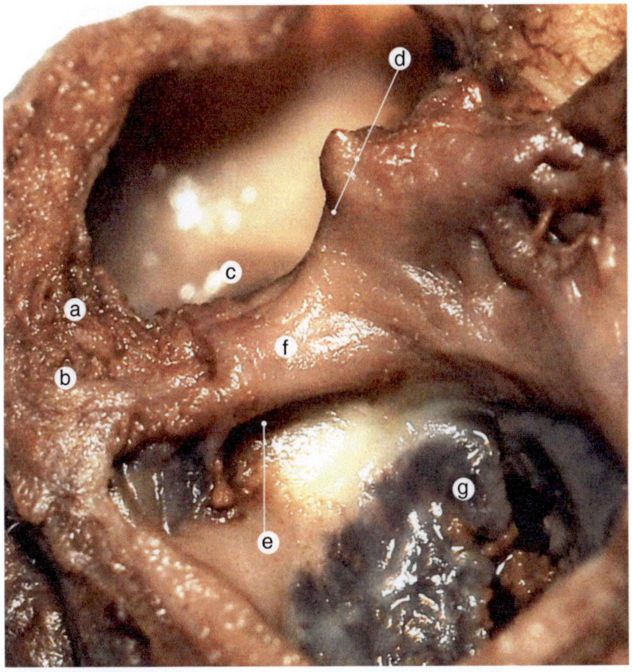

Fig. 2.28 Postero-superior view of interatrial septum base, after removal of the atria. A 5 months old heart. Notice the dissociation from the base of the interatrial septum. Two mesenchymal axes enter the septal base. The most obvious one (the right one) arises from the sinus septi thickness, then enters the septum secundum base. Its origin may lay in the extracardial mesenchyme of the dorsal mesocaridum, sequestered in the sinus septi mass. This axis will become the Todaro tendon. The less proeminent axis, situated to the left, follows the direction of the " spina vestibularis"-item of information introduced by Hiss- today holding an ambiguous meaning. It might represent mesenchyme which has migrated from the dorsal mesocardium following the direction of the right pulmonary edge of the septum primum. *a* Mesenchymal axis, *b* mesenchymal axis, *c* dissociation, *d* septum secundum, *e* ostium of the coronary sinus, *f* sinus septi, *g* septal cusp of the tricuspid valve

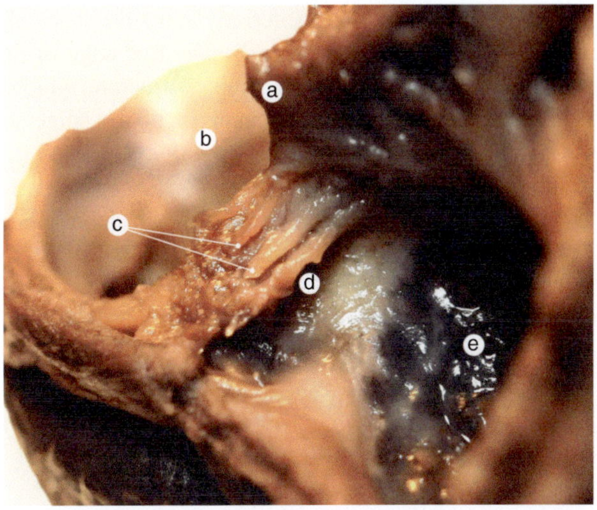

Fig. 2.29 Detail of the previous image, in which the two mesenchymal axes are well visible at the base of the interatrial septum. The left axis followed the base of the septum primum, while the right one the septum secundum base. Both are inserting on the tendinous center. These two neighbouring structures formed as a condensation of extracardiac mesenchyme, which are rather hard to identify, explains the extremely frequent confusion between the spina vestibularis and the tendon of Todaro. *a* Septum secundum, *b* left atrium, *c* mesenchymal axis, *d* ostium of the coronary sinus, *e* septal cusp of the tricuspid valve

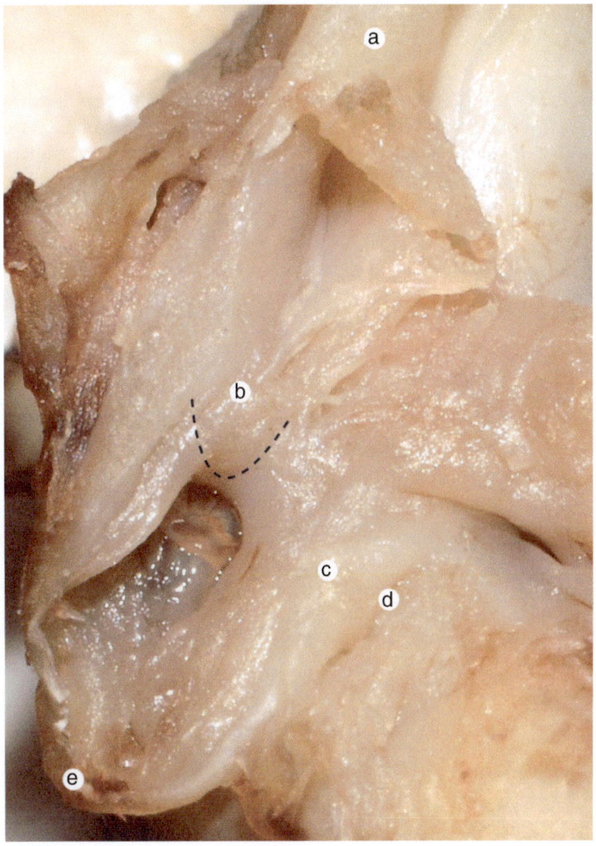

Fig. 2.30 Two and a half months old heart. The right side of the interatrial septum. The intervenous Lower tubercle protrudes on the superior edge of the septum secundum. *a* Superior vena cava, *b* the intervenous tubercle on the septum secundum edge, *c* sinus septi, *d* ostium of the coronary sinus, *e* inferior vena cava

Septum secundum evolves inferiorly. It has the shape of a reversed "U" also facing posteriorly. The free edge of this septum covers on the right side a complex structure, which is the result of fusion of septum primum, vestibular spine and left valve of the sinus venosus.

For conformity:

the edges of fossa ovalis are anterior-superior delimited by septum secundum and posteriorly my a atrial wall fold that continues septum secundum (muscular structure). This fold is considered to be part of septum secundum. These margins will become the limb of fossa ovalis.

the bottom of the fossa is partially formed by septum primum and partially by the complex structure formed by the fusion of septum primum, vestibular spine and left valve of sinus venosus – towards inferior (Figs. 2.33 and 2.34).

In fetus, the fossa ovalis isn't closed. It is just the entrance to an inter-atrial communication. Due to this fact, it is often called foramen ovale, which continues the fossa ovalis and opens in the left atrium. We consider that using the term fossa ovalis in this case is inadequate.

In previous lines we stated that left limb of septum primum faces towards left and there is a space between it and septum secundum.

This statement becomes essential in order to understand that through the vicinity of the fossa ovalis we can enter into a different conduit that is located within interatrial septum. It stretches between septum primum (membranous) and septum secundum (muscular). This conduit exits through an opening delimited by falx septi, atrial wall and septum secundum. This conduit is practically and oblique opening (not a fossa ovalis), which stretches between septum primum

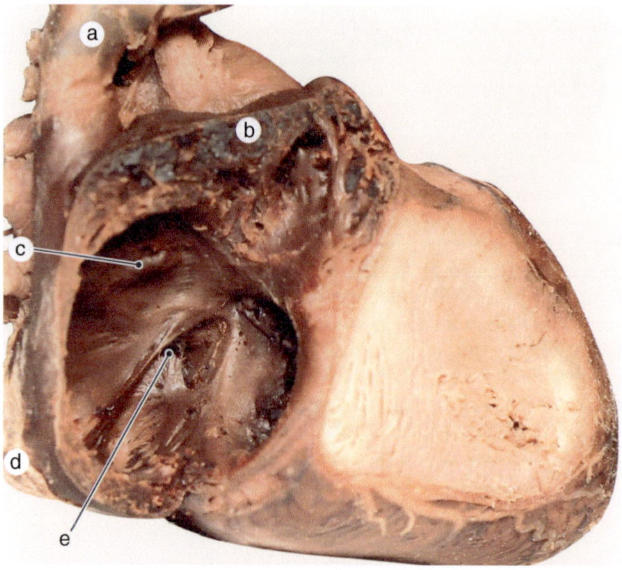

Fig. 2.31 A 7 months old heart with Norwood syndrome – left heart hypoplasia. Interatrial communication is prematurely interrupted. Fossa ovalis is bordered superiorly by the intervenous tubercle. *a* Superior vena cava, *b* right auricle, *c* intervenous tubercle – lower on the margin of the septum secundum. Fossa ovalis is closed, *d* inferior vena cava, *e* coronary sinus ostium

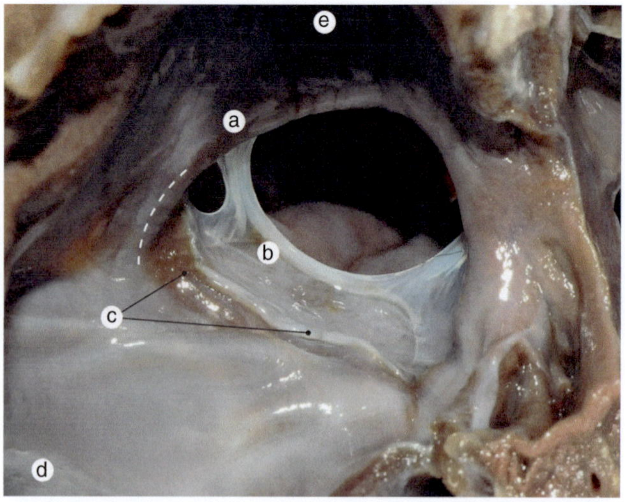

Fig. 2.32 Detailed view of the left valve from the heart in figure 2.20. The fold represented by the posterior limb of the septum secundum bulges in the left valve which has already merged with the septum secundum (*dotted line*). *a* Septum secundum, *b* septum primum, *c* left valve of the sinus venosus, *d* inferior vena cava, *e* superior vena cava

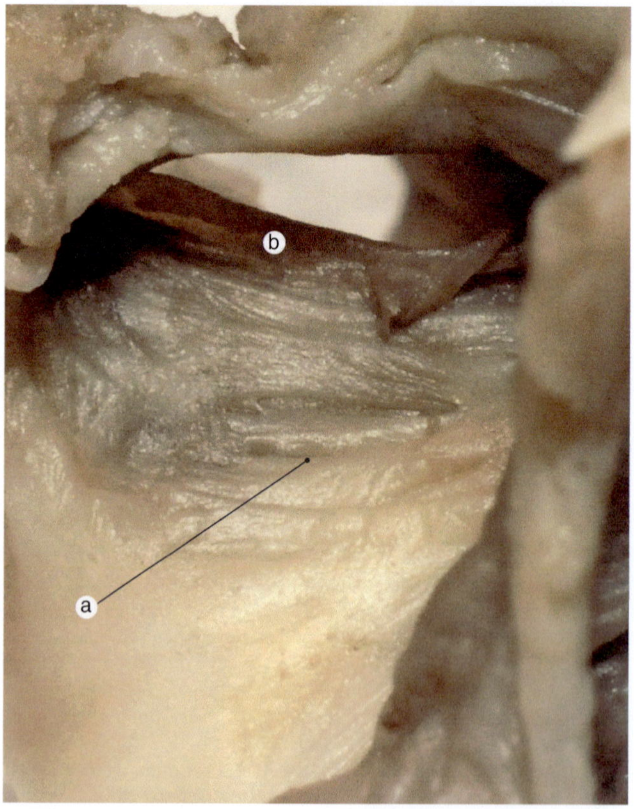

Fig. 2.33 The complex resulted from the fusion of the left valve with the extracardiac mesenchyme and the septum primum is displayed in a normal evolution, in the course of muscularization. *a* Left valve of the sinus venosus, merged with the septum primum, *b* septum primum

and septum secundum. Therefore, due to a higher pressure in the right atrium the falx sepi occurs like an enlargement of the atrial septum within left atrium (Fig. 2.34).

The oblique configuration of this conduit solves the blood dynamic problem we states before: the increased pressure in the left atrium (generated by the functioning pulmonary circulation) compresses falx septi upon septum secundum and the communication between both atria closes. Depending on the fusion grade of structures, a communication conduit between both atria may remain or not (Figs. 2.35 and 2.17).

The concave margin of septum secundum will become the limb of fossa ovalis (in the right atrium) and flax septi in the left atrium (see further – Internal aspect of atria).

Final development of atria is made by a strengthening of the posterior-inferior aspect of fossa ovalis and dorsal sinusal space.

This strengthening takes place along with the development of the extraembrionic mesenchyme, fusion between left valve and septum primum, coalescence of septal-oval recess and folding of right atrial wall.

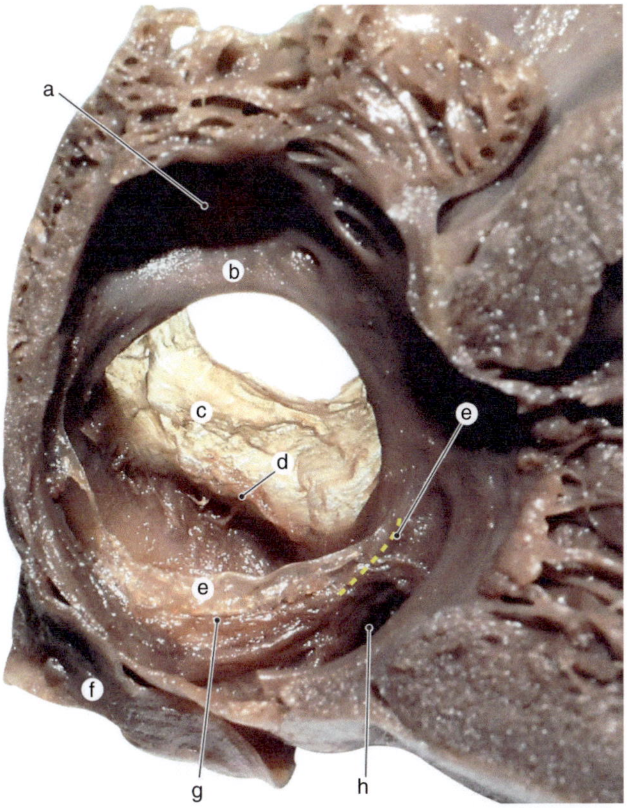

Fig. 2.34 A 4 months old heart. Detailed view of figure 2.21. Both valves of the sinus venosus in evolution can be detected simultaneously. The sinus septi bulges in the base of the right valve dividing it into the eustachian and thebesian valves. *a* Superior vena cava, *b* septum secundum, *c* septum primum, *d* left valve of the sinus venosus merged with the septum primum, *e* right valve, *f* inferior vena cava, *g* marginal fold, *h* coronary sinus ostium, *i* sinus septi

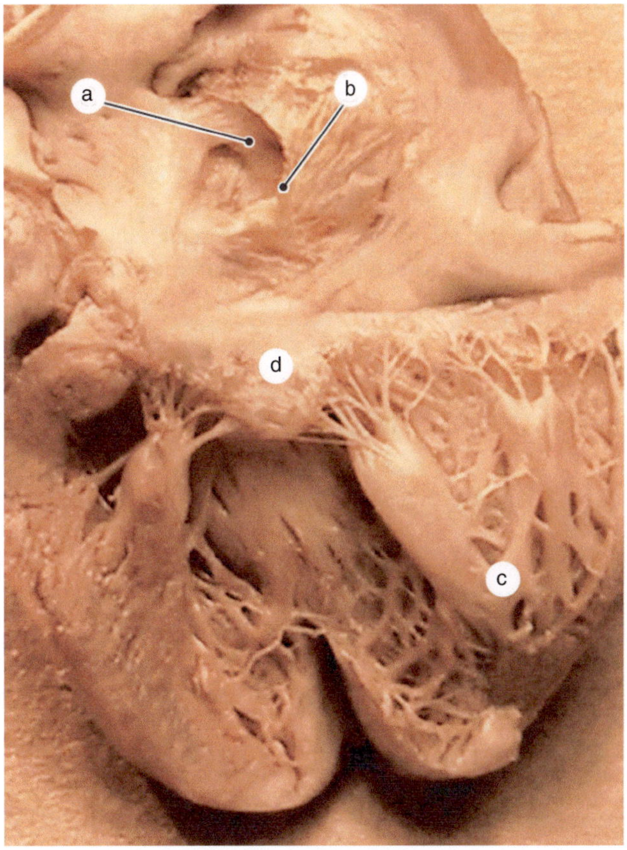

Fig. 2.35 A 4 months and a half old heart. The valve of the fossa ovalis – falx septi seen from the left atrium. *a* Septum secundum, *b* falx septi, *c* posterior papillary group, *d* anterior mitral cusp

2.2 Interatrial Septal Defects

Lack of dorsal mesoderm development may lead to the persistence of foramen primum, with an endocardial cushion fusion defect and a defect of the anterior mitral cusp. The interventricular septum still develops and this malformation is classically known as foramen primum defect. Therefore this type of defect occurs at the base of the interatrial wall and is accompanied by a partial fusion of endocardial cushions and defects of the anterior mitral cusp.

If septum intermedius does not forms due to a complete lack of endocardial cushion fusion, then an unique atrium with a small partial septum primum communicates with an unique ventricle partially septated. Therefore we can state that there is a persistence of the atrio-ventricular canal. This canal has its' own valves (five in number) (Figs. 2.36, 2.116 and 2.117).

It is often used "fossa ovalis persistence type defect". In our opinion this definition refers to a mistake we are going to talk about. The definition is based on a variable and persistent communication between left and right atria, communication located between septum secundum and falx septi. We consider that the definition should be: "interatrial persistence conduit defect associated with a lack of fusion with falx septi" (Fig. 2.37).

"Foramen secundum defect type" is based on the presence of at least one septal defect within fossa ovalis area or posterior to it. There is falx septi that can be fused or not with septum secundum (Figs. 2.19 and 2.20). There are parts of the fossa ovalis that can be used for differential diagnosis.

This lack of fusion might be due to a larger foramen secundum that couldn't be closed by a posterior-inferior development of septum primum or due to a lack of development of septum primum (most probably by a lack of fusion of left valve of sinus venosus) (Fig. 2.38). There can also be apoptotic regions within septum primum that can lead to a foramen secundum outside fusion area between septum primum and left valve of sinus venosus. These defects can be called "fossa ovalis perforation defects".

Septum secundum is incompletely closed by falx septi. It happens due to a lack of development of septum primum or

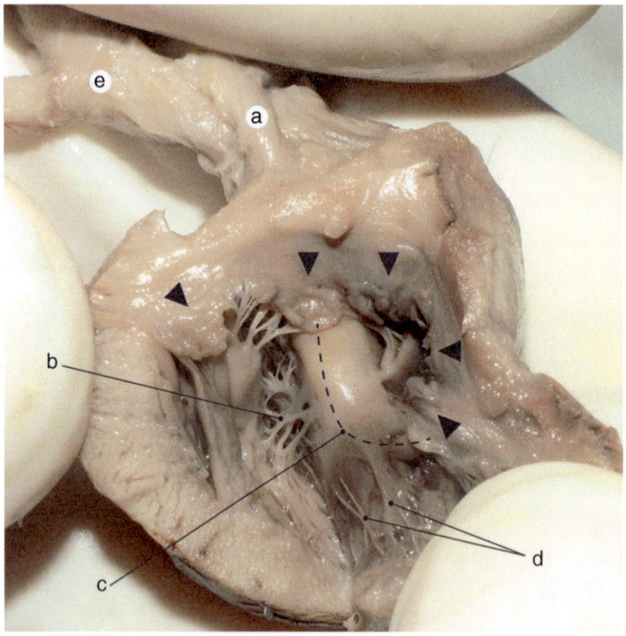

Fig. 2.36 A 6 months old heart. In a left isomerism syndrome we can identify an incompletely divided ventricle and an atrioventricular canal which is bordered by five cusps (indicated by the *arrowheads*). The detailed view of the image is found in the laterality disorders section. The dotted line indicates the muscular interventricular septum with the superior and the inferior limb. *a* Atresic pulmonary artery, *b* left branch of Hiss bundle, *c* muscular interventricular septum with superior and inferior limb, *d* right branch of Hiss bundle, *e* aorta with its origin in the right ventricle

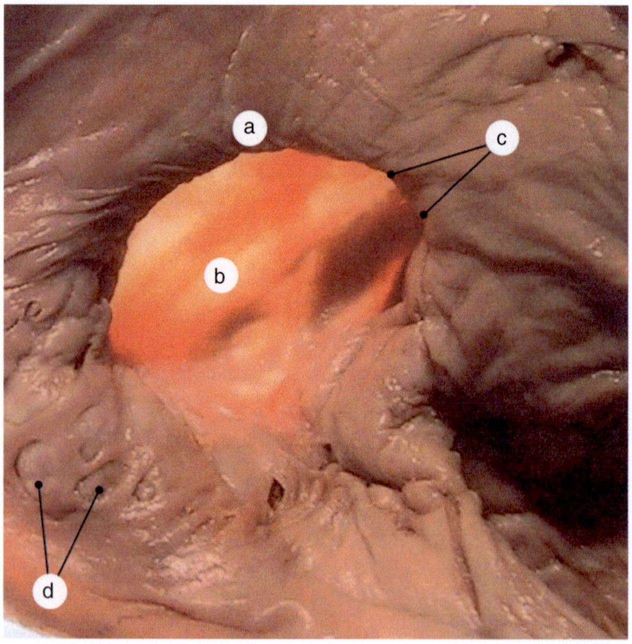

Fig. 2.37 Adult heart. View from the right atrium. Transillumination. Patent foramen ovale through the lack of fusion between falx septi and the septum secundum. *a* Patent interatrial communication, *b* the floor of the fossa ovalis is formed by the septum primum, *c* septum secundum, *d* reminiscences of the left valve

an excessive resorption of septum primum anterior to foramen secundum or a septum secundum development defect [5] (from Chap. 1). This type of defect is called "fossa ovalis floor development defect". This kind of defect has the shape of a fossa ovalis without its floor due to a lack of development. Calling this defect "persistence of oval foramen defect" was just a small step forward. A real oval foramen never existed during development therefore the "persistence of oval foramen" was misattributed to a patent intraseptal conduit.

Sinusal interatrial septal defect is located in the vicinity of sinus venarum.

These defects might be superior caval or inferior caval due to vicinity of caval orifices.

Superior caval sinusal defect is due to a lack of strengthening of interatrial septum in the posterior-superior part of fossa ovalis. This is a secondary orifice that is not compensated by fusion of the septum primum with posterior-superior limb of septum secundum. In this case, the superior right pulmonary vein opens in the right atrium.

Inferior caval sinusal defect represents a lack of strengthening of the posterior-inferior part of fossa ovalis. It is a secondary orifice due to a lack of fusion between septum primum and left valve of sinus venosus (Fig. 2.39).

If we consider the coronary sinus as an extension of the right atrium we can describe another defect – a pathologic interatrial communication due to defects of the coronary sinus roof and the coronary sinus opens in the left atrium.

A premature closing of interatrial communication, before birth, is followed by right heart hypertrophy and left heart hypoplasia. Figures 2.40, 2.41, 2.42 and 2.43 represents Norwood syndrome aspects (left heart hypoplasia).

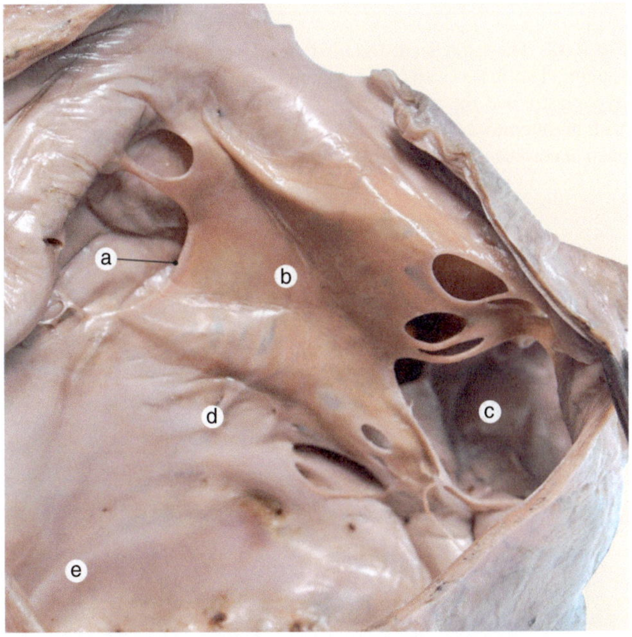

Fig. 2.38 Adult heart. View of the interatrial septum from whithin the left atrium. Falx septi is not merged with the septum secundum, so the interatrial conduit is patent. The orifice secundum has not been compensated and is still patent. Muscularised and rectangular shaped septum primum. The bottom of the inferior limb of the septum primum is correctly merged with the septum intermedium, so there is no ostium primum. *a* falx septi, *b* septum primum, *c* uncompensated ostium secundum, *d* former septum intermedium, *e* left atrium

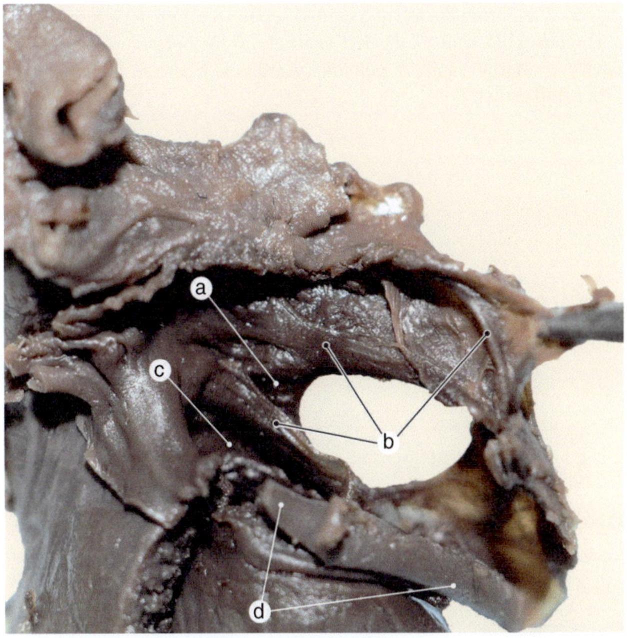

Fig. 2.39 A 4 months old heart. View of the interatrial septum from whithin the left atrium. Interatrial septal sinusal defect that involves the inferior vena cava. The coronary sinus venosus is merged with the inferior vena cava. The posteroinferior side of the interatrial septum has not been yet consolidated. We can distinguish the main elements of the septum primum. *a* Septum secundum, *b* septum primum, *c* mitral orifice, *d* coronary sinus opened in the inferior vena cava

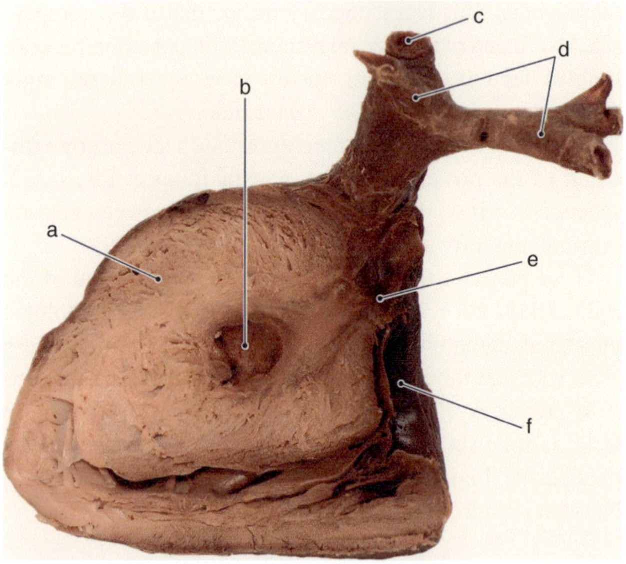

Fig. 2.40 A 8 months old heart. Norwood syndrome (left heart hypoplasia). View from the *left* of a sagittal section through the left ventricle. *a* Hypertrophic wall of the left ventricle, *b* hypoplastic left ventricle cavity, *c* arterial canal, *d* pulmonary arteries, *e* atresic aortic valves, *f* tricuspid orifice

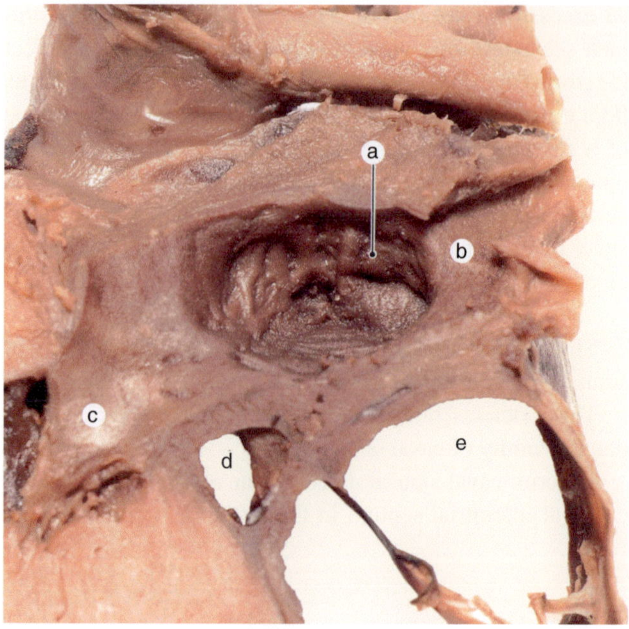

Fig. 2.42 The same heart. Detailed view from the left of the interatrial septum. The fossa ovalis is prematurely obturated. The left atrium is hypoplastic and the mitral valve is atresic. *a* Hypoplastic left atrium with no interatrial communication, *b* pulmonary veins, *c* atresic mitral cusp, *d* coronary sinus, *e* right atrium

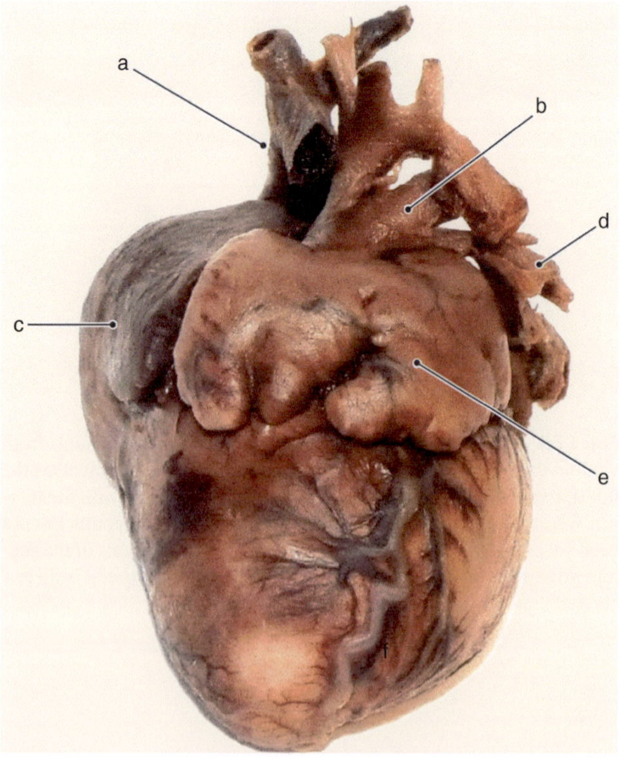

Fig. 2.41 The same heart. Anterior view. *a* Superior vena cava, *b* arterial canal, *c* right auricle, *d* left pulmonary artery, *e* giant left auricle

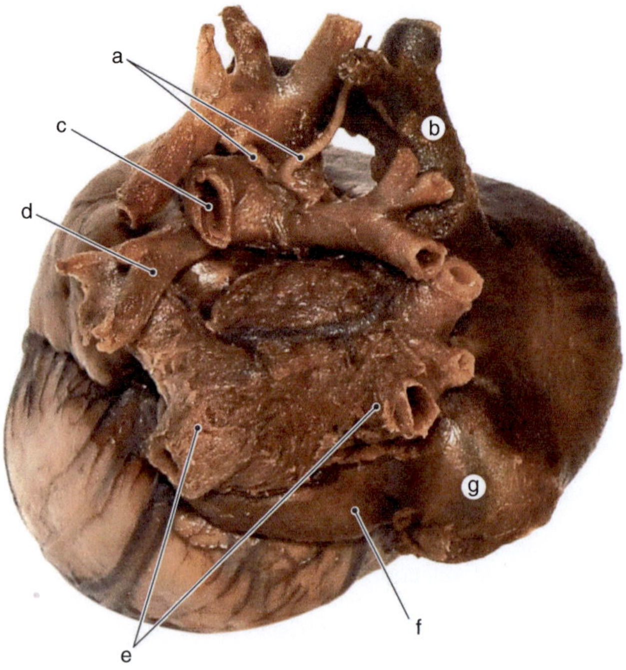

Fig. 2.43 The same heart. Posterior view of the base of the heart. Notice the incompletely developed coronary sinus, very suggestive for the expression: the sinus is an exteriorized right atrium. *a* Reminiscences of bronchial arteries, *b* superior vena cava, *c* arterial canal, *d* left pulmonary artery, *e* left atrium with pulmonary veins, *f* left horn of the sinus venosus, *g* inferior vena cava

2.3 Evolution of the Right Atrium and of the Sinus Venosus

2.3.1 Incorporation of the Right Horn of Sinus Venosus in the Atrial Wall

The main veins of the embryo (umbilical vein, vitelline vein and common cardinal vein) fuse in order to build a venous canal (Cuvier) called sinusal horn (on each side).

Both sinusal horns (right and left) fuse in order to form the primitive sinus venosus (Fig. 2.43).

These horns fuse inferiorly where a crest is formed and is called sinus septi (sinusal septum) (Fig. 2.56).

In the superior part, both horns fuse with the primitive atrium building the sinoatrial part. This part is delimited by the two valves of sinus venosus, that occur in the atrium as two endocardial folds. They are similar with the one from which the septum primum develops.

In the primitive cardiac tube, the sinusal valves are located at the sino-atrial border and are lateral structures. Evaluation of the congenital defects should consider the atrial involvement of the sinus and the lateral position of the valves.

Along with the atrial septation, the left umbilical vein involves, therefore the left atrium becomes smaller than the right one. It follows hemodynamic fall of the left atrium, followed again by an atrial asymmetry and the sinus venosus opens in the right atrium.

The primitive sinus venosus is involved in certain "movements" during development:

A. The sino-atrial junction suffers a translation movement and changes its position. From an almost transverse position on the longitudinal axis of the cardiac tube it reaches a final position in a frontal plane. In this new position the anterior commissural area is oblique, in contact with the inferior endocardial cushion. The posterior commissure is oblique and faces towards superior and to the right.

   Septum spurium is an endocardial fold raised by the fusion of the two valves at the superior commissure. The superior commissure is in contact with the superior endocardial cushion through this structure.

   In this position:

   The inferior extremity of the right valve fuses with the inferior endocardial cushion;

   The inferior extremity of the left valve fuses with the vestibular spine and with the inferior endocardial cushion [6].

   The superior parts of these valves fuse, but the inferior parts do not completely fuse at the level of the free margin of septum secundum (in Fig. 6.17, a Chiari network suggests the development of the right valve). They reach this part due to the fusion of both endocardial cushions.

   The traction of the sinus venosus valves along with the protrusion of the aorta within the superior endocardial cushion might play an important role in septum secundum formation (as an atrial wall fold).

B. Translation is accompanied by a right lateralization. Therefore the sinus becomes posterior to the right atrium.

C. In the next step, the sinus suffers a clockwise rotation and the left valve fuses with the septum primum.

D. In the next stage of development, the primitive sinus venosus protrudes towards the atrium and the sinus septi becomes anterior (from a posterior position) and partially fuses with the right valve. Following this step, the dorsal-sinusal space strengthens and the valves of the coronary sinus and of the inferior vena cava are formed. (see the internal aspect of right atrium).

   Along with these complex developmental movements, the right horn of the sinus venosus fuses with atrial wall. Therefore, most part of the right horn becomes sinus venarum, the smooth part of the atrial wall in between the two vena cavae.

   During the evolution of the sinus venosus, recesses within the sinusal wall occur and they later disappear due to coalescence processes. Some of these recesses are not cited in the literature and are first described now. They have been named according to their components.

   The evolution of these recesses increases the heterogeneity of the atrial wall.

2.3.2 Sinusal Recesses and Their Evolution

Next we shall present these recesses and their evolution.

1. Septal-valvular recess is located in the atrial wall between the left valve of the sinus venosus and the septum primum. This is the first recess that disappears and by this the left valve of sinus venosus strengthens the posterior-inferior part of the inter-atrial septum. The following evolution of the fused area (the inferior half of the fossa ovalis) is towards myocardization. The septum secundum starts developing after the beginning of the fusion process and is associated with the fusion process of the left valve.

   We can say that the left valve evolves and disappears way faster than the right valve. In Fig. 2.32 there can be noticed the fusion between left valve and the septum primum.

2. Terminal-marginal recess (new described recess) – is represented by the sinus venosus wall in between the terminal muscular fasciculus of the primitive atrium and the marginal fold (new term that is going to be explained in the following lines). It disappears throughout the fusion of the delimiting structures (Figs. 2.44 and 2.45).

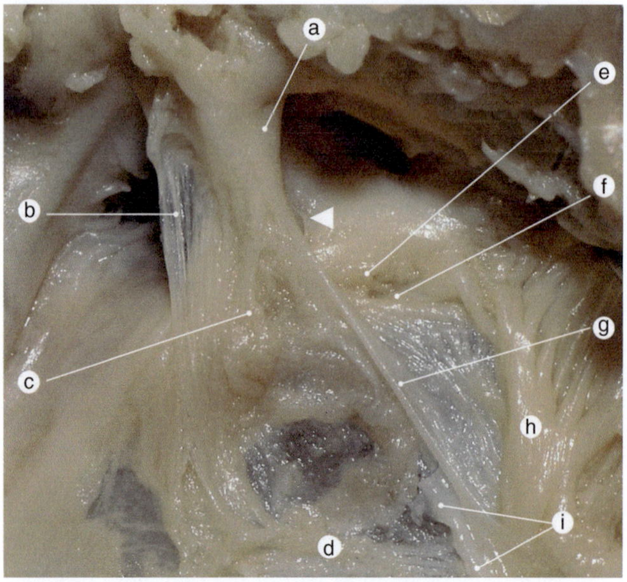

Fig. 2.44 A 4 months old heart. Posterosuperior view after removal of atrial walls. Terminal- marginal recess, between the terminal fascicle and the marginal fold. *a* Septum secundum, *b* septum primum, *c* reminiscence of the left valve, *d* inferior vena cava, *e* coronary sinus ostium, *f* sinus septi, *g* marginal fold, *h* terminal fascicle, *i* valve of inferior vena cava, The *arrowhead tip* indicates the inferior segment of the right valve

After its disappearance, the Eustachian valve (developed from the right valve of the primitive sinus) forms the complex named the terminal crest by using the fusion of marginal fold and the terminal atrial fasciculus. Formation of the marginal fold will be described in the following lines.

3. Sinusal recess (delimited by sinus septi and both sinusal horns). This recess is located outside the heart (Fig. 2.56).
   Initially, sinus septi represents a sagittal endocardial fold that separates right and left sinus venosus horns. Like any other horn it has two parts – right and left. In between these parts, but outwards the recess is delimited. From the venous sinusal horns the mesocardium develops anteriorly towards the transverse septum (Fig. 2.46) – this development is prior to the development of primitive sinus and specific for the mesocardium development. Posteriorly it forms the dorsal mesocardium that binds the primitive sinus and atrium to the primitive intestine.

Left rotation of the sinus venosus leads to a horizontal movement of the sinus septi. In order to understand the evolution and differentiation of the sinus septi we set as landmarks both anterior and posterior extremities of the sinusal fold together with the positions of both sides.

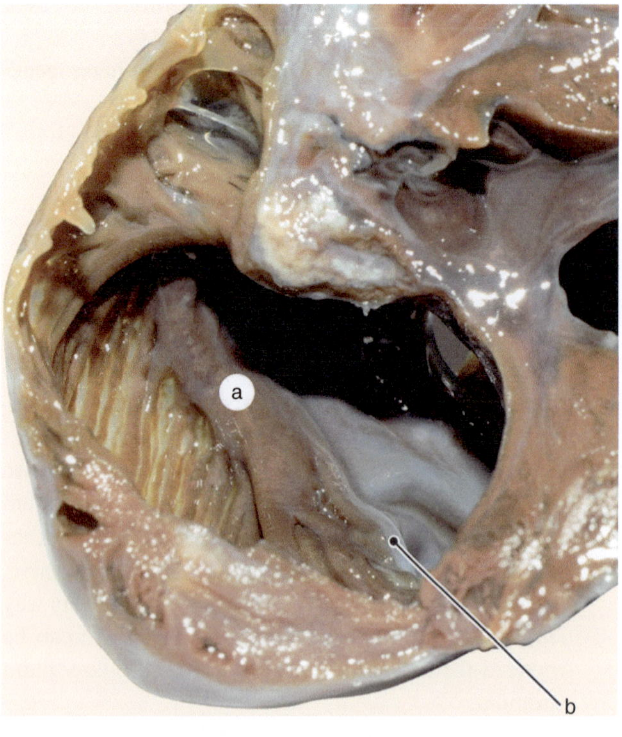

Fig. 2.45 Three and a half months old heart. View of the right atrium cavity through the tricuspid orifice. The terminal fascicle becomes the terminal crest. *a* Terminal fascicle, *b* valve of inferior vena cava

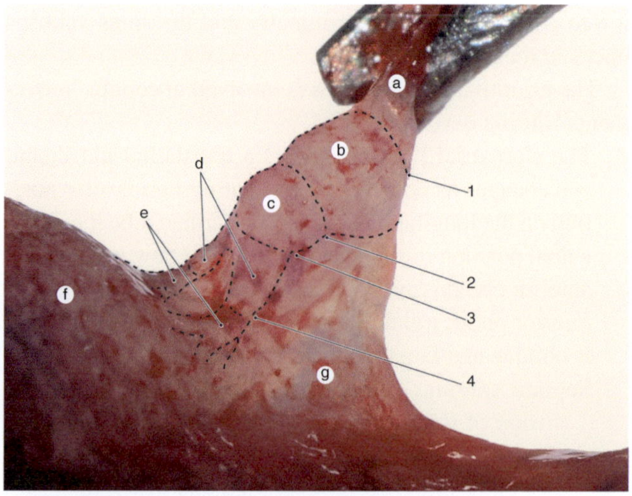

Fig. 2.46 Primitive cardiac tube from a 9 days old rat. Anterior and from the left view. The dorsal mesocardium pedicle remains only on the inferior side of the primitive cardiac tube. The sinus venosus is not yet formed. The reflexion of the venous mesocardium from the transverse septum to the anterior wall of the cardiac tube is suggestive for the final layout. The mesocardium segment between the primitive atria forms a recess which has not been described until now in specialized literature. *a* Dorsal aorta, *b* aortic bulb, *c* primitive bulb, *d* primitive ventricle, *e* primitive atrium, *f* transverse septum, *g*. reducing dorsal mesocardium, *1* bulbo-aortic sulcus, *2* inter-bulbar sulcus, *3* bulboventricular sulcus, *4* atrioventricular sulcus

The anterior extremity of the septal sinusal fold reaches the foramen of coronary sinus to the right and superiorly. The posterior extremity reaches a position superior and to the left to this foramen (Fig. 2.56).

The movement of the posterior extremity forms a fold of the sinusal wall called marginal fold. It is partially located at the base of the right valve of the primitive sinus venosus.

Sinus septi also protrudes in the primitive atrium.

Therefore, the marginal fold and sinus septi have a posterior – anterior development, partially raising the right valve (Fig. 2.47).

After the rotation, both parts of this fold are represented by the following parts:

Part of the atrial wall that stretches between the inferior vena cava and the base of interatrial septum (former right part);

The roof of the coronary sinus (former left part);

Fusion of these parts will build the dorsal-sinusal region.

In between the two parts of the fold a vascular embryonic remnant might remain, probably a remnant of an umbilical valve (see dorsal-sinusal region of the right atrium).

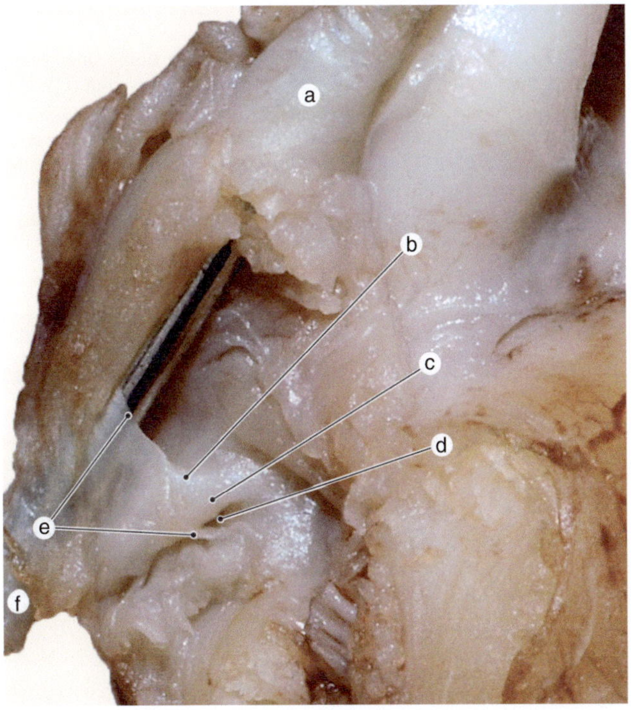

Fig. 2.47 A 2 months and a half old heart. Right valve of the sinus venosus. View from the right, after the resection of the atrial wall. The metalic needle loads the two venae cavae. *a* Superior vena cava, *b* marginal fold, *c* sinus septi, *d* coronary sinus ostium, *e* left valve, *f* inferior vena cava

2.4 A New Approach Upon Formation and Biologic Utility of Todaro's Tendon, Regarding the Evolution of the Primitive Sinus Venosus Recesses

2.4.1 Formation of Eustachian Margin and Evolution of Right Valve

Sinus venarum rotates towards the left side, therefore the left valve fuses with septum primum and the left horn of sinus venarum becomes inferior to the right one.

In order to understand the evolution of this region we make the following statements:

Anterior-superior part of the right atrial-ventricular junction becomes subauricular tricuspid vestibule;

Posterior margin of the primitive atrium (where it fuses with the sinus venarum) forms fasciculus terminalis that will become crista terminalis (Fig. 2.45).

The fold represented by sinus septi reaches a transverse position from an almost sagittal one. The former anterior part of sinus septi curves towards the coronary sinus and generates to the right the fold of Thebesius. The former posterior extremity of sinus septi also curves over the coronary sinus orifice, but superior and to the left. This part of sinus septi fuses with the inferior endocardial cushion, at the same level where both cushions fuse.

The complex rotation movement of the posterior part of sinus septi has another side effect: it raises a fold on the sinusal wall between the primitive atrium and the right valve of sinus venarum. This fold is called marginal fold (Figs. 2.44 and 2.47) and it will provide attachment point for the fusion between fasciculus terminalis and inferior vena cava valve. Following this fusion a complex structure is formed – the Eustachian margin (see the previous images).

In short: the Eustachian margin is build by three structures that fuse – fasciculus terminalis (that becomes crista terminalis), inferior vena cava valve (former right valve of sinus venarum that involutes) and marginal fold.

The marginal fold is formed between the fasciculus terminalis of primitive atrium and the right valve. This fold, along with sinus septi, rises the medial and inferior part of right valve therefore the right valve divides into Thebesian and Eustachian valves.

The caval-marginal recess can be considered a segment of the primitive sinusal wall that lies between the superior part of the right valve and the marginal fold. Through a coalescence process, the right valve fuses with the posterior part of the marginal fold (Figs. 2.48, 6.50 and 6.51). Remnants of this process can be noticed in adults (Fig. 6.12).

The right valve's part that does not participate in the coalescence process may occur in adults and rises over the Eustachian margin as the inferior vena cava valve.

Its shape is of a small membranous fold, with a free margin which runs along the crista terminalis until it reaches an anterior position to the superior vena cava foramen. This valve encircles the superior vena cava foramen.

Remnants of this valve may have various aspects, eventually taking the aspect of a Chiari fibrous network.

Another paradox can be solved after this exegesis: the coronary sinus foramen, in adults, seems to be aside to the right valve of the primitive sinus venarum and the intervalvular space. This might be impossible and this foramen should be located in between these valves or their remnants.

We must understand that initially, the coronary sinus foramen is covered by the inferior part of the right valve. This valve stretches between interatrial septum and the tricuspid vestibule. Most of the base of the right valve corresponds to the inferior endocardial cushion (Fig. 2.49).

Initially, the coronary sinus foramen lies between the inferior part of the right valve and the sinus septi. Next, sinus septi and marginal fold rise the inferior part the right valve. Part of the right valve involutes, where the pressure is at its maximum (where it passes over sinus septi). Therefore, the right valve divides into two parts – inferior vena cava valve (towards superior) and coronary sinus valve (towards inferior).

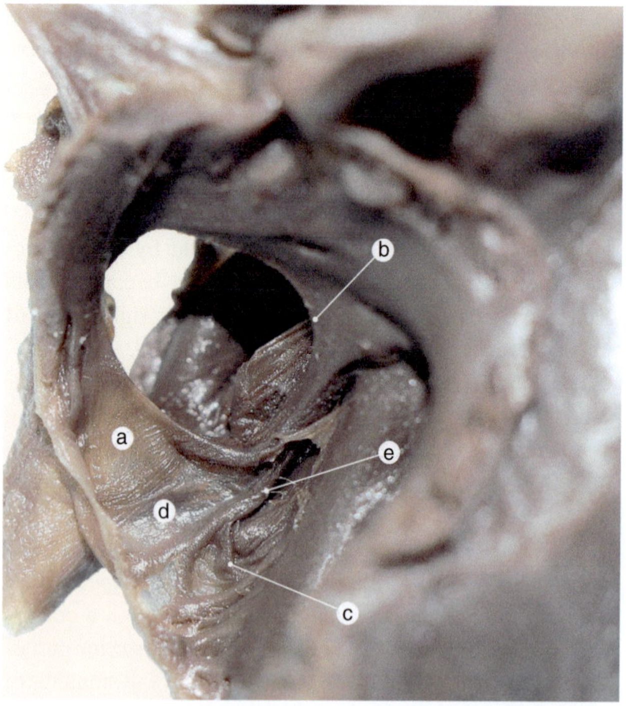

Fig. 2.48 A 4 months old heart. The left valve and the marginal fascicle border the cavomarginal recess. View from the right, after the removal of the atrial wall. *a* Right valve of the sinus venosus in the course of muscularization, *b* septum secundum, *c* subeustachian sinus, *d* cavomarginal recess, *e* marginal fold, merged with the terminal fascicle

Due to this evolution, the coronary sinus valve might be medial or lateral in accordance with the involved segment of the right valve. The coronary sinus valve might be also mistaken with the Thebesian margin of the sinus venarum (Fig. 2.50).

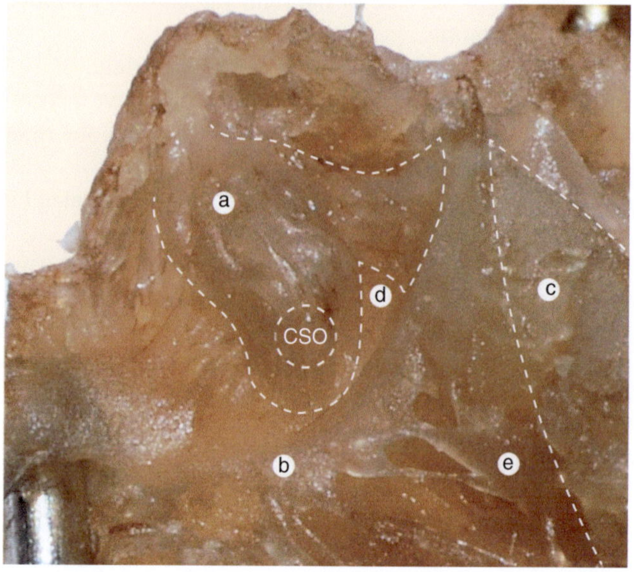

Fig. 2.49 An 8–9 months old heart. The right valve of the sinus venosus is confined by the dotted line. The coronary sinus ostium (*CSO*) is covered by the right valve. Its position is marked by *dotted line*. Sinus septi makes a loop in the right valve. Anterior view of the atrial cavity from the tricuspid valve, after removing the atrial wall. The tip of the needle points the primitive part of the right atrium. *a* Right valve of the sinus venosus, *b* septal cusp, *c* interventricular septum, *d* sinus septi, *e* posterior papillary muscle with tendinous cords

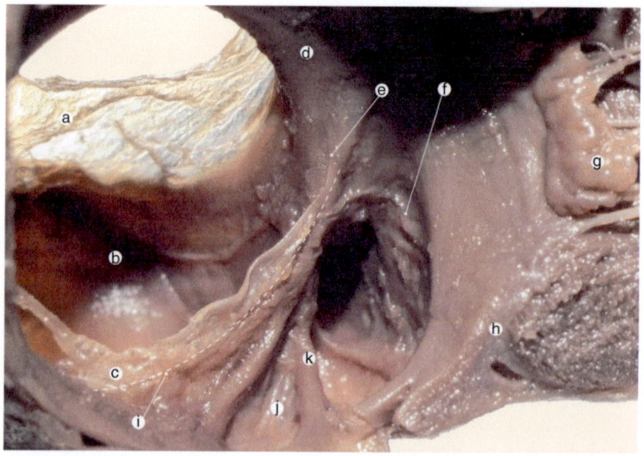

Fig. 2.50 A 4 months old heart. Interatrial conduit. Detailed view. Sinus septi makes a loop in the right valve. In the maximum pressure area the valve is divided in the valve of the inferior vena cava and the thebesian valve. *a* Septum primum, *b* left valve of the sinus venosus, *c* right valve of the sinus venosus, *d* septum secundum, *e* valvular process, *f* sinusal ostium valvule, *g* septal cusp, *h* atrioventricular junction, *i* marginal fold, *j* subeustachian sinus, *k* thebesian margin of the coronary sinus ostium

2.4.2 Formation of Todaro's Tendon

Early formation of Todaro's tendon as a connective tissue structure within marginal fold anchors the posterior part of the sinus septi to the tendinous part of the heart. This anchoring limits the rotation process of the sinus venarum and sinusal septum and the anchor is this tendon. The sinusal wall is tensioned between the tendon and both future caval veins, strengthening and defining the marginal fold and then, the Eustachian margin. The increased tension of the marginal fold between the two anchors represents a strongpoint that later generates the right valve segmentation (Fig. 2.47).

This tendon is, practically, a structure with a possible extracardiac origin, probably originating from the marginal fold extracardiac mesoderm. Therefore, in adults the final position of the tendon of Todaro is between the tendinous part of the heart and the dorsal-sinusal space (Fig. 2.51). If its origin was from the vestibular spine, then its trajectory should have been parallel with the interatrial septum, situation that does not match the reality, the tendon of Todaro lying oblique to the septum and passing through the marginal fold and disappearing in the dorsal-sinusal space.

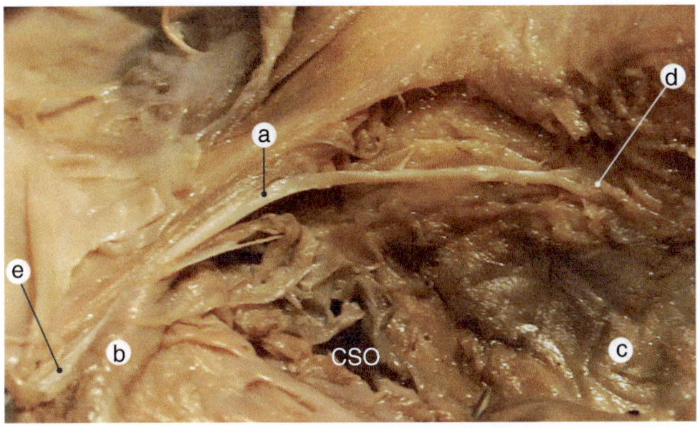

Fig. 2.51 Adult heart. Inside the right atrium. View from the right. The tendon of Todaro spreads from the dorsosinusal space to the tendinous centre. *CSO* Coronary sinus ostium. *a* Tendon of Todaro, *b* terminal crest, *c* septal cusp, *d* insertion of the tendon on the tendinous centre, *e* origin of the tendon in the dorsosinusal space

2.5 Evolutionary Significance of the Sinusal Valves and Horns

The sinusal valves guide the blood towards the left fetal atrium. The right valve has an extension within the right atrium and an anterior concave margin.

The evolution of the valves differs:

The left valve is rapidly pushed by the blood stream towards the fusion with the vestibular spine and septum primum.

The right valve is divided by the sinus septi and the marginal fold into the Thebesian and Eustachian valves.

The blood of the inferior part of the body is split in two parts by the septum secundum – crista dividens: towards the left atrium (most of it) and towards the tricuspid valve (a small part).

The blood of the superior part of the body is also divided by the intercaval tubercle – Lower (Fig. 2.31) (an inconstant prominence of crista dividens):

a small part runs towards tricuspid valve and the rest towards the left atrium.

We make again the statement that the blood flow from the right atrium towards the left atrium is made through an intraatrial conduit bordered by the right valve of the sinus venarum and by a complex structure built by the left valve of the sinus venarum that fuses with septum primum. This conduit has an oblique trajectory – intraseptal conduit.

The right valve and septum primum are pushed towards the right atrium by the blood flow.

The horns of the sinus venarum evolve differently:

The left horn has two parts – a proximal and a distal one. The proximal part evolves and forms the coronary sinus while the distal part evolves and forms the superior vena cava. It involutes afterwards and turns to fibrous connective tissue and forms the ligament of Marshall. The non-fibrous part that continues sinus venarum becomes the oblique vein of left atrium. The Marshall ligament forms a pericardial fold called triangular ligament (Figs. 2.52, 2.53, 2.54, 2.55 and 2.56).

The right horn (along with the septum between the two sinusal horns, called sinus septi) forms both the sinusal part of the right atrium called sinus venarum and the dorsal-sinusal

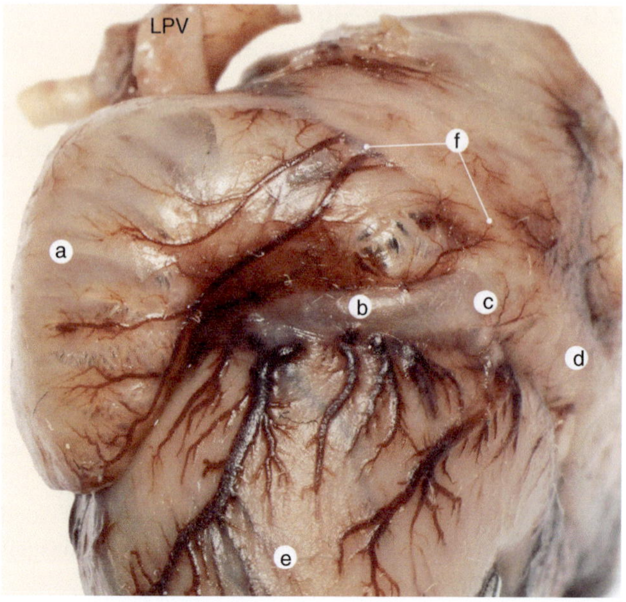

Fig. 2.52 A 5 months old heart. Posterolateral view of the left auricle. Under-developed fetus. Myocardisation of the left auricle. In the axis of each circular mesenchymal ribbon there is a vascular ramification. *a* Left auricle, *b* great cardiac vein, *c* myocardisation limit of the coronary sinus, *d* coronary sinus, *e* left ventricle, *f* oblique vein of the left atrium, *LPV* Left pulmonary veins

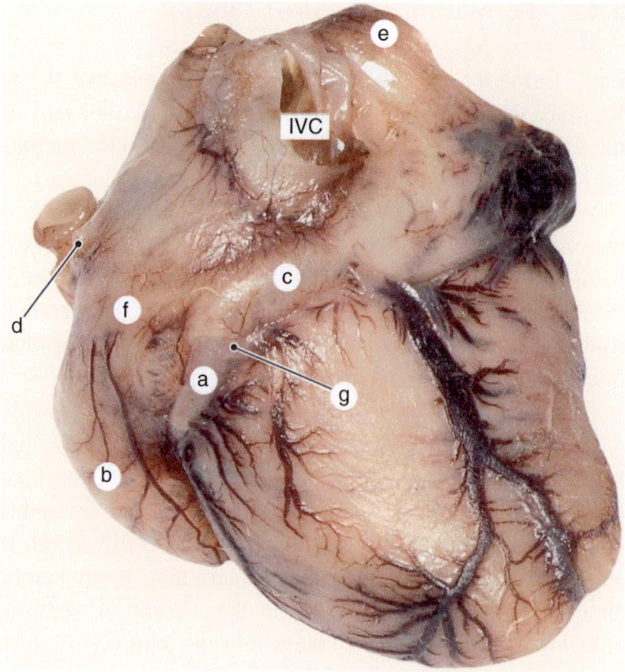

Fig. 2.54 The myocardisation of the coronary sinus is part of the atrial myocardisation process and it depends on vascular presence. View of the diaphragmatic surface of the heart. *a* Great cardiac vein, *b* left auricle, *c* coronary sinus, *d* left pulmonary vein, *e* right atrium, *f* oblique vein of the left atrium, *g* sinusal myocardisation limit

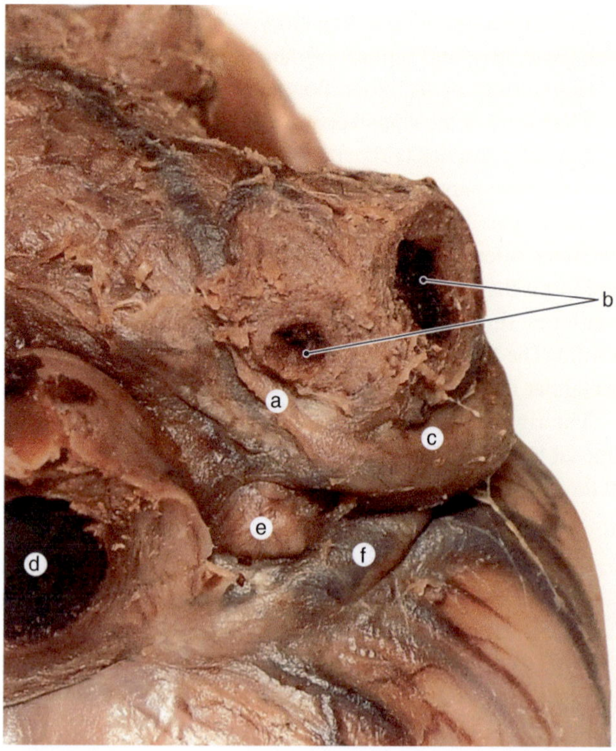

Fig. 2.53 A 7 months old heart. Reminiscence of the left superior vena cava continuing the coronary sinus. The part that drains into the sinus will become the oblique vein. View from the left. The left auricle has been resected in order to mark out the contents of the coronary sulcus. *a* Reminiscence of the left superior vena cava, *b* left pulmonary veins, *c* coronary sinus, *d* left auricle, *e* lymph node, *f* great cardiac vein

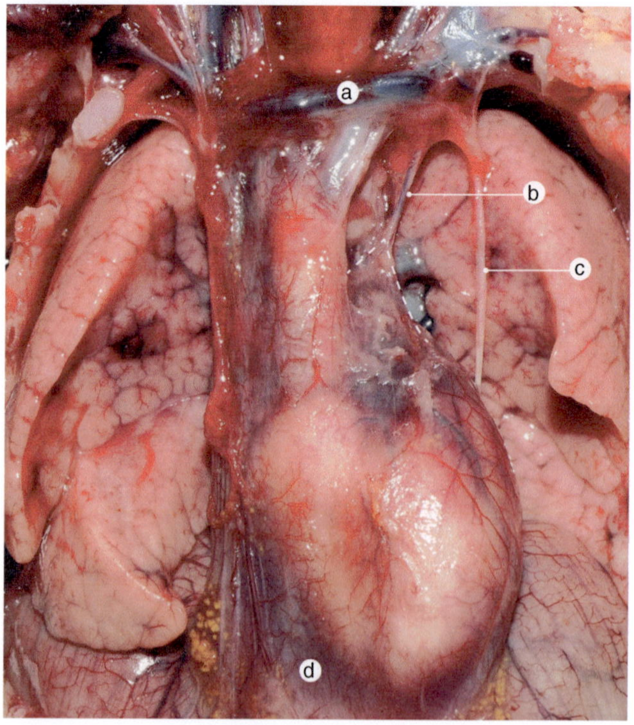

Fig. 2.55 A 7 months old heart. The left superior vena cava lifts a triangular pericardium fold at its origin. *a* Left brachiocephalic vein, *b* left superior vena cava, *c* left phrenic nerve, *d* pericardial sac

region (see right atrium). As we previously stated, the right atrium has a "primitive" part represented by the right auricle and the smooth region located superior and anterior to the tricuspid valve, called subauricular vestibule. It originates from the right half of the atrio-ventricular canal (atrioventricular junction).

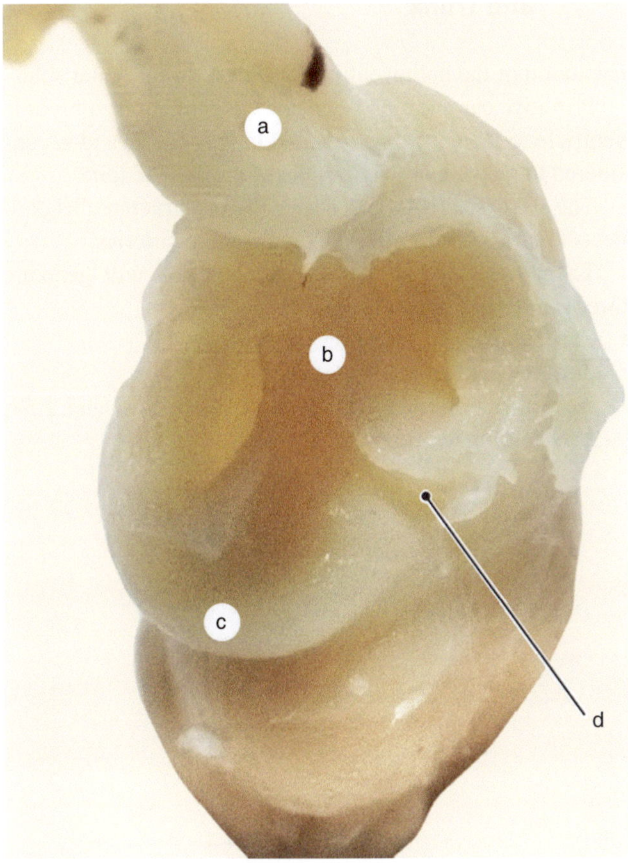

Fig. 2.56 Nine weeks old heart. The left horn of the sinus venosus is evident. Posterior view after removing the primitive atrium. *a* Aorta, *b* proper interatrial septum, *c* left horn of the sinus venosus, *d* sinus septi and the sinusal recess from the posterior

2.6 Evolution of the Left Atrium

The lung bud develops in early stages a vascular network that drains through the primitive pulmonary vein into the primitive atrium, just above the sinus venosus, between the two pulmonary ridges (or margins) (Fig. 2.57).

Resuming the way in which posterior atrial septation is finalized, we remind that the left valve merges with the vestibular spine, then with the septum primum, and the entire complex finally merges with the intermediate septum. As a result of atrial septation, the primitive pulmonary vein remains to open at the base and to the left of the posterior extremity of the interatrial septum. By atrial increase, the vein wall is included in the left atrium wall. The incorporation process is directed superiorly by the interatrial septum and an endocardial fold, represented by the posterior extension of the inferior endocardial cushion. Depending on the degree of primitive vein incorporation, between one and four pulmonary veins will open in the left atrium. Ultimately, the pulmonary veins ostia will remain in the center of a wider area resulting from the primitive vein incorporation.

The endocardial fold that was mentioned (extension of the inferior endocardial cushion) will be entirely or partially included in the interartial septum, reinforcing its base on the left side (see previous images).

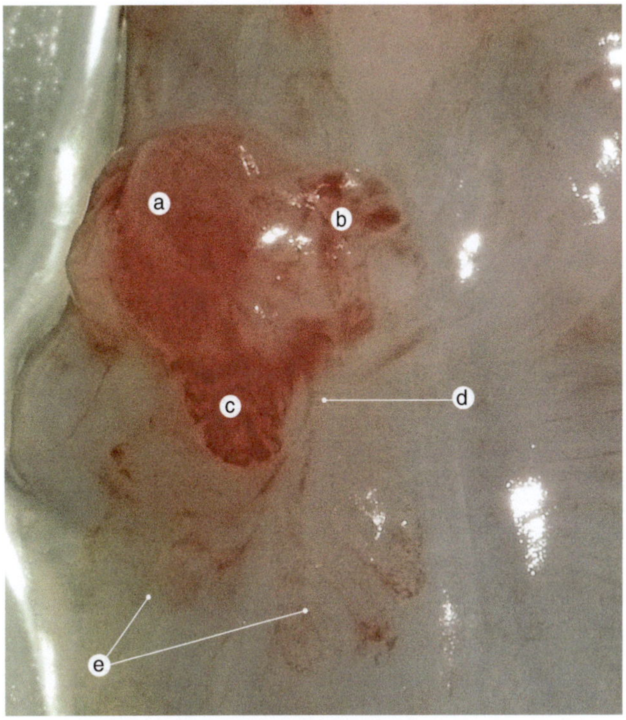

Fig. 2.57 Evidentiation of the primitive pulmonary vein. Ten days old rat heart. The heart is reversed and the diaphragmatic surface is visible. Notice the pulmonary vein that drains a primitive pulmonary vascular network. *a* Interventricular septum visible through transparency as a more light area, *b* left auricle, *c* right auricle, *d* primitive pulmonary vein, *e* primitive pulmonary vascular network

*The posterior extension of the inferior endocardial cushion into the left atrium was described by Licata [5] in 1954 (in an admirable article) as a "coronary sinus fold", considering it to be a fold elevated by the initial evolution of the coronary sinus, assumption that was not confirmed in time.

In conclusion the left atrial wall is composed of:

- left auricle that originates in the primitive atrium;
- most of the posterior wall, centered by the pulmonary veins ostia, results from the embedding the primitive pulmonary vein in the atrial wall;
- the subauricular vestibule arises from the atriventricular junction;
- the part corresponding to the mitral-aortic continuity arises from the superior endocardial cushion (after aortic protrusion);
- the future transverse pericardial sinus (the former atrial notch) originates in the primitive atrium;
- the left side of the interatrial septum results from the septum primum, septum secundum and endocardial cushions.

2.7 Evolution of the Cardiac Bulb and Truncus Arteriosus and Septation of the Primitive Ventricle

2.7.1 Defining Bulbus Cordis and Its Components – the Trabeculated Part of the Right Ventricle, Arterial Conus and Trunk

Evolution of the bulboventricular and conoventricular sulci

Primitive cardiac tube segment connecting the embryonic ventricle to the aortic sac is called bulbus cordis and is considered to be the exit tract or pole of the cardiac tube.

The aortic sac (bulb) is a mezenchymal structure that connects the truncus arteriosus to the branchial arteries.

The differentiation of the bulbus cordis will generate three main segments of the cardiac tube:

- trabeculated part of the right ventricle;
- the conus or the conal part;
- the truncus arteriosus (Figs. 1.11, 1.18, 7.35 and 2.58, 2.59 and Fig. 2.60).

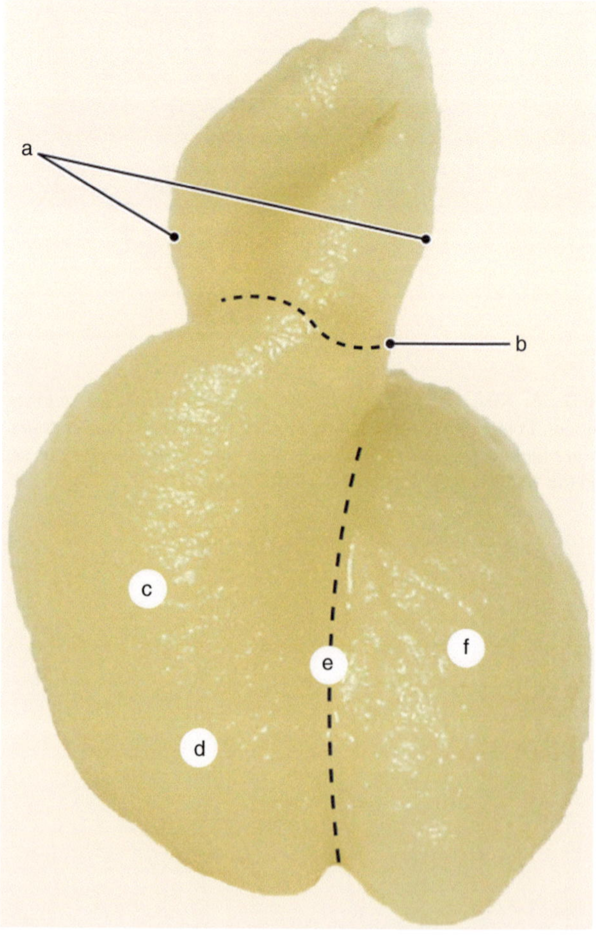

Fig. 2.58 An 8 months old heart. Inferior bulboventricular sulcus. *a* Arterial trunk, *b* conotruncal junction represented by the superior limit of conal muscularization, *c* conus, *d* trabeculate part of the right ventricle, e inferior bulboventricular sulcus, f primitive ventricle

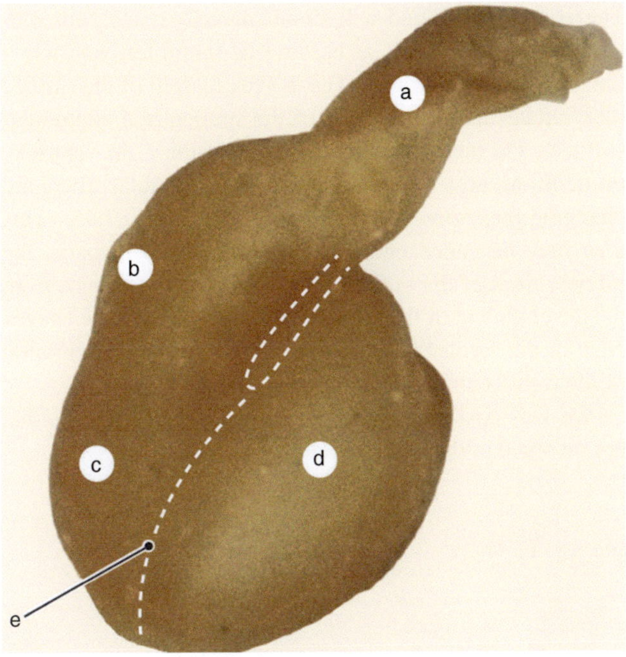

Fig. 2.59 An 8 weeks old heart. Inferior bulboventricular sulcus. Arterial trunk. Conoventricular fold indicated by the dotted line. *a* Arterial trunk, *b* conus, *c* trabeculate part of the right ventricle, *d* primitive ventricle, *e* inferior bulboventricular sulcus

The conal part will generate the subvalvular segments of the right and left ventricle.

The truncus arteriosus will differentiate into intrapericardial segments of the aorta and pulmonary artery.

The future trabeculated part of the right ventricle is delineated as follows: (Fig. 1.16)

- superior, between the future trabeculated part of the right ventricle and the conus it is forming a delicate sulcus named conal delineation sulcus or conoventricular sulcus
- inferior, separation from the primitive ventricle is due to the bulboventricular sulcus, that separates the future left ventricle from the future trabeculated part of the right ventricle.

During the cardiac tube folding, the bulb plies partially over the primitive ventricle. In fact, only the conal part of the bulb folds, producing a fold between the primitive ventricle and the conus, on the concave margin of the cardiac tube, known as the conoventricular fold (Fig. 2.66). Most of the bulboventricular sulcus remains captive in the depth of that fold after the merge of the conus and the primitive ventricle. A segment of the bulboventricular sulcus is again visible beyond the conoventricular fusion area, on the right side of the pulmonary conus, near the atrioventricular junction, known as the superior bulboventricular sulcus (Figs. 2.3, 2.60 and 2.61).

The concave margin diminishes and only on this edge the conoventricular and bulboventricular sulci meet and almost reach the atrioventricular canal (Figs. 1.11 and 1.18).

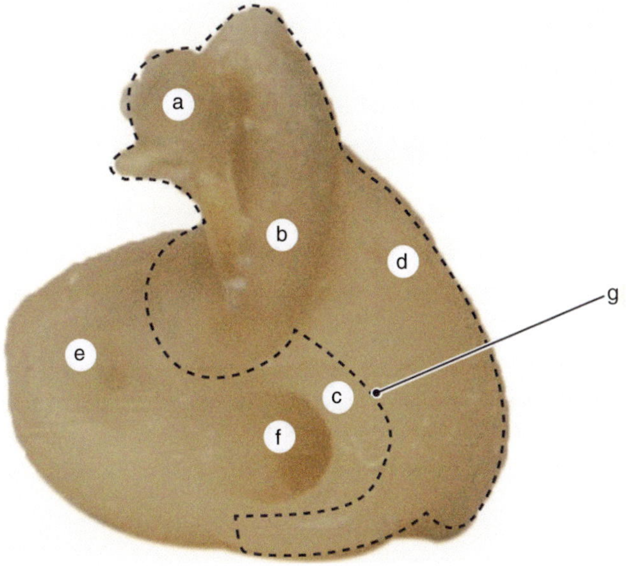

Fig. 2.60 A 7 weeks old heart. View of the base of the heart after removing the atria. The dotted line indicates the bulbary territory. *a* Pulmonary trunk, *b* aorta, *c* primitive ventricle territory near the bulboventricular junction, *d* conal territory, *e* mitral valve, *f* tricuspid valve, *g* superior bulboventricular sulcus

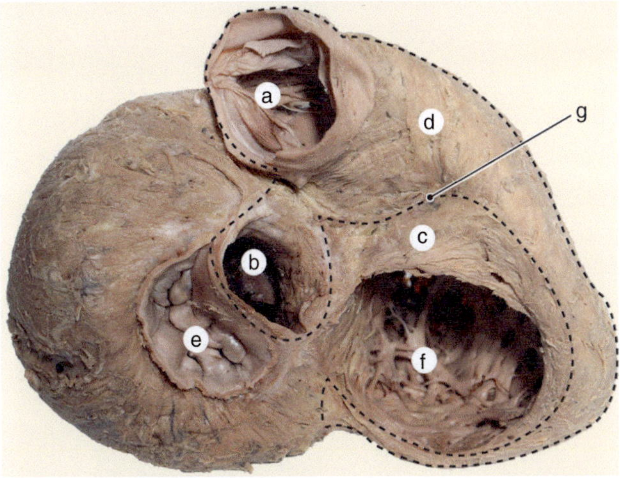

Fig. 2.61 View of the base of the adult heart after removing the atria. The dotted line indicates the bulbary territory. *a* Pulmonary trunk, *b* aorta, *c* primitive ventricle territory near the bulboventricular junction (three ostial isthmus), *d* conal territory, *e* mitral valve, *f* tricuspid valve, *g* superior bulboventricular line

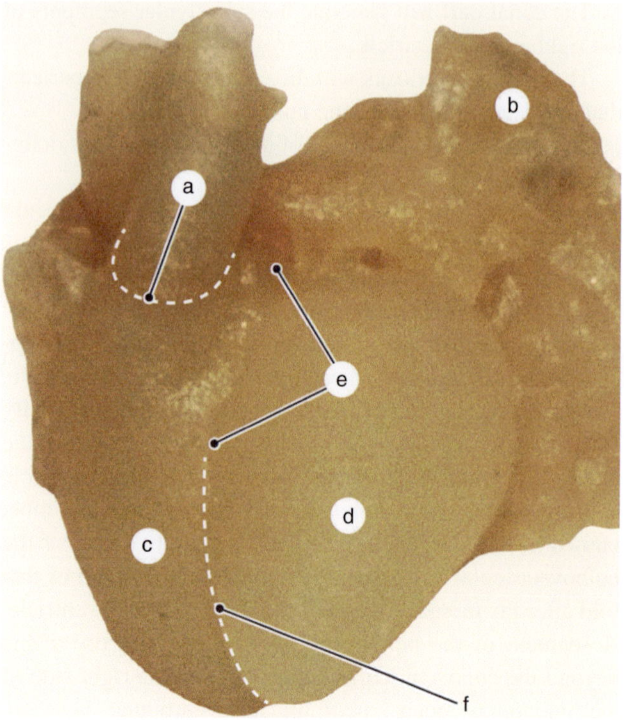

Fig. 2.62 An 8 weeks old heart. *a* Myocardisation at the conotruncal junction, b Atria, *c* conus, *d* primitive ventricle, *e* the myocardisation of the conoventricular junction leaves deep the superior part of the bulboventricular sulcus, *f* inferior bulboventricular sulcus

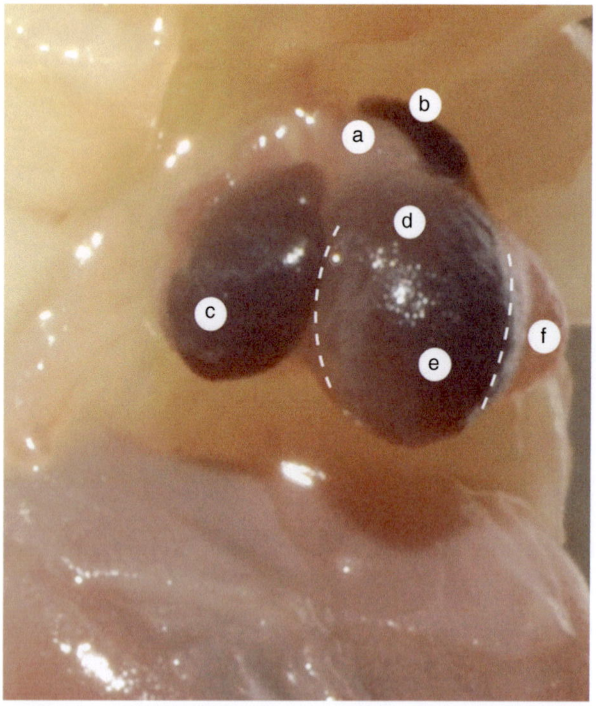

Fig. 2.63 A 12 days old rat heart. The superior and inferior bulboventricular sulci are indicated by dotted lines. The bulb grows into pars trabecularis, conus and trunk. Notice the existence of independent ventricular apices at the tip of the heart. *a* Arterial trunk, *b* left atrium, *c* right atrium, *d* cone, *e* pars trabecularis of the right ventricle, *f* primitive ventricle – apex

Therefore, atrial blood will simultaneously reach both ventricles, not sequentially as before (the future left ventricle – the future right ventricle). The convex margin of the cardiac tube inflates and forms most of the sternocostal ventricular surfaces. On the sternocostal surface of the right ventricle, on adult, an area where the superficial muscular fibers are changing their direction may be observed (Fig. 7.35). This area may be called conal boundary line and it marks the inferior limit of the pulmonary conus. The line comes from the development of the conoventricular sulcus on the convex edge of the cardiac tube (see also the external configuration of the right ventricle) (Fig. 2.64).

We will next try to systematize the complex events that are involved in the zonal development

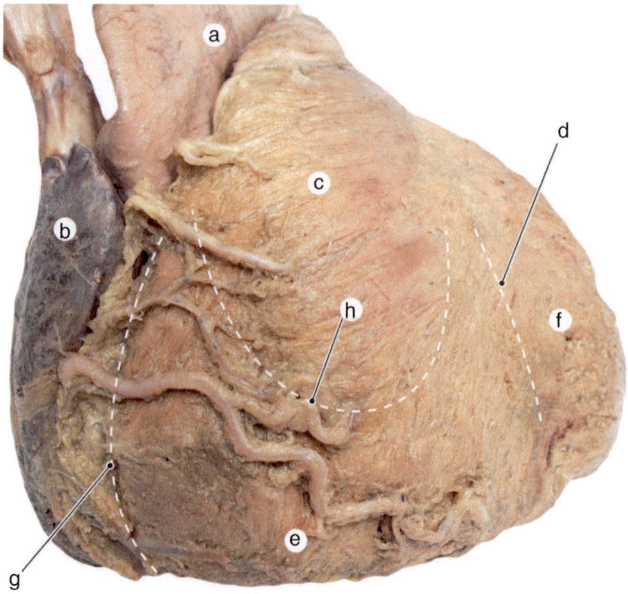

Fig. 2.64 In the adult heart, the change of direction of muscular fibers indicates the line that borders the conus. *a* Aorta, *b* right atrium, *c* conus, *d* inferior bulboventricular sulcus, *e* pars trabecularis of the right ventricle, *f* left ventricle, *g* hypothetical line on the direction of the superior bulboventricular sulcus, *h* line of conal delimitation

2.7.2 Spiral Septum Formation

Two endocardial proeminences are appearing along the lumen of the bulbus cordis, similar to the endocardial cushions (generated similar to those by accumulation of cardioglia) called bulbar ridge (sinistroventral and dextrodorsal) (Figs. 2.65, 2.66 and 2.69).

To the mesenchymal formation of the bulbar ridges also participate:

- Cells from the neural crest. Without their migration the bulbus cordis do not septate.
- Epicardial cells;
- Myocardial cells, their proliferation leads to myocardial formation of the output septum. Myocardial formation alteration translates into pathology of interventricular septation [7].

These bulbar crests, stretched along the bulb (actually in the conus and the trunk), unite to form the spiral septum, which, can be systematized topographically into three parts, although it is a continuous structure:

- A posterior and inferior part which participate to the formation of the interventricular membranous septum and the supraventricular crest [8]. In fact only the dextrodorsal crest fuses with the right extension of the superior endocardial cushion (from the atrioventricular canal) (Fig. 2.3). Completion of the septation and formation process and membranous septum formation process will be described below.
- An anterior and middle part – conal septum, that separates the subvalvular part of the pulmonary artery (pulmonary conus) from the subvalvular part of the aorta (aortic conus). So it also participates in the ventricular septation (Fig. 6.69).
- A superior part forming the aortico-pulmonary septum, a septum which will separate the aorta from the pulmonary artery in the intrapericardial portion. This septum will also disappear after a resorption process.

Note that the spiral septum does not separate the trabeculated part of the right ventricle from the left ventricle. These segments are separated by the interventricular septum.

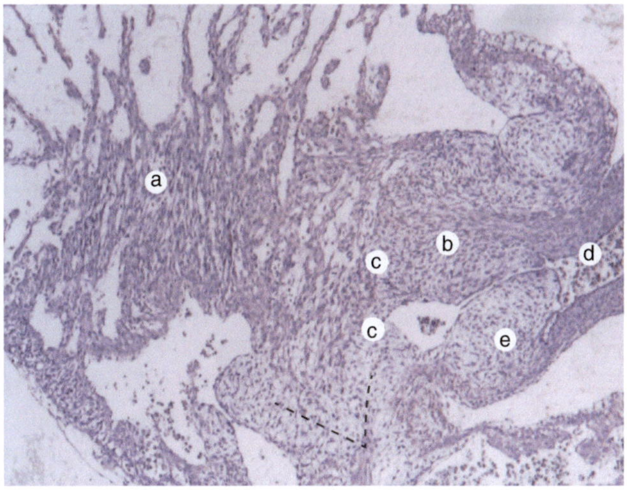

Fig. 2.65 A 11 days old rat heart. Sagittal section through the interventricular septum. The superior endocardial cushion is divided in a right and left extension (a *V* marked by *dotted line*). The right extension merges with the base of the spiral septum – the conal septum (resulted from the fusion of endocardial crests) as well as with the segment of the muscular interventricular septum (between the arms of the *V*). The conal septum also merges with the superior limb of the muscular septum. *a* Superior limb of the muscular interventricular septum, *b* sinistroventral endocardial crest, *c* conal septum, *d* arterial trunk, *e* dextrodorsal endocardial crest

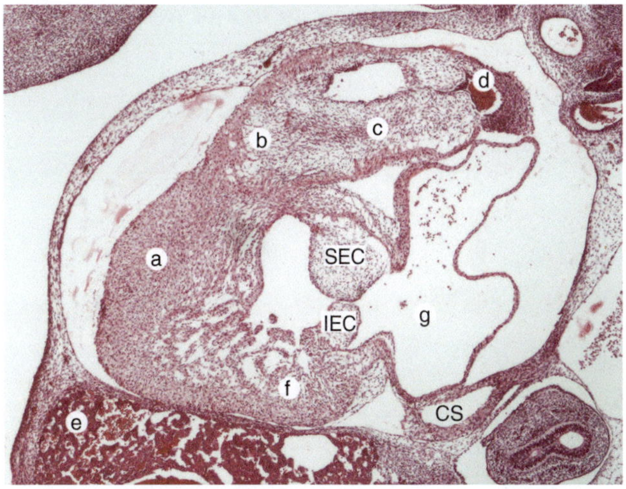

Fig. 2.66 A 7 weeks old heart. Sagittal section through the interventricular septum. The conal septum merges with the superior limb of the interventricular septum and with the right elongation of the superior endocardial cushion. *a* Superior limb of the muscular interventricular septum, *b* conal septum, *c* dextrodorsal endocardial crest, *d* arterial trunk, *e* liver inferior of the transverse septum, *f* inferior limb of the interventricular septum, *g* primitive atrium, *SEC* superior endocardial cushion, *IEC* inferior endocardial cushion, *CS* coronary sinus

2.7.3 Separation of the Primitive Truncus Arteriosus into the Aorta and the Pulmonary Trunk

The separation is made through the superior part of the spiral septum (aorticopulmonary septum). The evolution of this septum is marked by the appearance of a sulcus on both sides of the truncus arteriosus, at the margins of spiral septum. This sulcus gradually deepens into the septal mass, leading ultimately to disappearance (cleavage) of the septum and separation of the two vessels (Figs. 2.67, 2.68, 2.69 and 2.70). Basically, the walls facing each other of the two greater vessels originate from the differentiation of the spiral septum!

The primitive truncus arteriosus initially presents four endocardial prominences (which will eventually form the arterial valves) at the conotruncal junction: anterior, posterior, right and left. Aortico-pulmonary septum (but more precise the separation groove), divides the right and left prominences into two halves, so finally the two arterial ostia will present three valves each.

Valves are forming through a degeneration process of the central part of these prominences, which results in the valve sinuses (Figs. 2.71 and 2.76).

If case of valve atresia, the process of "cavitation" does not occur or it is incomplete and the valvules are fully or partially fused (probably due to lack of resorption of the corresponding part of the spiral septum).

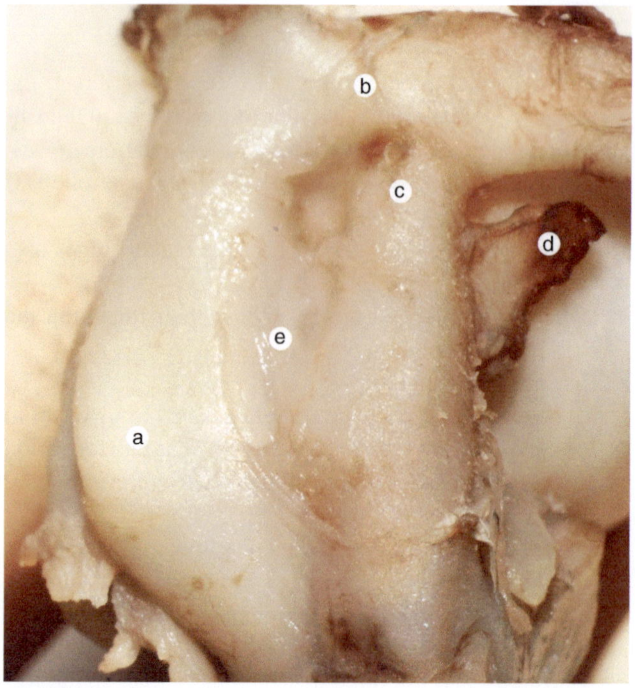

Fig. 2.68 A 3 months old heart. Anterior view of the arterial pedicle. After removing the pericardium, we notice the spiral septum in resorption. The arterial canal is well represented. *a* Aorta, *b* aortic cross, *c* arterial canal, *d* left pulmonary artery, *e* spiral septum in resorption

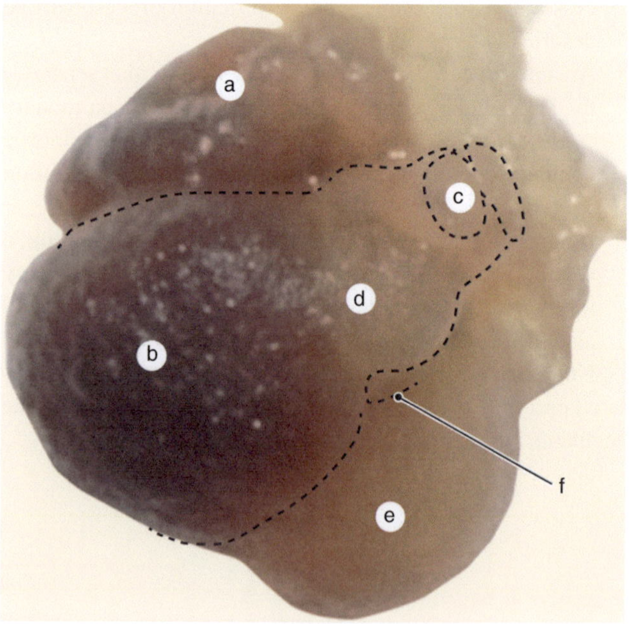

Fig. 2.69 A 7 weeks old heart. Notice the orientation of the spiral septum as well as the balloonisation from the bottom of the arterial trunk, near the bulb of the future pulmonary trunk. This balloonisation seems to be a stage of the septation process. *a* Right atrium, *b* conus, *c* arterial trunk in the course of septation, *d* initial dilation at the bottom of the pulmonary trunk, *e* left ventricle, *f* conoventricular fold

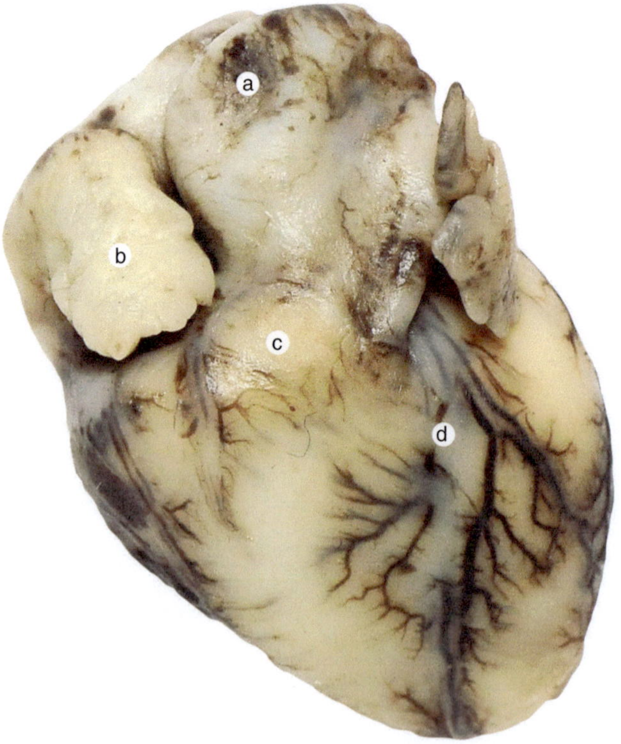

Fig. 2.67 A 3 months old heart. The arterial trunk is unseptate. The right auricle has the appearance of the left one, which suggests left isomerism. Also notice the fashion in which the myocardial bridges are formed. *a* Arterial trunk, *b* right auricle, *c* conus, *d* myocardial bridge

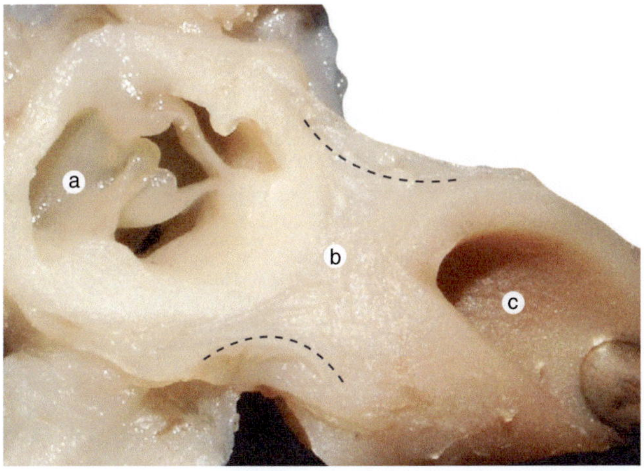

Fig. 2.70 A 3 months old heart. Spiral septum in the course of resorption. On the circumference of the arterial trunk we notice the existence of grooves (*dotted lines*) at the edges of the spiral septum. As they deepen, the aorta separates from the pulmonary trunk. *a* Pulmonary semilunar valves, *b* spiral septum, *c* aorta

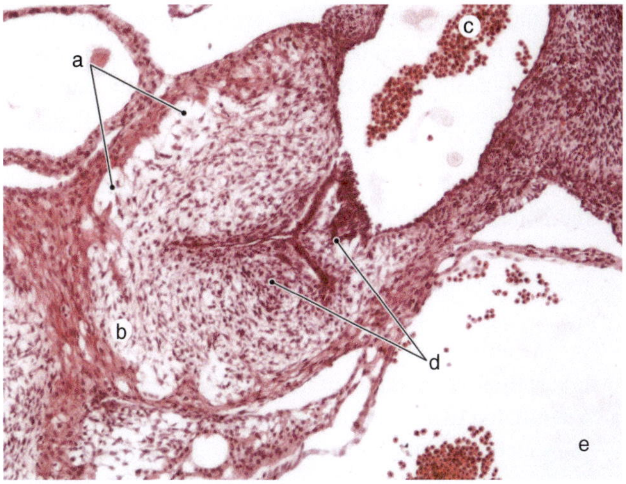

Fig. 2.71 An 8 weeks old heart. Formation of semilunar valves. *a* Cells migrated from the neural crests, *b* conal septum, *c* aorta, *d* endocardial prominence in the course of segmentation, *e* primitive atrium

Spiral path of the spiral septum explains the final relation of the intrapericardial parts of the aorta and the pulmonary trunk. It also explains why the membranous septum is situated posteriorly and not inferiorly to the conal septum.

Spiral septum formation does not interest the entire truncus arteriosus. The ductus arteriosus is forming in the region where the spiral septum does not exist, through which the pulmonary trunk communicates with the aorta in the intrauterine life.

Origin of the aorta is contained in the anterior interatrial notch and penetrates as a "splitting wedge" into the superior endocardial cushion mass of the intermediate septum, with which it partially fuses. The process is known as "aortic protrusion" [9] into the superior endocardial cushion.

Therefore the mesenchymal part of these cushions is incompletely divided into three parts: future mitral-aortic continuity (left extension), future tendinous center and right extension, which will merge with the spiral septum forming the future membranous septum. These structures are retained in adult in continuity with each other.

Protrusion of the aorta after septation favors establishing the continuity between the aorta and the left ventricle!

Delamination of the left extension of the superior endocardial cushion takes part in the formation of the anterior mitral cusp. On the other hand, the fusion of the left extension with the aortic wall will create the mitral-aortic continuity. That explains the relation between the aorta and the left atrium.

Also, as already shown, the diaphragmatic wall of the primitive cardiac tube does not fold, but, along with the convex margin, undergoes an expansion to the right.

This enlargement to the right also involves the right side of the atrioventricular junction, causing an extension to the right of the atrioventricular junction.

After septation, the extension to the right of the atrioventricular junction [9] will favor the possibility for the right atrium to align and to communicate with the right ventricle!

Reduction of the concave edge and conoventricular fold formation determines atrial blood to reach both ventricles simultaneously. In this way, after septation, each ventricle will be part of a distinct circuit!

2.7.4 Primitive Ventricle Septation and Interventricular Septal Defects

Ventricular septation is a process that essentially undergoes the following way: an endocardial fold arises on the infero-apical wall of the ventricle. Through growth and differentiation, this becomes the muscular interventricular septum. The fold has a falciform appearance and develops upwards (Fig. 2.36). This pleat derives from the intense multiplication of the cells located on the fusion line of the two endocardial tubes.

Its free margin and the intermediate septum delineate an orifice named foramen interventriculare. The orifice is bounded by an upper and a lower septal limbus.

Growth of the septum is accomplished at the insertion base by cardiomyocytes apposition, simultaneous with ventricular enhancement on the external margin [10].

Meanwhile, the interventricular orifice gradually shrinks.

Disorders in interventricular muscular septum formation are followed by the "muscular" type of ventricular septal defects.

As noted, the right dorsal crest of the truncus arteriosus (part of the spiral septum), merges with the upper endocardial cushion elongation and forms the membranous interventricular septum (see right ventricle).

The muscular interventricular septum grows, the interventricular foramen shrinks until it disappears and the disappearance of the orifice leads to the fusion of the muscular and membranous septa.

Interventricular septation is finalized by a simultaneous fusion of the:

- the conal septum (the middle part of the spiral septum) with the upper limbus of the interventricular septum. As a result, the pulmonary artery serves the right ventricle and the aorta serves the left one.
- the membranous interventricular septum with the muscular septum on the edges of the interventricular orifice. As a result, the two ventricles are separated.
- muscular interventricular septum with the intermediate septum (actually with the lower extensions of the two endocardial cushions). As a result, the two ventricles will engage with the corresponding atria. Correct coupling is favored, as we noted above, by the restriction of the concave margin of the cardiac tube and by conoventricular fold formation. That completes the interventricular septum formation in the fifth week.

Resuming:

- A small portion of the spiral septum base (septum separating the ejection ventricular compartments), merges with an extension to the right of the intermediate septum (prolongation that separates the aortic vestibule from the right atrioventricular canal). The future membranous septum and the supraventricular crest emerge from this fusion, and as a result, the right atrium aligns better with the right ventricle. Alignment is possible due to the initial expansion to the right of the atrioventricular junction and concave edge contraction.

Failure of this merge leads to a lack of membranous septum formation and the development of the interventricular septal defect, known as persistent interventricular foramen – Roger (Figs. 2.72 and 2.73).

Simultaneously, in the same region, the upper limbus of the muscular septum merges with the conal septum on its dorsal side and with the membranous septum on its posterior side!

Following these junctions, myocardial formation probably occurs (with variable extension) in the conal septum, membranous septum and supraventricular crest and the ventricular septation is finalized [8].

Upper limbus will merge both with the membranous septum (posteriorly) and the conal septum (dorsally)! Please note that the upper limbus of the muscular interventricular septum develops toward the junction with the membranous septum, passing inferior to the conal septum, due to the coiled path of the spiral septum. If the upper limbus fails the posterior junction with the membranous septum, infracrestal perimembranous type of ventricular septal defects occur (Figs. 2.73 and 2.74).

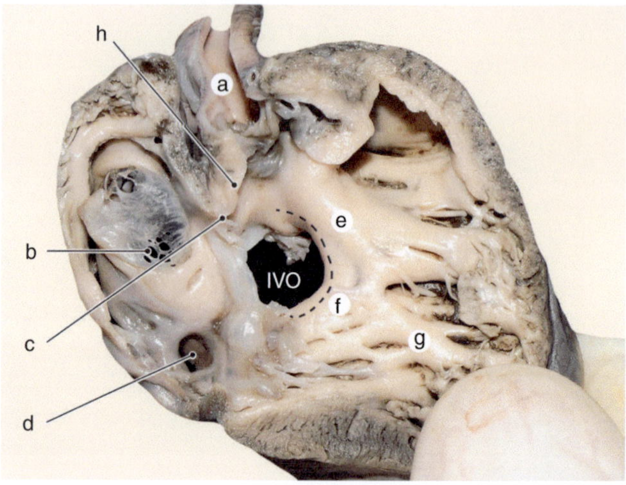

Fig. 2.72 A 7 months old heart. The right side of the interventricular septum. Tetralogy of Fallot. The aorta is 'riding' the septum. Between the aortic valves and the tricuspid orifice lies a fibrous structure " aortic curtain" type, which is inserted on an "aortic-tricuspid continuity", similar to the mitral-aortic continuity. We can notice very well the muscular interventricular septum with its two limbs that border the interventricular orifice (*IVO*). *a* Aorta, *b* orifice secundum, *c* aortic-tricuspidian continuity, *d* coronary sinus orifice, *e* superior limb, *f* inferior limb, *g* muscular interventricular septum, *h* " aortic curtain"

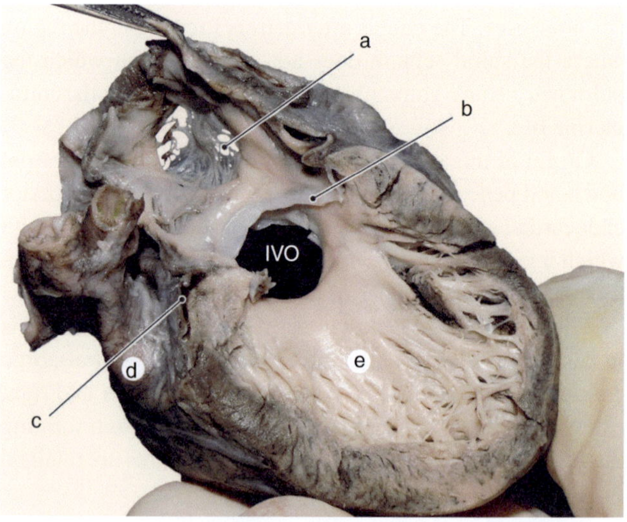

Fig. 2.73 The same heart. The left side of the interventricular septum. The origin of the aorta has the aspect of a cleft. *a* Orifice secundum, *b* mitral cusp, *c* the opening of the aorta in the left ventricle, *d* atresic pulmonary trunk, *e* left side of the interventricular septum

- Given the specific spiral septum disposition, the upper limbus of the muscular interventricular septum also junctions with the conal septum on its upper-dorsal side (Fig. 2.66). If the junction fails, the "supracristal" type of ventricular septal defects occurs.

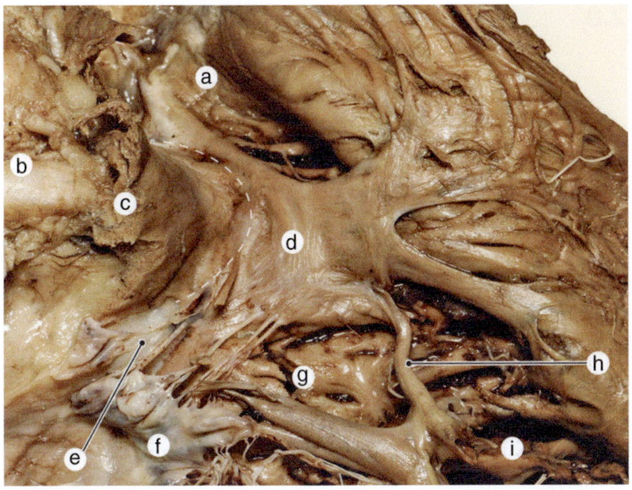

Fig. 2.74 The right surface of the interventricular septum in an adult heart. The supraventricular crest is indicated by dotted line in order to ease the localisation of supracristal and infracristal areas. *a* Subvalvular infundibulum, *b* right coronary, c supraventricular crest, *d* septomarginal trabecula, *e* membranous interventrivular septum, *f* septal cusp, *g* entry septum, *h* Moderator band, *i* trabeculated septum

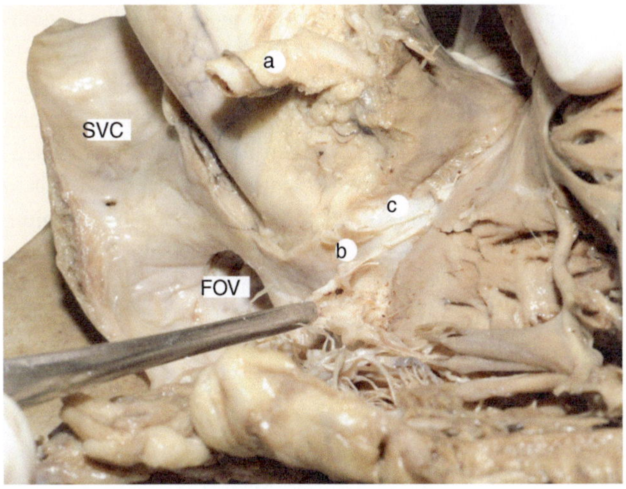

Fig. 2.75 View from the right of the membranous septum in an adult heart. This is an unique structure, with a ventricular and an atrial component. *a* Right coronary, *b* atrioventricular septum, *c* membranous interventricular septum, *SVC* superior vena cava, *FOV* fossa ovalis

- Following the junction with the upper limbus of the muscular interventricular septum, the supraventricular crest and the conal septum become muscular.

Failure of this process or disorders of conal septum formation are followed by conal interventricular septal defects and subvalvular defects (referring to the pulmonary valve).

Often the upper part of the septal defect is limited by an "aortic curtain" that is attached on a so called aortic-tricuspid continuity (Fig. 2.72). Highlighting this continuity can be a diagnostic criterion for perimembranos septal defects [11].

- Lower limbus of the interventricular septum merges with the intermediate septum (with its part representing the lower endocardial cushion) (Fig. 2.4). After this fusion process the "input" segment of the interventricular septum forms, just below the insertion of the tricuspid septal cusp.

If the junction does not take place, ventricular septal defects of "perimembranar – subvalvular " type occur (referring to the tricuspid valve) or septal input defects).

As noted, the two limbi of the muscular interventricular septum mark the boundaries of the interventricular foramen (Fig. 2.73), that narrows gradually in a way that, in the end, the muscular interventricular septum junctions with:

- the middle part of the spiral septum (conal septum). Therefore, ventricular outflow parts are separated. The conal septum (and the supraventricular crest) becomes muscular.
- membranous septum. Therefore, interventricular orifice disappears.

Each septum does its job of separating what they have to separate. Meanwhile, the three septal material merge into a small area in the perimembranous region.

Finally ontogenetically, the interventricular septum has several parts:

- The "input" part (muscular, subtricuspidian, arising from the inferior limbus)
- The trabeculated part (muscular, towards the ventricular apex, coming from the muscular septum);
- The conal part – subvalvular (which undergoes a complete muscularization process);
- The diaphragmatic part (with variable muscularization). ! The conal part of the interventricular septum is not visible from the side of the right ventricle, because it is an interventricular structure. A "conal" segment of the subvalvar infundibulum corresponds to it.

We want to specify that the pathology of the intermediate septum formation generates complex septal defects, after which a partially septated ventricle that communicates with both of the atrial cavities can be found (Fig. 2.36).

2.7.5 Atrioventricular Septum Formation

Atrioventricular septum separates the vestibule of the aorta from the vestibule of the right atrium. As already mentioned, the conotruncal junction (the area from where the arterial valves differentiate) joins the interatrial notch and the intermediate septum in the protrusion process. Two situations may arise as a result of this disposition:

- There may be no atrioventricular septum. In this hypothesis, tricuspidian vestibule of the right atrium it is closely attached, but separated from the aortic vestibule wall.
- There may exist an atrioventricular membranous septum. This hypothesis happens when the muscularization deficit of the membranous interventricular septum extends to the atrial extension of the superior endocardial cushion. Therefore, the membranous atrioventricular septum is forming (as a continuity of the interventricular membranous septum). The septum separates as a single wall the vestibule of the right atrium from the vestibule of the aorta.

The existence of a single wall is explained by the fusion of the aortic wall with the right extension of the superior endocardial cushion and the right atrial wall, during the aortic protrusion into the interatrial notch (Figs. 2.3 and 2.76). In fact, a similar process occurs in the genesis of the left mitral aortic continuity.

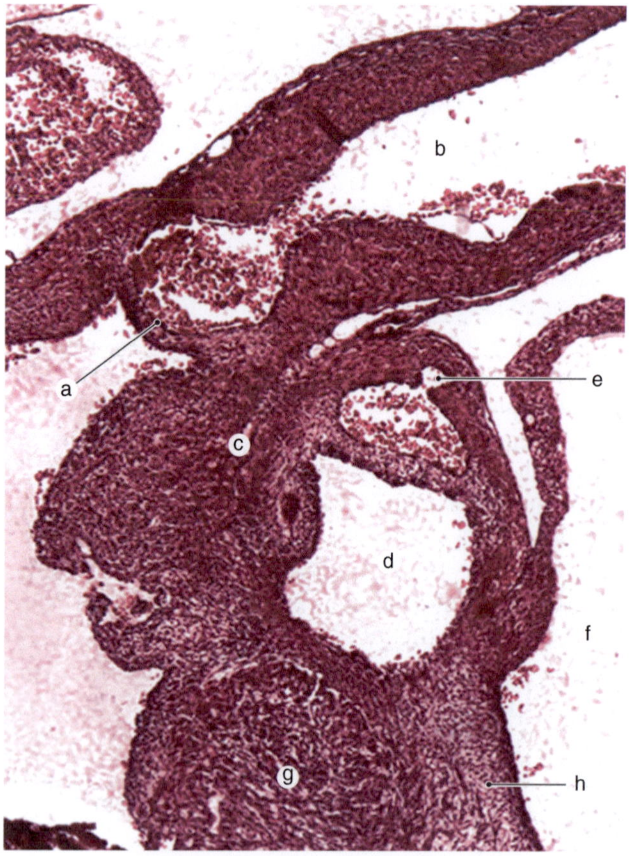

Fig. 2.76 A 2 months and a half old heart. In the left coronary sinus we notice the origin of the coronary artery. The right elongation of the superior endocardial cushion merges with the wall of the aortic vestibule participating to the formation of an unique wall that will become the atrioventricular septum. *a* Formation of the semilunar valve at the conotruncal junction, *b* pulmonary trunk, *c* spiral septum in the course of resorption, *d* aorta, e the bud of the left coronary artery in the coronary aortic sinus, *f* atrium, *g* supraventricular crest, *h* right process of the superior endocardial cushion

2.8 The Differentiation of the Myocardium, of the Valvular Apparatus, of the Vascularisation and the Extrinsic Nerve Supply of the Heart

2.8.1 Formation of the Working Myocardium

Working myocardium originates in the mesodermal cells of the myoepicardial plate (Fig. 2.77). It differentiates into two cell groups:

- A deep group, with spongy appearance that will form the muscular trabeculae, the papillary muscles and the chordae tendineae (last ones being devolved segments of the papillary muscles).
- The papillary muscles initially appear as prominences on the ventricular wall, with longitudinal grooves forming behind them on each side (Fig. 2.78). These grooves become deeper until they separate the muscle from the ventricular wall (Fig. 2.79).
- A compact group located superficially, which will differentiate into all the other myocardial territories.
- There are also extracardiac cell invasions in the superficial territory, coming from: the neural crest, the dorsal extracardial mesenchyme, the proepicardic body and angioblasts. Some of these cell types can develop into myocitary cell line.

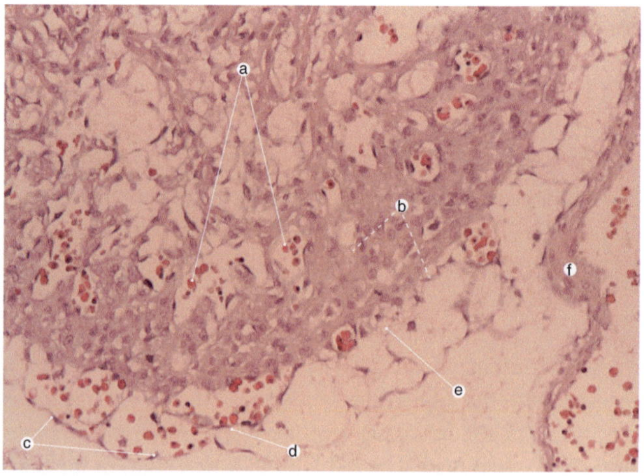

Fig. 2.77 A 10 days old rat heart. The epicardium is in the course of consolidation. The epicardial cells come together and border vascular lumina. *a* Intramyocardial sinuses, *b* myoepicardial ventricular plate, *c* epicardial cells, *d* subepicardial vessels in the course of formation, *e* cells from the neural crests, *f* atrial wall

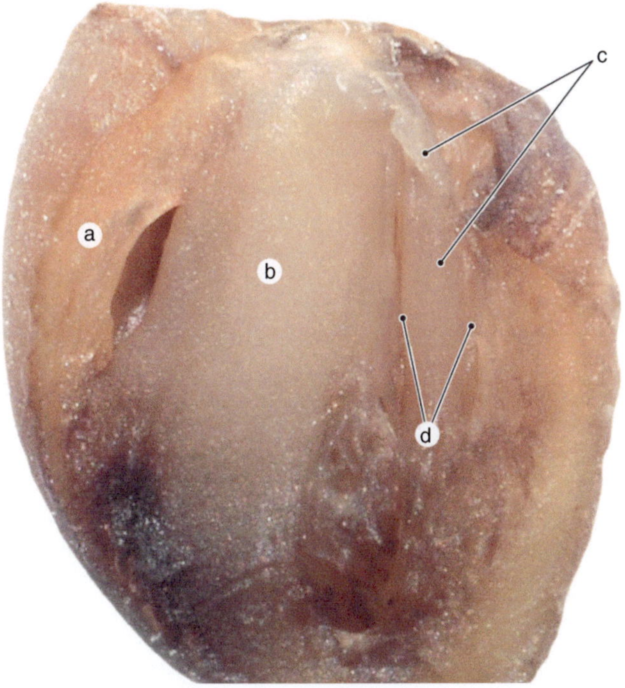

Fig. 2.78 A 2 months old heart. Frontal section through the ventricular pyramid. On both sides of the anterior papillary muscle we notice grooves that are parallel with it. These grooves deepen and separate the papillary fascicle from the wall. *a* Right ventricle, *b* interventricular septum, *c* papillary muscle continuing a cusp, *d* collateral grooves

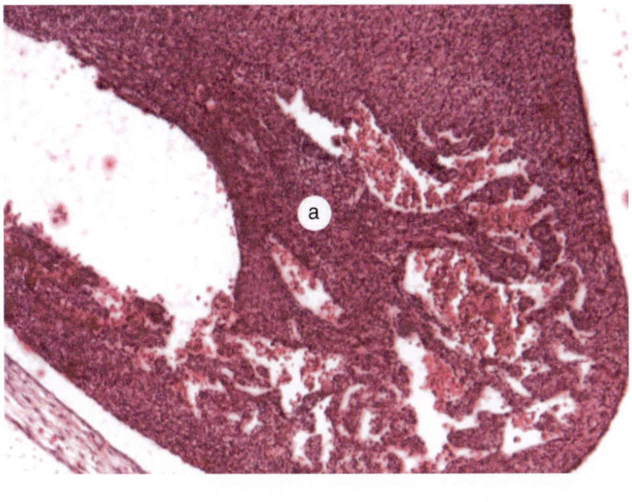

Fig. 2.79 A 2 months old heart. Sagittal section. The superior tip of the papillary muscle is still mesenchymatous. *a* Papillary muscle in the course of differentiation

2.8.2 Atrioventricular Valve Formation

Atrioventricular valves are formed as follows:

At the level of the atrioventricular canal, the wall reduces circularly more in the right side than in the left one, forming the atrioventricular junctions (Fig. 2.80).

Although, according to the microscopic sections (Fig. 2.81) we would be tempted to think that it is a process of clogging, folding or invagination of the wall, in fact it is a more complex change, based on complex resorptions and proliferation of the cell populations which will ultimately lead to atrioventricular junctions (Figs. 2.82 and 2.83).

Following these processes, endocardial folds are formed internally and endocardial coronary grooves are formed externally (Figs. 2.84 and 2.85).

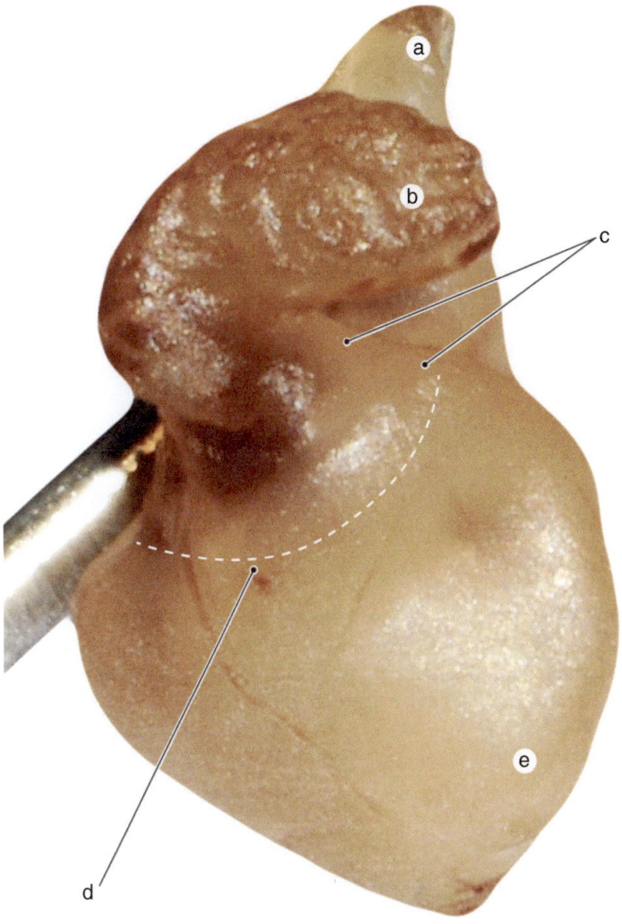

Fig. 2.80 A 7 week-old heart. Forming of the right coronary sulcus, at the level of the atrioventricular junction. The junctional mesenchyme contributes to the forming of the subauricular vestibule. The persistency of mesenchimal bundles in this area leads to the occurrence of abnormal atrioventricular muscular bundles (Kent) responsible for the WPW Syndrome. *a* Aorta, *b* right auricle, *c* subauricular vestibule, *d* atrioventricular junction, *e* right ventricle

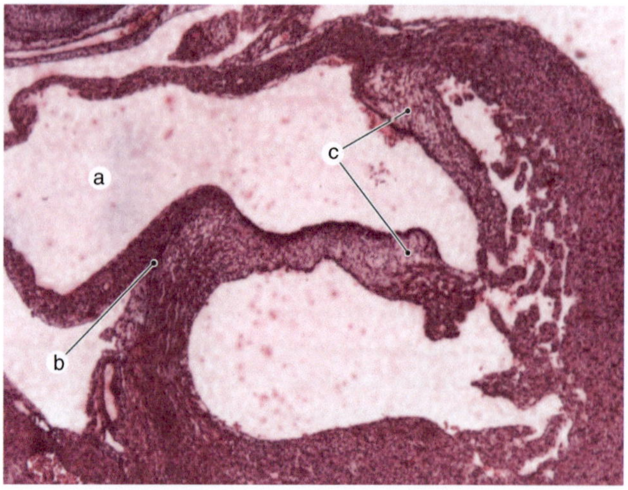

Fig. 2.81 Two and a half month-old heart. The cusps of the mitral valve during development. *a* Left atrium, *b* atrioventricular junction, *c* cusps during delamination

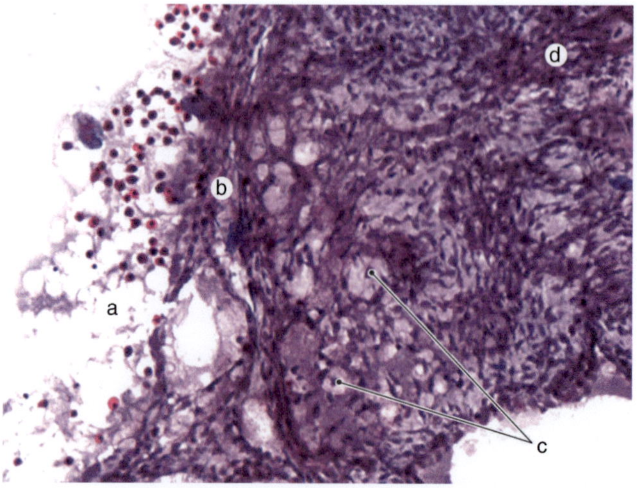

Fig. 2.83 A 2 month-old heart. Sagittal section by the anterior cusp of the tricuspid valve. Notice the diversity of cellular types in the ventricular mesechyme, *a* Right atrium, *b* atrioventricular junction, *c* cells from the neural crests, *d* right ventricle

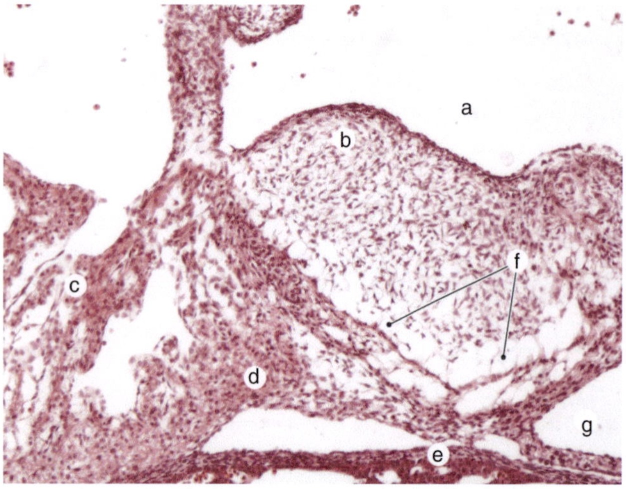

Fig. 2.82 A 2 month-old heart. The inferior endocardial cushion by the posterior cusp of the mitral valve. Sagittal section. Detail. Multiple cell populations. Notice that a segment of the inferior cushion remains in the atrium. *a* Left atrium, *b* inferior endocardial cushion – atrial section, *c* trabeculae carnae, *d* atrioventricular junction, *e* transverse septum, *f* cells from neural crests, *g* coronary sinus

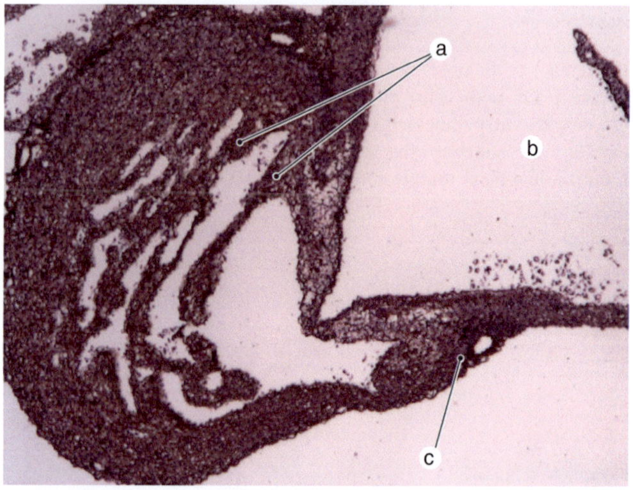

Fig. 2.84 A 2 month-old heart. Forming of the tricuspid valve. Cusps during delamination. Muscular bundles during differentiation into chordae tendineae. The right coronary artery is sectioned twice in the coronary sulcus. *a* Trabeculae carnae at the base of the cusp during delamination, *b* right atrium, *c* atrioventricular junction

One part of the atrioventricular junctions mesenchyme underwent a fibrous transformation, generating the atrioventricular ring (see fibrous skeleton of the heart) which electrically separates the atria from the ventricles.

Sometimes mesenchyme fascicles that do not suffer this transformation, continuing their evolution toward the myocitary cell line and generating muscular fascicles that are responsible for transmitting aberrant electrical impulse between the atria and the ventricles (fascicle of Kent), more commonly on the right side.

Regarding the cusps:

- The membranous part originates in the endocardial folds of the atrioventricular ostia.
- The fibrous part originates in the devolved muscular trabeculae.
- The septal tricuspid cusp and anterior mitral cusp formation involves fused material of the anterior and posterior endocardial cushions.

The formation process of the mobile parts of the cusps is called delamination (transformation in a lamina-type structure) and takes place between week 6 and week 12.

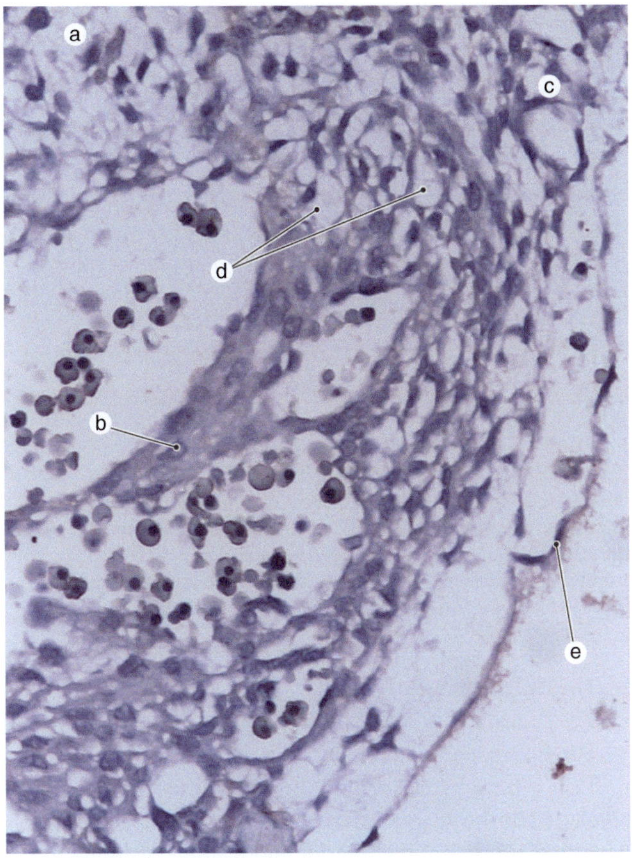

Fig. 2.85 A 10 day-old rat heart. Detail. Forming of the chordae tendineae. Sagittal section at the base of the posterior mitral cusp. The fibrous transformation of the trabeculae carnae is in connection with the invasion of the cells from the neural crests in these trabeculae. *a* Inferior endocardial cushion during delamination, *b* trabecula carna, *c* atrioventricular junction, *d* cells from the neural crests, *e* epicardial cells

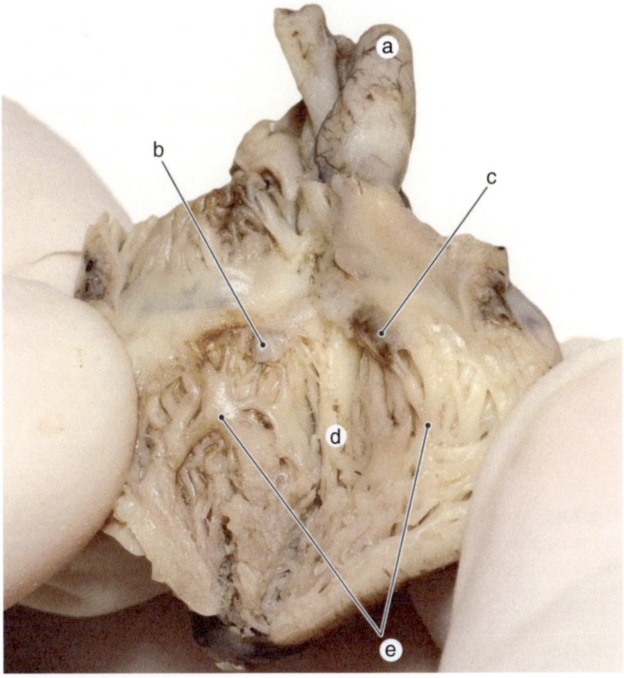

Fig. 2.86 Two and a half month-old heart. Forming of the tricuspid valve – Septal commissure. Papillary muscles and chordae tendineae during differentiation. *a* Aorta, *b* septal cusp, *c* anterior cusp, *d* right ventricle, *e* papillary muscles

The atrial and ventricular surfaces of the cusps have different origins.

The atrial surface comes from the endocardial crests and cushions, more specifically through the mesenchymal transformation of those structures into fibroblastic – fibrocyte cell line.

The ventricular surface forms as follows: inferior surfaces of the tricuspidian narrow pass and of the neighbouring endocardial structures are initially invaded by the ventricular myocytes. Soon after that, a fibrous transformation occurs resulting

2.8.3 Tricuspid Valve Formation

The inside of the right atrioventricular junction has the appearance of a narrow gullet, bordered in the fifth week by the inferior and the superior endocardial cushions (which form the intermediate septum) but also by the lateral endocardial cushion.

- The anterolateral cusp is formed by the union of the superior endocardial cushion extension and the dextrodorsal endocardial ridge, in other words, it originates from the delamination and muscularization of the supraventricular ridge.
- The inferior cusp is formed by the delamination process of the lateral endocardial cushion from the tricuspidian gullet and the adjacent ventricular myocardium.
- An interesting observation is that along phylogenetic evolution, in some reptiles and birds, the inferior and the anterosuperior cusps form a single structure named "the great mural cusp" [8].
- In humans the two cusps move together, simultaneously with the free ventricular wall.
- The septal cusp is formed by the fusion and delamination of the inferior and superior endocardial cushions (Figs. 2.1, 2.2 and 2.3), as well as the adjacent part of the interventricular muscular septum (Fig. 2.86).
- The anterior papillary is formed between the fifth and the seventh week (Figs. 2.87, 2.88 and 2.89)
- The medial papillary is formed between the 8th and the 12th week
- The posterior papillary is formed late, between the fifth and the seventh week
- The commissures start forming only after the cusps are structured [8].

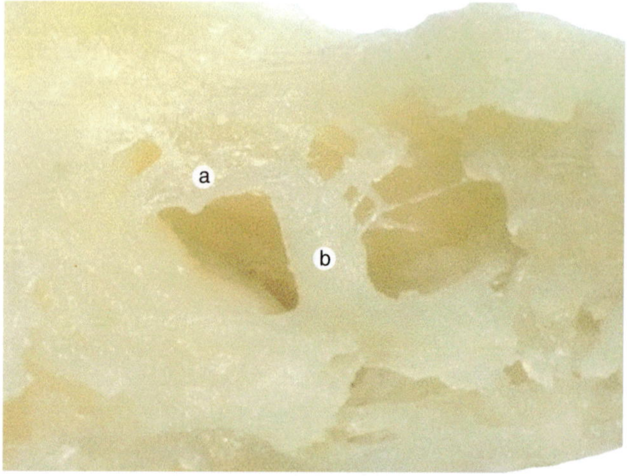

Fig. 2.87 A 6 week-old heart. Forming of the anterior papillary muscle in the right ventricle. Posterior view. *a* Cusp, *b* anterior papillary muscle in the right ventricle

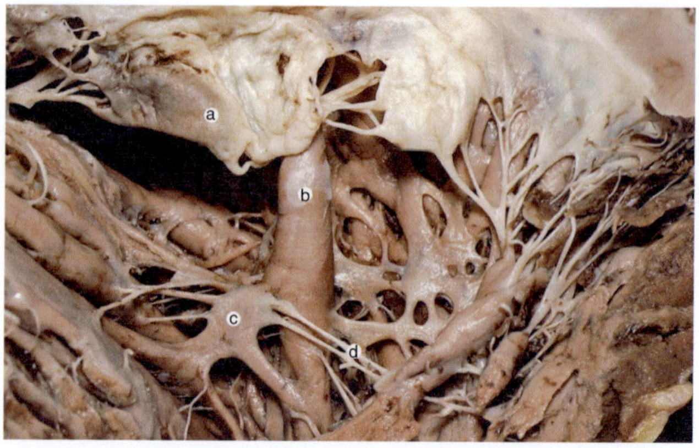

Fig. 2.89 Adult heart. Detail: anterior papillary muscle in the right ventricle. In comparison with the first image of the series (Fig. 2.87), in which the embryonic tissue (mesenchyme) has an identical aspect for the cusps, chordae tendineae and papillary muscles, in the adult heart the same structures are differentiated in various tissues. *a* Anterior cusp, *b* anterior papillary muscle, *c* moderator band, *d* Purkinje fibers

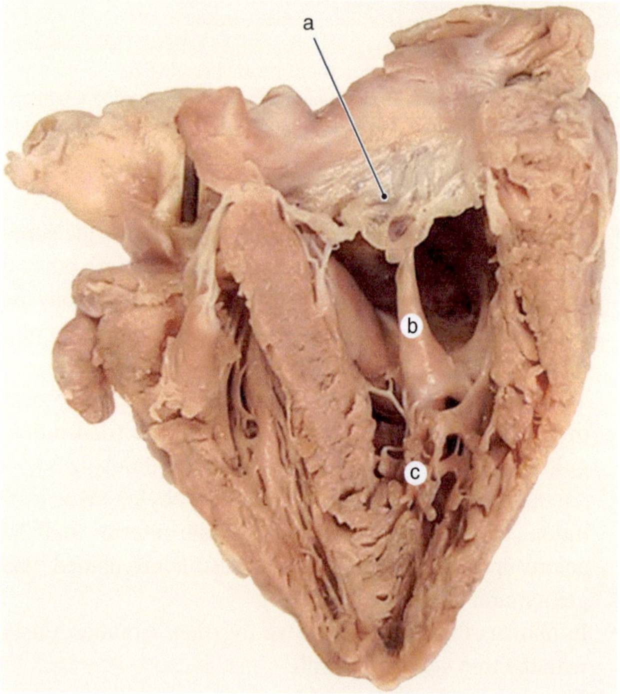

Fig. 2.88 A 8 month-old heart. Frontal section, posterior view. Anterior papillary muscle in the right ventricle. Its tip is still muscular, but during transformation into chordae tendineae. *a* Anterior cusp, *b* anterior papillary muscle with its tip during degeneration, *c* right ventricle

2.8.4 Mitral Valve Formation

The fact that there is mitroaortic continuity, at the mitral valve, in which the aortic cusp is inserted, causes the formation of the left cusp to differ from the right one.

As we have shown, the protrusion of the aortic origin in the superior endocardial cushion divides its matter into:

- The right extension;
- The future mitroaortic continuity;
- The future tendinous center (Fig. 2.3).

The mesenchyme of the future mitroartic continuity results from the fusion of the superior endocardial cushion with an extension of the inferior endocardial cushion.

The anterior (aortic) **cusp** of the mitral valve is formed through the delamination of the mesenchymal mass. In other words the aortic cusp is the result of the delamination of the two endocardial cushions fusion area, after the preliminary and incomplete division of this area from the remaining intermediate septum. This division occurs due to the aortic origin protrusion in the septum (Figs. 2.2, 2.90, 2.91 and 2.92).

The mitroaortic continuity is completed by way of the aortic protrusion process and requires the fusion of the aortic wall with tissue of the superior endocardial cushion and the left atrium wall (Fig. 2.93).

The posterior (mural) **cusp** is formed through the delamination of the lateral endocardial cusp (the cushion appears at the end of the fifth week) (Fig. 2.94).

The papillary muscles come from the differentiation of the ventricular trabeculae which molds on the ventricular floor and ends at the level of the lateral endocardial cushion and the intermediate septum. Trabecular ends are gradually separated from the ventricular wall by the appearance of grooves between them and the wall. The deepening of the grooves leads to the separation of the cranial ends from the wall. Thus the apparatus for the valvular tensioning is formed.

In the sixth week the mitral valvular primordium is fully present (Figs. 2.95 and 2.96). The differentiation of the valve is established in the eighth week, when the valve is well- structured.

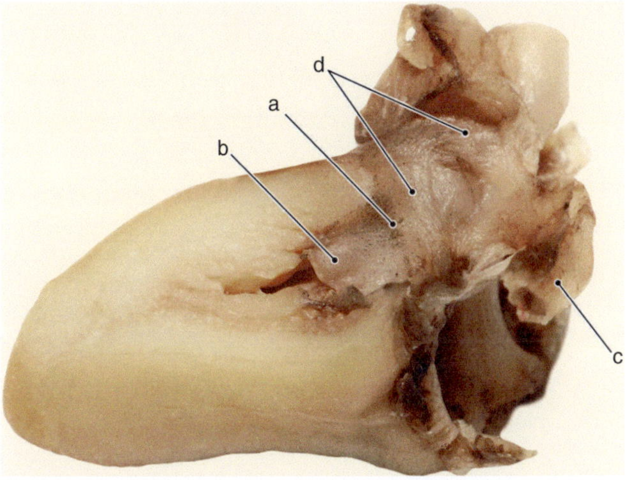

Fig. 2.90 A 12 week-old heart. The material of the superior endocardial cushion can be observed being organized in a circular fascicle, on the anterior wall of the left atrium. At the base of this fascicle, the endocardial delaminated material forms most of the anterior cusp of the mitral valve. Another fascicle from the endocardial material contributes to the forming of the interatrial septum. *a* Mitral-aortic continuity, *b* anterior cusp of the mitral valve, *c* fascicular part of the septum primum, *d* circular fascicle

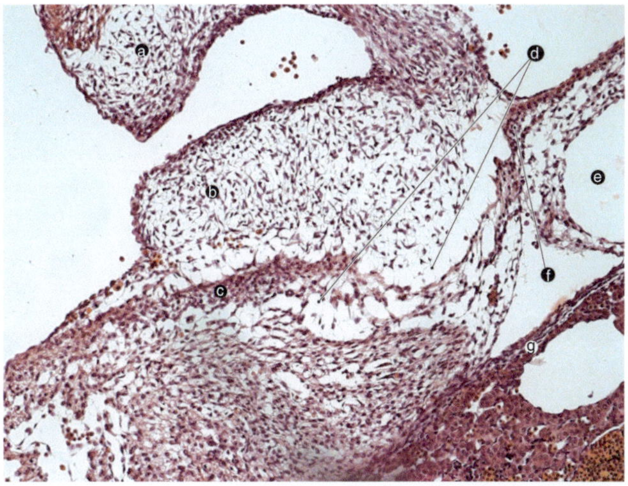

Fig. 2.92 A 2 month-old heart. The posterior cusp of the mitral valve during delamination. Basically, the atrioventricular junction divides the inferior endocardial cushion into a superior segment (see Fig. 2.82) and an inferior segment, which will delaminate. *a* Superior endocardial cushion, *b* inferior endocardial cushion, *c* muscular bundle (cardiomyoblasts) – future chordae tendinea, *d* bands of cells from the neural crests, *e* coronary sinus, *f* atrioventricular junction, *g* transverse septum

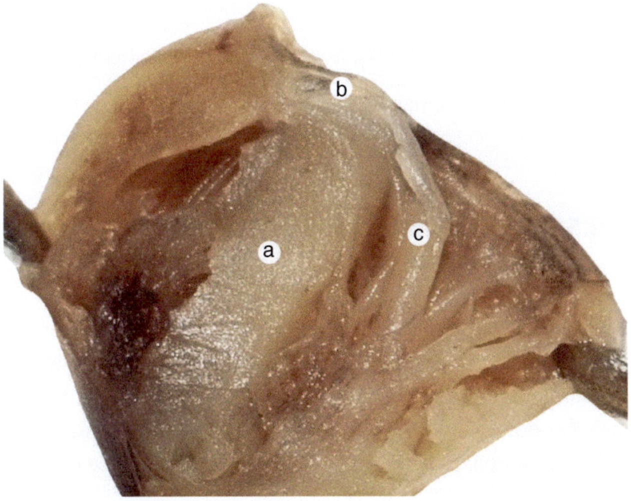

Fig. 2.91 A 2 month-old heart. In the posterior part of the aortic vestibule, the material from the superior endocardial cushion contributes to the forming of the anterior cusp of the mitral valve. *a* Interventricular septum, *b* aortic vestibule, *c* papillary muscle in continuity of the anterior cusp

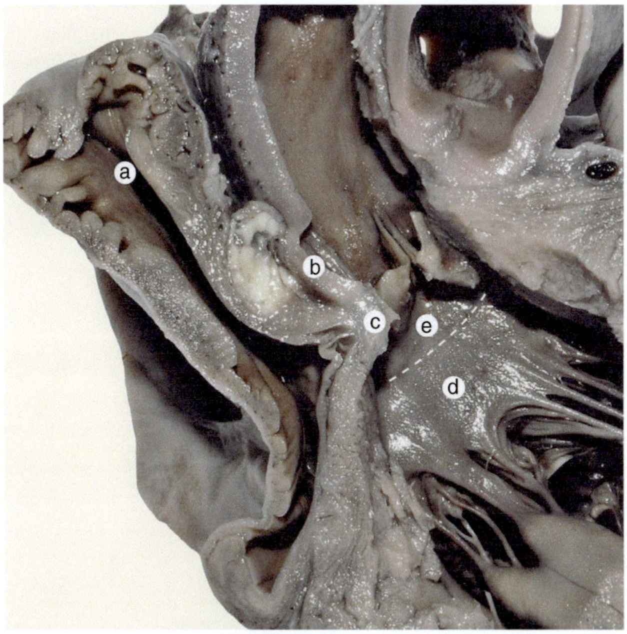

Fig. 2.93 A 7 month-old heart. Sagittal section. View from the right side. The mitral-aortic continuity is found at the place where the wall of the left atrium merges with the aortic curtain (see the aortic root). The anterior cusp of the mitral valve is inserted on this merger zone. The anterior left extention of the tendinous center penetrates in the continuity. *a* Left atrium, *b* aortic wall, *c* the anterior, left extention of the tendinous center, *d* anterior mitral cusp, *e* aortic curtain

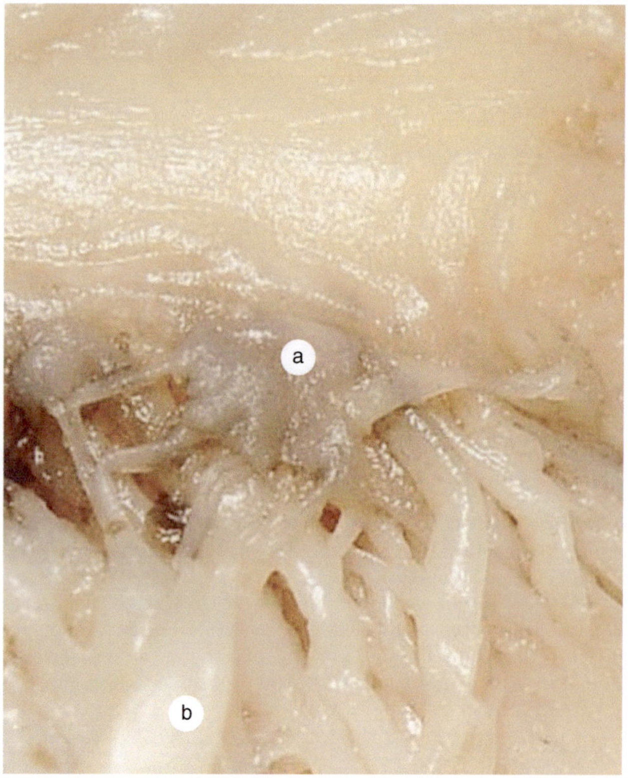

Fig. 2.94 A 2 month-old heart. At the same age as the heart in Fig. 2.92. The posterior cusp of the mitral valve is much better differentiated. The ontogenetic development is marked by individual variability. *a* Posterior mitral cusp, *b* posterior papillary group

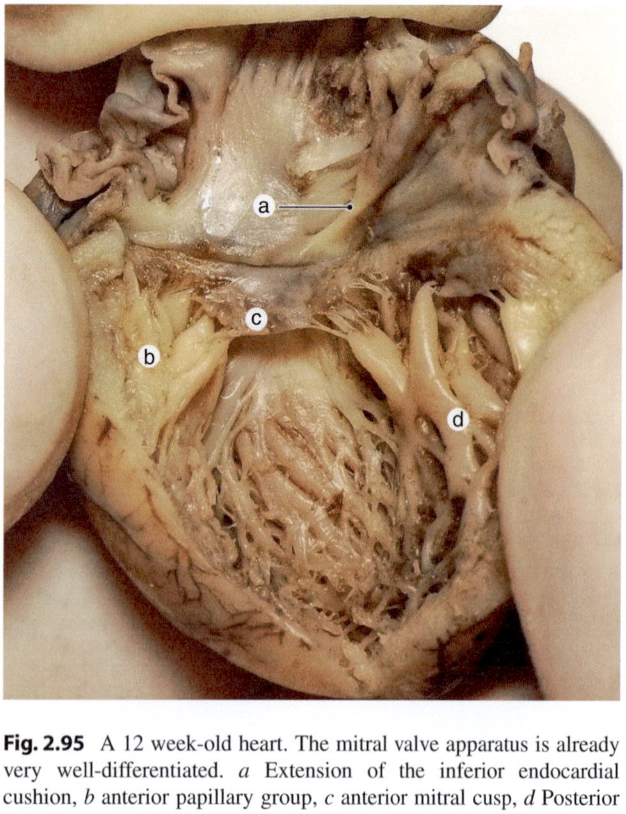

Fig. 2.95 A 12 week-old heart. The mitral valve apparatus is already very well-differentiated. *a* Extension of the inferior endocardial cushion, *b* anterior papillary group, *c* anterior mitral cusp, *d* Posterior papillary group

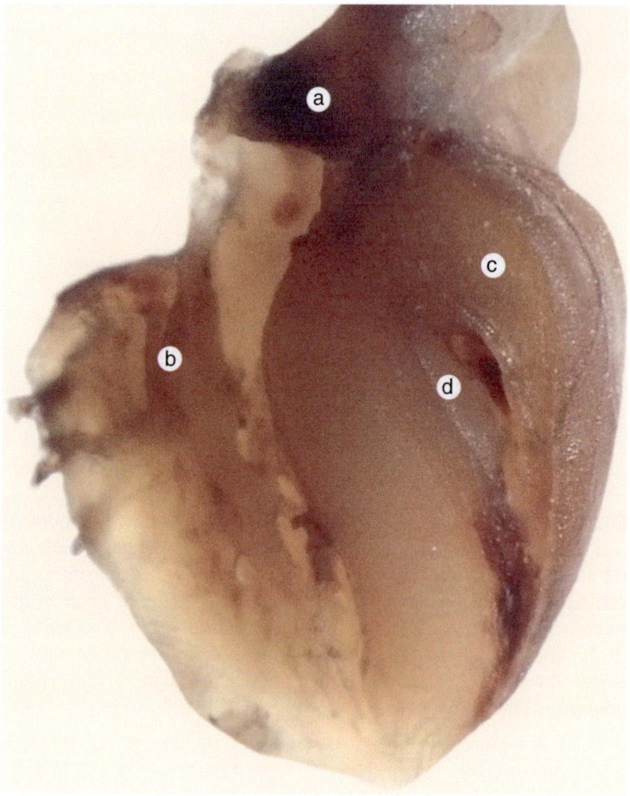

Fig. 2.96 An 11 week-old heart. Frontal section, view from posterior. Transillumination. *a* Aorta, *b* papillary muscle in continuity of the anterior cusp, *c* right ventricle, *d* Septomarginal trabecula – limit of the bulbar territory on the interventricular septum

2.8.5 Aortic Semilunar and Pulmonary Valve Formation

The aortic semilunar and pulmonary valves are formed on the appearance of the endocardial flaps at the level of the pulmonary and aortic ostium. By way of increasing in height and the occurrence of concavities on the parietal side, the valves change into semilunar valves. The appearance of flaps is conditioned

by the population with cells derived from neural crest. The apoptosis of these cells generates the cavitation phenomenon followed by the forming of the valvular sinuses (Figs. 2.76 and 2.97).

2.8.6 Epicardium and Coronary Vessels Formation

The epicardium is formed from the invasion of cell groups with different origin in the superficial layer of the cardiac tube wall: in the proepicardial organ (pericardial villosities) an probably in the aortic sac [12]. Thus, the myoepicardial mantle is formed through the alignment of these cell groups at the surface of the cardiac tube.

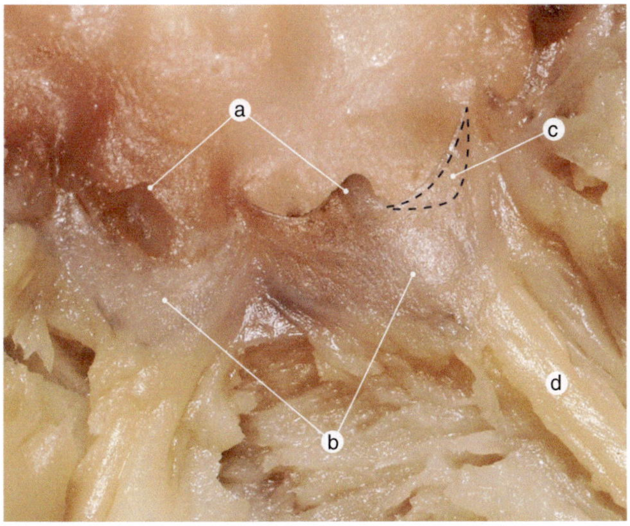

Fig. 2.97 A 10 week-old heart. The aortic semilunar valves are well formed. Observe the well represented muscular fascicles which are inserted on their base and which will suffer an involution. *a* Valvular nodules, *b* semilunar valves, *c* lunula, *d* muscular fascicle with valvular insertion

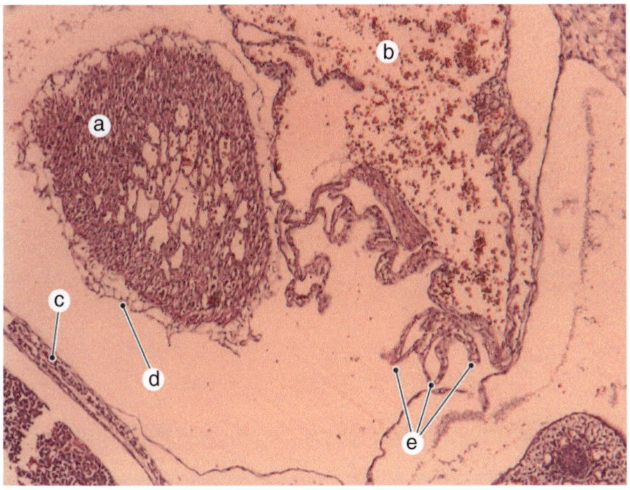

Fig. 2.98 A 10 day-old rat heart. Epicardial villi between the right atrium and the transverse septum. Objective 10×. *a* Ventricle, *b* atrium, *c* transverse septum, *d* epicardium during formation, *e* epicardial villi

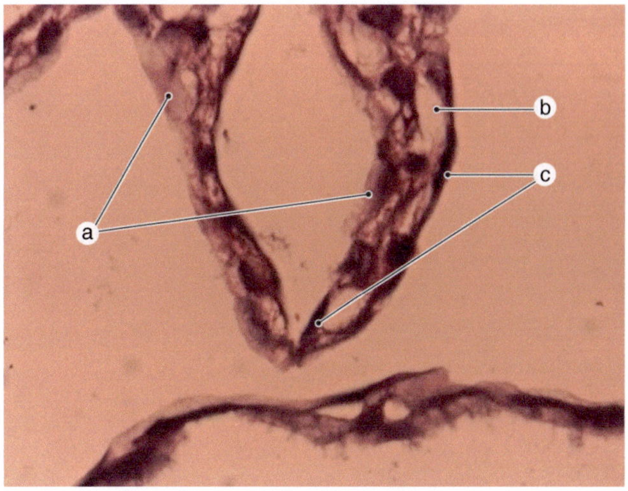

Fig. 2.99 Detail of the previous image. Objective 40×, Observe the presence of many cellular types. *a* Epithelial surface cells, *b* large cells with clear cytoplasm, *c* flattened cells

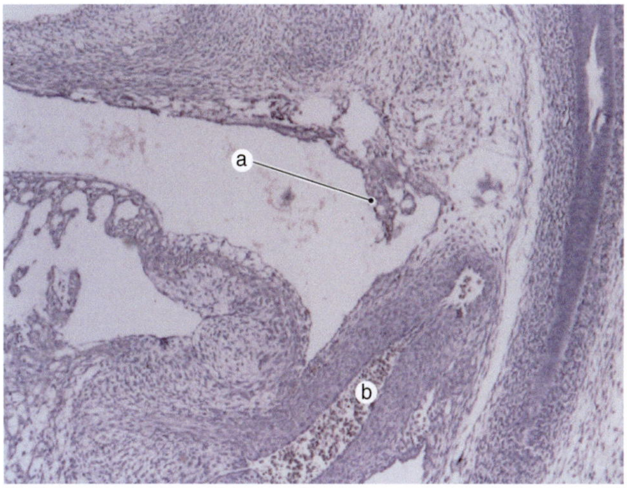

Fig. 2.100 Pericardial villi in the vecinity of arterial pedicle. *a* Pericardial villi in the vecinity of the arterial mesocardium, *b* arterial trunk

The proepicardial organ represents a structure that appears transient and early (fourth week) near the sinus venosus as an accumulation of villosities of the pericardial mesothelioma (Figs. 2.98, 2.99 and 2.100).

The cells, which originate from this "organ", align in a single row at the surface of the future myocardium, forming the epicardial primordium. The epicardial cells remain captive between the future myocardium and the epicardial primordium. These join and form the primordium of the subepicardial vessels. In this process the cells from the neural crest are also involved. Once initiated, the vascular network proliferates and enters the mesenchymal mass where it connects with the intramesenchymal endocardial spaces (sinuses). As a result of this process a vascular plexus is formed which stretches all the way to the subendocardial territory (Figs. 2.101, 2.102, 2.103 and 2.104).

This plexus will junction with both the coronary sinus venosus and the coronary vascular primordia, which sprout in the aortic sinuses (Fig. 2.76).

- The vessels are responsible for the debut of the myocardium penetration process in the endocardial tube. In close connection with the vascular pattern, the penetration of the myocardium is carried out in circular bands and then it extends until the muscular layers cover the entire endocardial tube. During this exuberant process of myocardization the vessels remain captive between the muscular fascicles and only the large trunks remain in a subepicardial position [13] (Fig. 2.105).

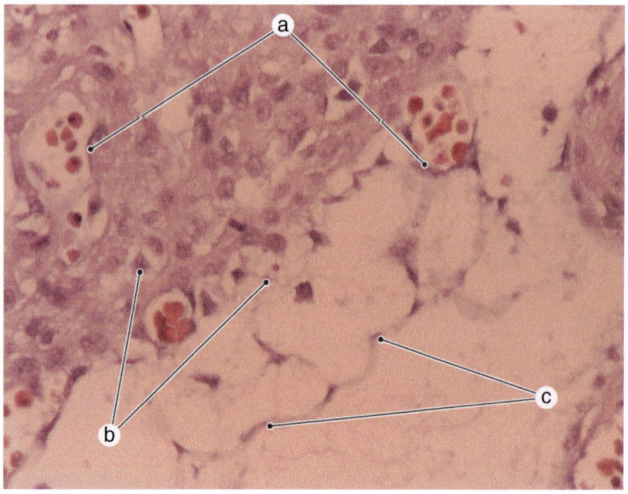

Fig. 2.101 Ten day-old rat heart, two types of cells (flattened and large) contribute to the forming of the epicardium and the subepicardial vessels. Large cells with clear cytoplasm are also found in the myocardial mass. *a* Primary vascular wall, *b* large cells probably from the neural crests, *c* epithelial cells junctioned during the formation of the epicardium

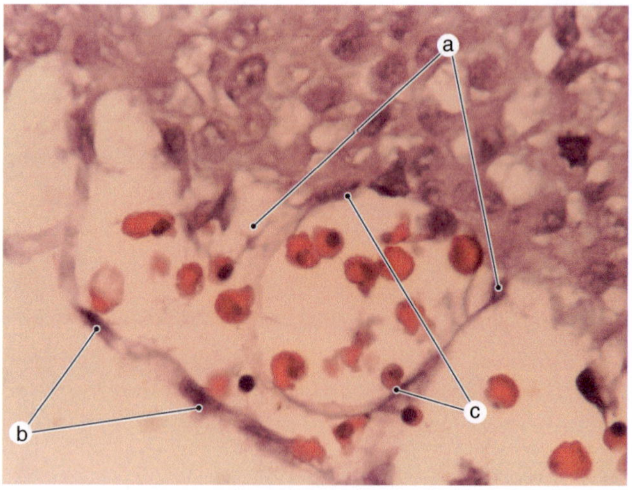

Fig. 2.103 Detail of a subepicardial vascular primordium. The primary vessel is formed by the initial junction of the epicardial flattened cells and the contribution of some large cells. *a* Cells from the neural crests, *b* epicardial single-layered cells, *c* primary vascular wall with single-layered cells

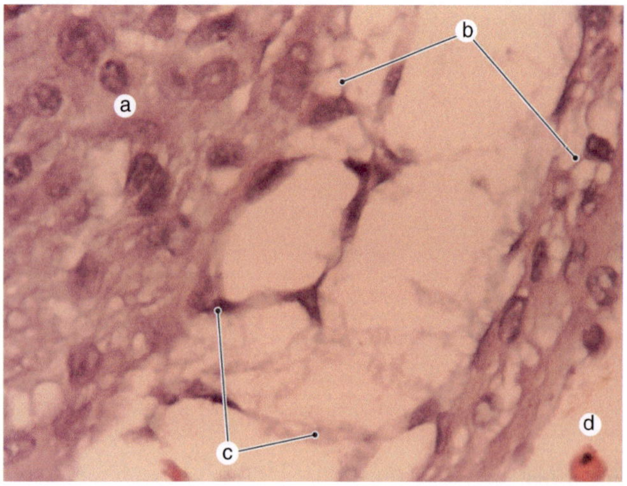

Fig. 2.102 In the angle between the atrium and the ventricle, the epicardial cells are united through cytoplasmic extentions, proof of their plasticity. *a* Ventricle, *b* cells from the neural crests, *c* epicardial cells with intercellular cytoplasmic bridges, *d* atrium

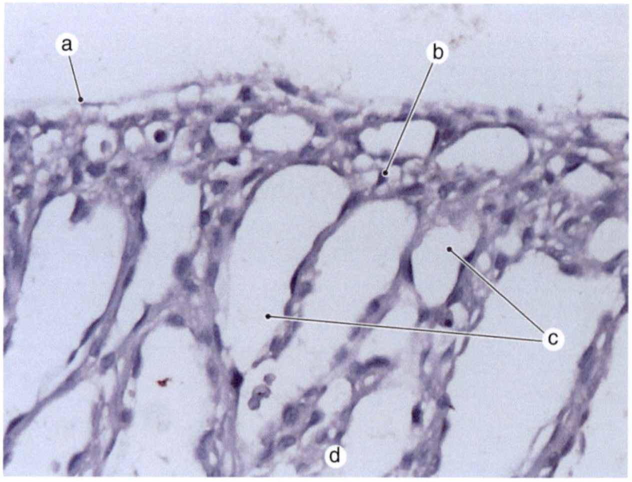

Fig. 2.104 In the ventricular wall can be seen large endocardial sinuses in connection with the future intertrabecular spaces; there are also visible endocardial primordia of intramyocardial vessels. *a* Epicardial cells, *b* cells from the neural crests, *c* vascular sinus lined with a single layer of cells, *d* ventricular wall

However the villosities of the pericardial mesothelioma are present in all vertebrates at embryonic stages. In humans, these pericardial villous accumulations were named the proepicardial organ and it represents a source of epicardial cells, subepicardial mesenchymal cells and the precursor vascular cells (angioblasts). These cells also invade the atrioventricular valvular primordium (Perez-Pomares) [14].

In humans, the mechanism for the transfer of these cells to the heart tube has not been properly clarified. Two ways are possible:

- Through vesicles which detach from the villous component and then adhere to the hearts surface.
- Through an assumed temporary sinoventricular ligament, which connect the left coronary sinus to the coronary sulcus and would disappear afterward. This ligament and the apical ligament of the heart (gubernaculum cordis) normally exist in reptiles.

Outside the proepicardial organ, small accumulations of pericardial villosities may also exist near the top of the heart.

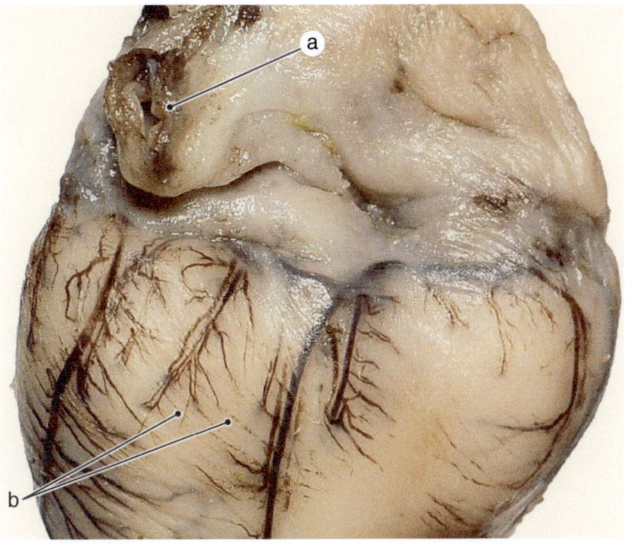

Fig. 2.105 A 2 months old heart. Diaphragmatic surface. Blood vessels form in the parallel spaces between the muscle fibres. There are many transverse anastomoses of small caliber between the main trunks. Although initially they are patent, these vessels lose their permeability so that in the adult heart the vascularization is of terminal type. In chronic coronary obstruction, some of these remaining anastomoses may regain their permeability, explaining one of the ways of adapting to ischemia. *a* Inferior vena cava, *b* vascular anastomoses

Excessive development of these structures can be correlated with the intrapericardial vessels formation.

In the fourth week, the vagus nerve will reach the heart, which in this way gains an extrinsic innervation. The sympathetic innervation develops later [15].

The embryonic heart is active since the third week.

2.9 The Differentiation of the Fibrous Skeleton of the Heart and of the Pacemaking and Conduction Tissue

In the second month, the cardioglia condenses and forms the fibrous skeleton of the heart [16], fact that finalizes the cardiac septation (Fig. 2.106). The only electric link between the atria and the ventricles remains the atrioventricular (His) bundle. The tendinous center is structured during the second month, from the mesenchyme of an intermediate septum part. It doesn't muscularize, but suffers a fibrocystic evolution. The sinoatrial node will differentiate into the right wall of the sinus venosus and later it will embed in the right atrium (Figs. 2.107, 2.108, 2.109, 2.110 and 2.111).

A well-known controversy is disputed about the origin of the cells from the conduction tissue:

- An opinion states that the conduction tissue has a neuroectodermal origin, coming from the neural crest. The neuroectodermal cells enter the arterial and venous mesocardium and invade the heart's wall. Their purpose is to gather in the known fascicles and nodules.
- The second opinion, which is more plausible, states that the conduction tissue originates from the embryonic cardiomyocytes. This was proven through the retroviral tracing of a single myocardial embryonic cell. It generated multicellular clones, which contained working myocardium as well as conduction cells.

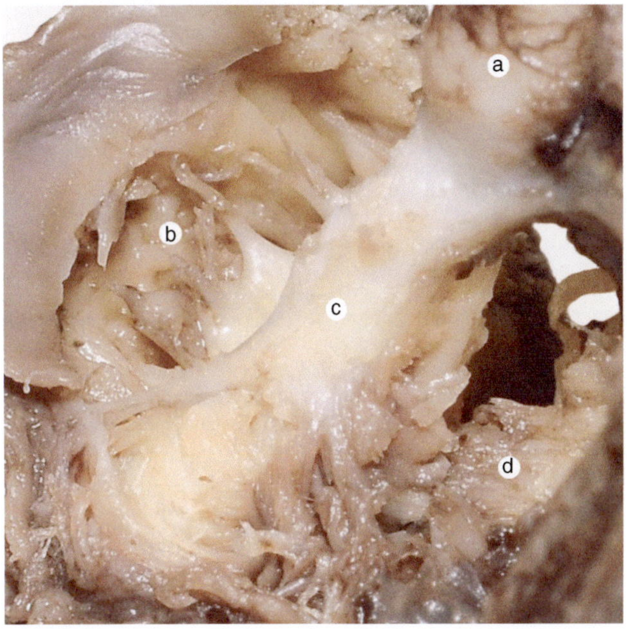

Fig. 2.106 Two and a half months old heart. Cardioglia during a condensing process forms the tendinous center of the heart. Upper – superior view, after removing the atria. *a* Aortab, *b* left ventricle, *c* the tendinous center of the heart, *d* right ventricle

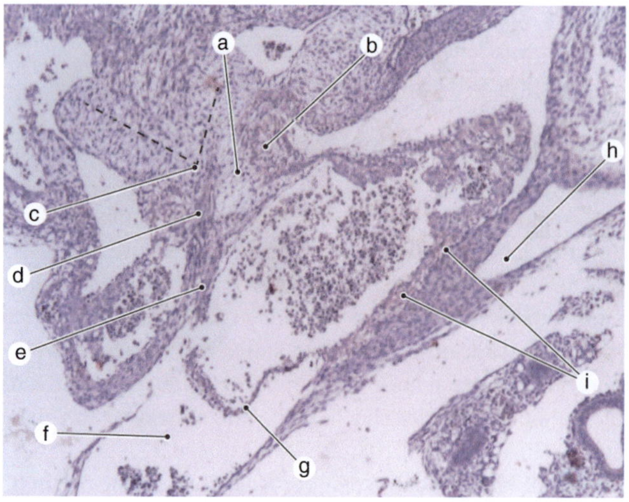

Fig. 2.107 An 11 days old rat heart. The right atrium, the sinoatrial junction, the area in which the sinoatrial node will be differentiated. Notice the vestibular spine and the tendon of Todaro, with parallel trajectory in the basis of the future interatrial sept (see Fig. 2.29). *a* Future tendinous center, *b* the area of the atrioventricular node, *c* superior endocardial cushion, *d* vestibular spine, *e* tendon of Todaro, *f* inferior vena cva, *g* right valve, *h* superior vena cava, *i* sinoatrial junction

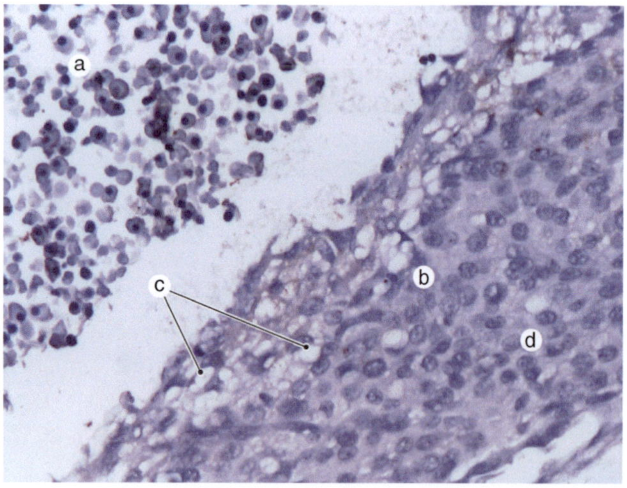

Fig. 2.108 Detail of the previous image. At the junction between superior vena cava and the right atrium, the myocardium has an obvious multitude of cellular types. *a* Right atrium, *b* sinoatrial junction, *c* cells of the neural ridges, *d* superior vena cava

Tracing cells from the neural crest and the proepicardial organ lead to the conclusion that they do not end within the control system, but have a strong bond with its elements [17].

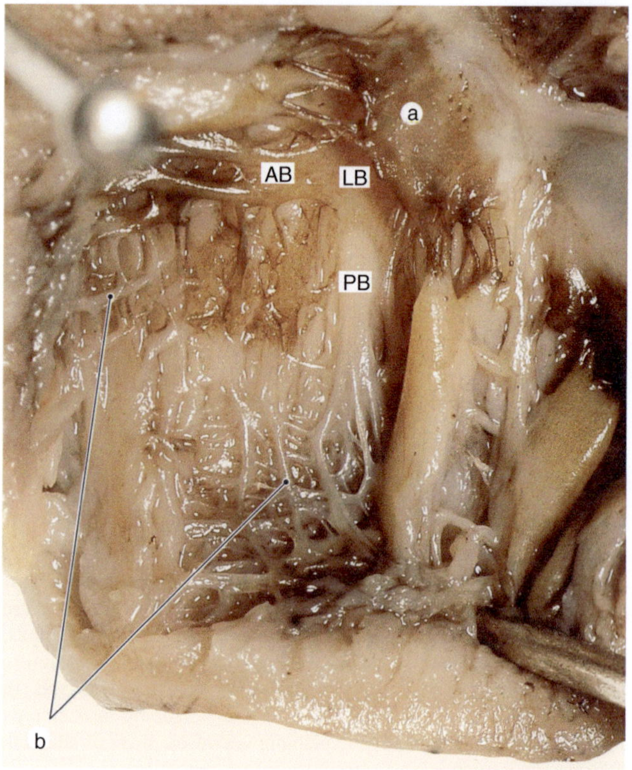

Fig. 2.109 Two and a half months old heart. The left surface of the interventricular septum. The left branch ("lata") of Hiss bundle bulges under the endocardium in the left ventricle and divides in an anterior and a posterior segment. There are also visible segments from the trabeculaecarneae which protude under the endocardium. *a* Anterior mitral cusp, *b* trabeculaecarneae. *LB* "lata" branch, *AB* anterior branch, *PB* posterior branch

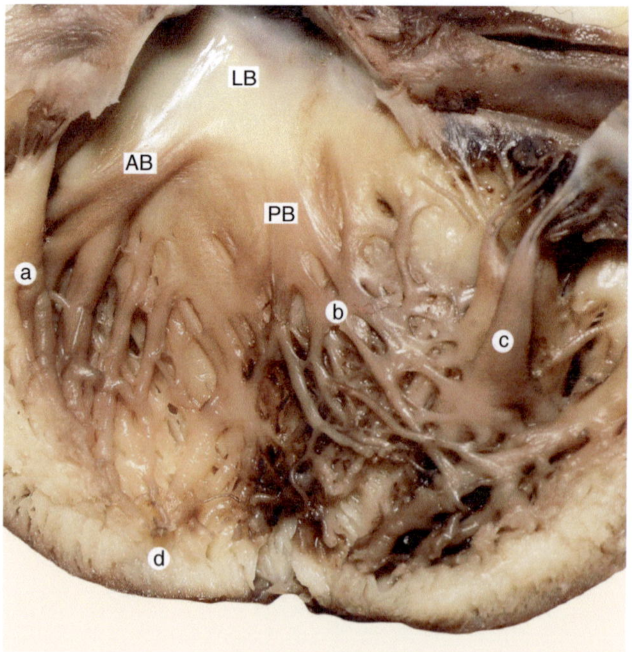

Fig. 2.110 The left branch of Hiss bundle and its divisions in another two and a half month old heart. *a* Anterior papillary muscle, *b* trabeculaecarneae, *c* posterior papillary muscle, *d* left ventricle. *LB* "lata" branch, *AB* anterior branch, *PB* posterior branch

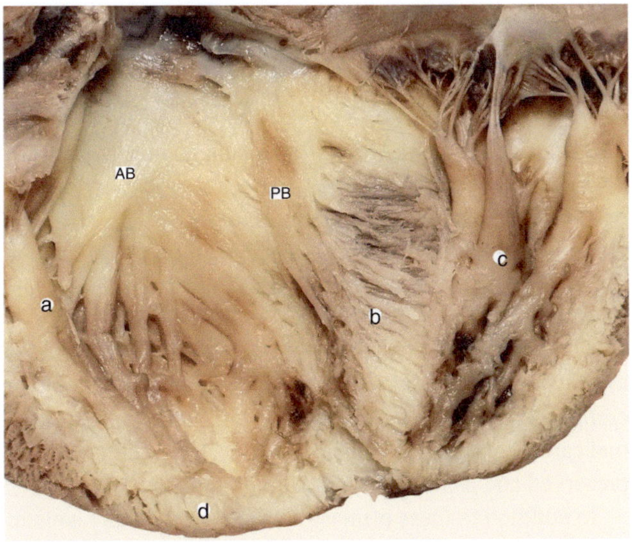

Fig. 2.111 Detail of the previous image after removing the endocardium and dissection of the posterior segment. *a* Anterior papillary muscle, *b* trabeculaecarneae, *c* posterior papillary muscle, *d* left ventricle. *AB* anterior branch, *PB* posterior branch

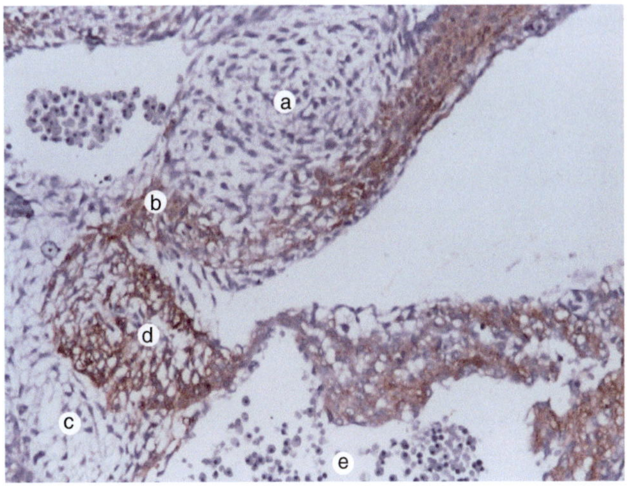

Fig. 2.112 An 11 days old rat heart. Imunohistochemistry. Within the area of the atrioventricular node there are cells with a positive reaction to antiactina antibodies. *a* Dextrodorsal crest in the arterial trunk, *b* the future membranous sept, *c* the future tendinous center, *d* the area of the atrio-ventricular node, *e* primitive atrium

2.9.1 Extracardial Cellular Contributions to the Consolidation of the Pacemaking and Conduction System [18]

Two groups of cells are strongly linked to the development of the conduction system:

- Migrated cells from the neural crest at the level of the venous pole. These get near the elements of the conduction system and then suffer an apoptosis process. The ablation of the neural crest leads to the loss of the atrioventricular node assembly and its electric isolation. These observations suggest an indirect role of the migrated neural cells in the differentiation of the conduction tissue.
- Another way for the migration of the cells, from the neural crest to the pacemaking territory, is at the arterial pedicle level, as shown in Figs. 2.112 and 2.113. Figure 2.114 reveals heterogenic populations of cells in the anterior atrial wall.
- The cells, which migrated from the proepicardial organ, have played an important role in the induction of the Purkinje fibers differentiation. Growth inhibition of the proepicardial organ leads to hypoplasia and unnatural Purkinje fibers.

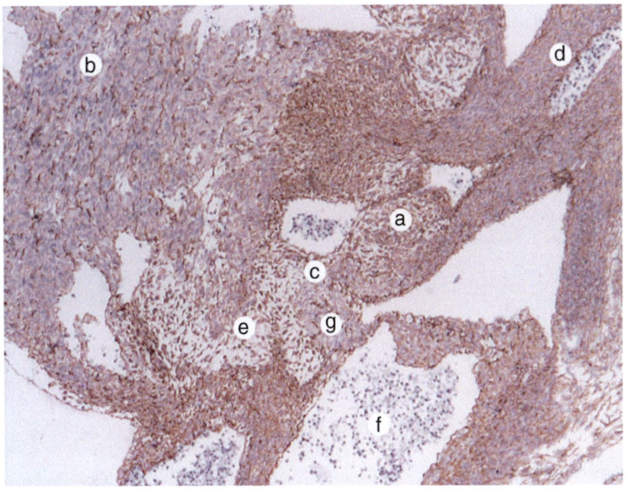

Fig. 2.113 The same heart as in the previous image. In the area of the atrio-ventricular node there are cells with a reaction to antivimentina antibodies. The multitude of cell populations in the nodal area is in this way proven. *a* Dextrodorsal crest in the arterial trunk, *b* muscular interventricular sept, *c* future membranous sept, *d* arterial trunk, *e* future tendinous center, *f* primitive atrium, *g* the area of the atrioventricular node

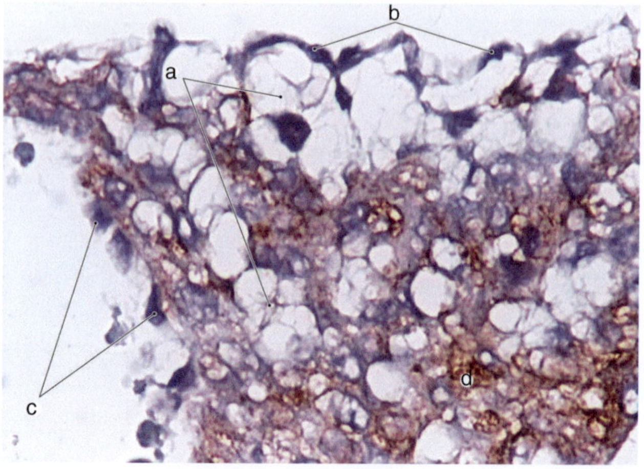

Fig. 2.114 Detail of a segment from the wall of the primitive atrium. Coloration for actin. Large cells with clear cytoplasm are evident under the epicardium which do not couple antiactin antibodies. There are cells migrated from the neural ridges. Similar cells are also found in the atrial mass, among the myoblasts. *a* Cells from the neural ridges, *b* epicardial cells, *c* endocardial cells, *d* cardiomyoblasts

2.10 The Left-Right Axial Asymmetry Determinism in the Heart Development [19]

The heart's development relies on a sum of factors (most of which unknown), which act to impose the organ asymmetry on the general symmetry pattern. These factors are involved not only in the breaking of the general symmetry, but also in the orientation of the organ towards the craniocaudial and anteroposterior axis.

Cellular and molecular differences, as compared to the bilateral symmetry axis, are present very early in the embryonic disc, at the level of the left and right mesodermal cardiogenic fields (primary fields). These differences are preserved and are emphasized during ontogeny.

In addition to these primary areas, there are other sources of mesodermal cells, called secondary cardiogenic areas, which participate in normal asymmetric differentiation of the heart tube. These areas are located in the primitive pharynx floor and in the mesoderm around the aortic bulbus, which extends to the branchial arches. In order to be successfully incorporated, the cells originating from the secondary fields depend on the migrated cells from the neural crest.

The regression of certain cellular groups (apoptosis), in their different development stages, plays an important role in determining the asymmetry.

But it seems that the cardiac asymmetry is mainly determined by the expression of some genes that control the development on the left-right axis (Pitx2c, BMP4 and flectin).

Creatine kinase B and Pitx2c are expressed in the interatrial septum cells, these genes being expressed in the left atrium and not in the right. This fact marks an asymmetry, which is present in the common atrium before the septal process.

According to this observation, we expect the atrial isomerism to have important interatrial septum pathology or even to be absent. Although they are called inferior and superior endocardial cushions, they are located on the left and right side of the atrioventricular canal.

The differences in the left-right expression of the Pitx 2c gene suggest the existence of a lateralization of the atrioventricular canal, but also of a conotruncal region. As a consequence, laterality defects will be accompanied by valvular and outflow pole defects.

The observation, which states that cardiac laterality defects are accompanied by laterality defects in one or more organs, suggests a causal link that precedes the organogenesis. Affecting the determinism of the left-right axial symmetry leads to the appearance of clinical entities:

- Situs inversus is present when all organs are arranged according to the craniocaudal symmetry, but positioned such as viewed in a mirror.
- Situs solitus refers to the reverse positioning of a single organ (dextrocardia).

- Situs ambiguus – a situation in which numerous laterality anomalies are present in varied combinations. Among the malformations encountered in situs ambiguus, at cardiac level, some are to be remembered: transposition of the great vessels, septal defects and great vessel malformations.

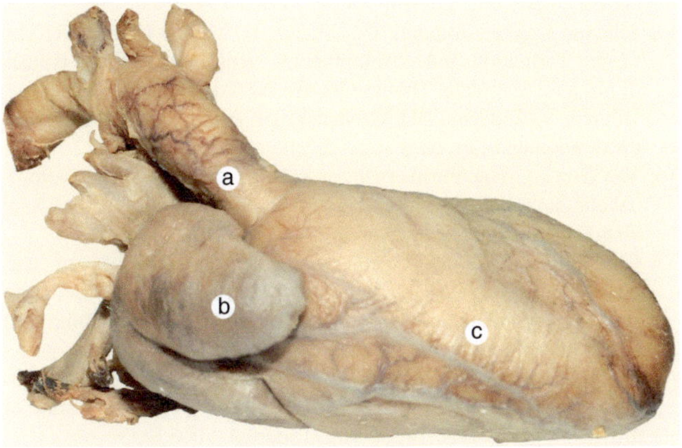

Fig. 2.115 A 6 months old heart. Left atrial isomerism. Right auricle looks like a bent finger, that is a characteristic look for the left auricle. *a* Aorta with right ventricle origin, *b* right auricle which looks like a hook, similar to the left auricle, *c* right ventricle

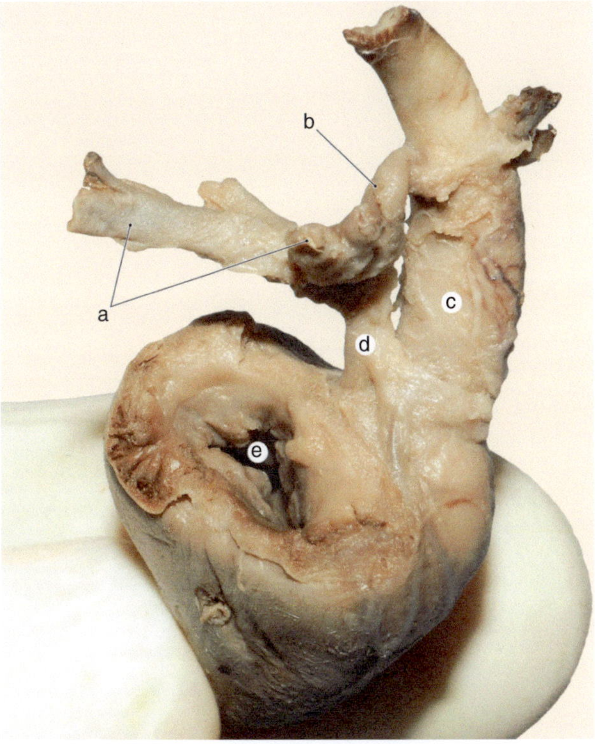

Fig. 2.116 The same heart after removing the atria. The aorta leaves the region of the right ventricle. The pulmonary trunk is atresic. Through the permeable arterial canal the blood reaches the pulmonary trunk. *a* Pulmonary arteries, *b* arterial canal, *c* "riding" aorta, *d* atresic pulmonary trunk, *e* unique atrioventricular orifice

- situs ambiguus including isomerism – a situation in which organs, which are different in structure in their right and left side, develop according to the model existing on a single side (e.g. the right pulmonary isomerism: the left lung has as well as the right one three lobes; in the hepatic isomerism we have the median liver, with two lobes almost identically developed).
- The right atrial isomerism – both auricles have the pyramidal form of the right one.
- The left atrial isomerism – both auricles have the hook form of the left one (Figs. 2.36 and 2.115, 2.116 and 2.117).

In the Ivemark syndrome (asplenia with atrial isomerism), also called the asplenia polysplenia syndrome [20], the following are aspects are encountered:

- Right or left cardiac isomerism (asplenia or polysplenia)
- Atrioventricular canal, defects of the endocardial cushions, atrial septal defect, pulmonary stenosis, ventricular septal defect.
- Visceral heterotaxy: median liver, common mesentery, agenesis of the corpus callosum, abnormal pulmonary lobation.

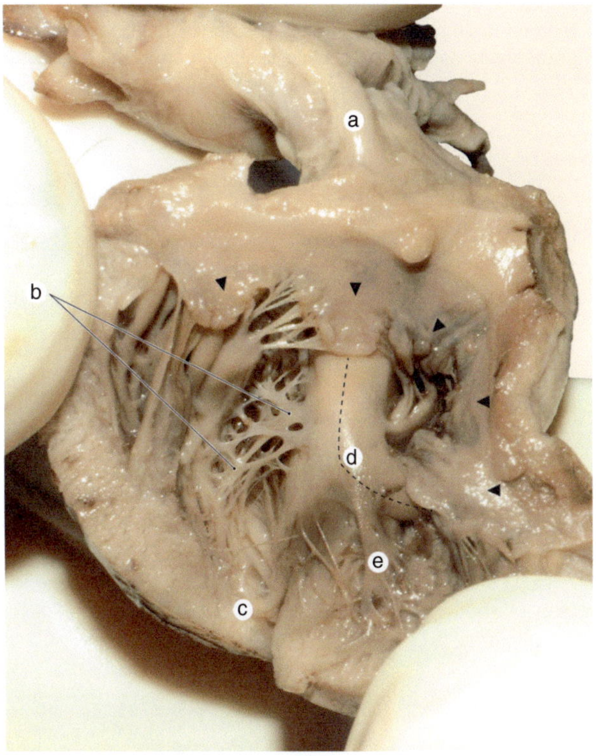

Fig. 2.117 The same heart. An unique atrium communicates with partially-septed ventricle. The atrioventricular communication has five functional and well-differentiated cusps (*arrows*). Purkinje network has an intraluminal course. The right branch of Hiss bundle has a direction corresponding to the left ventricle. *a* Atresic pulmonary trunk, *b* the left branch and Purkinje network, *c* left ventricle, *d* intraventricular muscular sept, *e* right branch of the Purkinje network situated in the left ventricle

References

1. Gittenberger-de Groot AC, Vrancken Peeters MPFM, Mentink MMT, Gourdie RG, Poelmann RE. Epicardium – derived cells contribute a novel population to the myocardial wall and the atrioventricular cushions. Circ Res. 1998;82:1043–52.
2. Odgers PNB. The formation of the venous valves, the foramen secundum and the septum secundum in the human heart. J Anat. 1935;69(Pt 4):412–22.
3. Franklin J, Thomas CC. Cardiovascular studies. Springfield: Blackwell Scientific Publications; 1948. xvi + 306 pp.
4. Moorman AFM, Christoffels MV. Development, genes, and evolution. Physiol Rev. 2003;83:1223–67.
5. Moorman A, Webb S, Brown NA, Lamers W, Anderson RH. Development of the heart: (1) formation of the cardiac chambers and arterial trunks. Heart. 2003;89:806–14.
6. Licata RH. The human embryonic heart in the ninth week. Am J Anat. 1954;94:73–125.
7. Van den Hoff MJB, Moorman AFM, Ruijter JM, Lamers WH, Bennington RW, Markwald RR, Wessels A. Myocardialization of the cardiac outflow tract. Dev Biol. 1999;212:477–90.
8. Lamers WH, Virágh S,Wessels A, Moorman AFM, Anderson RH. Formation of the tricuspid valve in the human heart. Circulation. 1995;91:111–21.
9. Lamers WH, Wessels A, Verbeek FJ, Moorman AF, Viragh S, Wenink AC, Gittenberger-de Groot AC, Anderson RH. New findings concerning ventricular septation in the human heart. Implications for maldevelopment. Circulation. 1992;86:1194–205.
10. De La Cruz MV, Castillo MM, Villavicenzio G, Valencia A, Moreno-Rodriguez RA. Primitive interventricular septum, its primordium, and its contribution in the definitive interventricular septum: in vivo labelling study in the chick embryo heart. Anat Rec. 1997;247(4):512–20.
11. McCarthy KP, Ho SY, Anderson RH. Categorisation of ventricular septal defects: review of the perimembranous morphology. Paediatr Cardiol. 2000;3:24–40.
12. Pomares JM, Phelps A, Chápuli R, Wessels A. The contribution of the proepicardium to avian cardiovascular development. Int J Dev Biol. 2001;45(S1):S155–6.
13. Männer J. The origin and course of coronary vessels: embryological considerations. Cardiol Young. 1998;8:534–5.
14. Männer J, Pérez-Pomares JM, Macías D, Muñoz-Chápuli R. The origin, formation and developmental significance of the epicardium: a review. Cells Tissues Organs. 2001;169(2):89–103.
15. Hildreth V, Anderson RH, Henderson DJ. Autonomic innervation of the developing heart: origins and function. Clin Anat. 2009;22:36–46.
16. Van Gils FA. The fibrous skeleton in the human heart: embryological and pathogenetic considerations. Virchows Arch A Pathol Anat Histol. 1981;393(1):61–73.
17. Christoffels CM, Moorman AFM. Development of the cardiac conduction system. why are some regions of the heart more arrhythmogenic than others? Circulation: Arrhythmia and Electrophysiology. 2009;2:195–207.
18. Jongbloed MRM, Mahtab EAF. Development of the cardiac conduction system and the possible relation to predilection sites of arrhythmogenesis. Scientific World Journal. 2008;8:239–69.
19. Wessels A, Markwald R. Cardiac morphogenesis and dysmorphogenesis. Normal development. In: Tuan RS, Lo CW (eds.). Methods in Molecular Biology, Vol. 136. Development Biology Protocols. Totowa, NJ: Humana Press; 2000; pp. 239–59.
20. Peeters H, Devriendt K. Human laterality disorders. Eur J Med Genet. 2006;49(5):349–62.

3 Concepts of Clinical Anatomy of the Heart: Definition, Location and Position

3.1 Definition

The heart is a thoracic musculocavitary, intrapericardial organ, situated in the middle mediastinum. Its main function is that of a suction pump which works simultaneously on two almost independent circuits. The heart has also a paraendocrine function due to some polypeptides production. The heart has a specific autonomy, justified by the presence in its structure of the cardiac conduction system. At the same time the heart is an organ which is under the central nervous control (both nervous and endocrine), perfectly integrated in the entire body economy and placed under the influence of the great regulating reflexes. Not least, the heart represents a vast territory of pharmacological reception, with varied receptors which can be manipulated in a specific manner.

- We mentioned earlier about "two almost independent circuits" because:
  - in the pulmonary circuit interpose the so-called arterial segments of control (arterio-arterial anastomoses between branches of the pulmonary arteries and that the bronchial arteries) through which, in a small percent, the two circulation systems (greater and lesser) are connected at the level of the bronchial wall.
  - someseptal defects may exist, connecting the two circuits, but due to their small dimensions presents no significant hemodynamic effects.

F.M. Filipoiu, *Atlas of Heart Anatomy and Development*,
DOI 10.1007/978-1-4471-5382-5_3, © Springer-Verlag London 2014

3.2 Location

The term of location refers to the heart placement into an anatomical circumstance, in relation with the neighboring organs.

The heart is situated in the middle mediastinum (Fig. 3.1). This is a topographical region limited by:

- anterior, by a coronal plane tangential to the pericardium
- posterior, by a coronal plane which passes posterior and tangential to the tracheal bifurcation, the pulmonary veins and the pericardium covering the left atrium.
- superior, by a transverse plane passing through the T4 vertebra and the sternal angle. This plane is situated inferiorly to the aortic arch and the azygos arch.
- inferior, the middle mediastinum is limited by the diaphragm, more precisely the heart sits on the diaphragmatic central tendon (Fig. 3.2).
- lateral, the middle mediastinum is bordered by the mediastinal pleurae of the lungs, that mold the heart (Figs. 5.6).

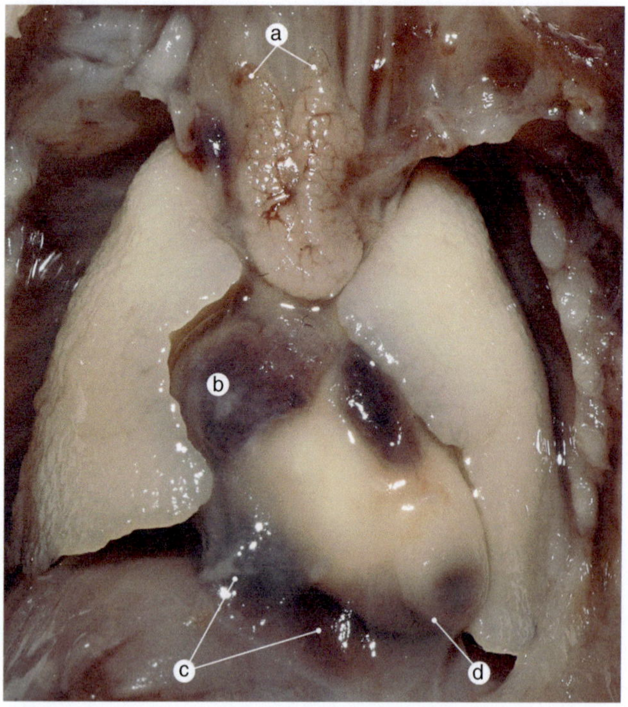

Fig. 3.1 Four months old heart, situated in the middle mediastinum. We may observe the transparent membranous pericardial sac and also the aspect of the thymus. *a* Thymus, *b* right atrium, *c* pericardial sac, *d* apex

Beyond this didactic presentation there are some aspects related with the mediastinum which have to be outlined:

- The mediastinum is an inhomogenous topographical region which contains varied organs connected by the conjunctive tissue. This isn't just a simple connective tissue. It contains multiple glomic-typed structures and baroreceptors which transforms the mediastinum into a sensitive space to the pressure changes and vibration.
- In this context, we mention that the movement or the 'balance' of the mediastinum (involving the heart also) triggers some vegetative reflexes which may lead to heart rhythm disorders and finally to cardiac arrest.
- The mediastinum contains transitional typed organs which are in close relation with the heart. The volume or temperature changes of these organs may have an influence on the heart activity.
- The mediastinum presents some declive spaces which represents the place for early accumulation of fluids with consecutive effects on the heart.
- The mediastinal tumors may exert compression over the heart.

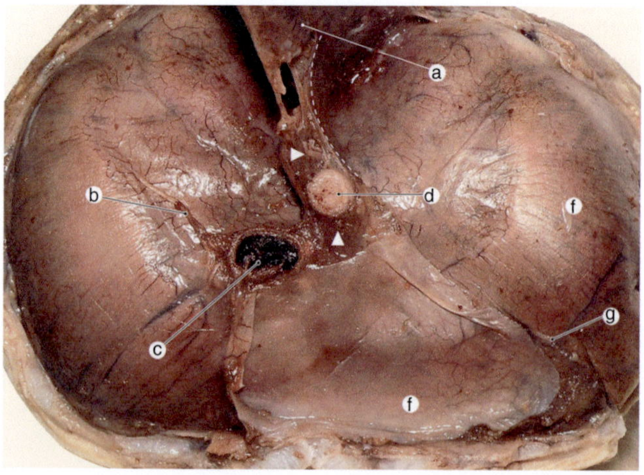

Fig. 3.2 Seven months old fetus. Anterosuperior vision over the diaphragm. The pericardial sack attaches to thetendinous center. Notice the aortic-esophageal recess (*dotted line*) covered by the mediastinal pleura, anterior and posterior vagal trunks (*arrows*) around the esophagus, as well as the different regions in which the two phrenicnerves approach the diaphragm. *a* Thoracic aorta, *b* right phrenic nerve, *c* inferior vena cava, *d* pericardium on the central tendon, *e* esophagus, *f* left hemidiaphragm, *g* left phrenic nerve

3.3 Position

The term of "position" refers to the organ placement along the standard anatomical axis and planes.

The heart is a pyramidal in shape organ, with its fixed base situated posteriorly, to the right and superior. Its long axis is oblique towards the left, inferior and anterior, uniting the center of the base with the apex of the heart. The apex is mobile during the heart contractions but also is mobile depending on the position and physiological status (Fig. 3.3).

The positioning of the heart longer axis varies accordingly to:

- in deep inspiration, the long axis tends to rotate towards right, so becoming more anterioposterior. We call this anteroposterior axis an arrow-like axis.
- in deep expiration, the axis orientates towards left and posterior. We call this a transverse axis. This situation occurs in the newborn, in children, in obese or in picnic constitutional typed individuals (Fig. 3.4).
- when the axis tends to be vertically orientated, with its apex inferiorly, we say that this is a drop-like type of heart. This situation is common in longilin type of individuals.

During the heart contractions, the apex of the heart touches the thoracic wall. This movement may be felt though palpation and is called the apexian shock. In the left dorsal decubitus position, the apex of the heart no longer projects on the midclavicle line, but move towards the anterior axillary line. Also the apex of the heart descends from the fifth left intercostal space (where it projects in dorsal decubitus) towards the sixth left intercostal space (where it projects in upright position). We say that the apex of the heart is mobile accordingly to the position of the body.

The apex of the heart ascends in the forth left intercostal space during a deep inspiration and descends in the sixth left intercostal space during a deep expiration. The apex of the heart is mobile with the breathing.

The heart can be studied using successive, perpendicular, transverse cross-section on the longer axis of the heart. These represent the anatomical cross-section of reference. For this cross-sections a global transverse axis can be described or one for each cavity (Fig. 3.5).

However, successive cross sections, perpendicular to the vertical axis of the thorax can be achieved. These are sections usually made by imaging means.

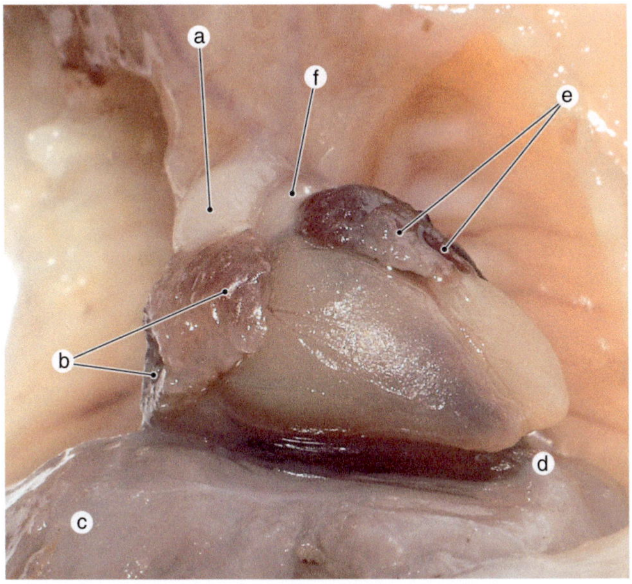

Fig. 3.3 Eleven weeks old heart. The heart location, after the lungs were removed. We may observe that the organ is held in place due to its attachment to the great vessels. All forces resulting in the autonomous contraction of the myocardium finally finds the support in the great vessels attachment. *a* Aorta, *b* right atrium and its auricle, *c* diaphragm, *d* apex, *e* left atrium and its auricle, *f* pulmonary trunk

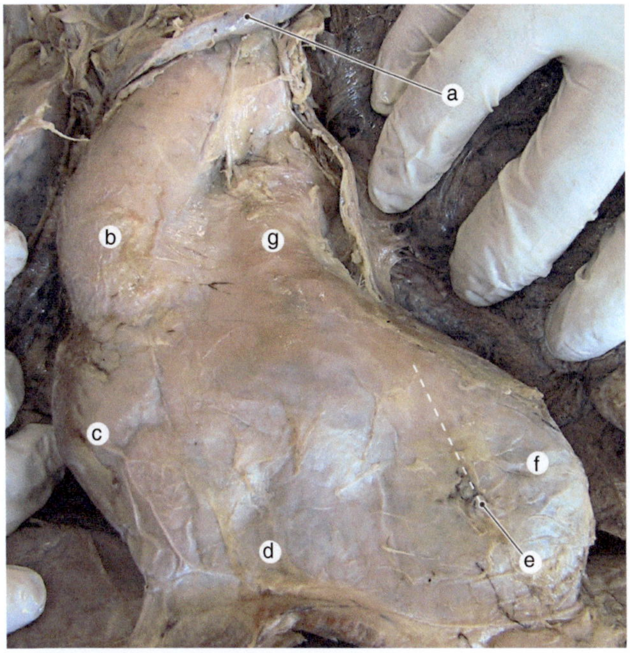

Fig. 3.4 Intrapericardic heart, with the long axis transversely orientated. *a* The left brachiocephalic vein, *b* the ascending aorta, *c* the right atrium, *d* the right ventricle, *e* correspondent to the anterior interventricular groove, *f* the left ventricle, *g* the pulmonary trunk

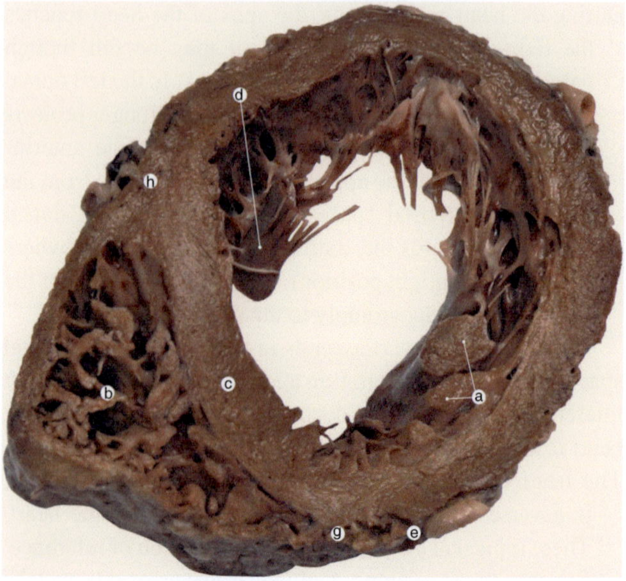

Fig. 3.5 Transverse cross-section of the heart and through the ventricular mass. The difference between the two ventricular cavities is obvious. *a* Anterior papillary group, *b* the right ventricle, *c* interventricular septum, *d* posterior papillary group, *e* anterior interventricular sulcus, *f* the left ventricle, *g* an anterior projection of the right ventricle, *h* a posterior projection of the right ventricle

The clinic tends to use the term "inferior" for the diaphragmatic orientation, the term "posterior" for basic orientation and the term "apical" for apex orientation.

Attention!

Defining the heart position is complex and requires always multiple parameters. This complexity can be a source for many confusions and contradictions.

The External Configuration of the Heart

4

4.1 The General Presentation

Classically, the heart size is compared to the size of the individual's right fist. This comparison is more suggestive than true, the heart size varying with the constitutional type, age, physiological status and possible pathology (Fig. 4.1).

Accordingly to the classical view, the heart presents a sternocostal surface, a pulmonary surface, a diaphragmatic surface, a right border, a base and an apex.

The sternocostal surface is named that way because of its relation with the sternum and the ribs (Figs. 4.2–4.10).

At this surface the atria are partially visible (in the superior one-third) but also the ventricles participate (in the inferior two-thirds). The ventricular component is represented in most of its part by the right ventricle and the rest by the left ventricle, the two ventricles being separated by the anterior interventricular groove (we say that the right heart is situated anteriorly to the left one). In this groove (in general at its left side) passes the anterior interventricular artery and the great cardiac vein. The groove finishes at about 1–2 cm to the right of the cardiac apex, inducing the appearance of the apexian notch at the right border of the heart. Its depth is highly variable.

The apex of the heart is orientated towards inferior and to the left and represents the region comprising both ventricles, separated by the apexian notch. Its appearance is variable and will be treated in detail+-z\z\ to the general architecture of the myocardium chapter.

The right ventricle extends superiorly and to the left with a region which presents an aspect compared with a truncated cone named the pulmonary conus. This region continues with an almost cylindrical segment with a variable presence and aspect, named the pulmonary infundibulum. Its distal part is the subvalvar infundibulum which finishes at the pulmonary valve as the last segment of the right ventricle having a muscular wall. Beyond the pulmonary valve, the right ventricle continues with the pulmonary trunk.

The atrial component of the sternocostal surface remains mostly hidden behind the emergence of the two great arteries, the aorta and the pulmonary artery.

The atria are separated from the ventricles by an anteriorly incomplete circular groove, the coronary groove. In its right side, the coronary groove contains the right coronary artery and the small cardiac vein, while its left side contains the circumflex artery, the great cardiac vein and the coronary sinus.

Towards the base of the heart, on the sternocostal surface, there are two arterial projections named the right and the left auricles. The auricles covers the anterior extremities of the atrio-ventricular groove and looks like it covers the origin of the two great vessels, the aorta and the pulmonary trunk. The whole ensemble is known as the "corona cordis". Inside the corona cordis, the aorta is situated to the right and posterior while the pulmonary artery to the left and anterior. These vessels give the impression that twist one inaround each other (Figs. 4.11, 4.12 and 4.13).

The pulmonary surface is represented by a large portion of the left ventricle (Figs. 4.14, 4.15, 4.16, 4.17, 4.18, 4.19,

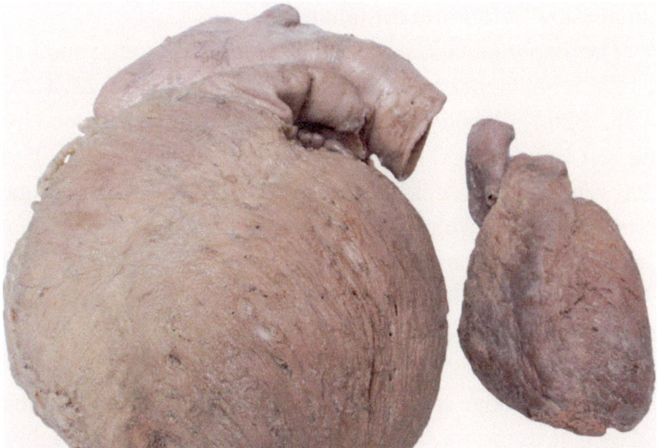

Fig. 4.1 Ventricular pyramids of different size

F.M. Filipoiu, *Atlas of Heart Anatomy and Development*,
DOI 10.1007/978-1-4471-5382-5_4, © Springer-Verlag London 2014

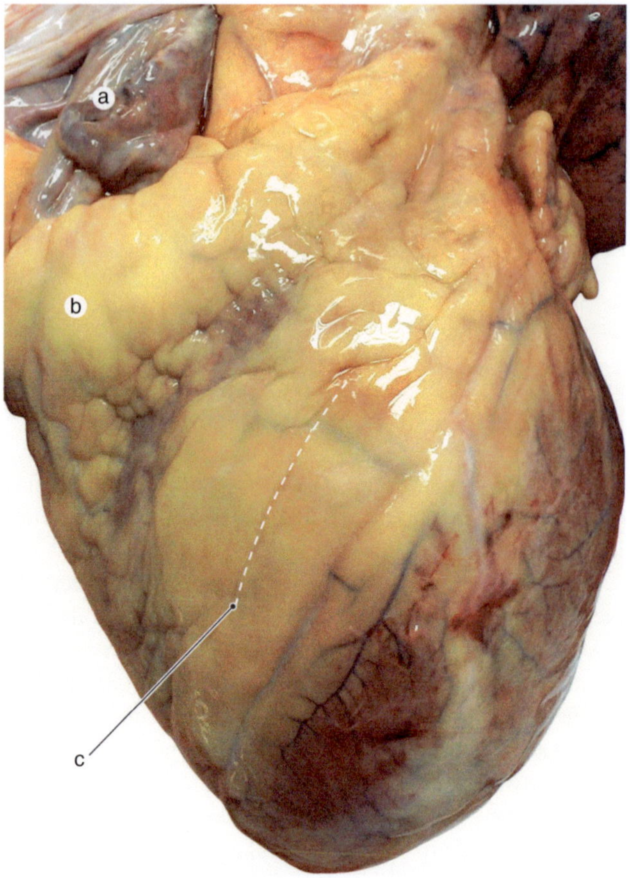

Fig. 4.2 Non-formaldehyded heart. Notice the different consistence of the atrial wall (flaccid) in comparison with the ventricular one (firm). *a* Right atrium, *b* fat deposits in the right coronary groove, *c* positioning of the anterior interventricular groove

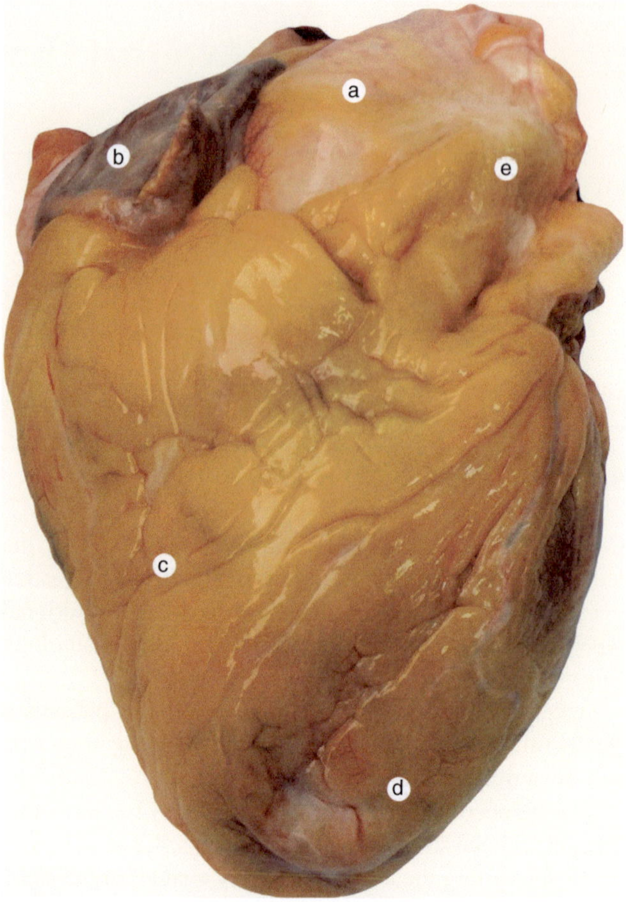

Fig. 4.3 Non-formaldehyded heart. Massive subepicardic fat accumulation. *a* Ascending aorta, *b* right atrium, *c* right ventricle, *d* left ventricle, *e* pulmonary trunk

4.20 and 4.21). This surface also presents the name of the obtuse border of the heart (margo obtusis). The name of pulmonary surface occurs due to the intimate relation with mediastinal surface of the left lung which marks the cardiac impression (inferior to the hilum).

The diaphragmatic surface is relatively horizontal and lies on the central tendon of the diaphragm Figs. 4.22, 4.23, 4.24, 4.25, 4.26, 4.27 and 4.28). Most of this surface is formed by the left ventricle and the rest of it by the right ventricle. The two ventricles are separated by the posterior interventricular groove through which passes the posterior interventricular artery and the middle cardiac vein. The place situated on the diaphragmatic surface where the coronary groove intersects the posterior interventricular groove is named the cross of the heart (crux cordis).

The percentage in which one or the other of the ventricles takes part in the formation of the cardiac surfaces is highly variable. Not infrequently times, the percentage of distributions are more balanced or are even reverse in comparison with the described situations.

The right border, named the acute or the sharp border, separates towards the right the sternocostal surface of the right ventricle from the diaphragmatic surface belonging to the same ventricle (Figs. 4.29, 4.30, 4.31, 4.32, 4.33, 4.34, 4.35, 4.36 and 4.37). It's more obvious in the corpse than in the living individual. Starts in right inferior vena cava and ends at the apex of the heart, being interrupted by apexian notch. At the level of the notch, the interventricular grooves may continue to each other and interventricular arteries can anastomose.

Confusions can be made between the anatomical and radiological term of right border. Radiologically, the right border is that segment of the right atrium situated between the ends of the two vena cava, visible on the chest radiography (Fig. 4.38).

The base of the heart is represented in most of it by the posterior aspect of the left atrium in which drains the four pulmonary veins and in small percent by the sinusal part of the right atrium. The limit between the two atria barely identifies and carries the name of the interatrial groove (Waterstone) (Figs. 4.39, 4.40, 4.41, 4.42, 4.43, 4.44, 4.45 and 4.46).

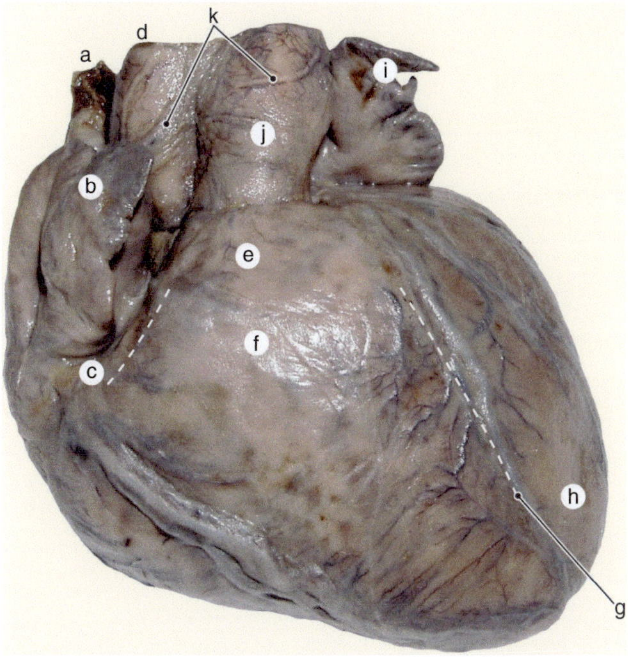

Fig. 4.4 Fetal heart of 7 months of age. Notice the total absence of subepicardic fat deposits. *a* Superior vena cava, *b* right auricle, *c* right coronary groove, *d* aorta, *e* right ventricle's infundibulum, *f* right ventricle's conus, *g* anterior interventricular groove, *h* left ventricle, *i* left auricle, *j* pulmonary trunk, *k* periarterial nervous plexus

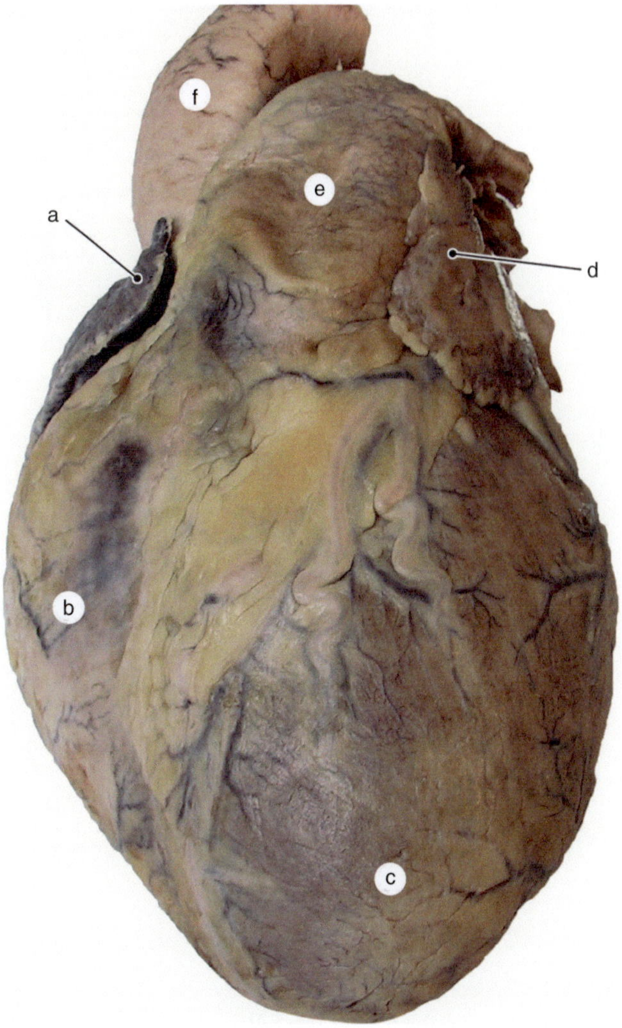

Fig. 4.5 Formaldehyde prepared heart. The fat depositing usually met in healthy individuals. *a* Right auricle, *b* right ventricle, *c* left ventricle, *d* left auricle, *e* pulmonary trunk, *f* ascending aorta

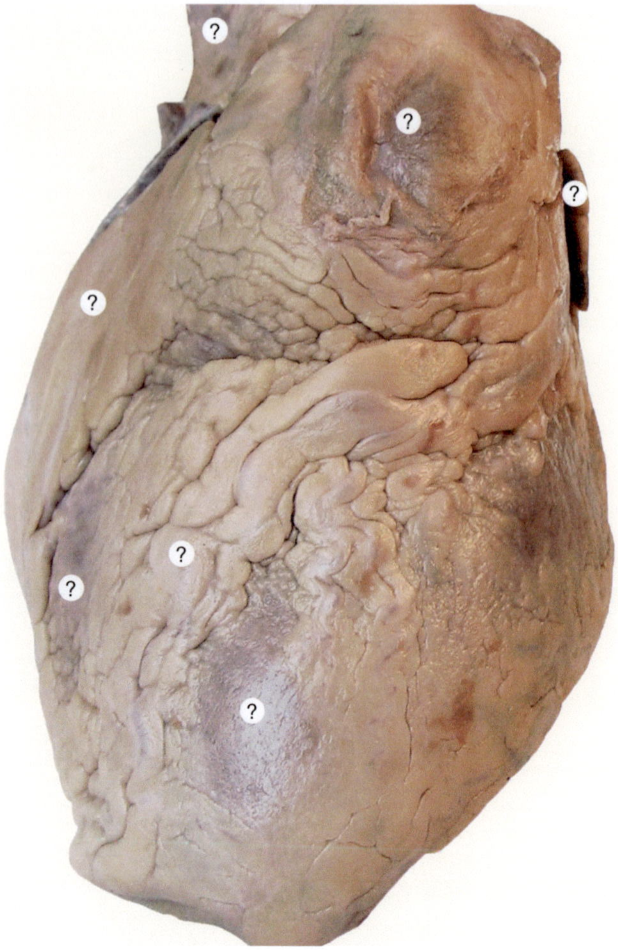

Fig. 4.6 Undissected heart. Plese identify the structers on the sterno-costal surface (same as the Fig. 4.5)

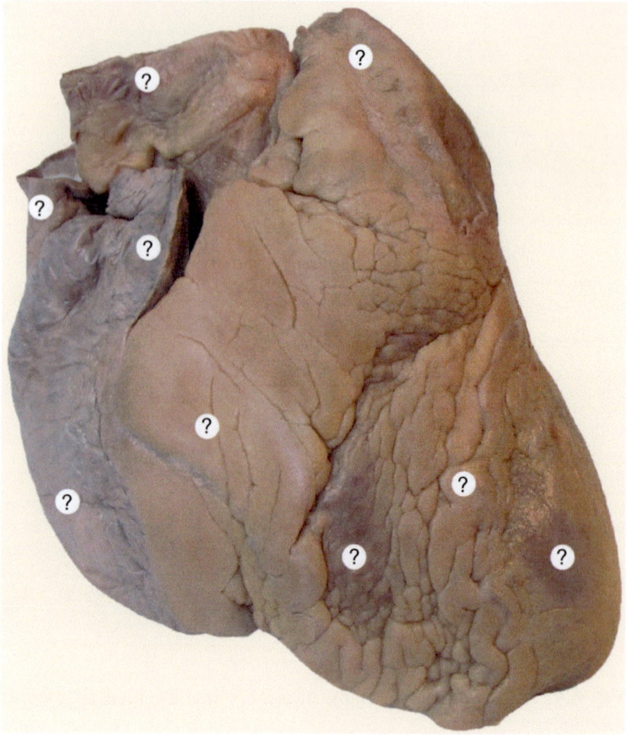

Fig. 4.7 Undissected heart. Plese identify the structers on the right surface (same as the Fig. 4.4)

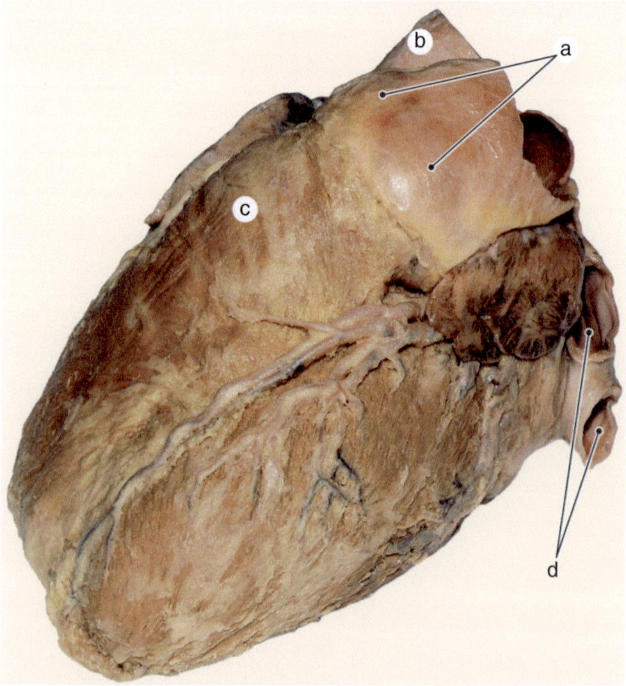

Fig. 4.8 The well structured subpulmonary infundibulum continues with an evident bulb at the origin of the pulmonary artery. *a* Pulmonary trunk's bulb, *b* aorta, *c* subpulmonary infundibulum, *d* left pulmonary veins

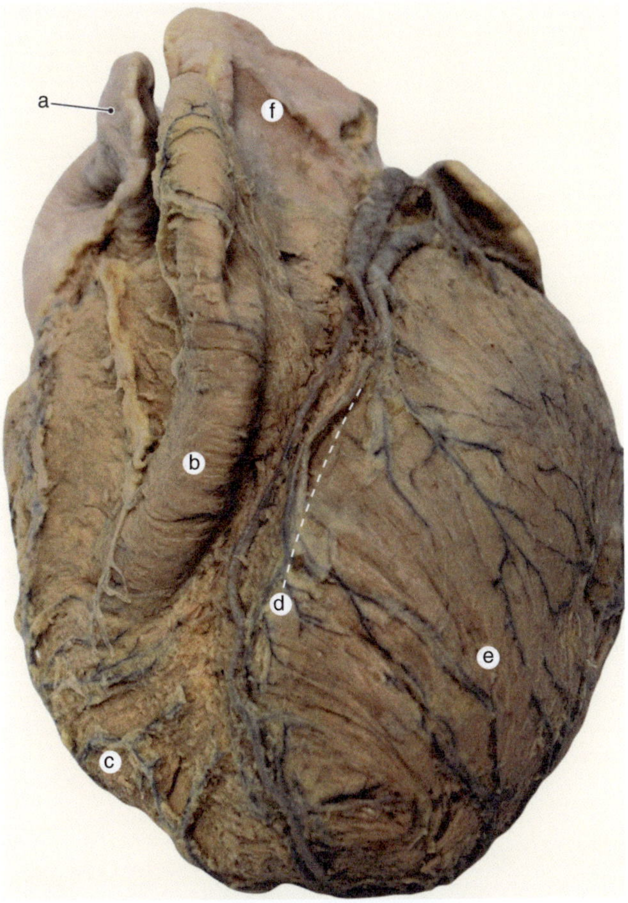

Fig. 4.9 The bulbus cordis from the embryological period kept the individuality of the conal region. The conus projects on the sternocostal surface like a well structured formation. *a* Right auricle, *b* conal region, *c* right ventricle, *d* anterior interventricular groove, *e* left ventricle, *f* pulmonary trunk

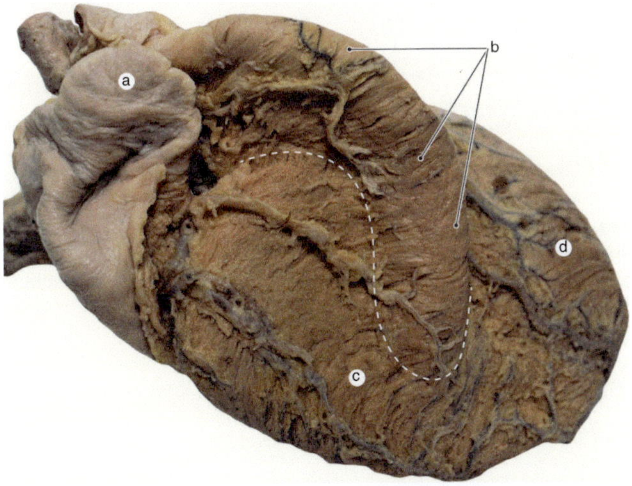

Fig. 4.10 The conus has its own vessels an presents a specific myocardial organization. The dotted line represents the conal limits. *a* Right auricle, *b* former region of the ventricular bulbus, currently the conoinfundibular region, *c* right ventricle, *d* left ventricle

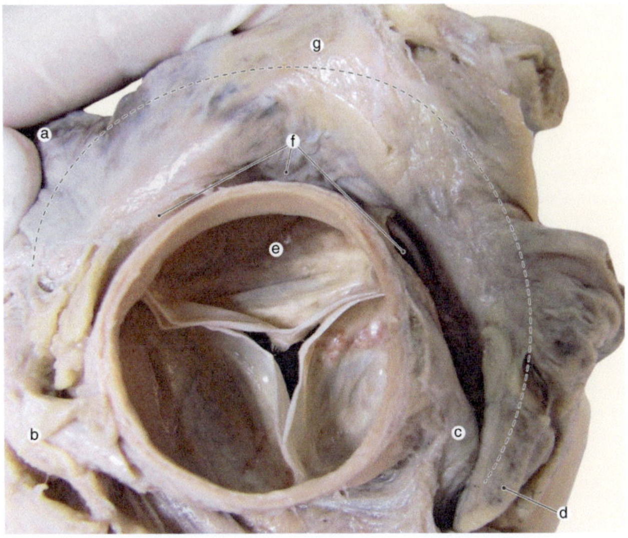

Fig. 4.11 Interatrial notch and corona cordis. *a* Right auricle between examiner's fingers, *b* right coronary artery, *c* left coronary artery, *d* left auricle, *e* aorta, *f* transverse pericardial sinus located behind the aorta, *g*. corona cordis

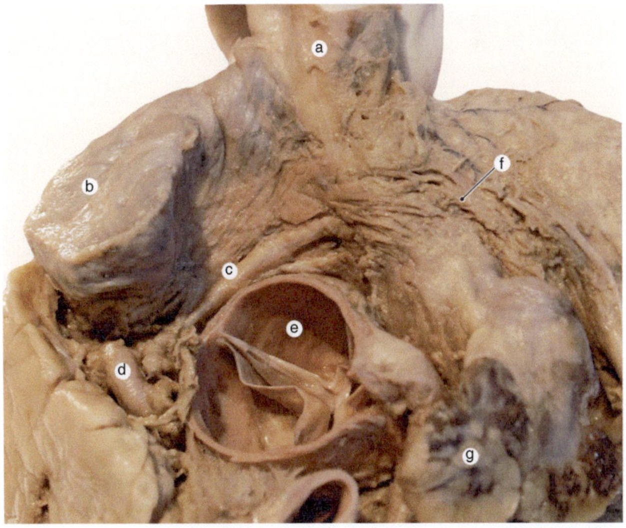

Fig. 4.12 The interatrial notch and a variant of the sinoatrial node artery. *a* Superior vena cava, *b* right auricle, *c* sinoatrial node artery, *d* right coronary, *e* aorta, *f* interatrial fasciculus

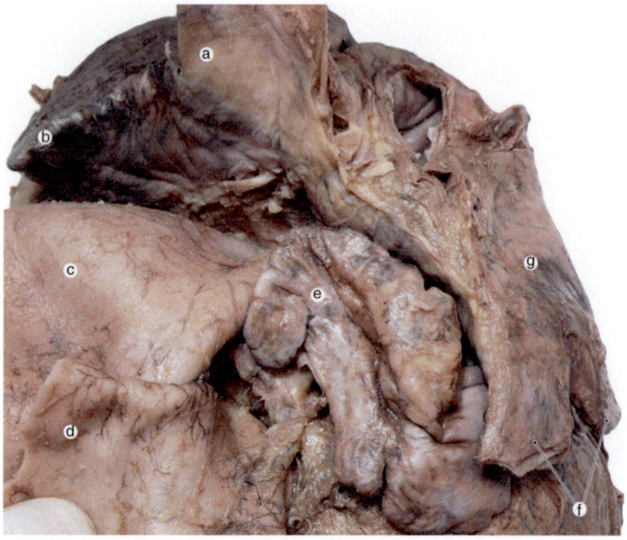

Fig. 4.13 The left auricle is prominent retroaortic. *a* Superior vena cava, *b* right auricle, *c* aorta, *d* pulmonary trunk, *e* left auricle, *f* left pulmonary veins, *g* left atrium

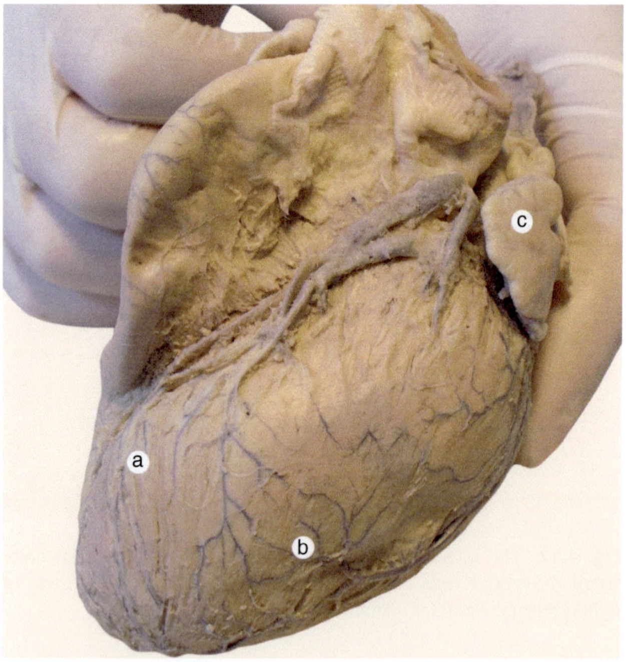

Fig. 4.14 Between the pulmonary and the sternocostal faces there is no precise limit. *a* Sternocostal face left ventricle, *b* pulmonary face left ventricle, *c* left auricle

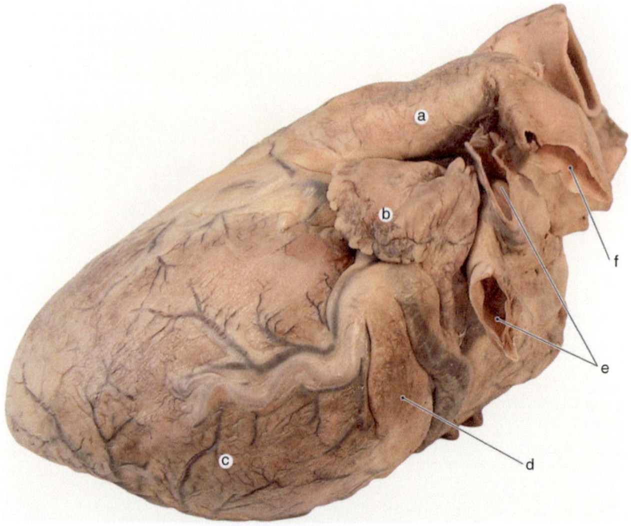

Fig. 4.15 Notice on the pulmonary surface, towards the ventricular base, the existence of an individualized ventricular muscle fasciculus. *a* Pulmonary trunk, *b* left auricle, *c* pulmonary surface of left ventricle, *d* ventricular muscle fasciculus, *e* pulmonary veins, *f* left pulmonary artery

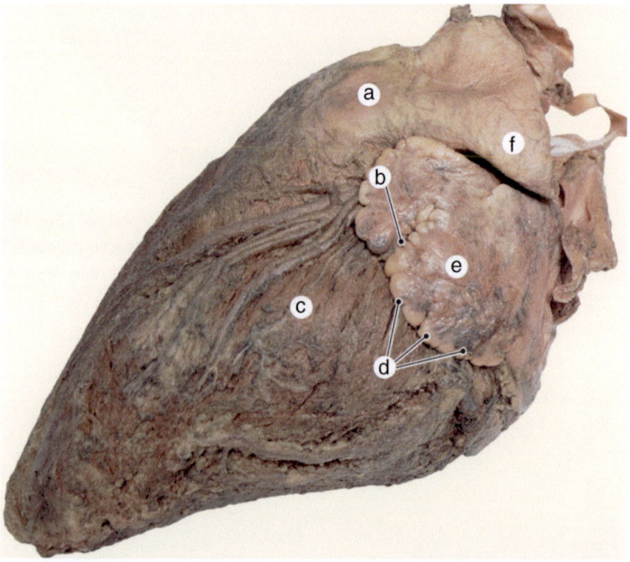

Fig. 4.16 The left auricle has crenelate borders and deep notches that completely separate unequal territories. *a* Pulmonary trunk, *b* auricular notch, *c* pulmonary face left ventricle, *d* crenelate border left auricle, *e* left auricle, *f* left pulmonary artery

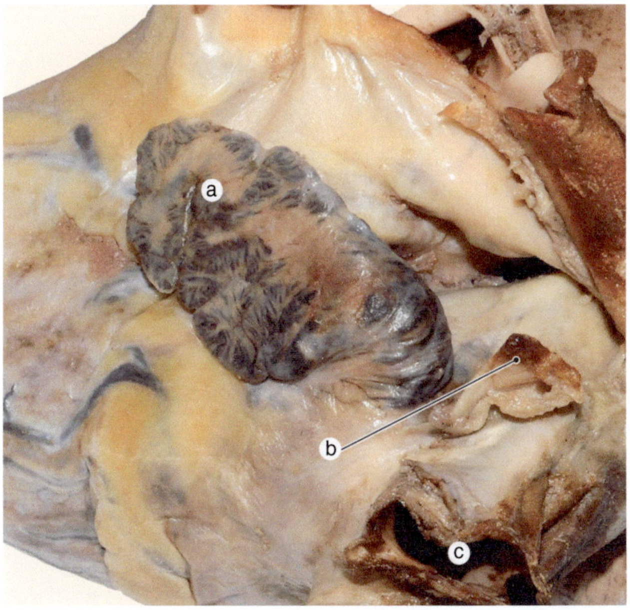

Fig. 4.17 Left auricle with bended finger aspect. *a* Left auricle, *b* triangular ligament of Marshall, *c* left pulmonary veins

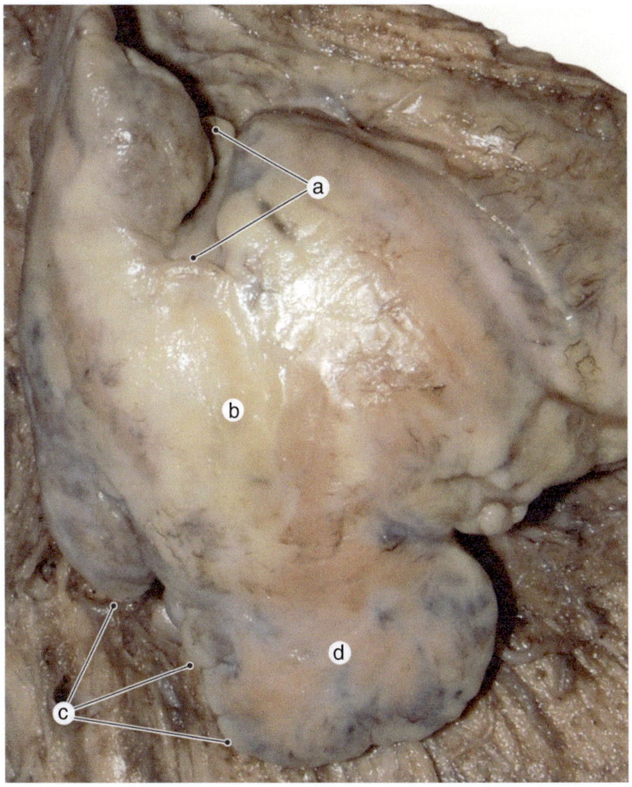

Fig. 4.18 Left auricle with well individualised lobules and the tip oriented posteriorly. *a* Notch, *b* left auricle, *c* crenelate border left auricle, *d* lobule

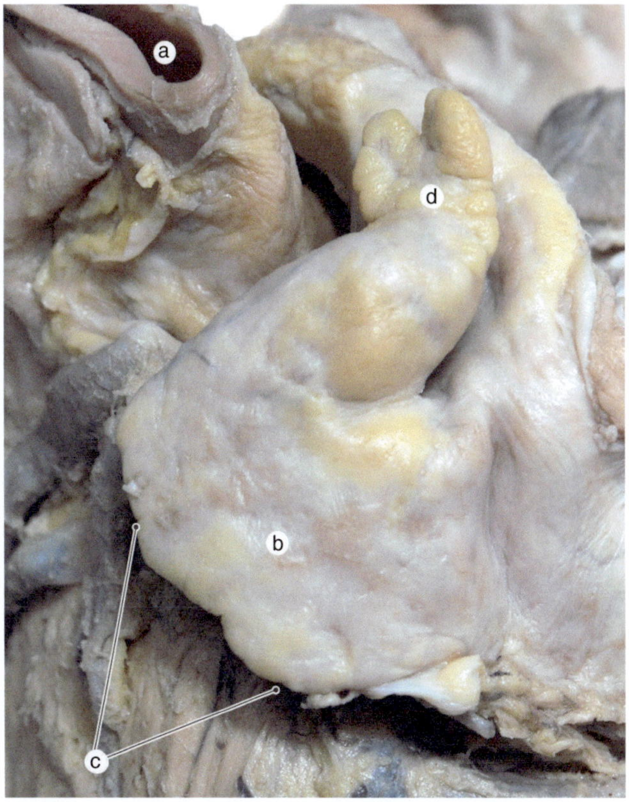

Fig. 4.19 Left auricle with bifid apex. *a* Aorta, *b* left auricle, *c* crenelate border of left auricle, *d* bifid apex oriented posteriorly

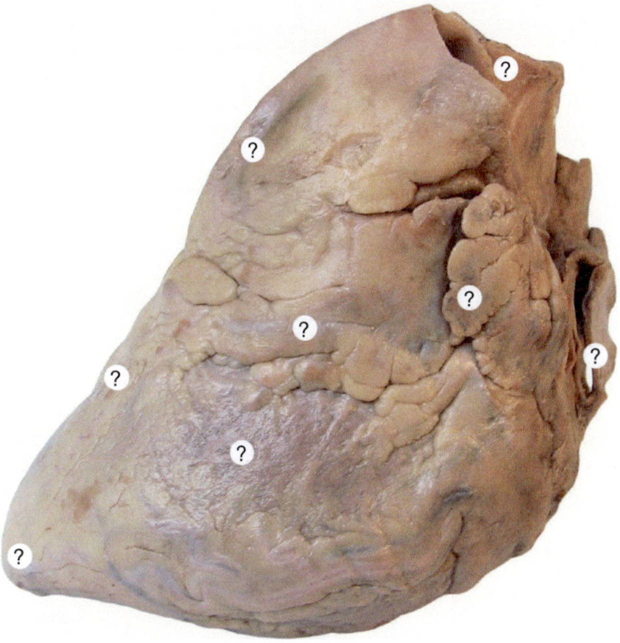

Fig. 4.20 Undissected heart. Plese identify the structers on the pulmonary surface (same as the Fig. 4.21)

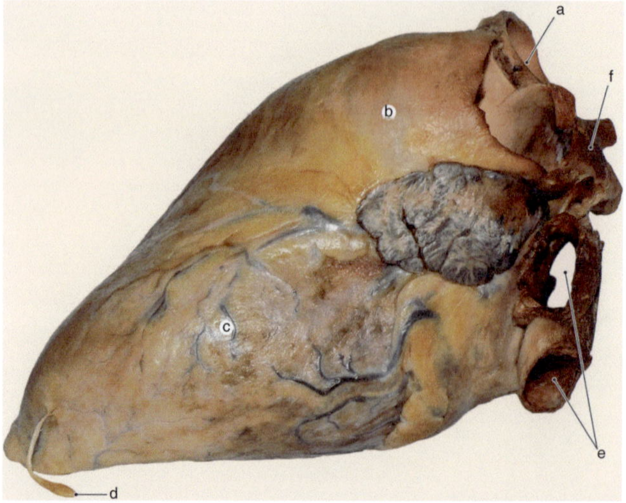

Fig. 4.21 Notice an epicardiac appendix on the pulmonary face, like the epiploic appendices of the colon. *a* Aorta, *b* trunk of pulmonary artery, *c* left ventricle, *d* epicardiac appendix, *e* left pulmonary veins, *f* right pulmonary artery

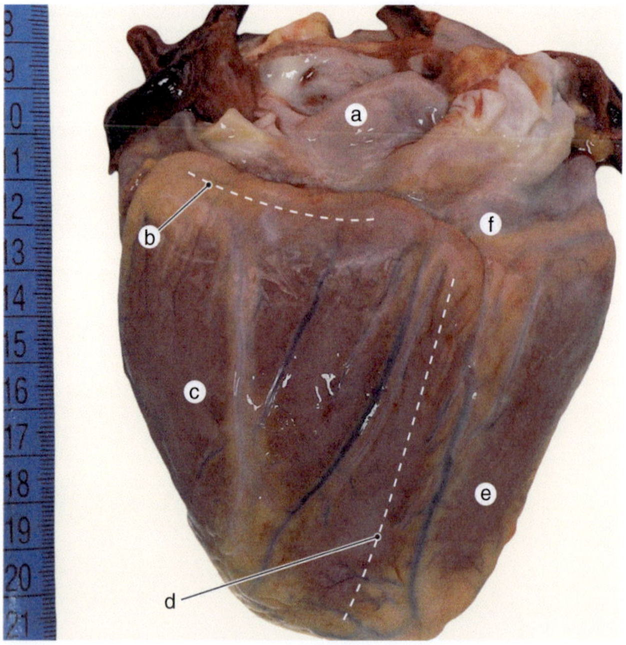

Fig. 4.22 Non-formaldehyded heart. Diaphragmatic face. *a* Left atrium, *b* left coronary groove, *c* left ventricle, *d* posterior interventricular groove, *e* right ventricle, *f* crux cordis

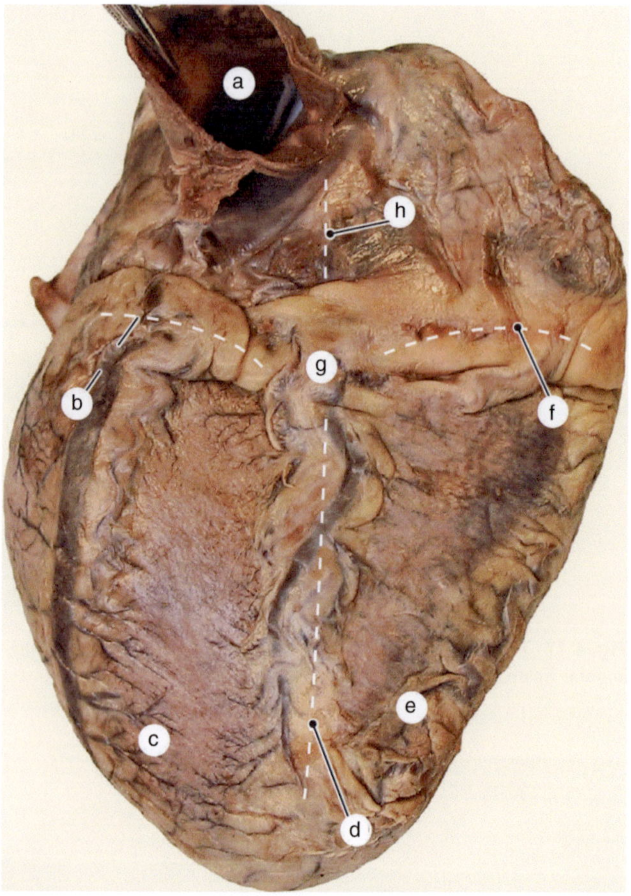

Fig. 4.23 Diaphragmatic face. The projection of the cavotricuspidian isthmus is extended. *a* Inferior vena cava, *b* left coronary groove, *c* left ventricle, *d* posterior interventricular groove, *e* right ventricle, *f* right coronary groove, *g* crux cordis, *h* the projection of the cavotricuspidian isthmus

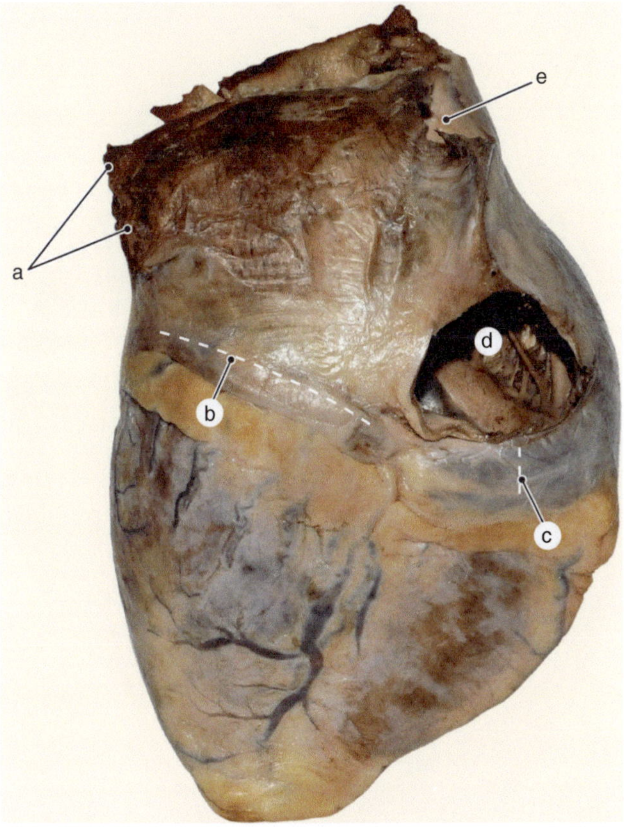

Fig. 4.24 Diaphragmatic face. The projection of the cavotricuspidian isthmus is small. *a* Left pulmonary veins, *b* coronary sinus, *c* projection of the cavotricuspidian isthmus, *d* inferior vena cava, *e* right pulmonary veins

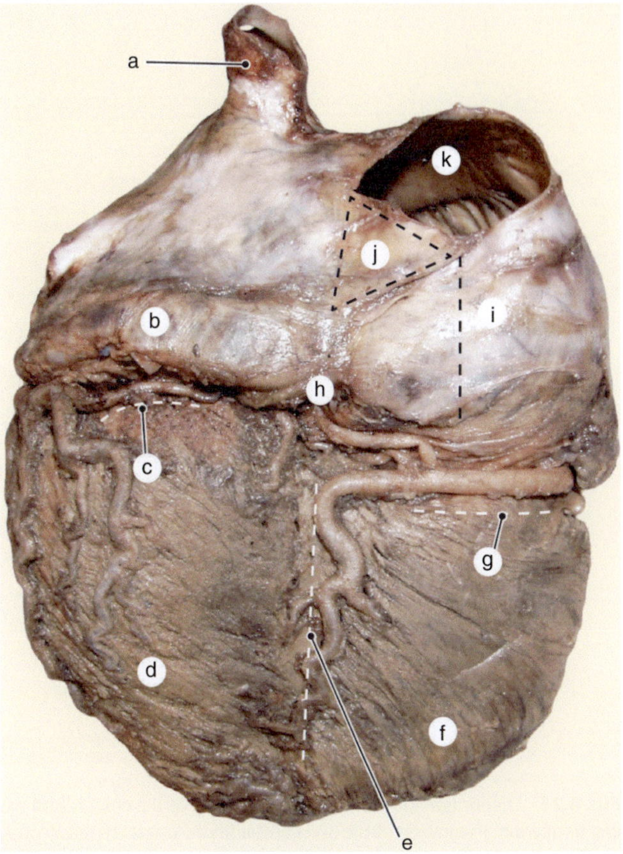

Fig. 4.25 The cross of the heart is represented by the intersection of the coronary groove with the posterior interventricular groove. *a* Inferior right pulmonary vein, *b* coronary venous sinus, *c* left coronary groove, *d* left ventricle, *e* posterior interventricular groove, *f* right ventricle, *g* right coronary groove, *h* crux cordis, *i* projection of the cavotricuspidian isthmus, *j* projection of the dorsosinusal space, *k* inferior vena cava

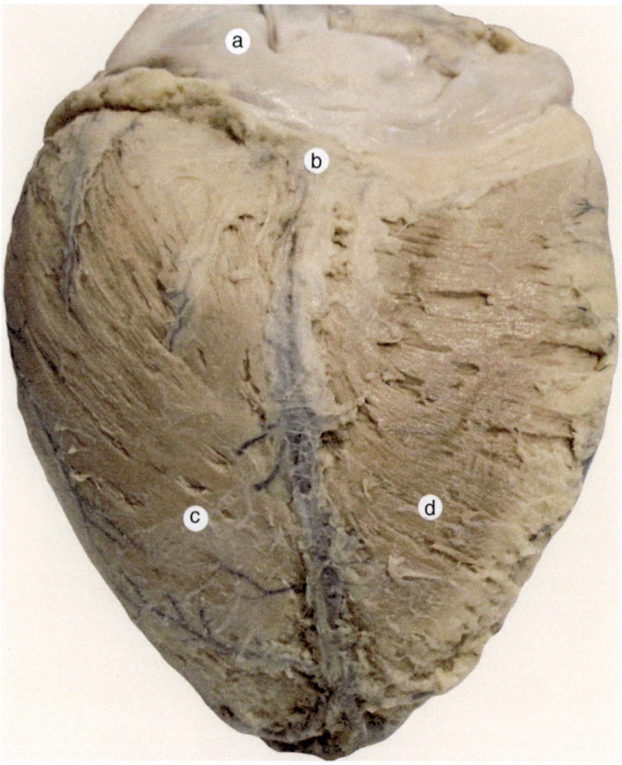

Fig. 4.26 Diaphragmatic face. After the removal of the epicardium we can notice the orientation of the myocardial fibers. *a* left atrium, *b* crux cordis, *c* left ventricle, *d* right ventricle

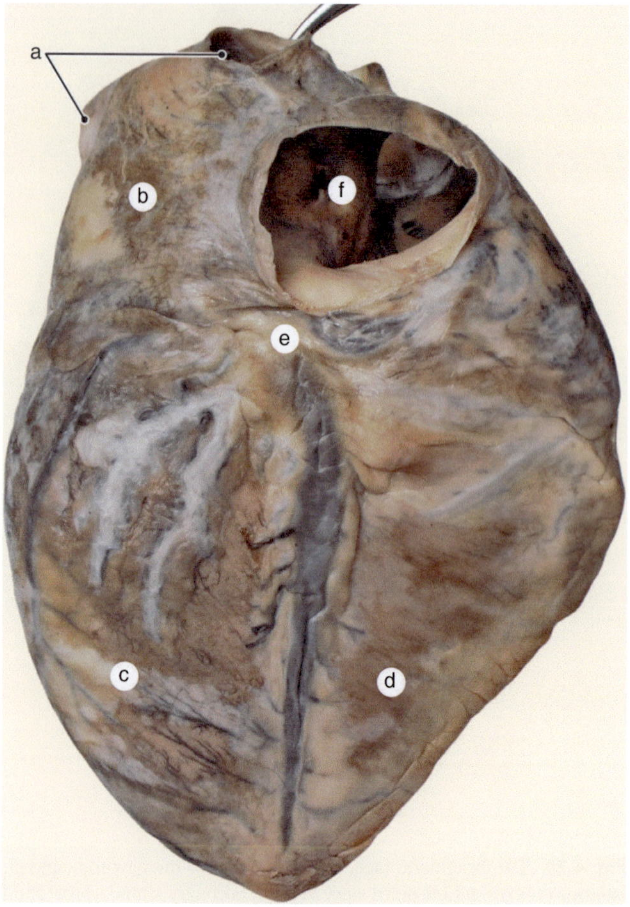

Fig. 4.27 The fatty tissue lies around the blood vessels on the diaphragmatic face also. *a* Pulmonary veins, *b* left atrium, *c* left ventricle, *d* right ventricle, *e* crux cordis, *f* inferior vena cava

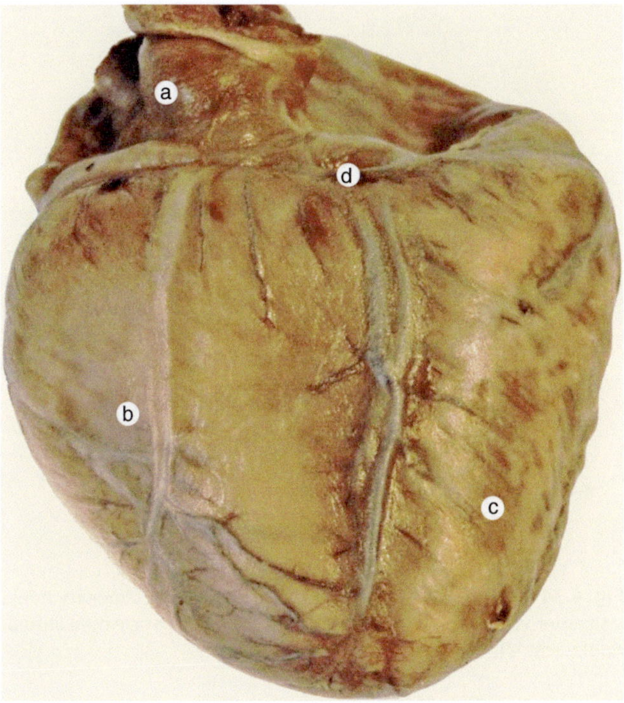

Fig. 4.28 At the 7 month heart there is no fatty deposit on the diaphragmatic face. *a* Left atrium, *b* left ventricle, *c* right ventricle, *d* crux cordis

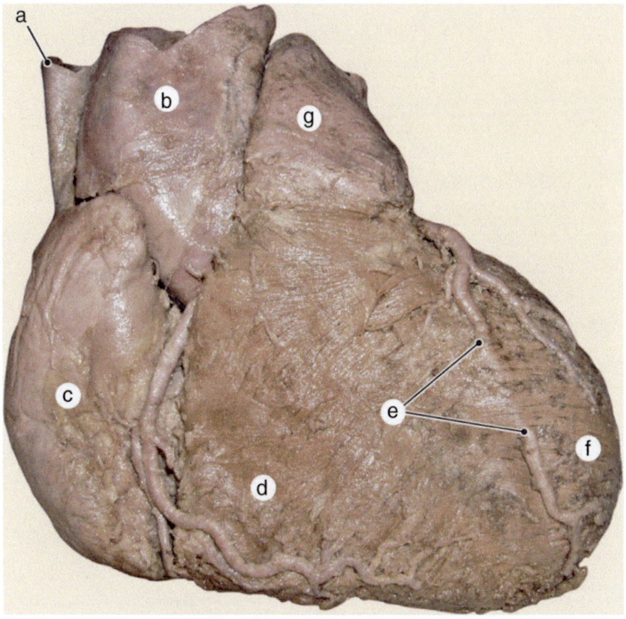

Fig. 4.30 Right auricle with a blunt tip and a broad base. *a* Superior vena cava, *b* ascending aorta, *c* the right atrium with its auricle, *d* right ventricle, *e* myocardial bridge, *f* left ventricle, *g* pulmonary trunk

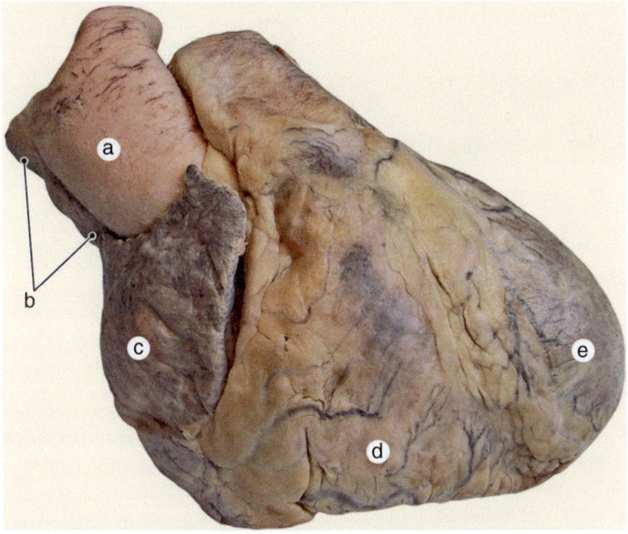

Fig. 4.29 The notion of right border generally refers to the ventricle. It obviously interests the right atrium also. *a* Ascending aorta, *b* superior vena cava, *c* right atrium, *d* right ventricle, *e* left ventricle

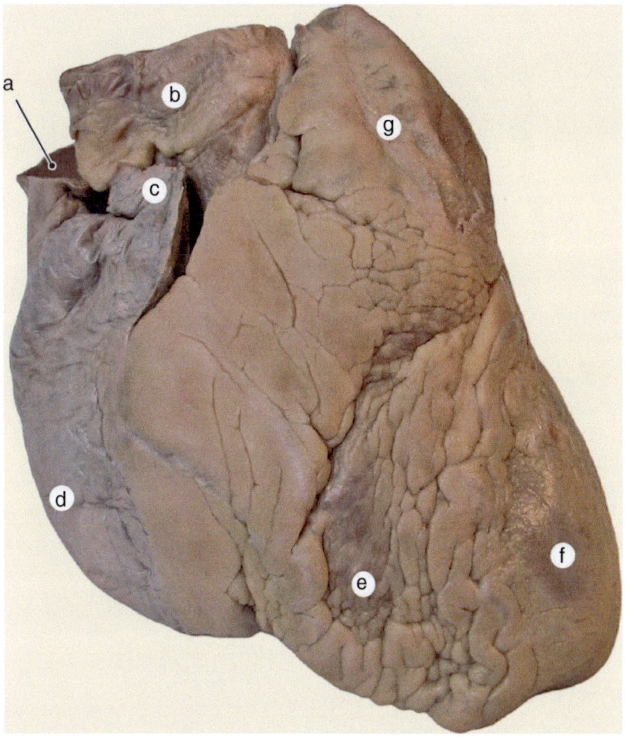

Fig. 4.31 Right auricle with the tip curved posteriorly. *a* Superior vena cava, *b* ascending aorta, *c* right auricle, *d* right atrium, *e* right ventricle, *f* left ventricle, *g* pulmonary trunk

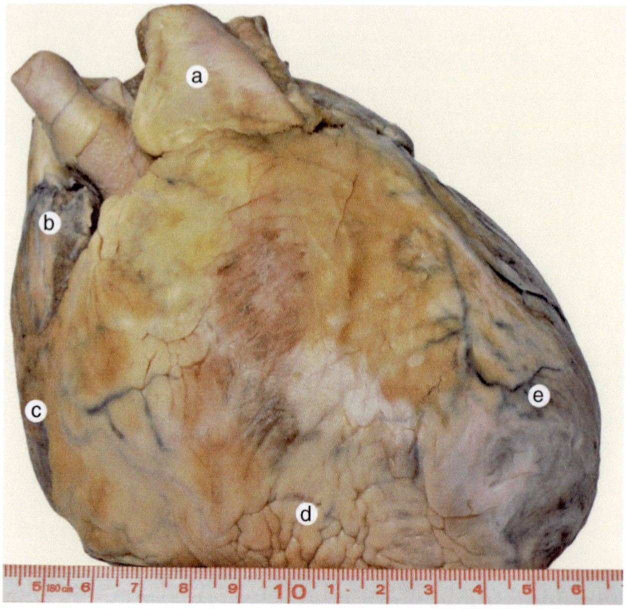

Fig. 4.32 Length of the right border. *a* Pulmonary trunk, *b* right auricle, *c* right atrium, *d* right ventricle, *e* left ventricle

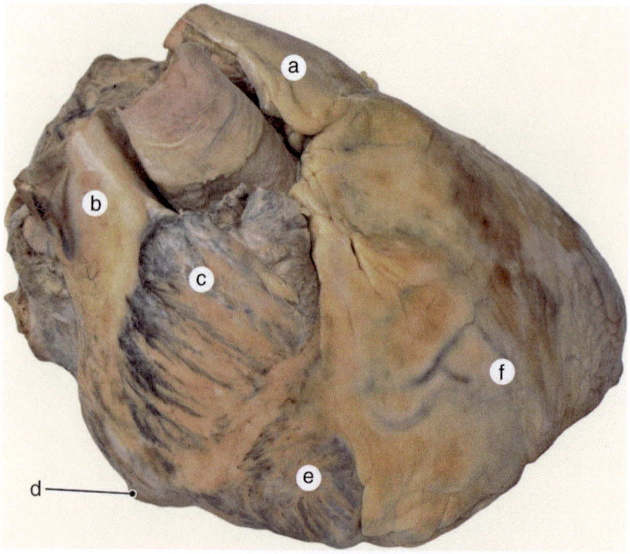

Fig. 4.34 The classical aspect of the right auricle. *a* Pulmonary trunk, *b* superior vena cava, *c* right auricle, *d* Inferior vena cava, *e* right atrium, *f* right ventricle

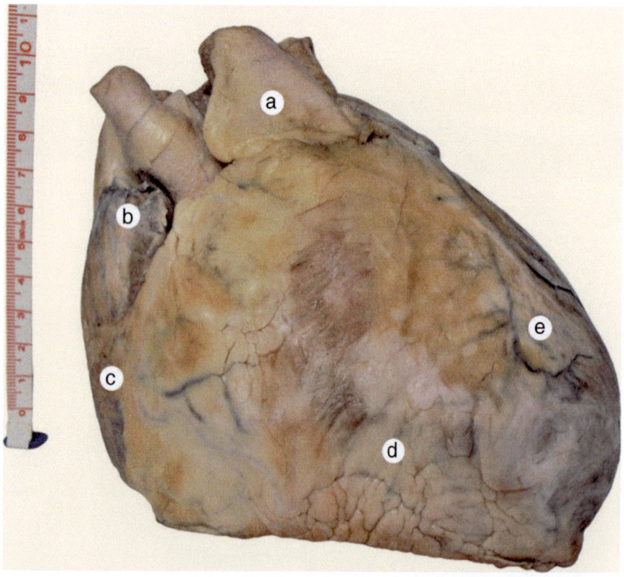

Fig. 4.33 The hight of the heart at the base. *a* Pulmonary trunk, *b* right auricle, *c* right atrium, *d* right ventricle, *e* left ventricle

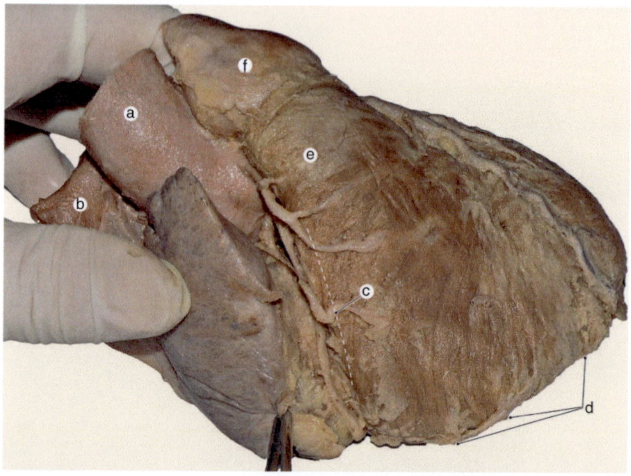

Fig. 4.35 The right coronary groove intersects the acute border. *a* Aorta, *b* superior vena cava, *c* right coronary groove, *d* acute border, *e* infundibulum, *f* trunk of the pulmonary artery

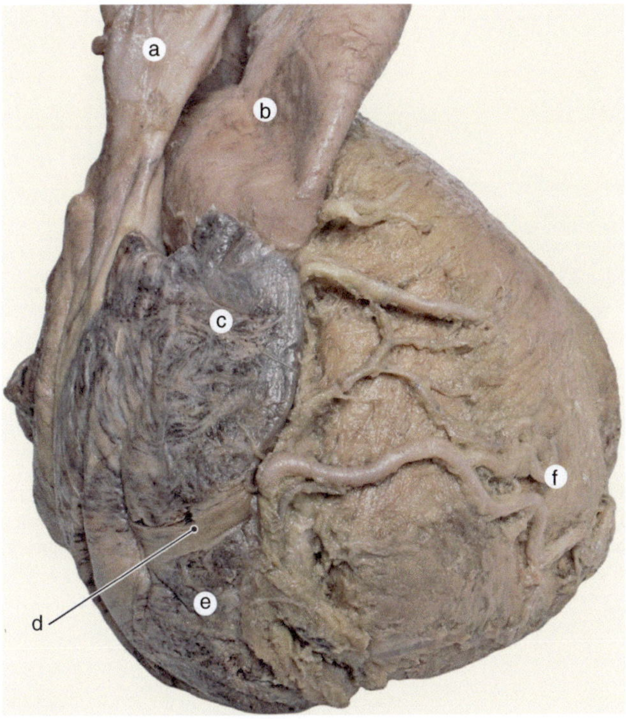

Fig. 4.36 Right auricle with blunt tip. *a* Superior vena cava, *b* ascending aorta, *c* right auricle, *d* subepicardial muscle fasciculus, *e* right atrium, *f* right ventricle

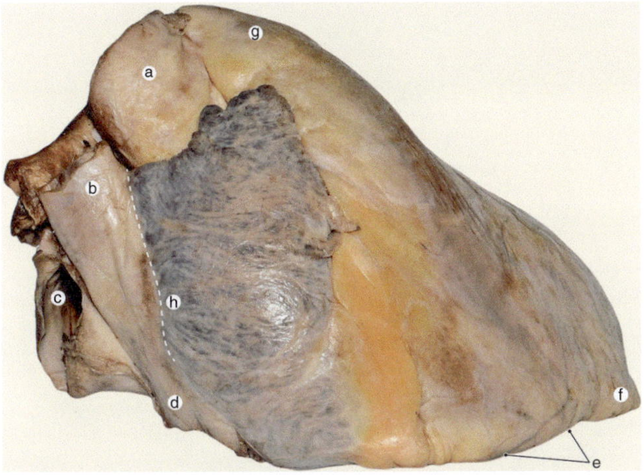

Fig. 4.37 Very well-defined right border and enhanced throughout its length, from the inferior vena cava towards the tip. *a* Aorta, *b* superior vena cava, *c* right pulmonary veins, *d* inferior vena cava, *e* right border, *f* apex, *g* trunk of the pulmonary artery, *h* terminal groove (*dotted*)

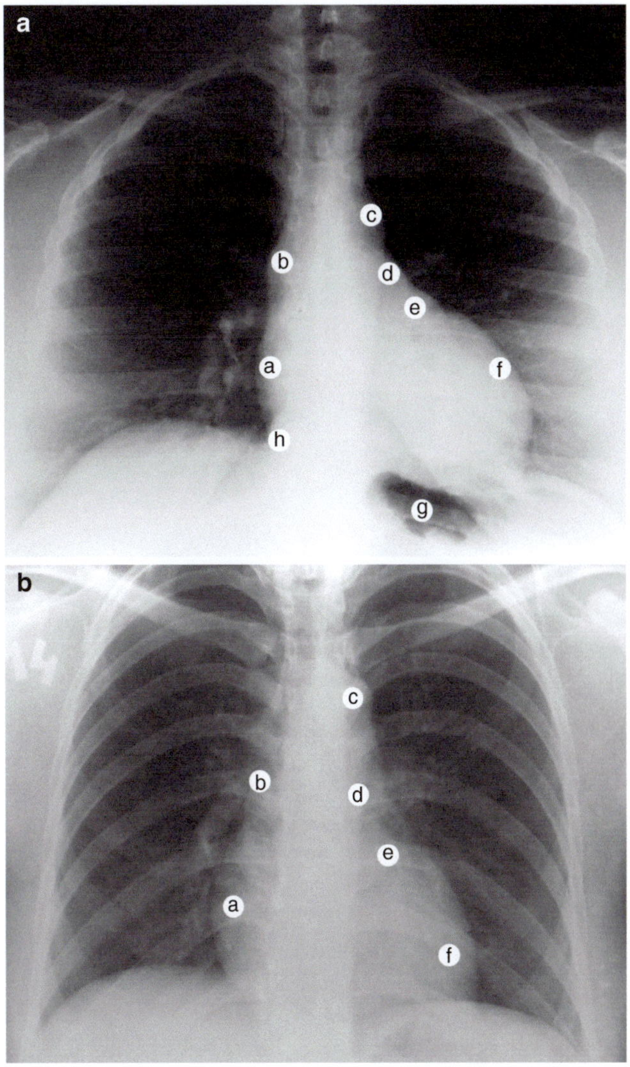

Fig. 4.38 (**a**) Thoracic X-Ray. The parts of the heart that form the contours of the heart on the right and left side are highlighted. *a* Right atrium, *b* superior vena cava, *c* the aortic knob, *d* left pulmonary artery, *e* left auricle, *f* left ventricle, *g* the airchamber of the stomach, *h* inferior vena cava. (**b**) Thoracic X-Ray. The parts of the heart that form the contours of the heart on the right and left side are highlighted. *a* Right atrium, *b* superior vena cava, *c* the aortic knob, *d* left pulmonary artery, *e* Left auricle, *f* left ventricle

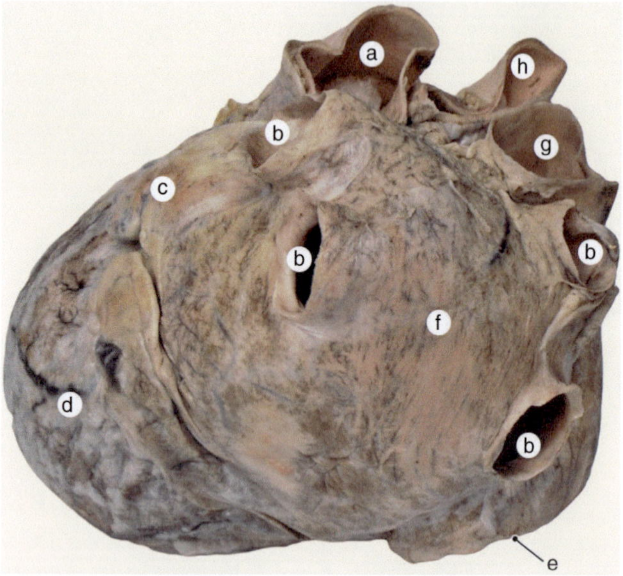

Fig. 4.39 Left-posterior view of the base of the heart. The area between the pulmonary veins (the interveno-pulmonary space) is not primitive atrium but pulmonary primitive vein inserted in the atrial wall and later covered by miocardium. The left pulmonary veins are located slightly superior than the right ones. *a* Pulmonary trunk, *b* pulmonary veins, *c* left auricle, *d* left ventricle, *e* inferior vena cava, *f* left atrium – interpulmonary segment, *g* superior vena cava, *h* aorta

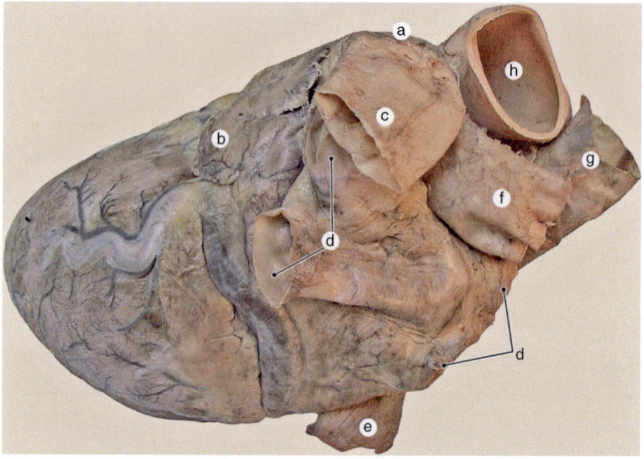

Fig. 4.41 The great vessels at the base of the heart. *a* Posterior view from the left side. Pulmonary trunk, *b* left auricle, *c* left pulmonary artery, *d* pulmonary veins, *e* inferior vena cava, *f* right pulmonary artery, *g* superior vena cava, *h* aorta

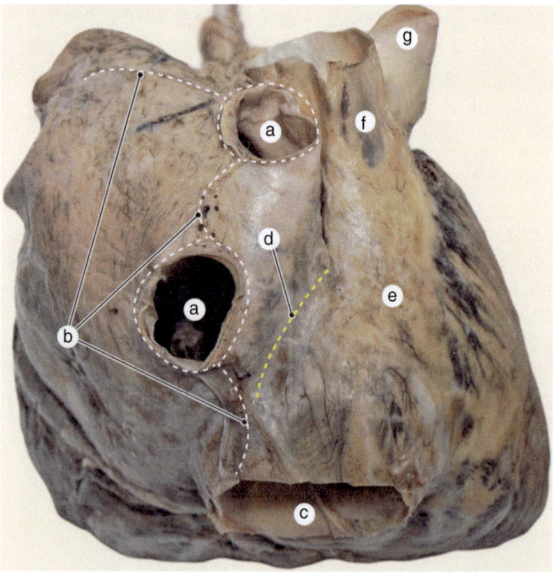

Fig. 4.40 Right-posterior view of the base of the heart. *a* Right pulmonary veins, *b* reflection line of the pericardium, *c* inferior vena cava, *d* interatrial groove, *e* right atrium – intercaval segment, *f* superior vena cava, *g* aorta

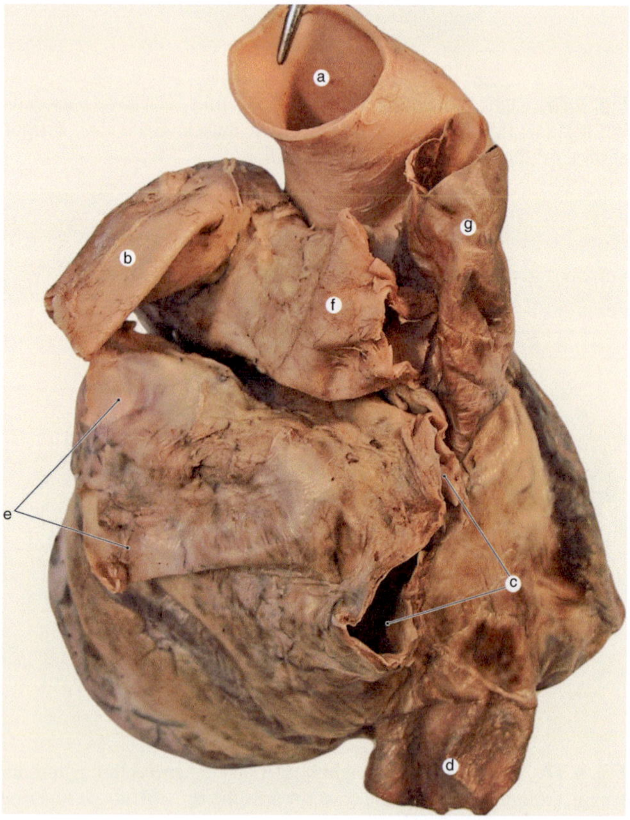

Fig. 4.42 The great vessels at the base of the heart. Posterior view from the right side. The intercaval space derives from the incorporation of the right horn of the sinus venosus within the atrial wall. Subepicardic fatty tissue lies within its area. It is not usually covered by muscle or it may have a few muscular fascicles structured in the intercaval muscular fascicle (see the atrial miocardium). *a* Aorta, *b* left pulmonary artery, *c* right pulmonary veins, *d* inferior vena cava, *e* left pulmonary veins, *f* right pulmonary artery, *g* superior vena cava

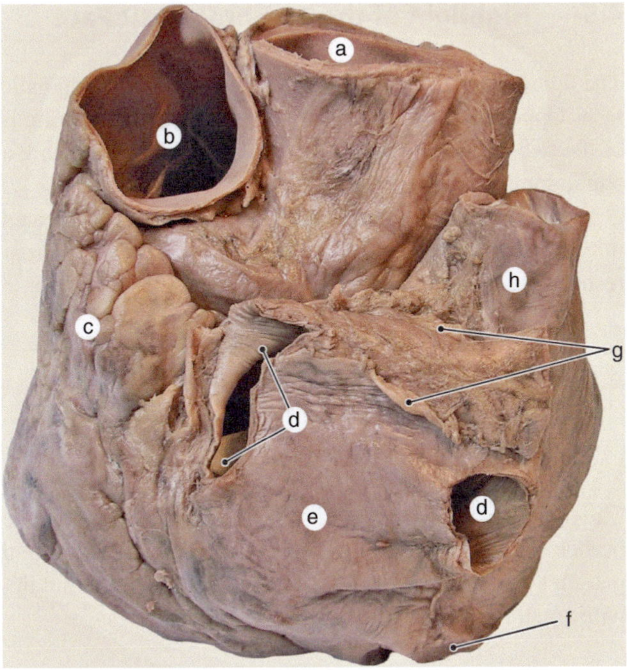

Fig. 4.43 The reflexion line of the parietal pericardium in the visceral pericardium. *a* Aorta, *b* pulmonary trunk, *c* left auricle, *d* pulmonary veins, *e* left atrium – interpulmonary segment, *f* inferior vena cava, *g* pericardium reflexion line, *h* superior vena cava

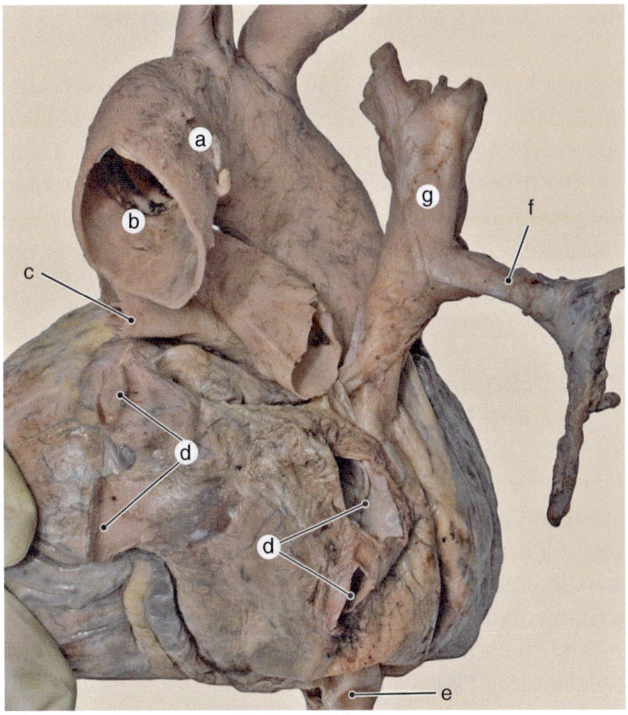

Fig. 4.45 View of the structures at the base of the heart. *a* Bronchial arteries, *b* aorta, *c* left pulmonary artery, *d* pulmonary veins, *e* inferior vena cava, *f* arch of the azygos vein, *g* superior vena cava

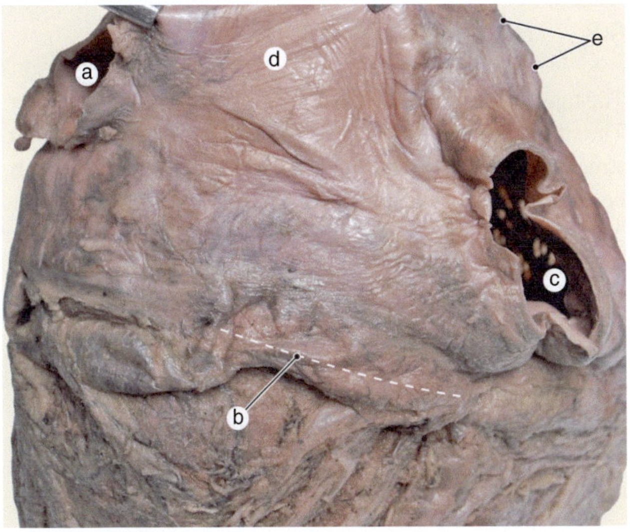

Fig. 4.44 The interveno-pulmonary space and its relation with the coronary venous sinus. *a* Left pulmonary veins, *b* coronary venous sinus, *c* inferior vena cava, *d* intervenous-pulmonary atrial segment, *e* right pulmonary veins

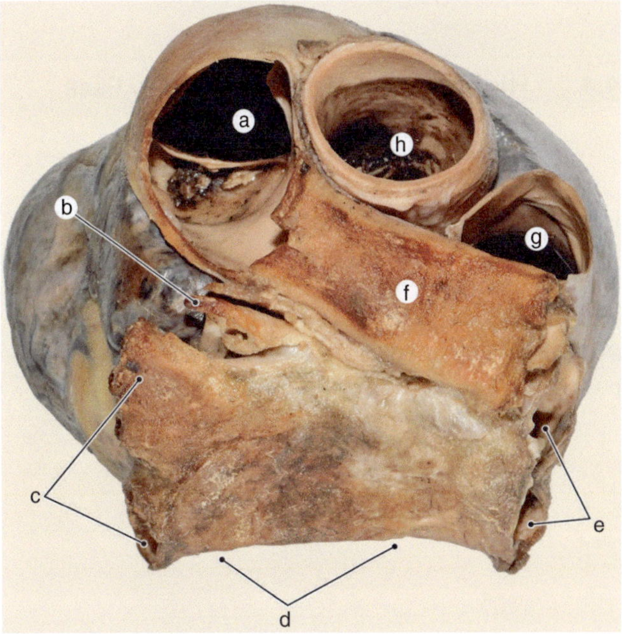

Fig. 4.46 The relation between the pulmonary arteries and veins. *a* Pulmonary trunk, *b* Marshall triangular ligament, *c* left pulmonary veins, *d* intervenous-pulmonary segment, *e* right pulmonary veins, *f* right pulmonary artery, *g* superior vena cava, *h* aorta

4.2 Views of the Sternocostal Surface

Figures between 4.2 and 4.10 are views of the sternocostal surface of hearts of different age and different clinical situations. As shown, individual variability is very large, starting from the way in which the fat deposits and reaching the proportions of different segments, the appearance and distribution of vessels, the general shape, the depth of the grooves, etc..

4.3 Highlighting the Interatrial Notch and the Corona Cordis

Figures between 4.11 and 4.13 exemplify the interatrial notch and promote understanding of the concept of corona cordis. Recall that the notch is formed from interatrial aortic wall protrusion towards the primitive atrium and towards the territory of the superior endocardic cushion.

The interatrial notch is generally concave in aspect and is determined by the anterior wall of the two atria, centered by the base of the interatrial septum and related with the aorta.

Correspondent to it, sometimes there is a small fibrous fold on the midline connecting the aorta with the atria. Between arterial pedicle and the notch is delimited the transverse pericardial sinus.

4.4 Highlighting of the Pulmonary Face and the Identification Pattern of the Left Auricle

Figures between 4.14 and 4.21 present the pulmonary face.

For the left auricle, the identification pattern consists of crenelate borders, notches that limit auricular lobules, auricular tip with bended finger aspect, oriented anteriorly or posteriorly to the arterial pedicle.

4.5 Highlight of the Diaphragmatic Face

The figures between 4.22 and 4.28 present the diaphragmatic face. Opposing to the classical statements, the distributions of the two ventricles on this face are relatively equal, with a slight dominance of the left ventricle.

Attention! The diaphragmatic face of the heart is located inferiorly and not posteriorly. The diaphragmatic face is represented mainly by the ventricles.

4.6 Highlight of the Right (Acute) Border of the Heart and of the Identification Pattern for the Right Auricle

The figures between 4.29 and 4.37 present the right or acute border of the heart. For the right auricle, the identification pattern assumes the existence of a broad base and a blunt tip, with small bulges.

4.7 Highlight of the Radiological Contours of the Heart on a Postero-anterior X-Ray (Fig. 4.38)

4.8 Highlight of the Base of the Heart

The figures between 4.39 and 4.46 present the base of the heart. The structures located here are easily compressible by extrinsic structures and a lot less mobile than the rest of the heart, because they are connected to the great vessels. The relations between them and the extracardiac structures are very close.

5 Boundaries of the Heart

All boundaries of the heart are mediated by the fibrous pericardium. In Figs. 5.1, 5.2, 5.3, 5.4, 5.6, 5.7 and 5.22, different aspects of the rapports between the heart and pericardium are revealed.

5.1 The Border with the Sternocostal Surface

This face is partially covered by the right and left costomediastinal recesses of the pleura. The anterior margins of the recesses are partially overlapped and they outline the thymic and cardiac triangles (Figs. 5.6, 5.7 and 5.8).

Keep in mind!
Any instrumental access to the heart on its sternocostal surface must avoid puncturing the pleural recesses and opening of the pleural cavities.

5.1.1 Highlighting the Internal Thoracic Arteries

On the posterior face of the anterior thoracic wall, one centimeter from the sternum, the internal thoracic arteries descend (Fig. 5.9).

Keep in mind!
To avoid perforating the left internal thoracic artery during cardiac punctures, the needle must be perpendicular to the thoracic wall and tangent on the sternum in the interspace between the fifth and sixth ribs.

Internal thoracic arteries are frequently utilized in coronary surgery. We consider that a minimum knowledge of the anatomy of these arteries is necessary.

The right internal thoracic artery is the first branch on the inferior face of the right subclavian artery. It descends in the thorax passing behind the brachiocephalic vein and intersects the right phrenic nerve under the clavicle. In its upper third it divides into the pericardiacophrenic and mediastinal branches. In the intercostal spaces it divides into the anterior intercostal and sternal branches (Figs. 5.10 and 5.11).

Both internal thoracic arteries end with a musculophrenic artery for the diaphragm and a superior epigastric artery. The latter perforates the rectus sheath and anastomoses in the rectus abdominis muscle with branches of the inferior epigastric artery (branch of the external iliac artery). This

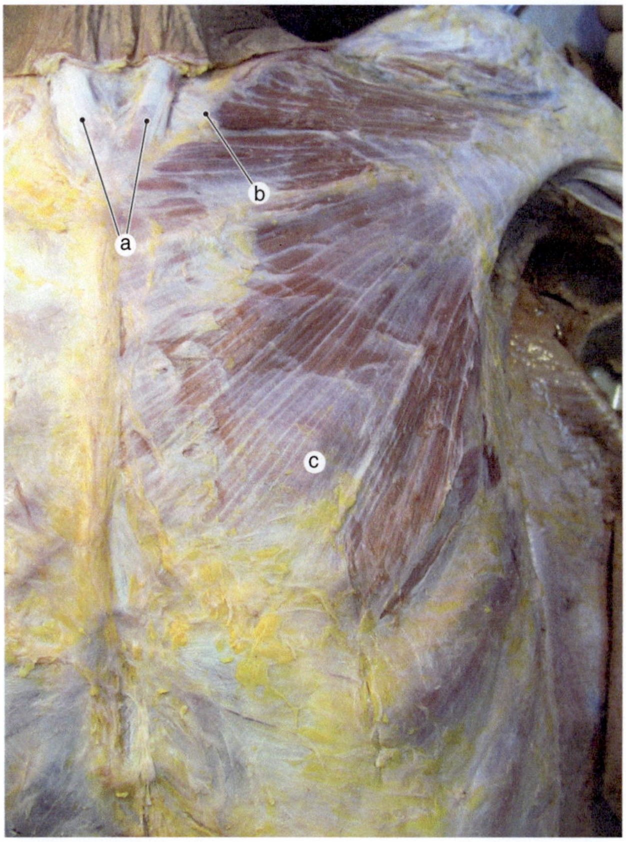

Fig. 5.1 Aspect of thoracic wall after removal of tegument. In the intercostal spaces, the thoracic wall is thin and can be easily perforated. *a* Insertion of the sternocleidomastoid muscles in the sternal notch, *b* clavicle, *c* pectoralis major muscle

F.M. Filipoiu, *Atlas of Heart Anatomy and Development*,
DOI 10.1007/978-1-4471-5382-5_5, © Springer-Verlag London 2014

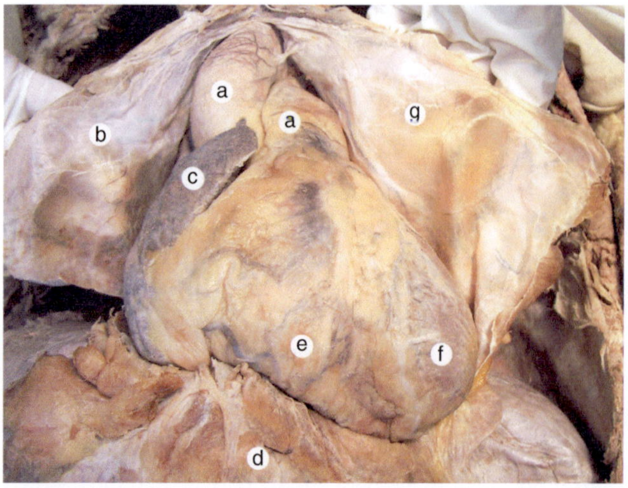

Fig. 5.2 The pericardium has been sectioned and removed. Observe its location in relation to the greater vessels. *a* Arterial pedicle, *b* fibrous pericardium, *c* right auricle, *d* diaphragm, *e* right ventricle, *f* left ventricle, *g* fibrous pericardium

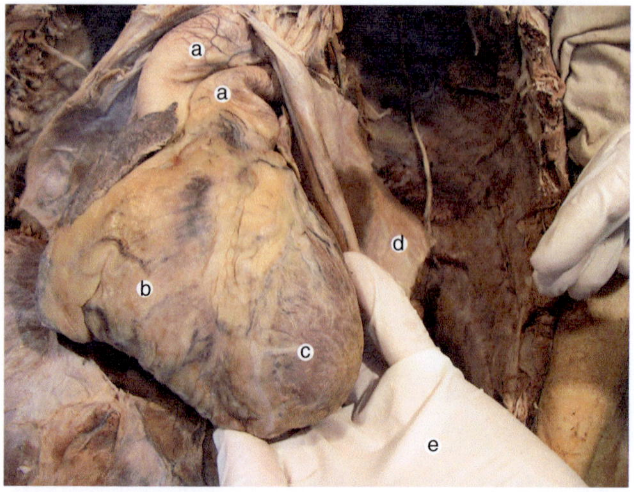

Fig. 5.4 Examiner's hand is introduced in the oblique pericardial sinus. *a* Arterial pedicle, *b* right ventricle, *c* left ventricle, *d* fibrous pericardium, *e* examiner's finger into oblique pericardial sinus

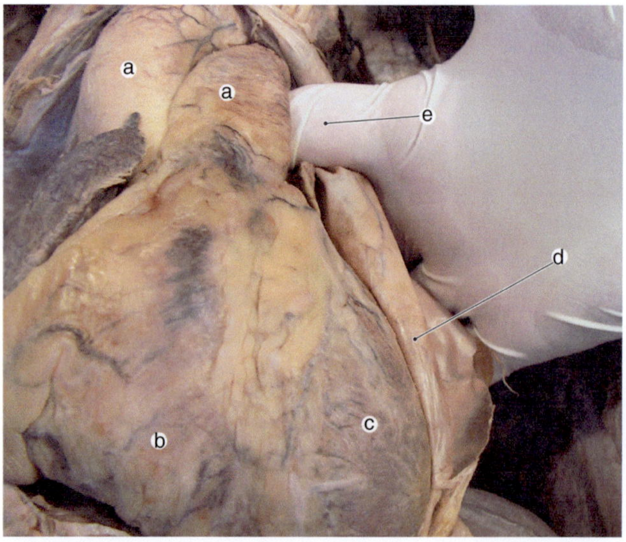

Fig. 5.3 Examiner's finger is introduced behind the arterial pedicle, in the transverse pericardial sinus. *a* Arterial pedicle, *b* right ventricle, *c* left ventricle, *d* fibrous pericardium, *e* examiner's finger into transverse pericardial sinus

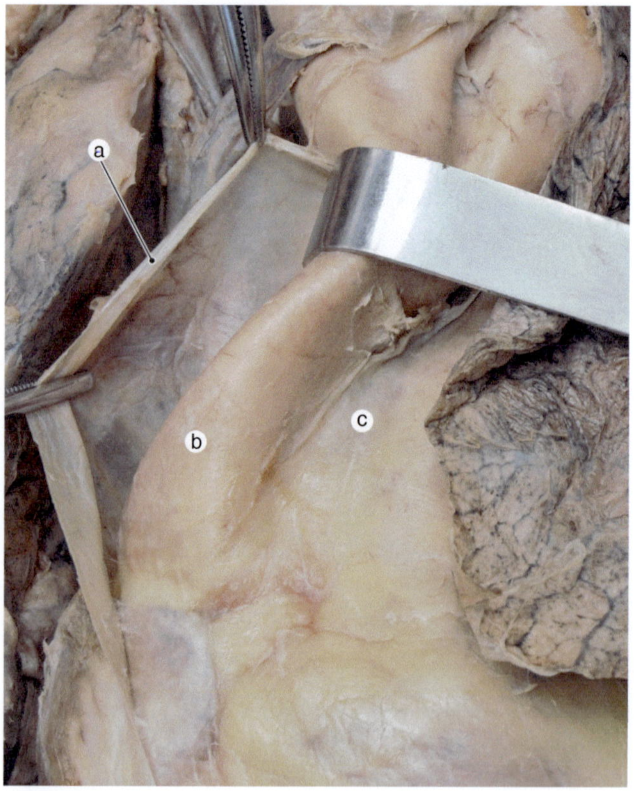

Fig. 5.5 Line of fusion of pericardium to aorta. *a* Fibrous pericardium ascends on the arterial pedicle to reach the origin of the brachiocephalic trunk, *b* aorta, *c* arterial pedicle

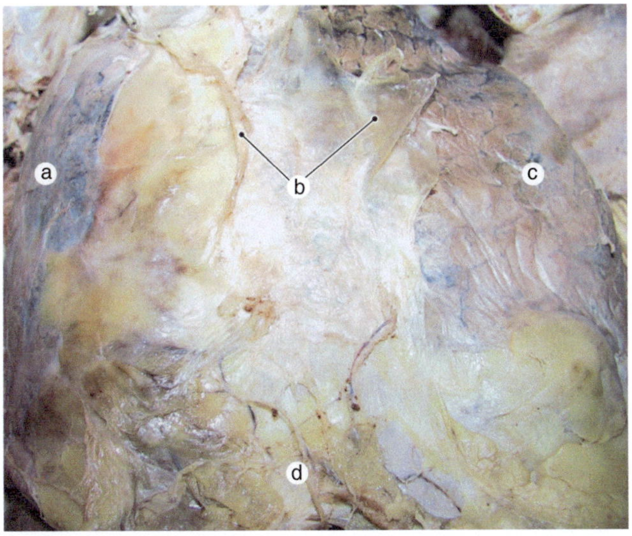

Fig. 5.6 Aspect of thoracic organs after removal of the rib cage. Remark the difficulty in the indentification of the pulmonary and cardiac limits. *a* Right lung, *b* sectioned parietal pleurae, *c* left lung, *d* adipose tissue and retrosternal vascular network

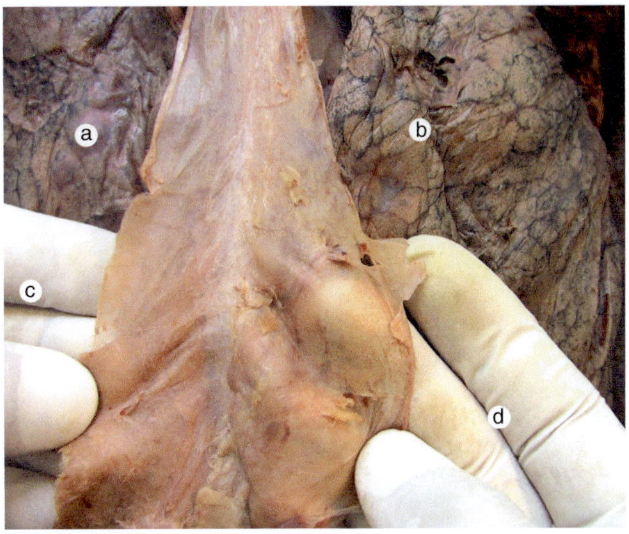

Fig. 5.8 Examiner's fingers are introduced in the costomediastinal pleural recesses. The recesses are strengthened with loose connective tissue that, sometimes, can be hardly dissected. *a* Right lung, *b* left lung, *c* examiner's fingers into right costomediastinal recess, *d* examiner's fingers into left costomediastinal recess

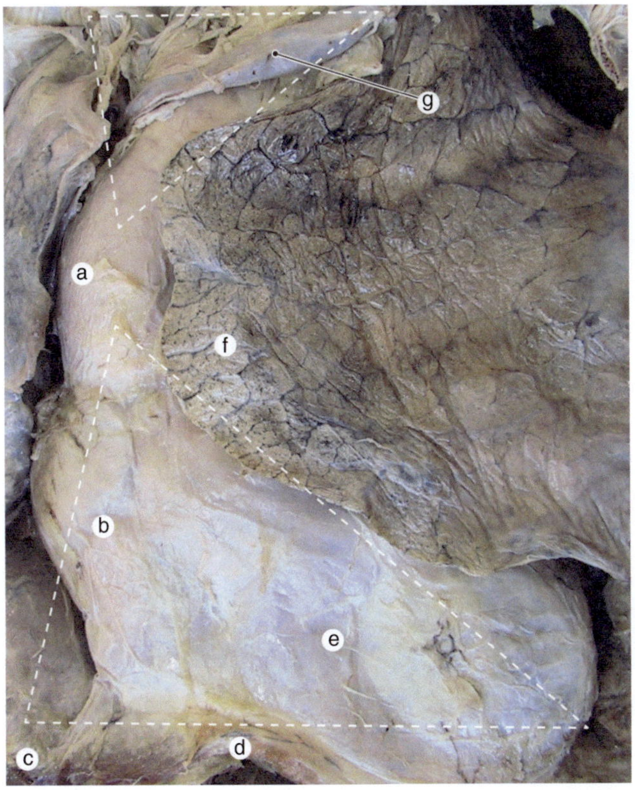

Fig. 5.7 Pulmonary borders outline better the thymic trigon (superior) and cardiac trigon (inferior). *a* Ascending aorta, *b* right atrium, *c* inferior vena cava, *d* diaphragm, *e* heart in pericardial sac, *f* lingula, *g* left innominate vein

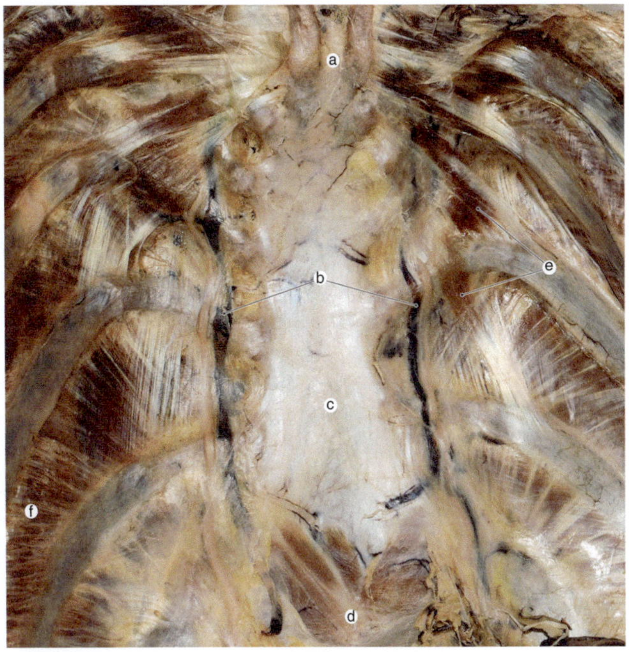

Fig. 5.9 Thoracic cage opened in the superior part. The internal thoracic vessels can be observed on both sides of the sternum. *a* Xiphoid process of sternum, *b* internal thoracic artery and veins, *c* body of sternum, *d* sternohyoid muscle, *e* transversus thoracic muscle, *f* internal intercostal muscle

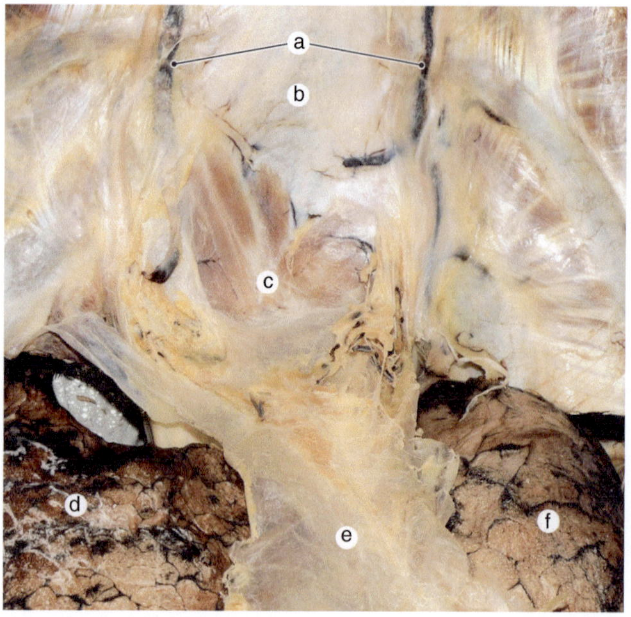

Fig. 5.10 Detail at the entrance of the internal thoracic arteries in the thorax. The ribcage is removed. The arteries descend between the pleurae and the sternocostal wall. *a* Internal thoracic arteries and veins, *b* sternum, *c* sternohyoid muscle, *d* right lung, *e* the costomediastinal pleural recesses, *f* left lung

anastomosis can bypass blood to the inferior limbs in case of aortic coarctation. In this case, the arterial pulse can be palpated in the rectus abdominis muscle area.

The left internal thoracic artery is situated initially behind the left brachiocephalic vein and in front of the phrenic nerve, descending on the posterior face of the anterior thoracic wall at 0.5–1 cm from the sternum.

Its anterior intercostal branches are accompanied by the intercostal nerve and vein. They perforate the intercostal space under the anterior intercostal membrane. The internal thoracic artery also divides into the pericardiacophrenic and mediastinal branches (Figs. 5.12, 5.13, 5.14 and 5.15).

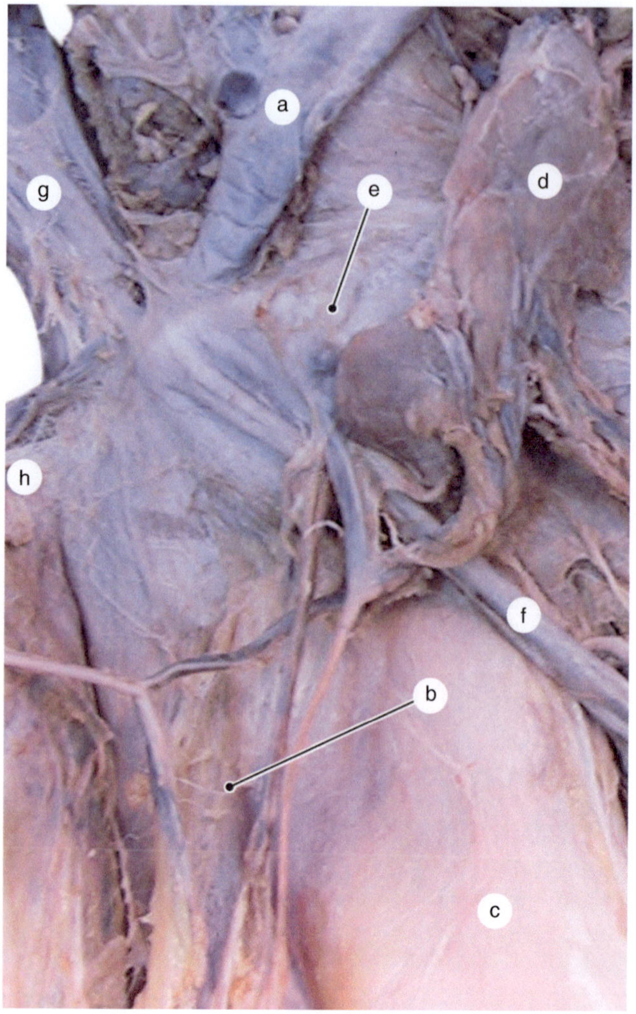

Fig. 5.11 Thymus remainings are included between the venous plane and the sternocostal wall. *a* Inferior thyroid veins, *b* superior vena cava, *c* ascending aorta, *d* thymus remaining, *e* left innominate vein, *f* pericardiophrenic vein, *g* right internal jugular vein, *h* right subclavian vein

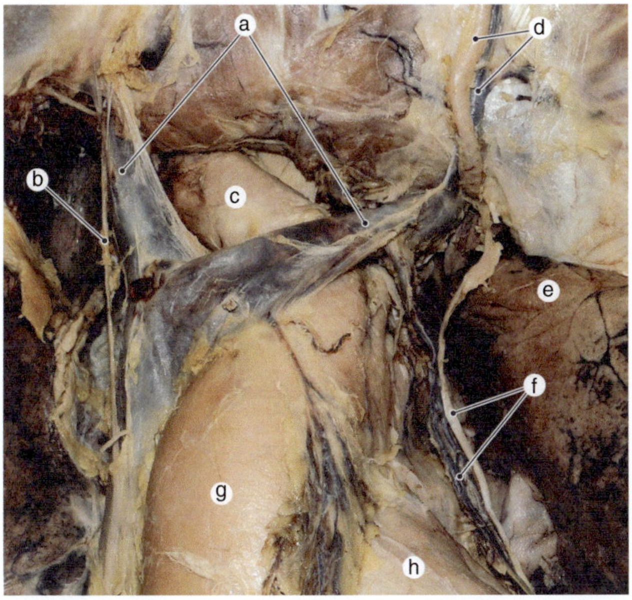

Fig. 5.12 The left internal thoracic artery enters the thorax included between the phrenic nerve and the left innominate vein. Notice the abundance of pericardial veins. *a* Innominate veins, *b* right phrenic nerve, *c* brachiocephalic trunk, *d* left internal thoracic arteries and veins, *e* left phrenic nerve and pericardiophrenic vessels, *g* aorta, *h* pulmonary trunk

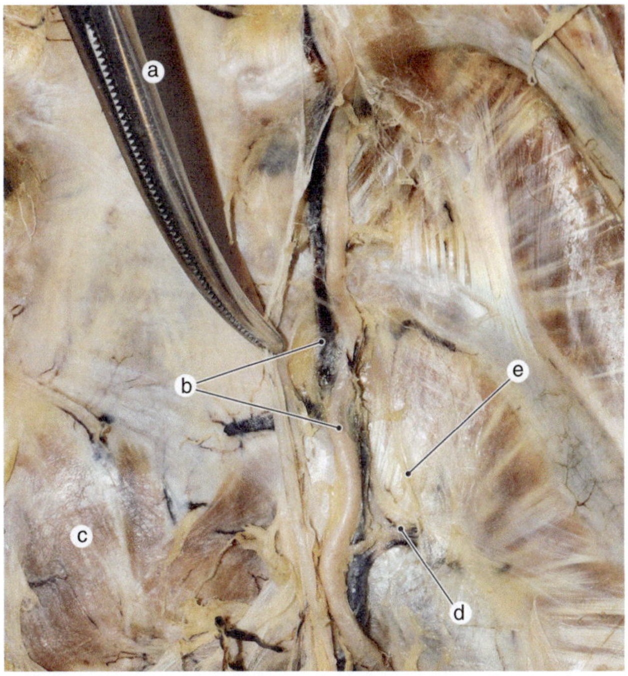

Fig. 5.14 Relations of the left internal thoracic vessels. The ribcage is retracted. *a* Within the clamp, the parietal pleura, *b* internal thoracic arteries and veins, *c* insertions of the sternohyoid muscles, *d* intercostal neurovascular bundle, *e* internal intercostal membrane

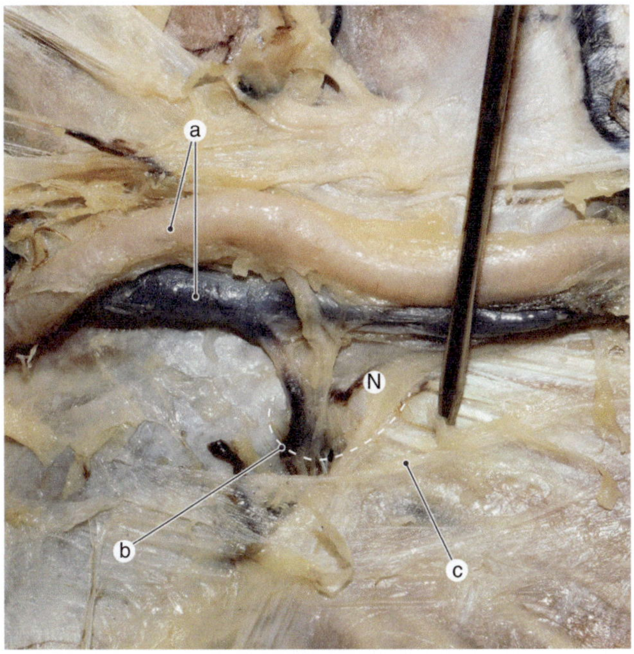

Fig. 5.13 Anterior intercostal neurovascular bundle. *a* Internal thoracic artery and vein, *b* intercostal neurovascular bundle, *c* internal intercostal membrane, *N* intercostal nerve

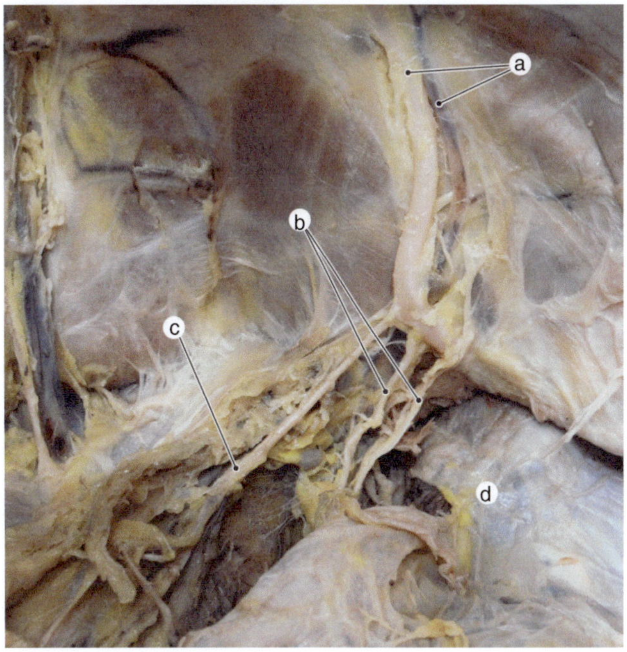

Fig. 5.15 Left internal thoracic artery branches. *a* Left internal thoracic artery and vein, *b* mediastinal artery, *c* pericardiophrenic artery, *d* apex of the left lung

5.2 Pulmonary Surface Boundaries

The pulmonary surface (Margo obtusis) is completely covered by the left lung (Fig. 5.7). The left phrenic nerve alongside the pericardiacophrenic vessels descend between the left ventricle and the mediastinal pleura of the left lung (Figs. 5.16, 5.17, 5.18, 5.19, 5.20 and 5.21).

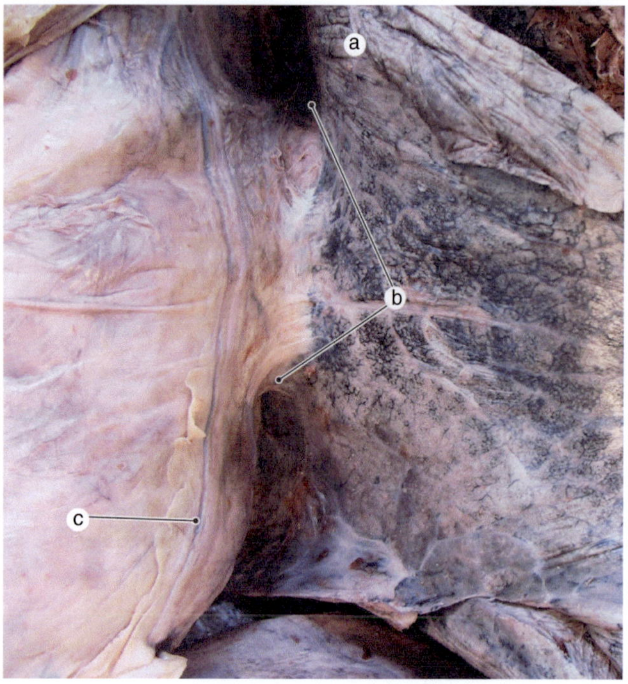

Fig. 5.16 Undissected left pulmonary pedicle. The phrenic nerve is noticed through the transparency of the mediastinal pleura which moulds the pericardium. *a* Left lung, *b* lung pedicle lined by pleura, *c* left phrenic nerve between the mediastinal pleura and heart

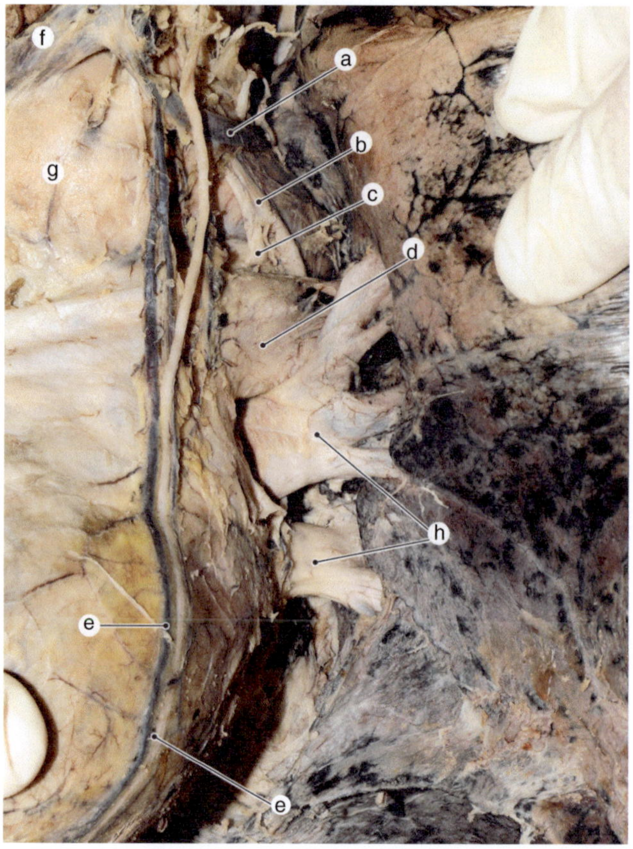

Fig. 5.17 Dissected left pulmonary pedicle. Notice the left supreme intercostal vein. *a* Left supreme intercostal vein, *b* left vagus nerve, *c* laryngeal recurrent nerve, *d* left pulmonary artery, *e* phrenic nerve and pericardiophrenic vessels, *f* left innominate vein, *g* aortic arch, *h* left pulmonary veins

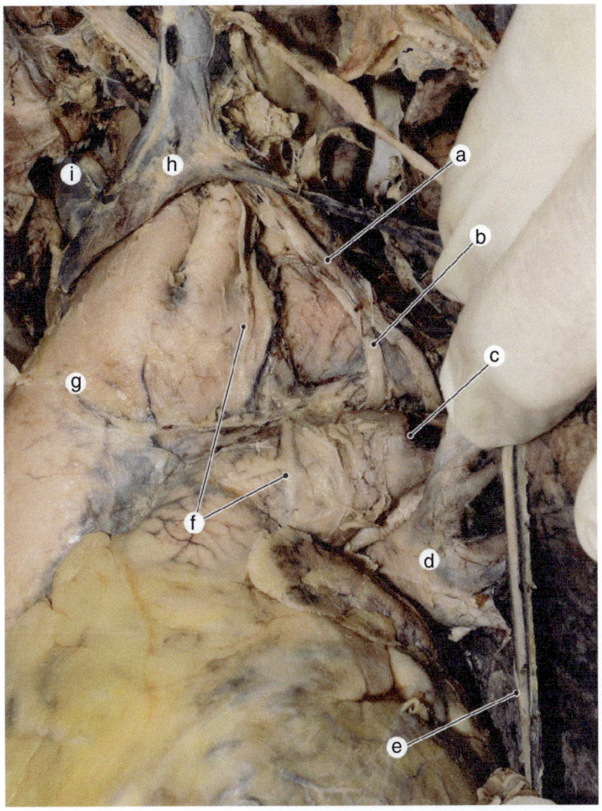

Fig. 5.18 Relations of the left pulmonary pedicle with the nervous trunks. *a* Left vagus nerve, *b* laryngeal recurrent nerve, *c* left pulmonary artery, *d* left pulmonary veins, *e* phrenic nerve and pericardiophrenic veins, *f* sympathetic cardiac nerves, *g* aortic arch, *h* left innominate vein, *i* right innominate vein

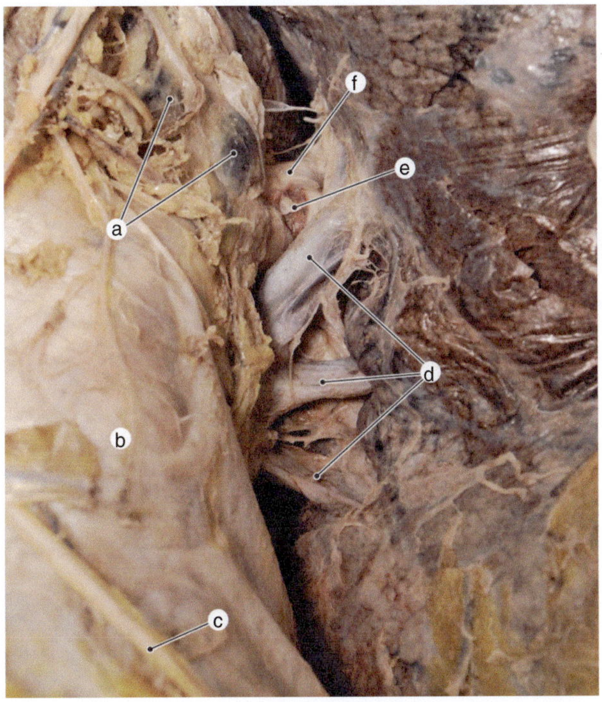

Fig. 5.19 Bronchopulmonary lymphatic ganglia in the left pedicle. *a* Lymphatic ganglia, *b* heart, *c* phrenic nerve, *d* left pulmonary veins, *e* left pulmonary artery, *f* left main bronchus

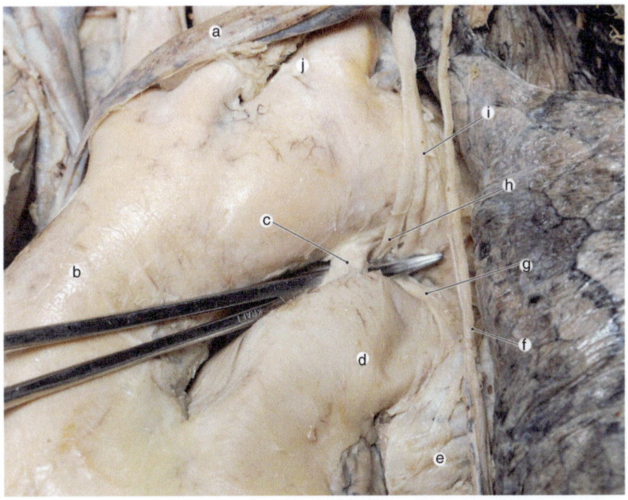

Fig. 5.20 Relation of the left laryngeal recurrent nerve with the arterial ligament. *a* Left innominate vein, *b* aortic arch, *c* arterial ligament, *d* pulmonary trunk, *e* pulmonary vein, *f* left phrenic nerve, *g* cardiac nerves, *h* laryngeal recurrent nerve, *i* left vagus nerve, *j* left subclavian artery

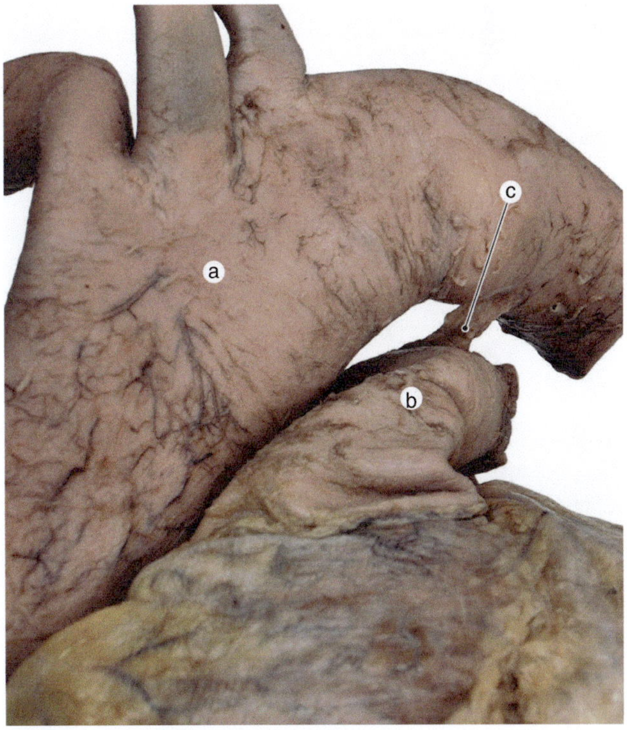

Fig. 5.21 Arterial ligament extends from the origin of the left pulmonary artery to the aortic arch. *a* Aortic arch, *b* pulmonary trunk, *c* arterial ligament

5.3 Diaphragmatic Surface Boundaries

Through the diaphragm (Fig. 5.22), the heart is bordered by the left hepatic lobe and the fundus of the stomach (Fig. 4.38a). The variations in volume (physiological or pathological) could affect cardiac activity. Very suggestive in postprandial aerophagia, the dilatation of the stomach's air pouch, associated with decubitus, compresses the heart and can provoke postprandial extrasystoles.

The points where the two phrenic nerves approach the diaphragm and the borders of these areas with the heart are highlighted in Figs. 5.23 and 5.24.

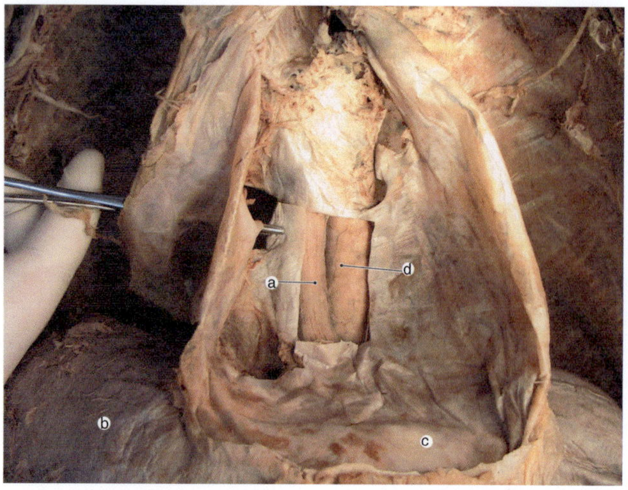

Fig. 5.22 The pericardial sac after removing the heart. Notice the relation with the diaphragm. *a* Esophagus, *b* diaphragm, *c* pericardial sac, *d* aorta

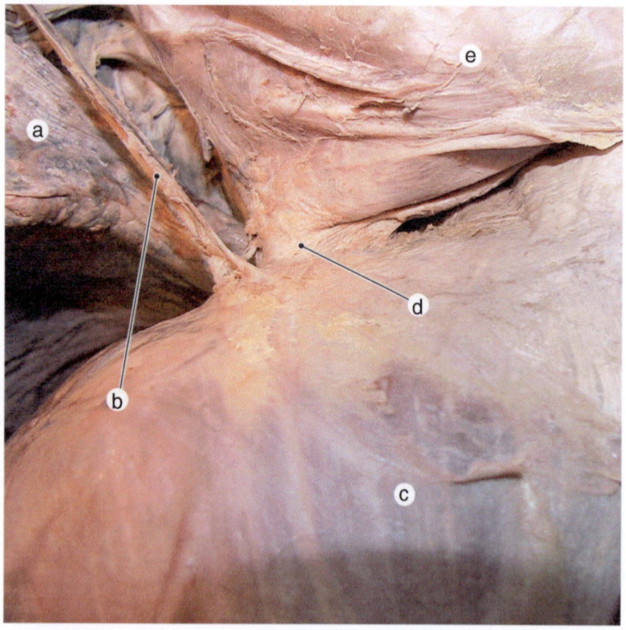

Fig. 5.23 Right phrenic nerve approaches the diaphragm anterior and to the right of the inferior vena cava orifice. *a* Left lung, *b* phrenic nerve and right preicardiophrenic vessels, *c* diaphragm, *d* inferior vena cava – supradiaphragmatic sector, *e* heart

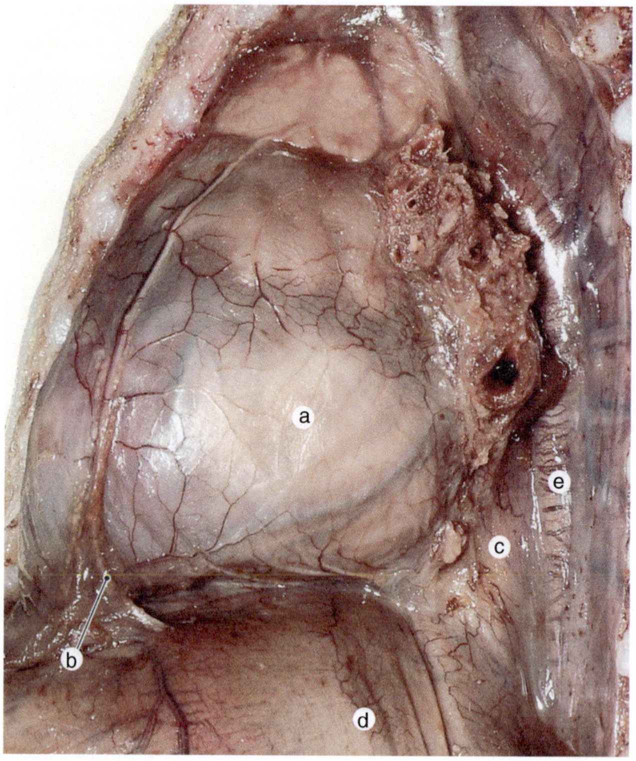

Fig. 5.24 View from the left of the pulmonary side. Seven months old fetal heart. Left phrenic nerve approaches the diaphragm in the proximity of the cardiac apex. *a* Heart – pulmonary side, *b* left phrenic nerve, *c* esophagus in the cardioaortic space, *d* diaphragm, *e* descending thoracic aorta

5.4 The Right Border Boundaries

The anatomical right border (the acute margin) separates the sternocostal and diaphragmatic surfaces. It is bounded in front by the thoracic wall represented by the posterior face of the sternum and the left sixth and seventh sternocostal articulations and the sixth left costal cartilage.

The radiologic left border (Fig. 4.38) is represented by the inferior vena cava, the right atrium and the superior vena cava and it is bounded by the left pulmonary hilum. Between the right border of the heart and the left pulmonary hilum there is a space radiologically called the inter cardio hilar space (this space disappears in pulmonary hypertension) (Figs. 4.38 and 5.25).

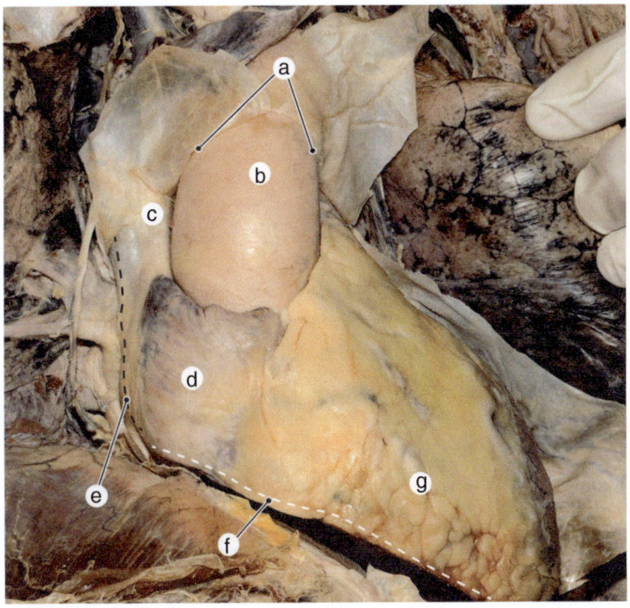

Fig. 5.25 Right anatomical edge comes in contact with the sternocostal wall. Radiologic edge is outlined by the base of the heart. *a* Line of reflection of the pericardium, *b* ascending aorta, *c* superior vena cava, *d* right atrium, *e* right radiologic edge, *f* right anatomical edge, *g* right ventricle

5.5 The Boundaries of the Hearts Base

These are the most complex of all boundaries of the heart. This complexity is reflected by the fact that we cannot separate the boundaries of the heart from those of the great vessels from the base of the heart.

Practically, the base of the heart is in the proximity of a large amount of elements from the posterior mediastinum, between the two mediastinal pleurae.

The boundaries of the base of the heart can be systematized in the upper border and lower border

The upper border of the base of the heart is bounded by the tracheal bifurcation, the pulmonary pedicles and posterior to them by the esophagus, descending aorta, thoracic canal, azygos veins, the thoracic sympathetic trunks and the vertebral column.

On the lower border the left atrium is in direct relation with the esophagus, the periesophageal vagal plexus, and posterior and to the left of the esophagus, with the thoracic part of the descending aorta and its posterior intercostal branches (Fig. 5.26).

This relation explains why the dilatation of the left atrium (in various valvular pathologies) compresses and deforms the esophagus. This relation also explains why the ingestion of very cold or very hot food could affect the cardiac function inducing, for example, extrasystoles.

When the descending aorta reaches the diaphragmatic surface of the heart, a triangle is formed between the aorta, the diaphragm and the base of the heart, called the cardioaortic triangle. It is in this area that we can find the thoracic esophagus (Figs. 5.24 and 5.28).

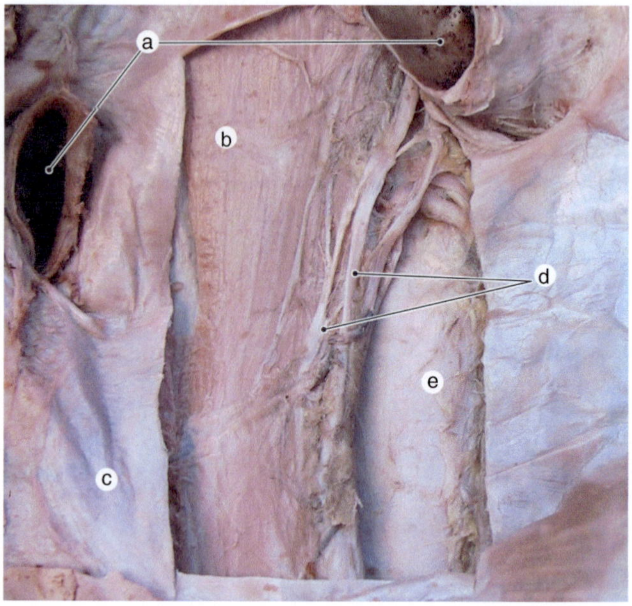

Fig. 5.26 The posterior relations of the left atrium are observed after cutting out an opening in the pericardium at the base of the heart. *a* Inferior pulmonary veins, *b* esophagus, *c* pericardium, *d* periesophageal vagus plexus, *e* thoracic aorta and interaortico-esophageal recess

5.6 The Intrinsic Boundaries of the Pulmonary Pedicles

The right pulmonary pedicle is bordered above and behind by the right main bronchus (this will rapidly divide in the superior lobar bronchus and the common trunk of the middle and inferior lobar bronchus). Immediately in front and below is the right pulmonary artery. Below the artery there can be found the superior right pulmonary vein, and under it the inferior right pulmonary vein.

In the left pulmonary pedicle, the intrinsic boundaries are as follows: superior is the pulmonary artery, inferior and posterior the left main bronchus, inferior and in front by the superior left pulmonary vein, and inferior to the bronchus by the inferior left pulmonary vein (Figs. 5.27 and 5.28).

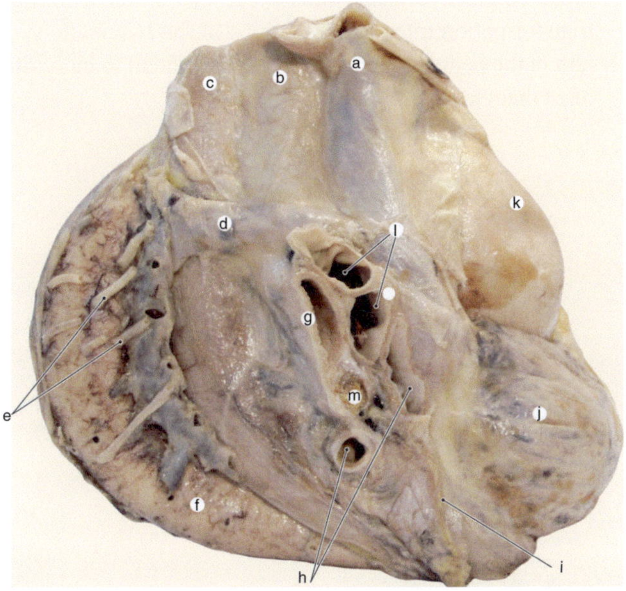

Fig. 5.27 The extrinsic and intrinsic relations of the right pulmonary pedicle. *a* Superior vena cava, *b* trachea, *c* esophagus, *d* azygos vein arch, *e* posterior intercostal arteries, *f* descending aorta, *g* right main bronchus, *h* right pulmonary veins, *i* pleural ligament, *j* right ventricle, *k* ascending aorta, *l* right pulmonary arteries, *m* lymphatic ganglion

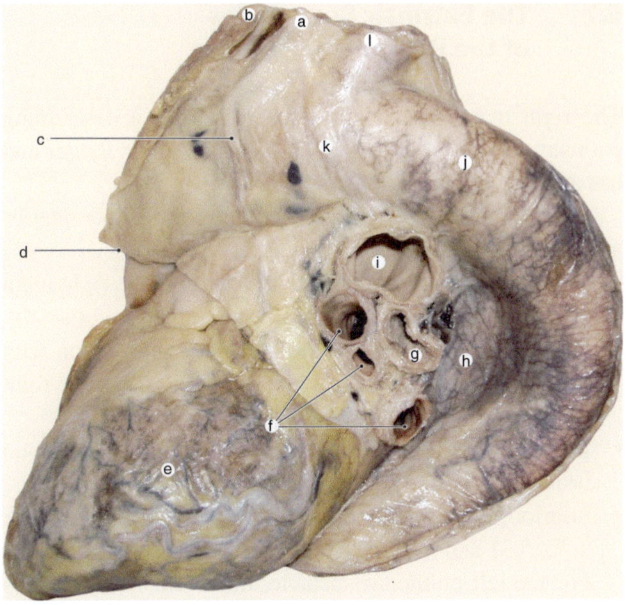

Fig. 5.28 The extrinsic and intrinsic relations of the left pulmonary pedicle. *a* Left common carotid artery, *b* brachiocephalic trunk, *c* left phrenic nerve, *d* sectioned pericardium, *e* left ventricle, *f* left pulmonary veins, *g* left main bronchus, *h* esophagus in the cardiac- aortic space, *i* left pulmonary artery, *j* aortic arch, *k* left vagus nerve, *l* left subclavian artery

5.7 The Extrinsic Boundaries of the Pulmonary Pedicles

The right main bronchus is shorter and has a descending pathway, unlike the left main bronchus which is longer and has a more horizontal trajectory.

For the right pulmonary pedicle, the extrinsic boundaries are as follows:

- superiorly (in close relation to the origin of the right main bronchus) lies the arch of the azygos vein
- anteriorly it lies the superior vena cava (in relation with the right pulmonary artery), the right atrium and the right phrenic nerve
- posteriorly is the esophagus (in relation with the main bronchus) and the right vagus nerve
- inferiorly is situated the pulmonary ligament (Figs. 5.29, 5.30, 5.31 and 5.32)

For the left pulmonary pedicle, the extrinsic boundaries are as follows:

- above the pedicle is the arch of the aorta (in close relation to the origin of the left main bronchus). The arterial ligament links the origin of the left pulmonary artery to the inferior terminal part of the aortic arch (Figs. 5.19 and 5.20 and Fig. 7.16). Under the ligament, the left vagus nerve gives off the left recurrent laryngeal nerve branches off from the left vagus nerve. This nerve passes directly under the aortic arch and ascends between the trachea and esophagus.
- In front is the left phrenic nerve
- Posterior lies the esophagus (in relation with the origin of the left main bronchus) and the left vagus nerve which branches into its cardiac branches.
- Below is the pulmonary ligament

Besides this type of systematization, for a correct understanding of the boundaries, there are a few more specifications:

- The tracheal bifurcation is flanked on its posterior surface and a little to the left by the esophagus. This explains why the origins of both main bronchi are bordered behind by the esophagus.
- Both the tracheal bifurcation and the esophagus are flanked to their right by the arch of the azygos vein and to their left by the arch of the aorta.
- The tracheal bifurcation is covered on its anterior surface by the origin of the right pulmonary artery.
- The main bronchi are accompanied both upper and lower by the superior and inferior tracheobronchial lymph nodes, as well as their lymph vessels. The adenopathy of these lymph nodes could compress nearby structures of the pulmonary pedicles.
- On the left lateral surface of the aortic arch lie, from anterior to posterior, the structures presented in Fig. 5.33.
- The bronchial arteries and veins (two left arteries and one right artery) usually accompany the main bronchi posterior to them.
- The pulmonary pedicles also contain nervous fibers from the vagus nerve and thoracic sympathetic trunks.
- The elements of the pedicle are closely united to each other and the related structures around them through loose connective tissue (this tissue can suffer a fibrous transformation after inflammations of the lymphatic system in the pedicle, therefore it can be difficult to individualize them surgically).

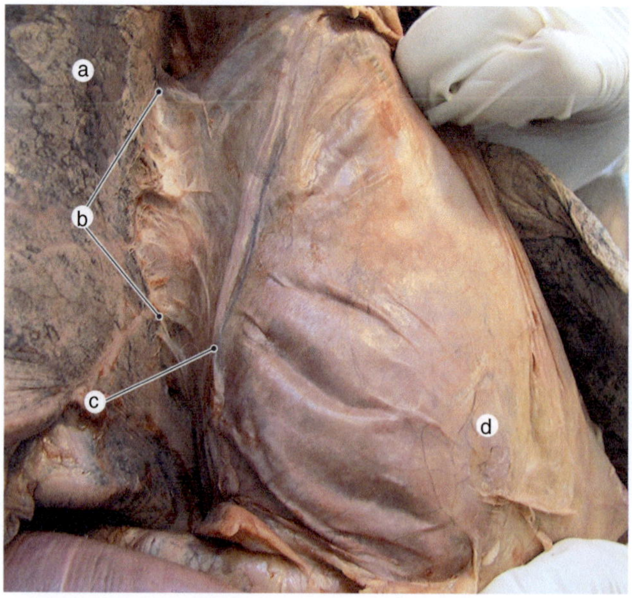

Fig. 5.29 Undissected left pulmonary pedicle. *a* Left lung, *b* right pulmonary pedicle, *c* right phrenic nerve between the pleura and the pericardium, *d* intrapericardial heart

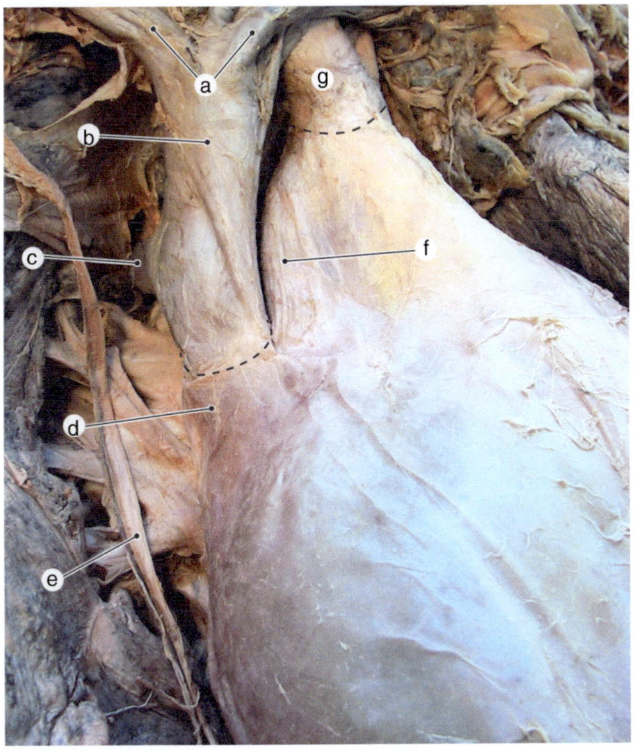

Fig. 5.30 Dissected right pulmonary pedicle. Notice the point and manner of insertion of the pericardium on the greater vessels. *a* Innominate veins, *b* extrapericardial superior vena cava, *c* azygos vein arch, *d* intrapericardial superior vena cava, *e* the phrenic nerve anterior of the right pulmonary pedicle, *f* intrapericardial ascending aorta, *g* arterial brachiocephalic trunk

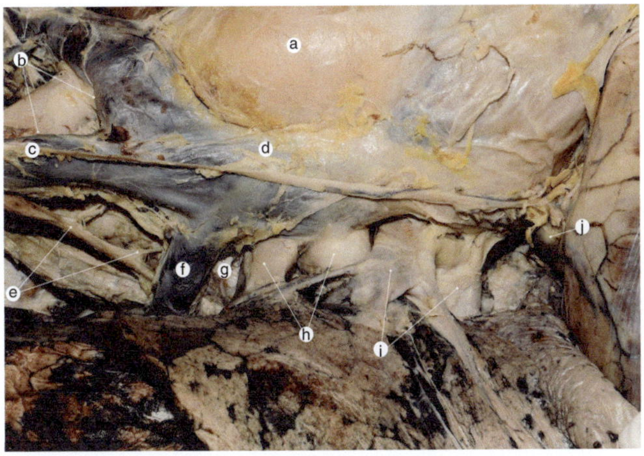

Fig. 5.31 Dorsal decubitus. Right side view. The relations of the pulmonary pedicle with the nervous trunks. Notice the cardiac branches of the right vagus nerve. *a* Ascending aorta, *b* innominate veins, *c* right phrenic nerve, *d* superior vena cava, *e* cardiac branches from the right vagus nerve, *f* azygos vein arch, *g* right main bronchus, *h* pulmonary arteries, *i* pulmonary veins, *j* superior vena cava

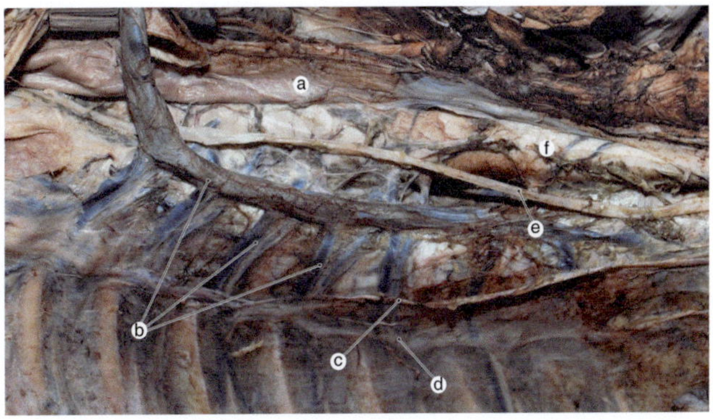

Fig. 5.32 Dorsal decubitus. Right side view. The relations of the viscera from the posterior mediastinum. *a* Thoracic esophagus, *b* azygos vein with the posterior intercostal veins and arch, *c* parietal pleura, *d* thoracic sympathetic chain, *e* thoracic canal, *f* descending thoracic aorta and the interaortic-esophageal and interazygo-aortic recesses

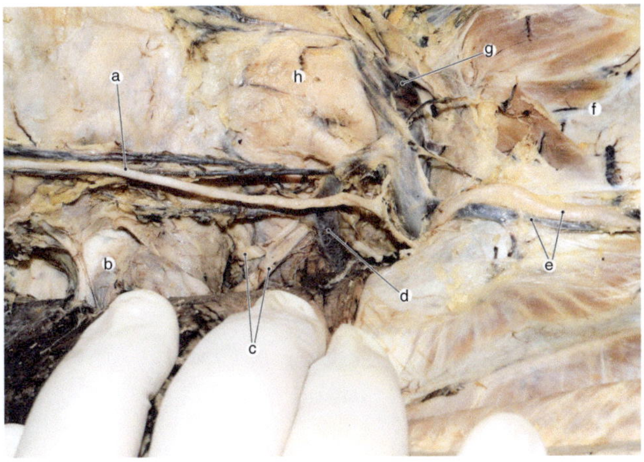

Fig. 5.33 Dorsal decubitus. Left side view. Highlighting of the formations which pass lateral to the aorta. *a* Phrenic nerve with pericardiophrenic vessels, *b* left pulmonary pedicle, *c* vagus and laryngeal recurrent nerves, *d* supreme intercostal vein, *e* internal thoracic artery and vein, *f* sternocostal plastron reflected upwards, *g* left innominate vein, *h* aortic arch

6 Internal Configuration of the Heart

6.1 Internal Configuration of the Right Atrium

The right atrium is situated in front and to the right of the left atrium. From the tricuspid orifice the right atrium is located further more behind than above (Fig. 6.1).

The right atrium has a globular aspect. It has an anterior extension called the right auricle.

The right atrium is where the superior vena cava, the inferior vena cava and the coronary sinus end. The anterior and small veins of the heart (also known as the thebesian veins) open in the right atrium through orifices called foramina thebesii. Through the right atrioventricular orifice – the tricuspid orifice, the blood from the right atrium passes into the right ventricle.

The internal surface of the right atrium has some specific areas:

- The right auricle is the anterior expansion of the right atrium, with a general conical shape, deriving from the primitive atrium. The conical shape with the blunt apex, relatively smooth margins and a large base, represent the elements which help in imagistic identification of the right atrium.
- The pectinate part is a segment in the wall of the atrium which has the pectinate muscles. They are arranged as muscular trabeculae like "the teeth of a comb". Actually, this part represents the base of the auricle (Fig. 6.2).

The aspect of the trabeculae in the lumen of the right auricle is highly variable. Frequently one sagital trabecula acts as a support for the insertion of other trabeculae arranged like "the ribs of a palm leaf". Figures 6.3, 6.4, 6.5, 6.6, 6.7, 6.8, 6.9 and 6.52 offer an exemplification of the variability of pectinate muscles.

In the internal configuration of the right atrium there is a second set of thin trabeculae, harder to identify, situated between the superior part of the crista terminalis and the membranous wall of the primitive atrium. These trabeculae are in continuity with the superficial muscular fibers of the atrium Fig. 6.10.

- The sinusal part – called sinus venarum is represented by the smooth surface between the ostia of the two venae cavae (Fig. 6.10).
- The tricuspid vestibule derives from the atrioventricular canal. It has an anterior part with smooth walls which can be named the subauricular vestibule.
- The floor of the atrium, the cavotricuspid isthmus. The subeustachian and subthebesian sinuses, Koch's triangle, represent the parts of the vestibule
- The atrioventricular septum is represented by the superior segment of the membranous septum
- The dorsosinusal space and the interatrial septum with their complex origin
- The oval fossa
- The valve of the inferior vena cava, which derives from the right valvule of the embryo's venous sinus
- The crista terminalis

Each of these regions alongside other elements present inside the atrium will be defined and described one at a time (Figs. 6.11 and 6.12).

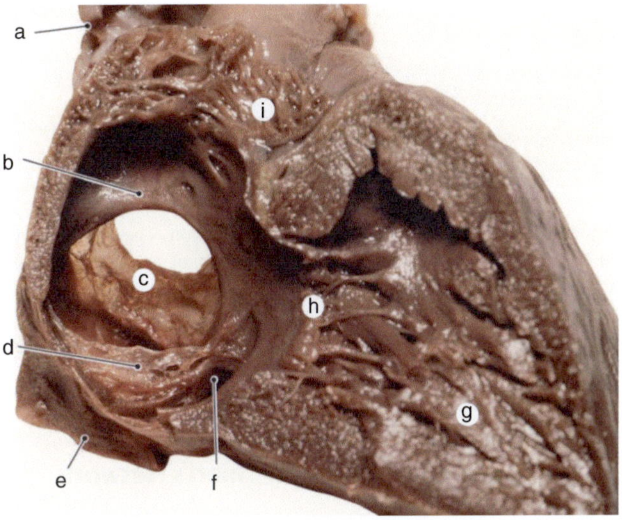

Fig. 6.1 Five months old heart. Sagittal paramedian section through the right heart. *a* superior vena cava *b* septum secundum, *c* septum primum, *d* inferior vena cava valve, *e* inferior vena cava, *f* sinus ostium, *g* right ventricle, *h* tricuspid valve, *i* right auricle

F.M. Filipoiu, *Atlas of Heart Anatomy and Development*,
DOI 10.1007/978-1-4471-5382-5_6, © Springer-Verlag London 2014

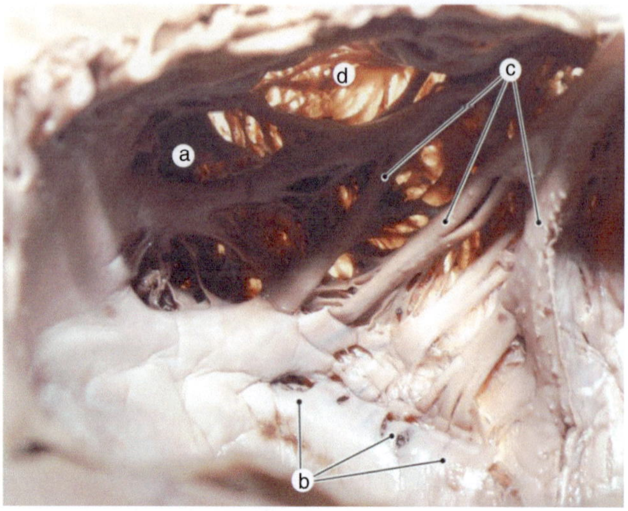

Fig. 6.2 Muscular trabeculae inserted on the inferior segment of the crista terminalis. In the subauricular vestibule a deep venous canal with incomplete wall is observed. *a* right auricle, *b* profound venous canal, *c* muscular trabeculae, *d* transparent membranous wall

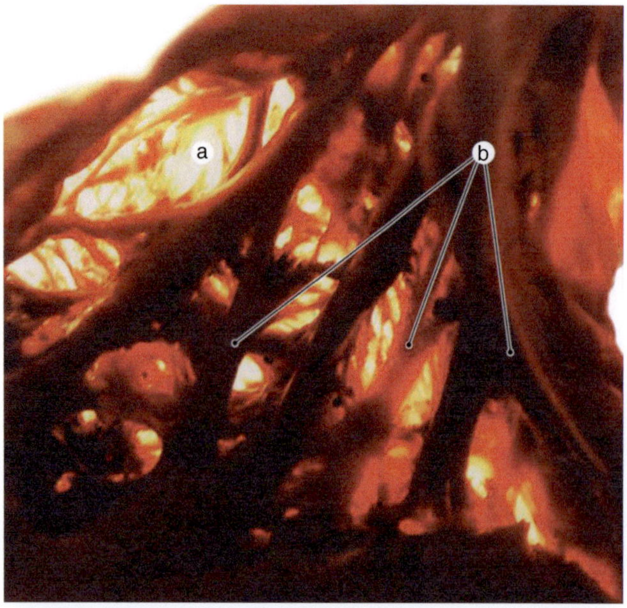

Fig. 6.3 The pectinate muscles – transillumination. The main muscular fascicles, disposed parallelly, like the teeth of a comb. Between these fascicles thinner fascicles anchor the atrial wall which has a membranous appearance. *a* Transparent membranous wall, *b* muscular trabeculae

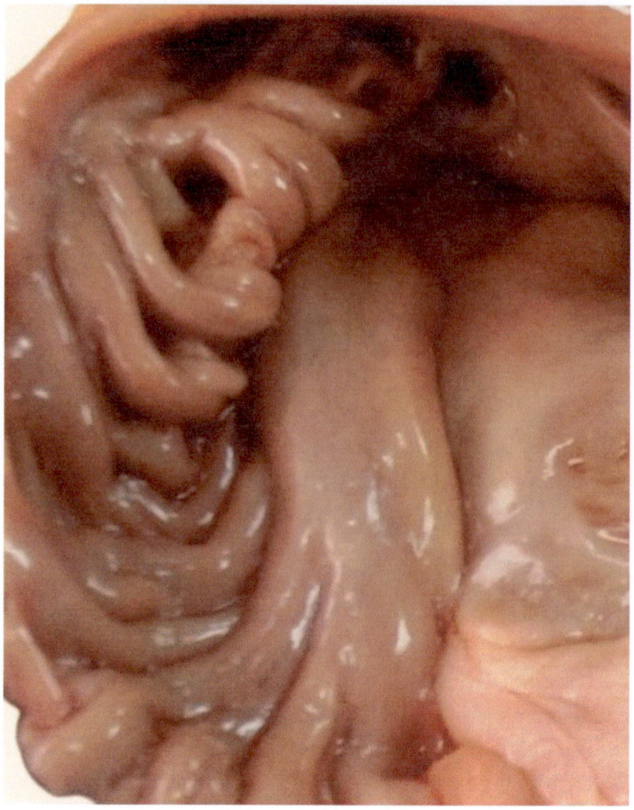

Fig. 6.4 The appearance of the pectinate muscles on a heart not preserved in formaldehyde

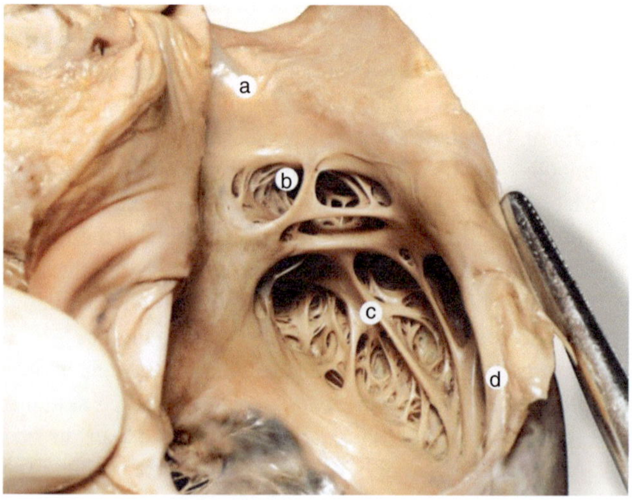

Fig. 6.5 Right atrium with the pectinate territory reduced. *a* superior vena cava, *b* right auricle, *c* muscular trabeculae, *d* terminal ridge

6.1.1 The Orifice of the Inferior Vena Cava, the Eustachian Valve, Chiari's Network

The orifice of the inferior vena cava is inconstantly bordered in its front part by an incomplete semilunar valve. This is called the valve of the inferior vena cava or Eustachio's valve and it derives from the right valve of the embryonic venous sinus (Fig. 6.14). This valve previously directed the venous blood to the interatrial communication, in fetal life.

The valve of the inferior vena cava has variable aspects and dimensions. It covers (and sometimes overlaps in the superior part) a ridge called the Eustachian margin (Figs. 6.13 and 6.14).

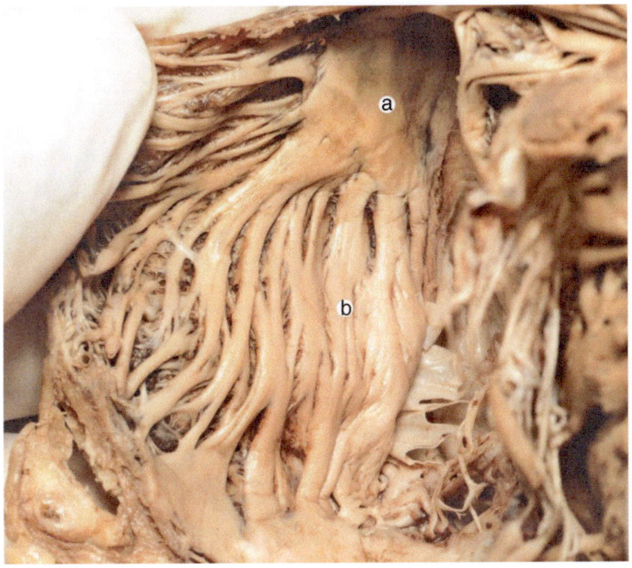

Fig. 6.6 Pattern of organization of the pectinate muscles without connection to the crista terminalis. The pectinate fascicles diverge fanwise, from a common muscular mass, located in the sinus area. *a* common muscular mass, *b* pectinate fascicles

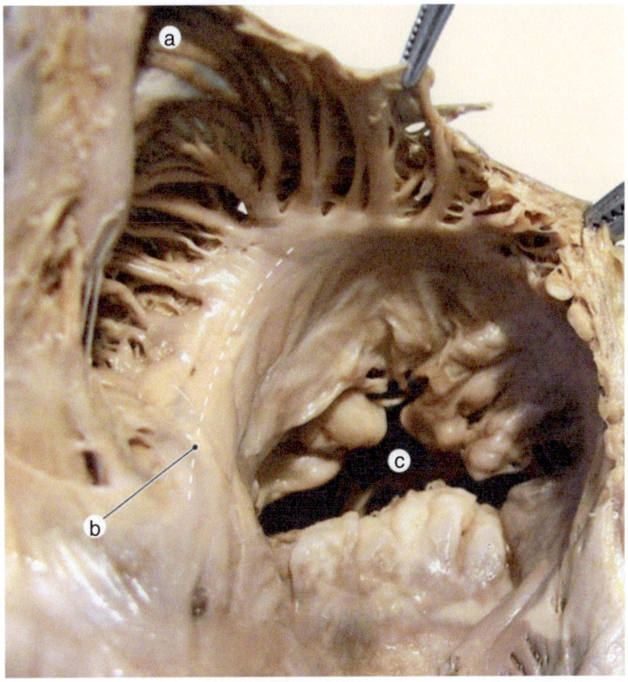

Fig. 6.8 The insertion of the pectinate muscles occupies approximatively half of the circumference of the tricuspid vestibule. The subauricular vestibule is individualized as a smooth area at the base of the auricle. *a* right auricle, *b* subauricle vestibule, *c* tricuspid valve

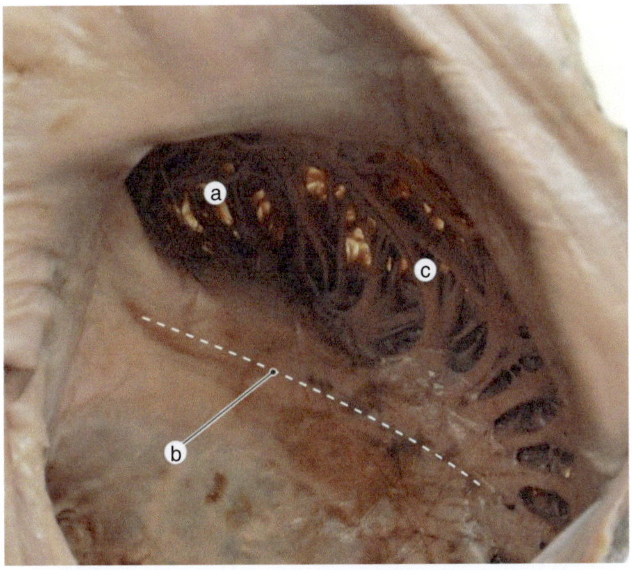

Fig. 6.7 Pattern of organization of the pectinate muscles, located backward to the previous case – muscular fascicles reunite on the lateral side of the atrial vestibule. *a* right auricle, *b* subauricular vestibule, *c* pectinate muscles

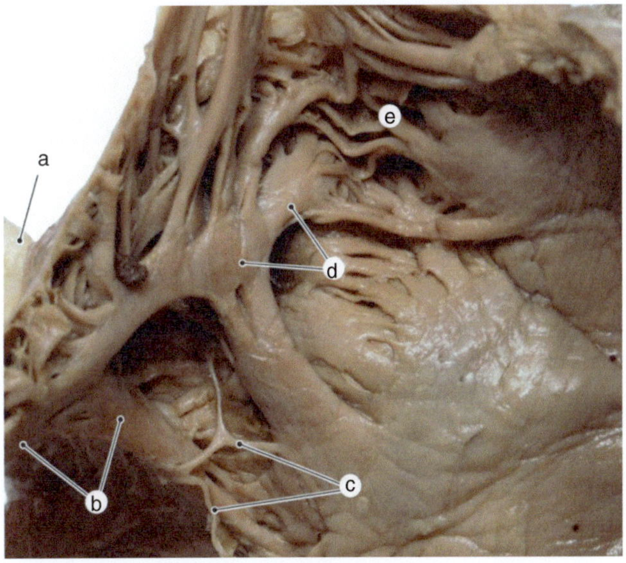

Fig. 6.9 Sagittal trabecula in the lumen of the right auricle. In the proximity of the crista terminalis remainings of the right valve of the primitive sinus venosus can be observed. *a* superior vena cava, *b* crista terminalis, *c* remainings of the right valve, *d* sagital trabecula, *e* right auricle

The valve of the inferior vena cava usually has a right horn oriented towards its superior part and a left horn oriented towards the septum (Fig. 6.1).

The right horn inconstantly follows the contour of the crista terminalis, and can be more or less individualized. Its extensions with a membranous aspect end before and to the right of the orifice of the superior vena cava (Figs. 6.16 and 6.27a).

In some cases some portions of the right valve of the venous sinus persist into adult life with variable shapes, like a perforated membrane, strips or anastomosed endocardic fascicles. This residual structure is called Chiari's network

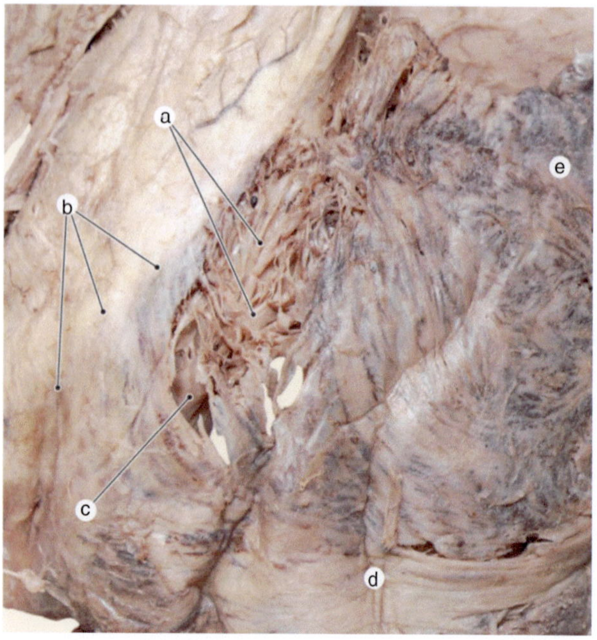

Fig. 6.10 Thin trabeculae diverge towards the atrial wall from the thickness of the crista terminalis, in the proximity of the sinus area. Some of them continue with subepicardial atrial muscle fibers. *a* thin muscular trabeculae, *b* terminal sulcus, *c* crista terminalis, *d* subepicardial muscular fibers, *e* right auricle

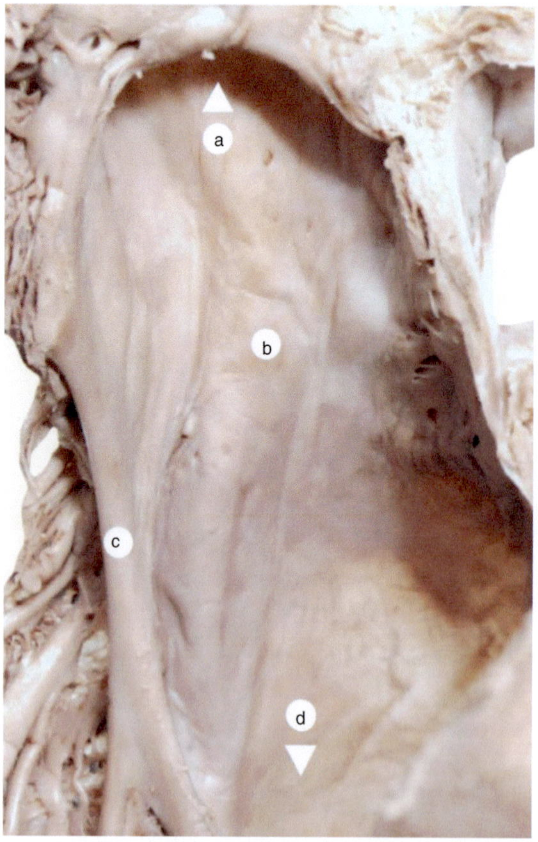

Fig. 6.11 Sinus venarum seen from the interior of the right atrium. *a* superior vena cava (*arrowhead*), *b* sinus venarum, *c* crista terminalis, *d* inferior vena cava (*arrowhead*)

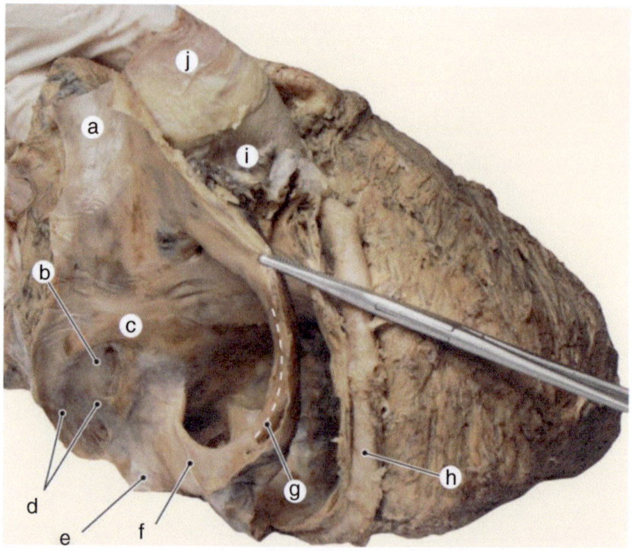

Fig. 6.12 Right atrium after removing the pectinate part. The inferior vena cava orifice is limited anteriorly by a fold with membranous aspect, named the inferior vena cava valvule. *a* superior vena cava, *b* fossa ovalis, *c* limbus, *d* remainings of the left valve, *e* inferior vena cava, *f* inferior vena cava valvule, *g* crista terminalis, *h* right coronary artery, *i* right auricle, *j* aorta

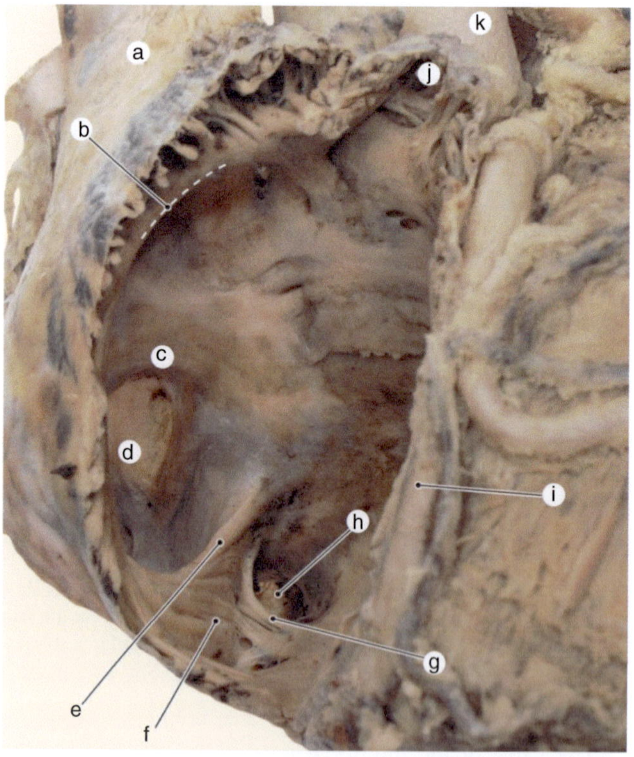

Fig. 6.13 Eustachian edge continues the crista terminalis in its inferior portion. *a* superior vena cava, *b* crista terminalis, *c* limbus, *d* fossa ovalis, *e* eustachian edge, *f* subeustachian sinus, *g* thebesian edge, *h* coronary sinus ostium, *i* right coronary artery, *j* right auricle, *k* aorta

(Figs. 6.15, 6.16, 6.17 and 6.18). Its insertion and rapport with the Eustachian margin offer indications about the embryological disposition of the right valve of the venous sinus.

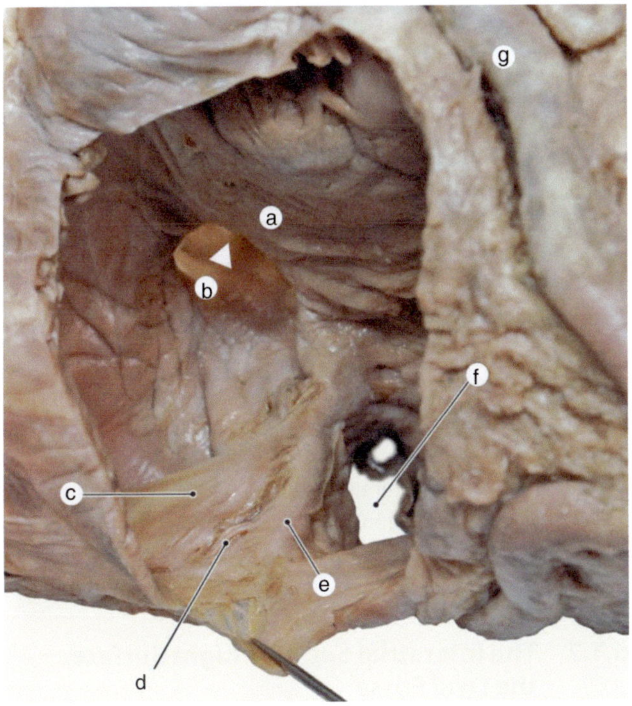

Fig. 6.14 The relation between the inferior vena cava valvule and the Eustachian edge. The pectinate atrial wall has been resected. *a* limbus, *b* patent interatrial orifice (*arrowhead*), *c* inferior vena cava valvule, *d* cristovalvular recess, *e* eustachian edge, *f* coronary sinus ostium, *g* right coronary artery

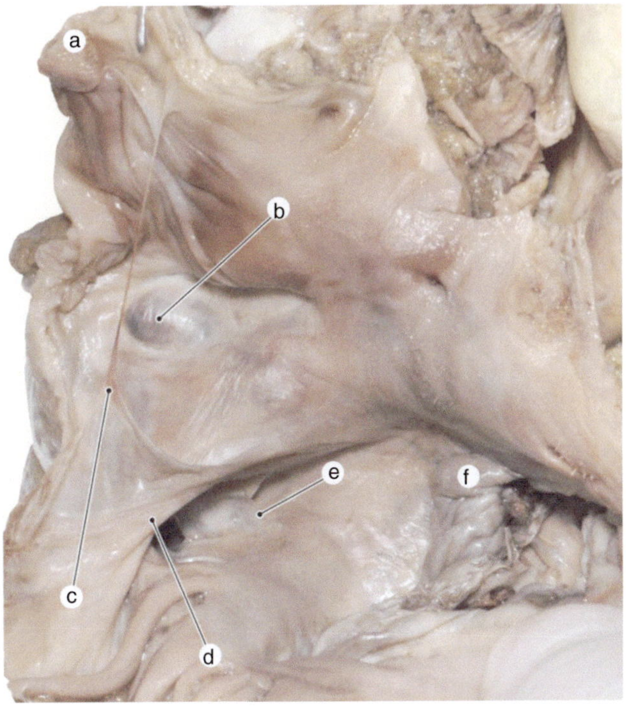

Fig. 6.16 In adult heart, the limits of insertion have been kept from the right valve of the sinus venosus, reunited by a fibrous bridle. Therefore, we have an image of the initial expansion of the right valve. *a* superior vena cava, *b* fossa ovalis with intraseptal tumor, *c* Chiari network – remaining of the right valve, *d* eustachian edge, *e* sinus valvule (Thebesian), *f* tricuspid valve

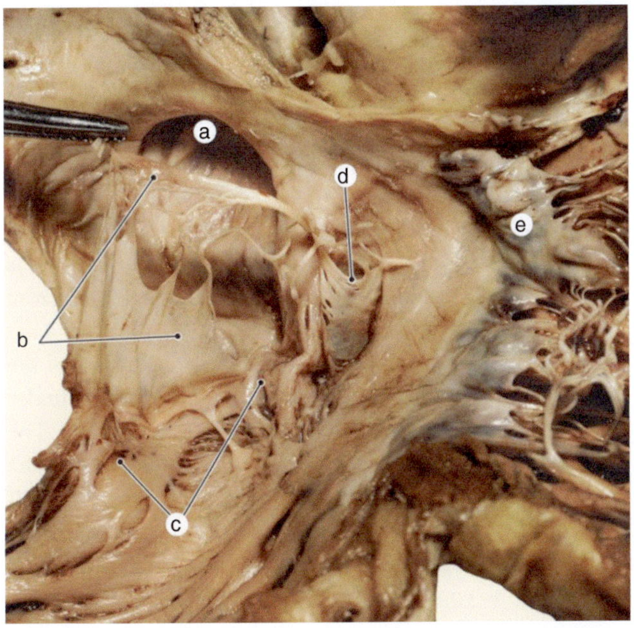

Fig. 6.15 Sinus valvule of muscular origine has been resected. At the point where the Eustachian edge passes under the former right valve a separation is produced between the two valvulae – caval valvula and sinus valvula. *a* fossa ovalis, *b* Chiari network – remaining of the right valve, *c* eustachian edge, *d* sinus valvule (Thebesian valvule), *e* tricuspid valve

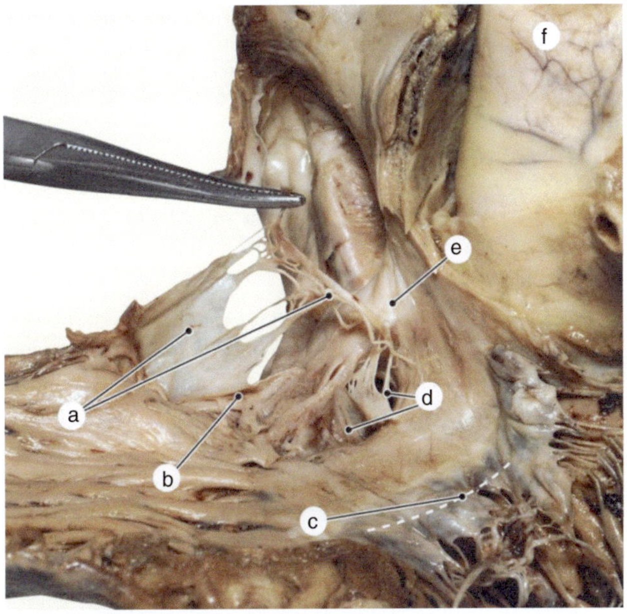

Fig 6.17 Inferior vena cava valvule with Chiari's network. Notice the fact that there are two valvulae of the coronary sinus, each one with clearly different origins. Notice the insertion of the network on the septum secundum. The atrial wall is removed. *a* Chiari's network – remaining of the right valve, *b* eustachian edge, *c* tricuspid valve, *d* 2 sinus valvulae, *e* insertion on the septum secundum, *f* aorta

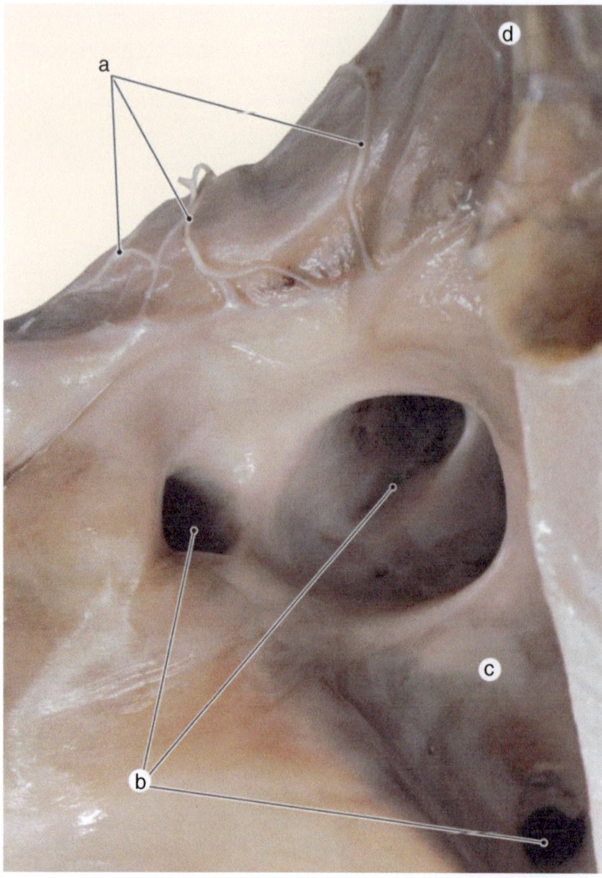

Fig. 6.18 Inferior vena cava is opened below and transdiaphragmatic. We can observe the line of insertion of a Chiari's network at the borderline between the venous endothelium and the atrial endocardium. *a* Chiari's network – remaining of the right valve, *b* hepatic veins orifices, *c* inferior vena cava, *d* right atrium

We also can observe that the right valve forms creases as it passes over the Eustachian margin, and its apex reaches the septum secundum.

Observing the continuity between the valve of the inferior vena cava and the valve of the coronary sinus, the common origin of the two structures is confirmed, both deriving from the right valve of the venous sinus (Figs. 6.15, 6.16, 6.17 and 6.18).

Keep in mind:

Chiari's network could represent the starting point of an intraatrial thrombus. Fragments from this thrombus could migrate to the left atrium through a interatrial septum defect, which is a frequent finding alongside Chiari's network. These fragments could give birth to paradoxical embolisms.

When the right valve has a great degree of remanence in the form of a fibromuscular membrane, it partially divides the right atrium into two sides, situation known as cortriatriatrum dextrum-34 (cortriatriatrum sinister is the situation when the left atrium is divided into two parts by a perforated fibromuscular membrane).

Between the valve of the inferior vena cava and the Eustachian crest there can be reminiscent parts of the cavomarginal recess.

The left horn of the valve of the inferior vena cava is sometimes in continuity with the valve of the coronary sinus (also see embryology).

The latter is represented by an endothelial fold that partially covers the ostium of the coronary sinus in its inferior and right part, preventing the reflux of blood into the sinus.

Sometimes the ostium of the coronary sinus is covered by a valve on its left side.

The valve of the coronary sinus is also a vestige of the right valve of the embryonic venous sinus.

Through the coronary ostium the coronary sinus, the largest collector of the venous coronary system, opens in the right atrium. The coronary sinus derives from the left horn of the embryonic venous sinus.

6.1.2 The Interatrial Septum: Right Surface, the Oval Fossa

The interatrial septum can be considered the left posterior-lateral wall of the right atrium (the right atrium is situated in front and to the right of the left atrium).

In the inferior and posterior part of the septum, at a distance from the atrioventricular orifice, a depression called the oval fossa can be observed.

Its surface is thinner that the rest of the interatrial septum and it is formed in its superior part by the septum primum and in its inferior part by the fusion of these structures:

- The septum primum (towards the left atrium)
- The vestibular spine
- The left valve of the left venous sinus

The fusion of the left valve and the septum primum is variable, and its contour gets more or less disengaged from the floor of the oval fossa.

Sometimes, more frequently in the superior part of the fossa, there is a small interatrial communication, under the form of an oblique orifice cut into the septum. The oblique aspect of the orifice permits the pressure from the left atrium to keep it closed, so that its presence in a small size does not have any hemodynamic significance.

The terms oval foramen or oval window are terms which usually lead to confusion.

Sometimes these terms are used to name an interatrial defect of the septum in the form of a unique orifice in the floor of the oval fossa. In this situation, when the septum primum has united correctly with the septum secundum and there is a relatively circular orifice at the level of the floor of the oval fossa, its correct name should be second orifice-type defect in the floor of the oval fossa (Fig. 6.29).

Other times it refers to the interatrial communication in embryonic life when the term oval foramen – Botallo – is used to name the normal gap between the septum primum and septum secundum, which ensures a shunt for pulmonary circulation. This space (also defined as an intraseptal conduct) is not oval and it does not correspond to the oval fossa, but to the space between the falx septi and septum secundum (Fig. 2.13). When falx septi does not fuse to the adult heart, we can speak of a patent interatrial communication, not an oval foramen (Fig. 6.30).

The oval foramen is a transitory appearance in embryonic life, appearing when the oval fossa does not yet have a well constituted floor, because either the septum primum or septum secundum, or both have reduced dimensions and are not yet overlapped (Figs. 2.12, 2.16 and 2.18) (also see embryology). We also emphasize on the fact that the oval aspect is an aspect given by summation, in reality it being an oblique gap and not an oval orifice.

The oval fossa is limited in its superior, posterior and anterior-inferior borders by a prominent margin called the isthmus or limbus of the oval fossa. The limbus has an anterior and a posterior rim. Sometimes the valve of the inferior vena cava extends to the anterior rim of the oval fossa. The limbus represents the margin of the previous septum secundum (Figs. 6.19, 6.20, 6.21, 6.22, 6.23, 6.24, 6.25, 6.26, 6.27, 6.28, 6.29 and 6.30).

The septum secundum is however a proper septum only in its anterior and inferior borders. Its posterior rim is actually a fold with a fibrous – adipose content derived from the atrium wall (also see embryology) (Fig. 6.31). Even though the posterior rim is initially constituted like a fold it suffers a process of consolidation. As a result, in the adult heart, this segment represents an anatomical and functional segment of the interatrial septum.

Subendocardially at the level of the limbus, there always is a more or less well-developed circular muscular fascicle of the limbus of the oval fossa (Fig. 6.25).

The limbus of the oval fossa is, however, incomplete in its inferior and posterior parts, where the inferior vena cava seems to be continuing the floor of the oval fossa. In this area, at the endocardial level, we can observe reminiscent parts of the left valve of the embryonic venous sinus with the septum primum. These reminiscent parts are the result of a defect in fusion between the two structures and they appear in variable forms, such as endocardial perforations, rudimentary network, fused membranes, and so on. However, the superior concave aspect of the left valve of the venous sinus can always be spotted. Sometimes, the inefficiency of the fusion between the valve and septum is so obvious that we can consider it a "real Chiari's network of the left valve" (Figs. 6.20, 6.21, 6.23, 6.24, 6.28 and 6.30).

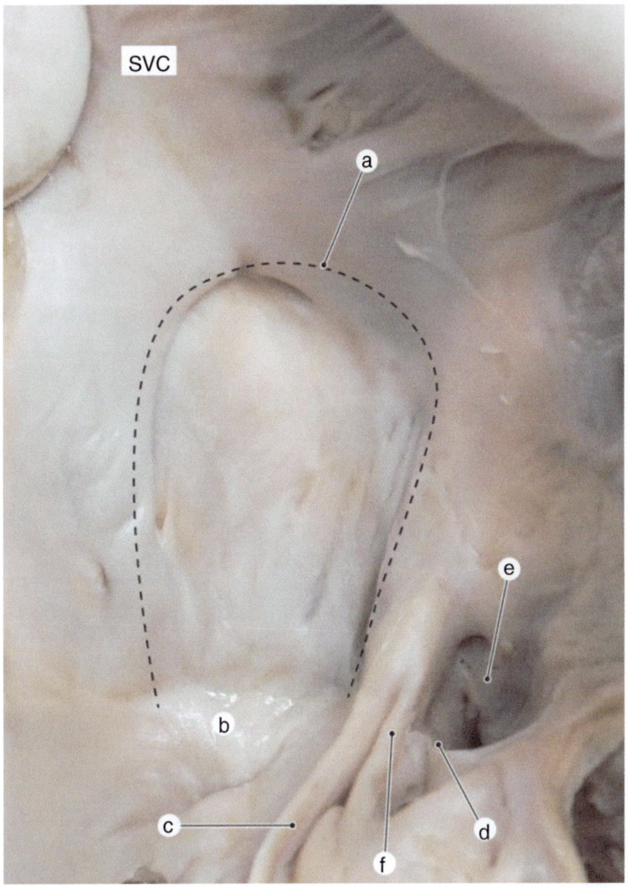

Fig. 6.19 Fossa ovalis. On the Eustachian edge is observed the differentiation between the marginal fold and the fold originating from the sinus septi. *SVC* superior vena cava, *a* limbus of the fossa ovalis, *b* dorsosinusal space, *c* eustachian edge (marginal fold), *d* membranous sinus valvule, *e* coronary sinus ostium, *f* sinus septi fold

6.1.3 The Dorso-Sinusal Region

The dorso-sinusal region is the part of the right atrium wall which lies dorsal to the terminal part of the coronary sinus. It derives from the incorporation of the right horn of the primitive venous sinus, the left valve and the sinus septi into the atrium wall.

The endocardium of this region continues the endocardium from the posterior- inferior part of the oval fossa.

The region is bounded in front by the Eustachian margin, behind by the ostium of the inferior vena cava and to its left by the interatrial septum, precisely the posterior inferior part of the oval fossa.

To its exterior, in the area of the crux cordis, it has a corresponding triangular space (the projection of the dorso-sinusal space – term proposition) which is bounded by the contour of the coronary sinus and the inferior vena cava (Fig. 6.32).

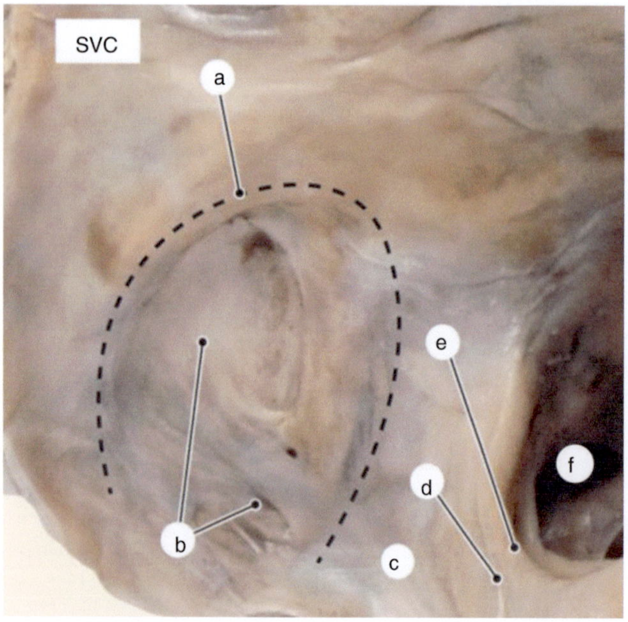

Fig. 6.20 Fossa ovalis with remainings of the left valve. The limbus does not continue with the Eustachian edge. *SVC* superior vena cava, *a* limbus of the fossa ovalis, *b* remainings of the left valve of the sinus venosus, *c* dorsosinusal space, *d* inferior vena cava valvule, *e* eustachian edge, *f* coronary sinus ostium

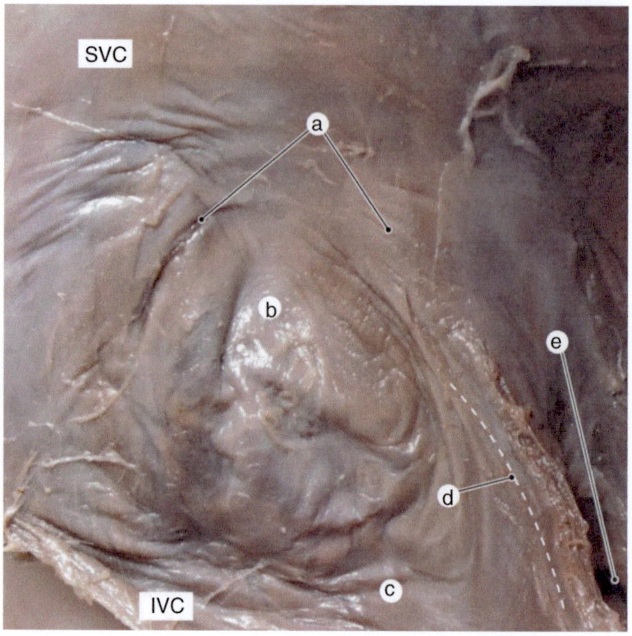

Fig. 6.22 Fossa ovalis with weak differentiation of the limbus. *SVC* superior vena cava, *IVC* Inferior vena cava. *a* limbus of the fossa ovalis, *b* floor of the fossa ovalis, *c* dorsosinusal space, *d* eustachian edge, *e* coronary sinus ostium

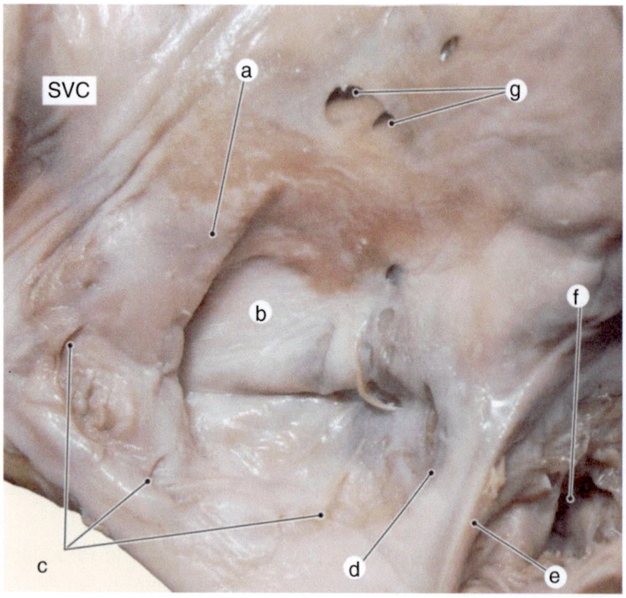

Fig. 6.21 Fossa ovalis with remainings of the left valve. Foraminae and foraminules in the superior part of the fossa. *SVC* superior vena cava, *a* limbus of the fossa ovalis, *b* floor of the fossa ovalis, *c* remainings of the left valve of the sinus venosus, *d* dorsosinusal space, *e* eustachian edge, *f* coronary sinus ostium, *g* foraminae

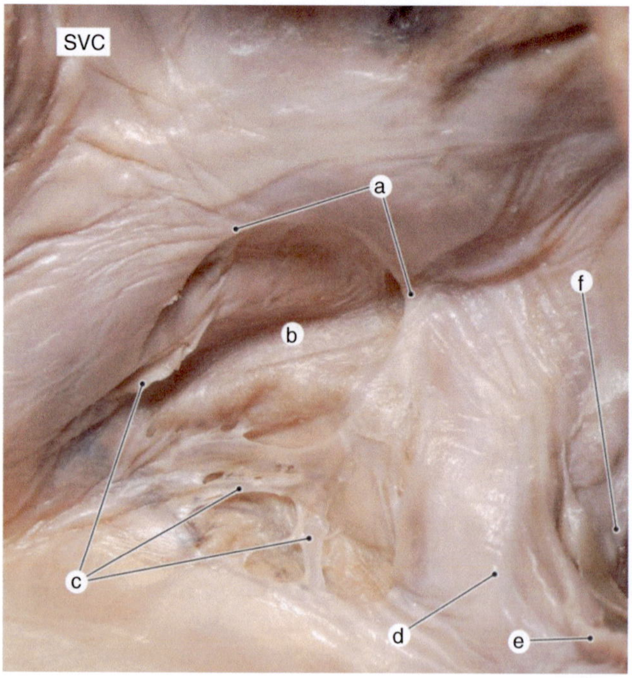

Fig. 6.23 Fossa ovalis with remainings of the left valve with coalescence deficiency. *SVC* superior vena cava, *a* limbus of the fossa ovalis, *b* floor of the fossa ovalis, *c* remainings of the left valve of the sinus venosus, *d* dorsosinusal space, *e* eustachian edge, *f* coronary sinus ostium

For better understanding of the dorsosinusal space anatomy, it is necessary to review the embryological concepts of the atrial division (also see embryology). Figures 6.33, 6.34 and 6.35 exemplify the dissection of the dorsosinusal region in successive layers.

In this area there are muscular fibers in the subendocardial space, which continue the ones in the limbus of the oval fossa and the muscular Eustachian margin.

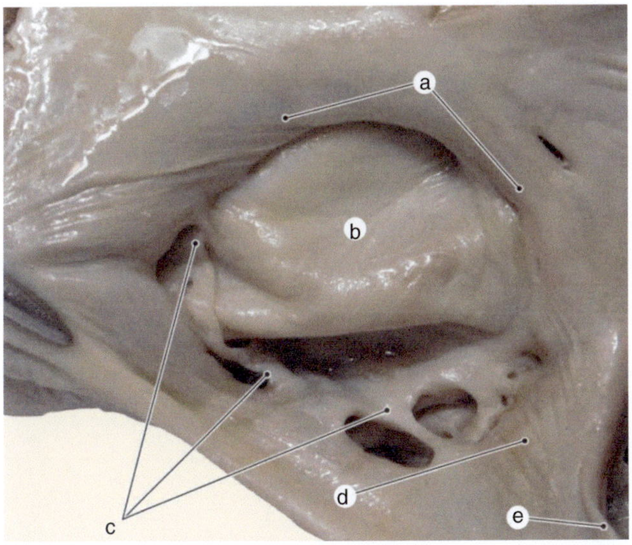

Fig. 6.24 Fossa ovalis with formation deficiency of the left valve and the dorsosinusal space. *a* limbus of the fossa ovalis, *b* floor of the fossa ovalis, *c* remainings of the left valve of the sinus venosus, *d* dorsosinusal space, *e* eustachian edge

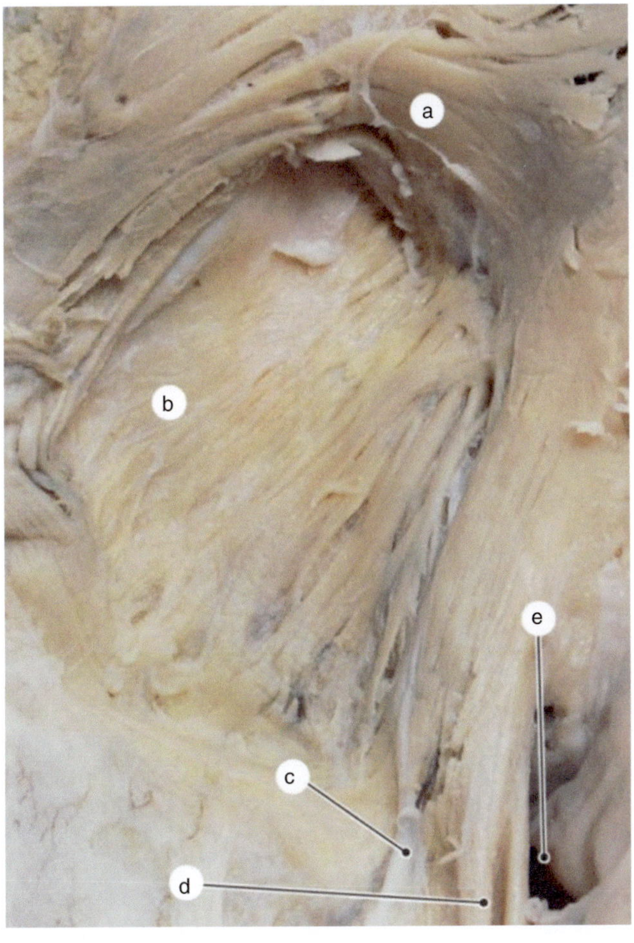

Fig. 6.25 Fossa ovalis with highlighting of the great limbic muscular fascicle. *a* circle-wise fascicle, *b* floor of the muscularized fossa ovalis, *c* inferior vena cava valvule, *d* eustachian edge, *e* coronary sinus ostium

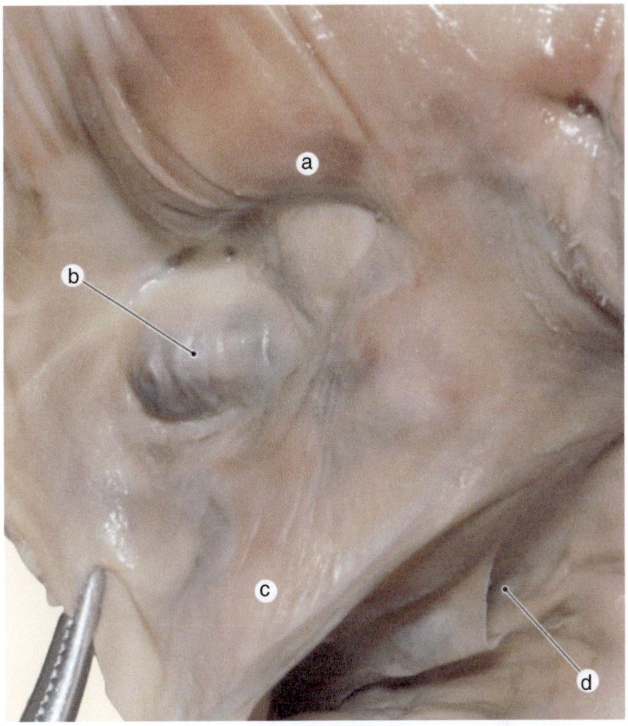

Fig. 6.26 Small tumor in the thickness of the fossa ovalis floor. *a* limbus of fossa ovalis, *b* small tumor in the thickness of the fossa ovalis floor, *c* dorsal sinus space, *d* the coronary sinus ostium

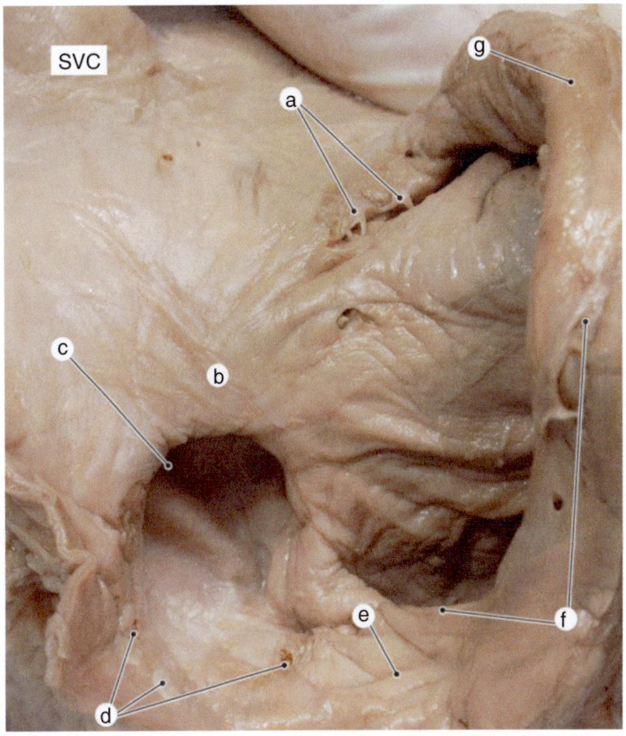

Fig. 6.27 Fossa ovalis arrangement in relation to the terminal crest. Patent interatrial communication. Reminiscences of the left valve. *SVC* superior vena cava, *a* right valve reminiscence of primitive sinus venosus, *b* limbus of fossa ovalis, *c* fossa ovalis with patent interatrial communication, *d* left valve reminiscence of primitive sinus venosus, *e* dorsosinusal space, *f* valve of the inferior vena cava, *g* atrial wall folded on the terminal crest

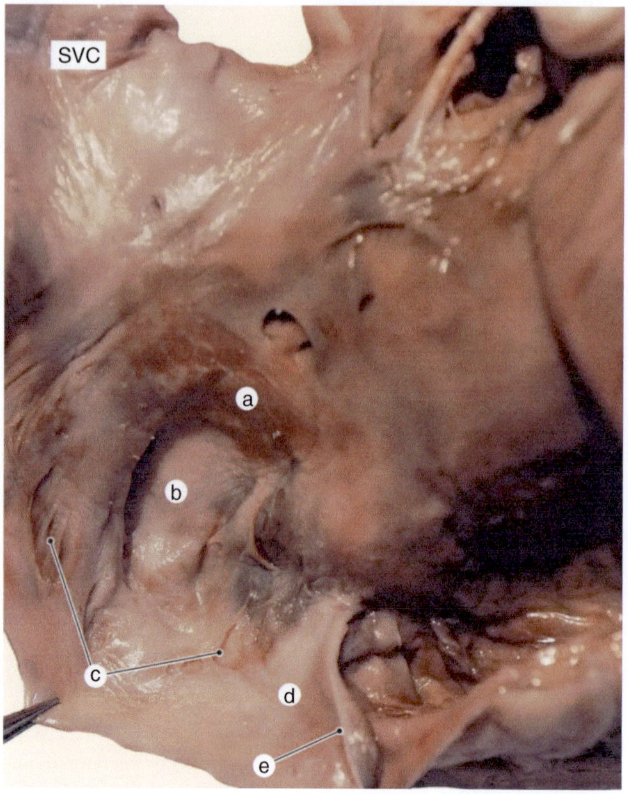

Fig. 6.28 Reminiscence of the left valve at the base of the fossa ovalis. *SVC* superior vena cava, *a* limbus of fossa ovalis, *b* fossa ovalis floor, *c* left valve reminiscence of the primitive sinus venosus, *d* dorsosinusal space, *e* eustachian edge

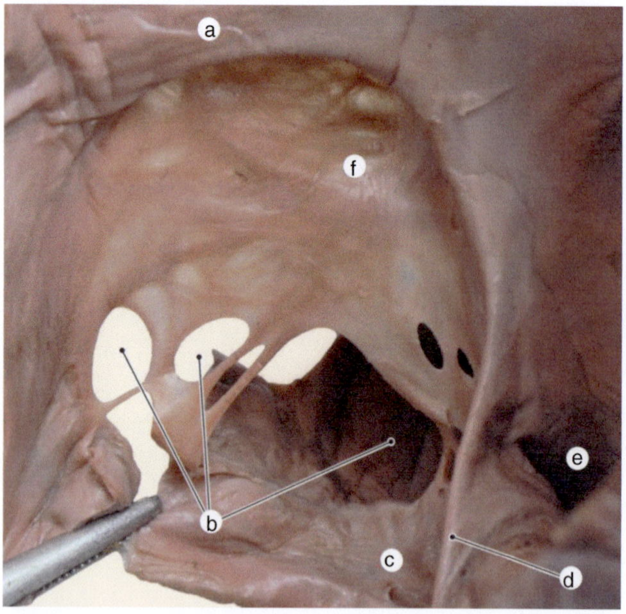

Fig. 6.29 Orifice secundum type of septal defect in the fossa ovalis floor. Notice the muscularisation of the floor and the fact that the eusctachian edge continues directly with the limbus of fossa ovalis. *a* limbus of fossa ovalis, *b* uncompensatede orifice secundum type of septal defect, *c* dorsosinusal space, *d* eustachian edge, *e* the coronary sinus ostium, *f* fossa ovalis floor partially muscled

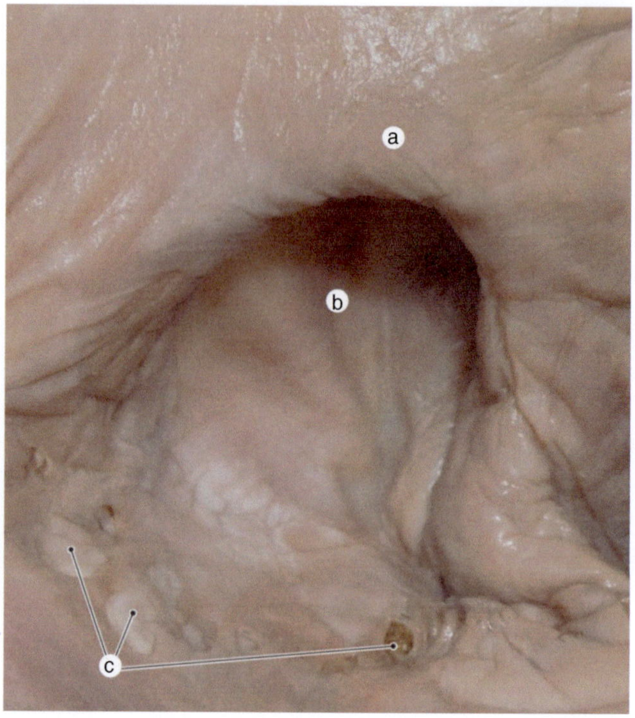

Fig. 6.30 Detail of the fossa ovalis that highlights both reminiscence of the left valve and the patent interatrial communication. *a* limbus of fossa ovalis, *b* the floor of the oval fossa with patent interatrial orifice, *c* left valve reminiscence of the primitive sinus venosus

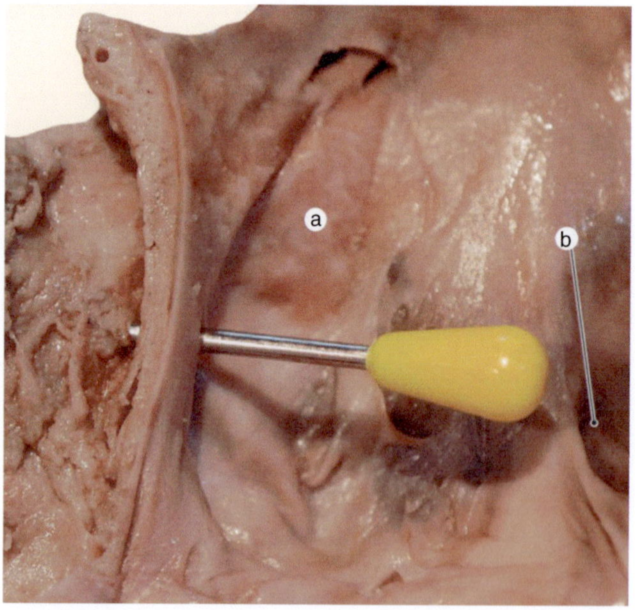

Fig. 6.31 Needle inserted into the limbus of the fossa ovalis through the right atrium, reacheas extracardiac tissue and then perforates the wall of the left atrium. In this way the fold character of the lower posterior part of the limbit is demonstrated. *a* floor of the fossa ovalis, *b* coronary sinus ostium

Under these muscle fibers, the left valve of the embryonic venous sinus has fused with the septum primum and septum secundum during the embryological period.

For this fusion to be possible, the left valve has attached itself over (probably) the vestigial part of the right umbilical vein (found as a cavernous vascular structure) and then over the terminal segment of the coronary sinus (vestigial part of the left horn of the venous sinus) (Figs. 6.33 and 6.34).

Before merging with to the septum primum, a coalescent process has taken place the septoalveolar recess (the space found in the first stages of cardiac development between the interatrial septum and the left valve of the embryonic venous sinus), which led to the disappearance of this recess.

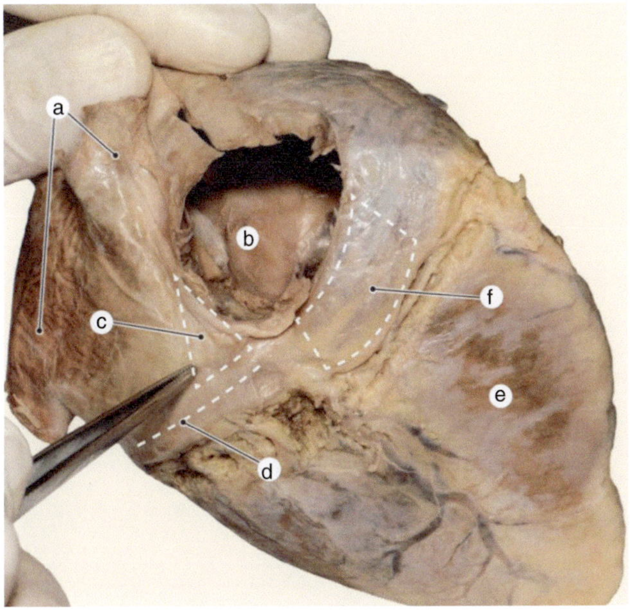

Fig. 6.32 Demonstration of the projections for the venous-tricuspid isthmus and dorsosinusal space. *a* inferior pulmonary veins, *b* inferior vena cava, *c* the projection of the dorsosinusal space, *d* coronary sinus, *e* right ventricle, *f* projection of the venous-tricuspid isthmus

Attaching itself to the septum primum, between the valve and the septum, a mesenchymal area of probable extracardiac origin was included, area known as the dorsal mesenchymal protrusion.

This mesenchymal segment suffers a muscular transformation, resulting in deep muscle fascicles which complete the limbus of the oval fossa on at its inferior side (fascicles related to the muscles of the pulmonary veins) (Fig. 6.35).

! These muscular fascicles can represent an additional pathway for conduction.

Deep in the dorsosinusal space, under all these successive structures, the sinus wall can be observed, and parallel to it the nervous fibers from the cardiac plexus (Figs. 6.36 and 6.37).

Review: in the structure of the dorsosinusal space from the luminal surface towards the deep surfaces we can find :

- Endocardium
- The subendocardial muscular layer
- The vestigial part of the left valve which covers the reminiscent septovalvular recess
- The vestigial part of the right umbilical vein (embryonic vascular-cavernous vestigial parts)
- The muscularization of the dorsal mesenchymal protrusion
- The sealing of the terminal segment of the coronary sinus (embedded in the atrium wall – chronologic stage in division).

We have made this journey in the embryogenesis of the area for understanding that the completion of atrial division is made through the consolidation of the posterior inferior part of the oval fossa and the dorsosinusal space!

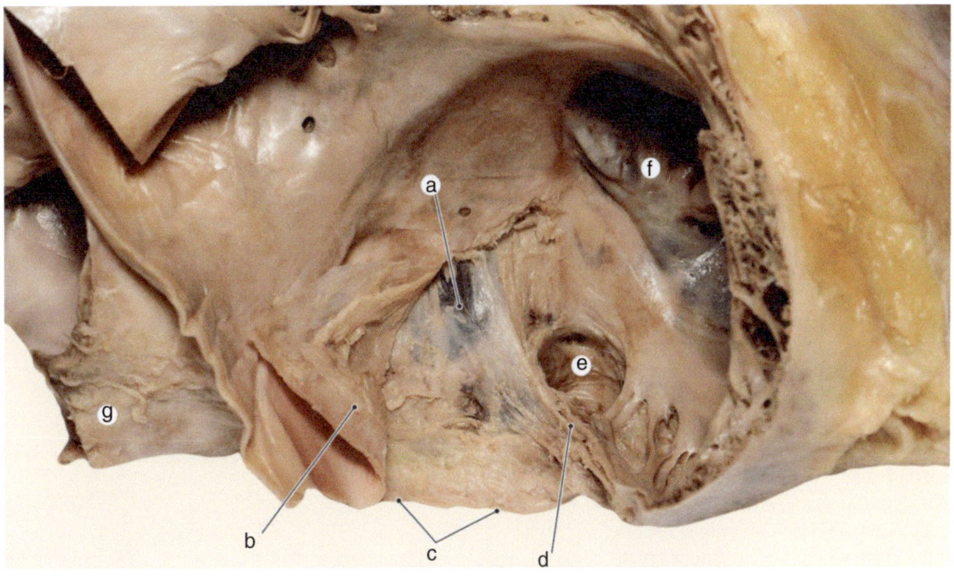

Fig. 6.33 Below the subendocardium muscle fibers we notice the reminiscences of the left valve which strengthen the floor of the fossa ovalis. The marginal fold is very well defined. *a* fossa ovalis, *b* endocardium and muscle fibers, *c* inferior vena cava, *d* eustachian edge, *e* Sinus ostium, *f* septal cusp of tricuspid valve, *g* right pulmonary veins

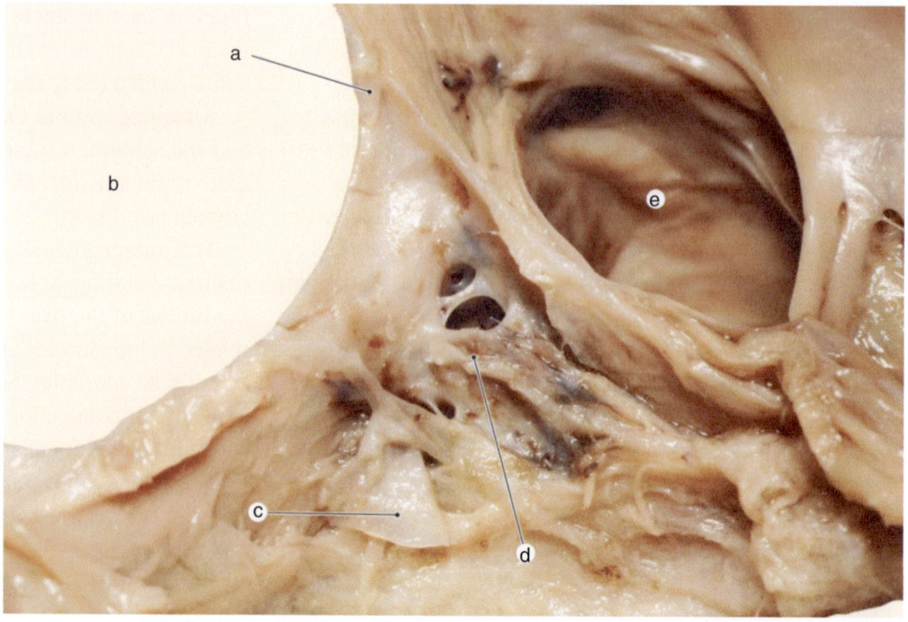

Fig. 6.34 Cavernous vascular structure in the depth of the dorsosinusal space. *a* primitive sinus valve commissure on the former septum secundum, *b* fossa ovalis, *c* left valve reminiscence, *d* cavernous vascular organ, *e* sinus ostium

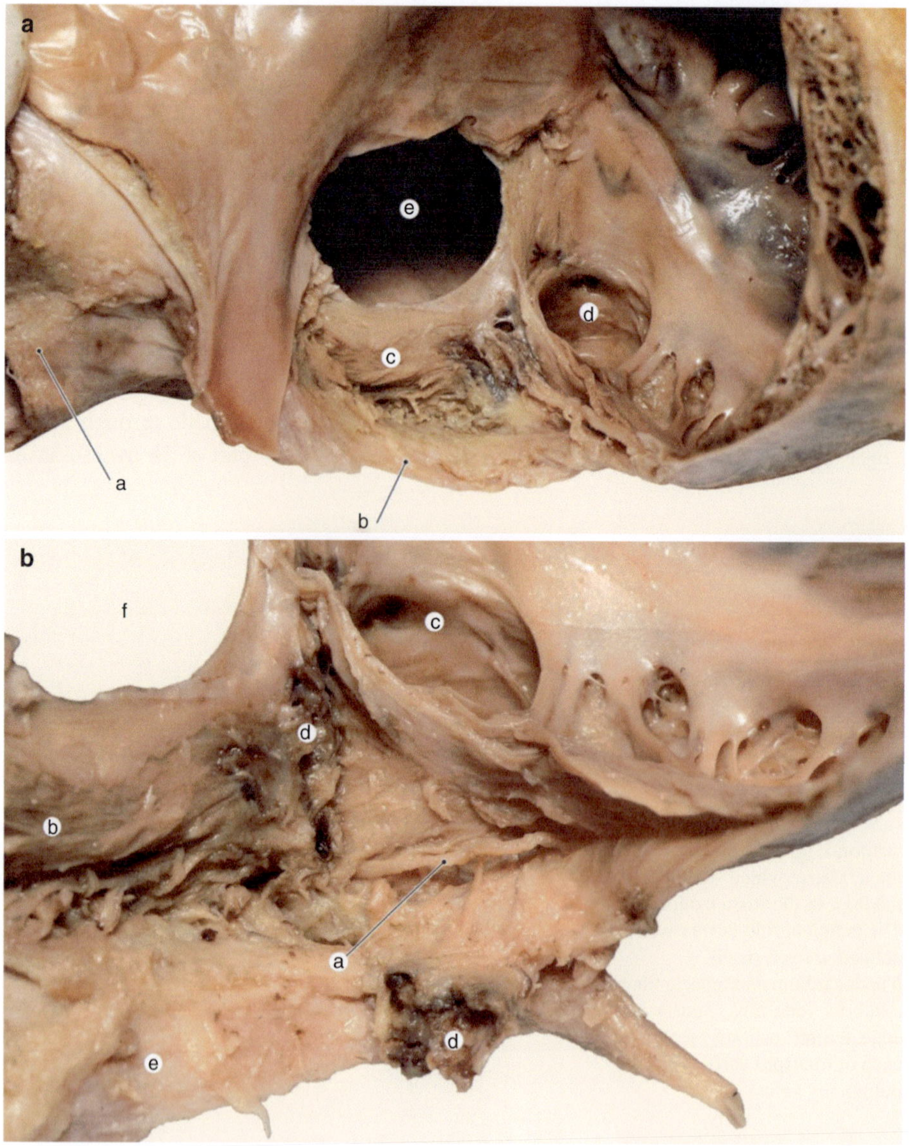

Fig. 6.35 (**a**) The muscular fascicle in the depth of the dorsosinusal space could reprezent an interatrial connection path for the electrical impulse. *a* inferior right pulmonary vein, *b* inferior vena cava, *c* profound muscular fascicle in continuation of the muscular fibres surrounding the pulmonary vein, *d* sinus ostium, *e* fossa ovalis. (**b**) A nerve trunk accompanies the sinus in the depth of dorsosinusal space. *a* nerve trunk, *b* deep muscular fascicle, *c* sinus ostium, *d* the place where the cavernous organ was resected, *e* inferior vena cava, *f* fossa ovalis

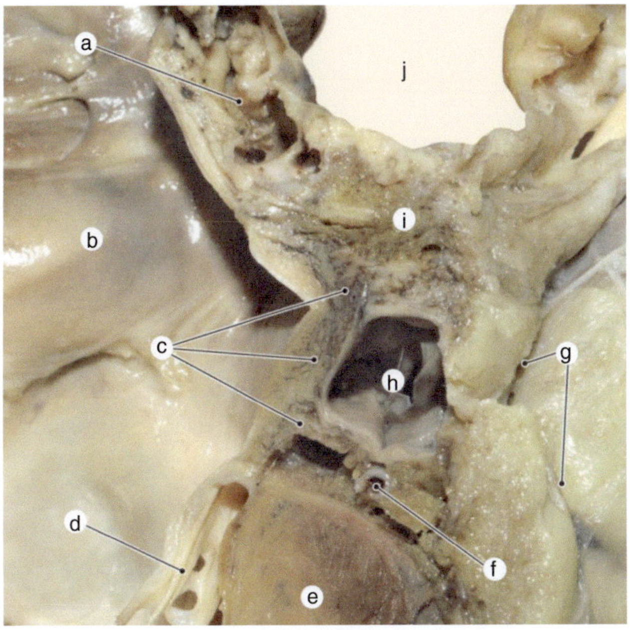

Fig. 6.36 Frontal section through the dorsosinusal space. View from the rear. Atrial septum does not reach the base of the ventricle. *a* cavernous organ, *b* left atrium, *c* perisinusal muscular fibers which continue the left atrium fibers, *d* posterior mitral cusp, *e* interventricular septum, *f* atrioventricular node artery in the pyramidal space, *g* epicardium, *h* coronary sinus, *i* dorsal sinus space, *j* right atrium

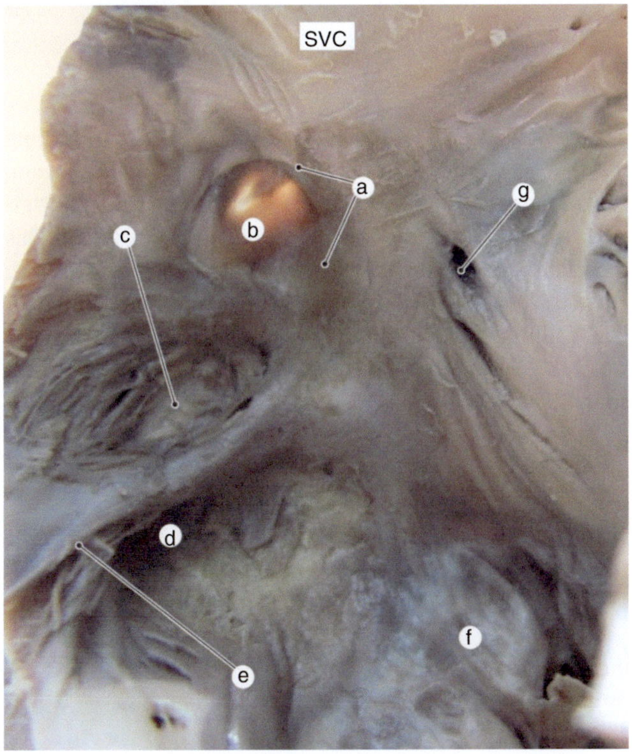

Fig. 6.37 Structural deficiency of the dorsosinusal space. View of the fossa ovalis from the right side. *SVC* superior vena cava, *a* limbus of fossa ovalis, *b* the floor of fossa ovalis, *c* structural deficiency of the dorsosinusal space due to lack of fusion of the left valve, *d* coronary sinus ostium, *e* eustachian edge, *f* septal cusp, *g* foramina

Damage to this consolidation leads to inferior interatrial-septal defects of a venous sinus type.

The protrusion of the extraembryonic mesenchyme from the dorsal mesocardium in the atrium wall is a relatively new embryological term (also see embryology).

The consolidation of the septum necessarily requires the protrusion of the extraembryonic mesenchyme, the fusion of the left valve to the septum primum, the coalescence of the septoalveolar recess as well as the formation of the posterior limbus of the septum secundum through the folding of the right atrium wall. Failure of any of these stages is followed by a specific type of interatrial defect.

For a long period of time, the importance of the dorsosinusal space for the anatomy, electrophysiology and clinical study of the heart has been underestimated. Alongside with the evolution of electrophysiological studies and development of the capacity to block reentry mechanisms, the clinical significance of this area has been reconsidered.

! The vascular cavernous structure from the depth of the dorsosinusal space has not been described until now in scientific literature. The caverns certainly communicate with the venous blood flow. This structure could have its own pathology (inflammation or thrombosis).

6.1.4 The Tricuspid Vestibule

The tricuspid vestibule is a segment of the atrial cavity that originates in the embryonic atrioventricular canal. It is represented by a circular area with smooth walls that surrounds the opening of the tricuspid valve (Fig. 6.38).

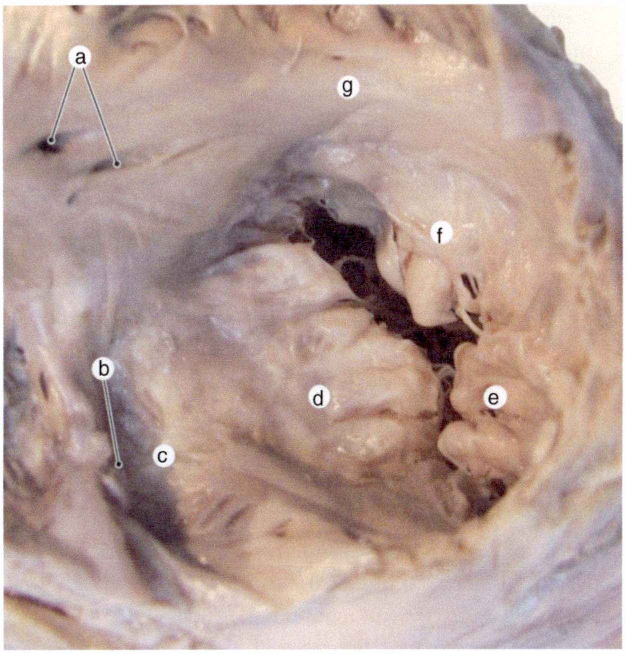

Fig. 6.38 Superior view of the tricuspid valve and tricuspid vestibule. *a* foramina, *b* coronary sinus ostium, *c* atrial floor, *d* septal cusp, *e* posterior cusp, *f* anterior cusp, *g* subauricular vestibule

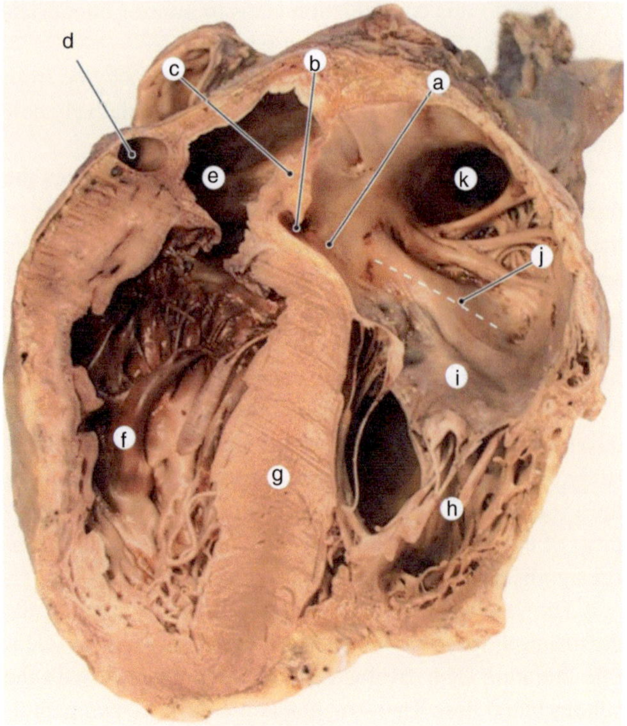

Fig. 6.39 Oblique section highlighting the four cavities. Posterior view. *a* atrial floor, *b* coronary sinus ostium, *c* interatrial septum, *d* coronary sinus, *e* left atrium, *f* left ventricle, *g* interventricular septum, *h* right ventricle, *i* anterior cusp, *j* subauricular vestibule, *k* right auricle

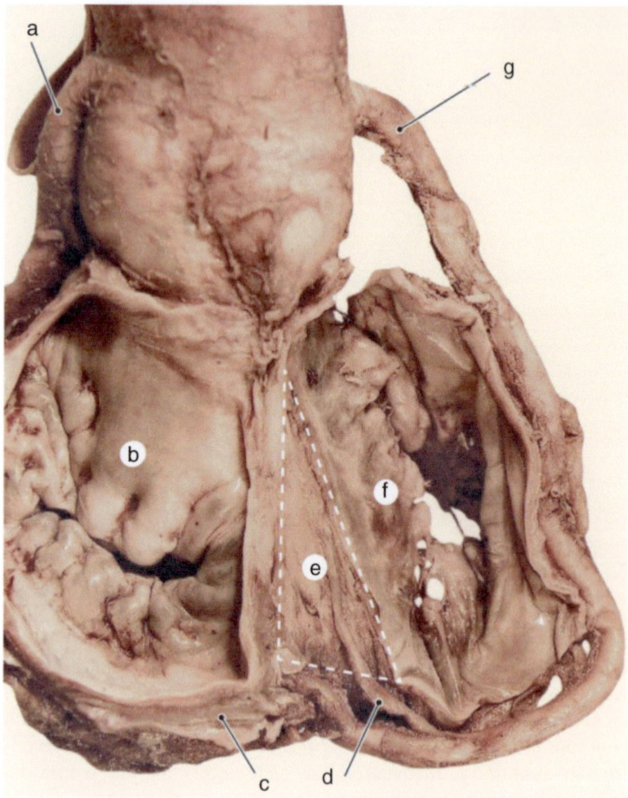

Fig. 6.40 After removal of the atria, the projection of the pyramidal space on the base of the interventricular muscular septum is highlighted. Superior and posterior view. *a* left coronary, *b* anterior cusp, *c* coronary venous sinus, *d* atrioventricular node artery, *e* floor of the pyramidal space, *f* septal cusp, *g* right coronary

The vestibule can be divided into several territories. The names of these territories are disputed and they are not adopted neither by the anatomical schools nor by nomina anatomica. We shall define these terms in the way that they are used in clinical anatomy.

These terms are: the atrial floor, the cavotricuspid isthmus, the subeustachian and thebesian sinuses, the Koch triangle, the subauricular part of the tricuspid vestibule.

6.1.5 The Floor of the Right Atrium

The floor of the right atrium is difficult to guess because the atrium is configured superiorly to the ventricle in many descriptions or representations. In these representations, the atrium has a floor located behind the tricuspid opening. In reality, the right atrium is located more to the posterior than superior to the right atrioventricular opening and the plane of the tricuspid opening is located on the anterior wall of the atrium. The term of "floor" is still kept and it refers mainly to the part of the atrial wall located between the attachment of the septal cusp, the eustachian border and the base of the interatrial septum (Figs. 6.39 and 6.40).

The ostium of the coronary sinus represents the opening of the biggest vein of the heart in the floor of the right atrium. It is bordered posteromedially by a muscular fold that originates from sinus septi and by the eustachian border. This muscular fold is often mistaken for the ostial valve. The valve is an endocardic fold that borders variably (medially or laterally) the ostium of the coronary sinus and it originates from the right valve of the primitive venous sinus. It can sometimes be absent or can have exaggerated dimensions (exuberant) (Figs. 6.41, 6.42 and 6.43).

The terminal crest unfolds inferiorly its muscular fibers like a fan, in a thin subendocardic layer.

These longitudinal subendocardic fibers reach the atrioventricular node forming the atrial floor (see excitoconductor system).

This thin subendocardic muscular layer is separated from the crest of the interventricular septum and the base of the right ventricle by a layer of connective-adipose tissue which continues the subepicardic adipose tissue from the crux cordis. The connective-adipose lamina enters between the right atrium and ventricle below and around the terminal segment of the coronary sinus.

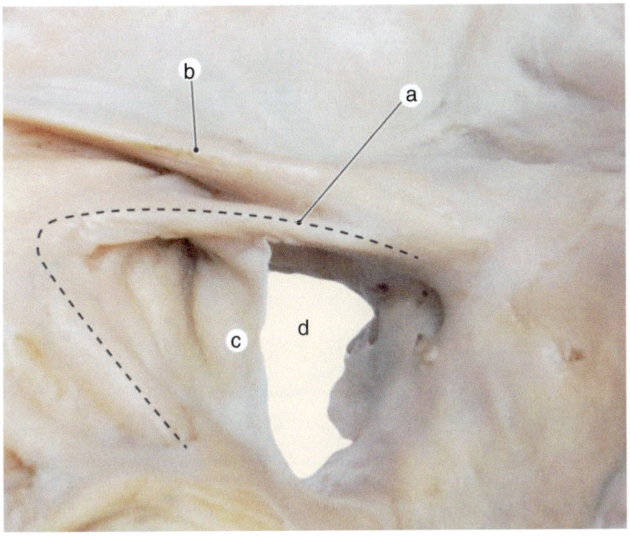

Fig. 6.41 Detail of the coronary sinus ostium, with explicit periosteal structures. *a* muscular edge from sinus septi, *b* Eustachian edge originating from the marginal fold, *c* Sinus valve originating from the right valve, *d* Coronary sinus ostium

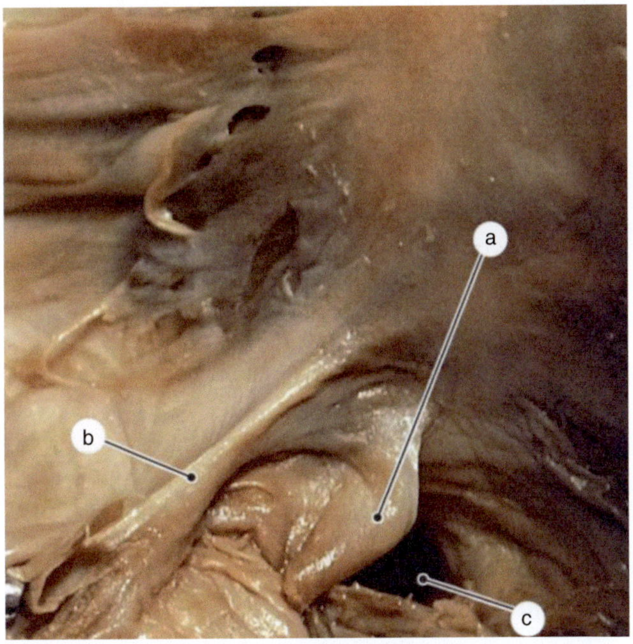

Fig. 6.42 An exuberant valve of the sinus ostium can make more difficult the catheterisation procedure. *a* exuberant valve sinus, *b* eustachian edge, *c* coronary sinus ostium

The artery of the node, the veins and the nervous fibers reach the atrioventricular node through this connective-adipose lamina.

The space occupied by this connective-adipose lamina, located in the fold between the atrial wall and the base of the ventricle is called the pyramidal space (Fig. 6.36).

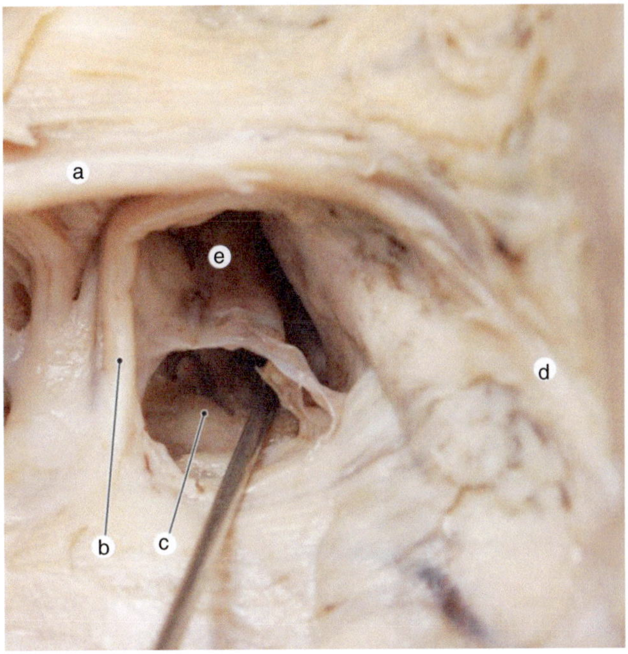

Fig. 6.43 When the medium vein is draining into the right atrium at the level of the sinus ostium, sinus catheterisation can be missed. *a* eustachian edge arising from marginal fold, *b* muscular edge arising from sinus septi, *c* medium vein ostium, *d* todaro tendon, *e* coronary sinus ostium

The performance of ablation procedures on the atrial wall presents the risk of injuring the nodal artery that crosses through this space either from the right coronary artery or from the left one.

In conclusion, if we insert a needle through the floor of the right atrium we first reach the pyramidal space, located extra cardially, and then enter the base of the right ventricle.

The division of the heart is not a process that results in symmetric chambers. While the vestibule of the left atrium is relatively symmetric, in the right atrium the vestibule is asymmetric. The floor of the right atrium coats a part of the base of the right ventricle and a part of the posterior segment of the crest of the interventricular septum (Fig. 6.39).

To have a correct image we remind you that the two atrioventricular rings are connected through the right fibrous triangle (the tendinous center). This triangle is located towards the left of the interventricular septum – it literally "floats" in the vestibule of the aorta (see the fibrous skeleton). The right triangle is a landmark for the base of the interatrial septum. We understand now that according to the width of the crest of the interventricular septum, the interatrial septum is moved towards the left and the floor of the right atrium lines the crest of the interventricular septum and the base of the right ventricle.

The left horn of the valve of the inferior vena cava is sometimes continued on the floor of the right atrium by the valve of the coronary sinus (these valves have a common

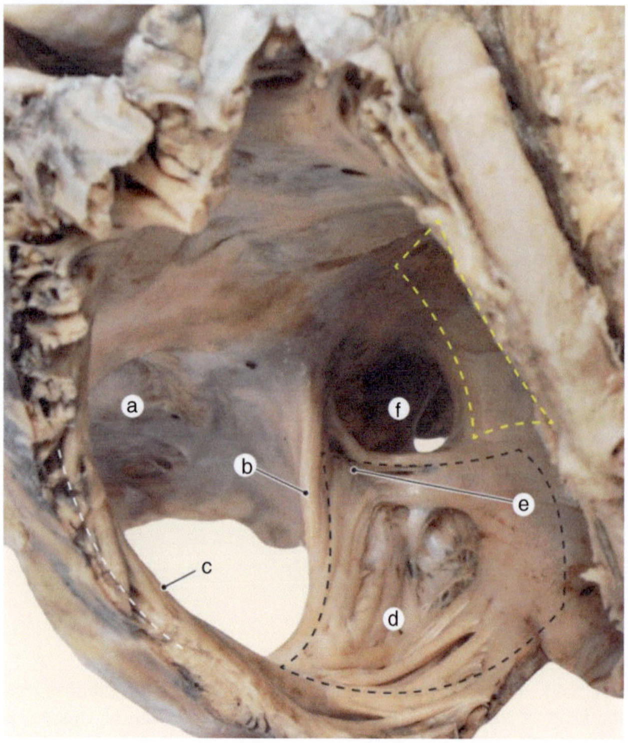

Fig. 6.44 Right atrium after the resection of the primitive wall. The position of the septal isthmus (*yellow line*) and the venous-tricuspid isthmus (*black line*). *a* fossa ovalis, *b* eustachian edge, *c* terminal crest, *d* subeustachian sinus, *e* subthebesian sinus, *f* coronary sinus ostium

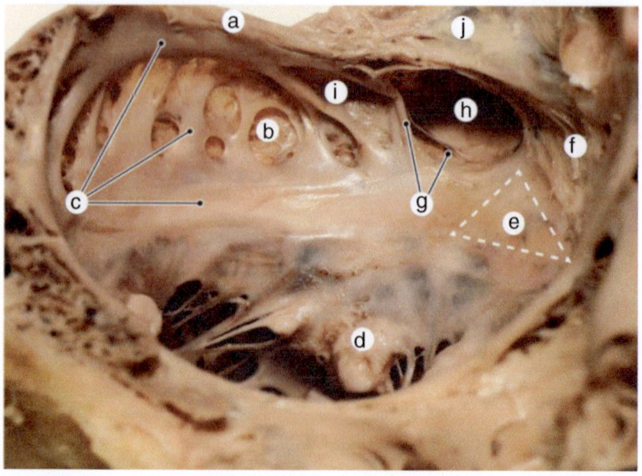

Fig. 6.45 Venous-tricuspid isthmus and vestibular topography. Anterior view. *a* eustachian edge, *b* subeustachian sinus, *c* venous-tricuspid isthmus (trabecular, central and anterior parts), *d* septal cusp, *e* Koch triangle, *f* septal isthmus, *g* thebesian valve, *h* sinusal ostium, *i* subthebesian sinus, *j* dorsosinusal space

embriological origin in the valve of the primitive venous sinus). In other cases, it is continued by the anterior extremity of the limbus of the fossa ovalis (this is also normal because at this level – of the septum secundum- the two valves of the primitive venous sinus have a merging area) (Figs. 2.48, 2.49 and 2.50).

6.1.5.1 The Spetal Isthmus and Cavotricuspid Isthmus

The septal isthmus is located on the floor of the right atrium, at the root of the interatrial septum, between the border of the coronary sinus and the insertion of the septal cusp. In the anatomical position of the heart, it is located superiorly to the cavotricuspid isthmus, for that being called the superior isthmus (Fig. 6.44).

This isthmus is crossed by the nervous impulse that follows the “slow path” in it’s way towards the atrioventricular node [1].

The cavotricuspid isthmus occupies most of the atrial floor.

It is bordered by the eustachian border and valve posteriorly and by the insertion of the septal cusp anteriorly; by the thebesian valve superiorly and inferiorly by a line that connects the opening of the vena cava with the insertion of the tricuspid valve.

It is also called the inferior isthmus, in order to be differentiated from the septal isthmus, located superiorly (Fig. 6.45).

The cavotricuspid isthmus is a major part of the circuit responsible for most types of flutter [2].

The cavotricuspid (or inferior) isthmus has three parts:

- The trabeculated part, represented by the eustachian border. It is also called the posterior sector. Its structure consists of a fibro-adipose component and muscular fibers (see the formation of the eustachian border).
- The central part, membranous, represented by the two subeustachian and subthebesian recesses (or the Keith sinus). Here its aspect is characterized by the presence of some muscular trabeculae that divide very thin membranous segments.
- The anterior part, vestibular, located in the vicinity of the insertion of the septal cusp. This part is smooth, nontrabeculated, its wall being formed entirely by thin atrial miocardium. The myocardial fibers that emerge from the terminal crest are generally parallel and lead towards the Koch triangle. However, in the vicinity of the sinusal opening there are still some crossings of muscular fibers.

6.1.5.2 The Tendon of Todaro

The tendon of Todaro is a fibrous subendocardic, inconstant cord, with variable development and aspect. It is about 0.5–1.5 cm long and 1–2 mm thick. Most frequently, after cutting and removing the endocardium, it appears as a thin connective cord, bright white, resembling a tendinous cord. Its insertion is on the right triangle, above the atrioventricular node. Its origin fades at the level of the left horn of the Eustachian valve, in the dorsosinusal space.

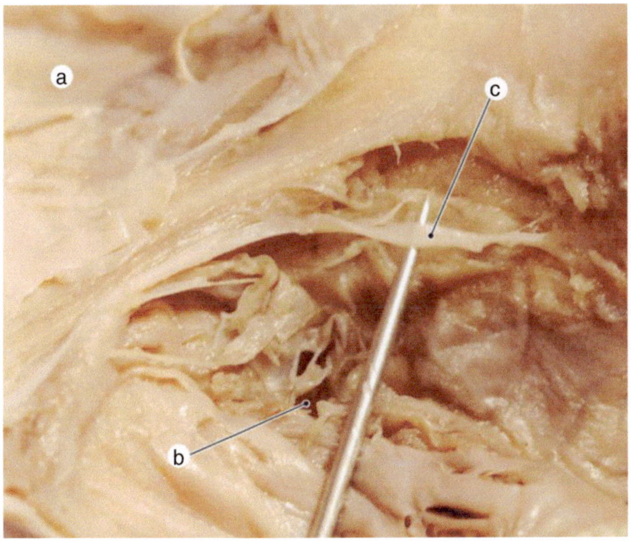

Fig. 6.46 Highlighting the tendon of Todaro. *a* dorsosinusal space, *b* coronary sinus ostium, *c* tendon of Todaro

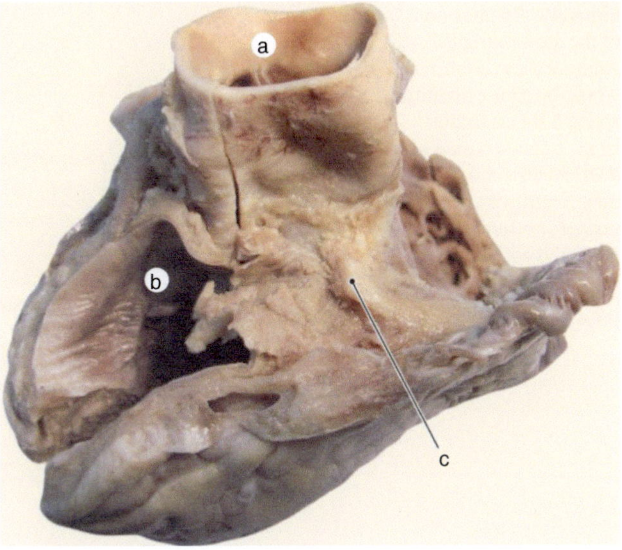

Fig. 6.48 Base of the ventricular pyramid after removing the atria. *a* aorta, *b* left atrium, *c* tendon of Todaro turned cartilaginous

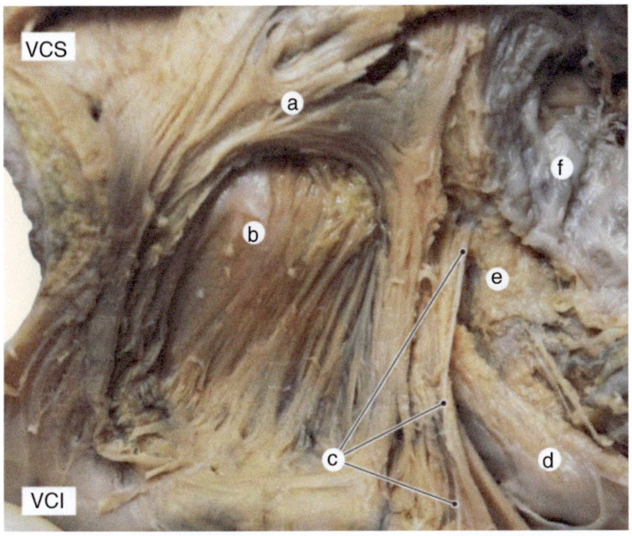

Fig. 6.47 The tendon of Todaro begins in the dorsosinusal space and inserts in the tendinous center, superior to the atrioventricular node. Posterior and lateral view. *a* limbic fascicle, *b* the floor of the muscled fossa ovalis, *c* todaro tendon, *d* coronary sinus ostium, *e* atrioventricular node, *f* septal cusp

The tendon of Todaro may have a fibro-cartilaginous appearance. It is sometimes replaced by a muscular trabecula that extends from the limbus of the fossa ovale, taking the name of the tendon of Todaro (Figs. 6.46, 6.47 and 6.48).

6.1.5.3 The Koch Triangle

The need for some topographical guidance for the location of the atrioventricular node led to the definition of the Koch triangle.

This is located in the left extremity of the floor of the atrium, in the angle between the base of the septum and the insertion of the septal cusp.

When subendocardially we can find and palpate the tendon of Todaro at the base of the interatrial septum, the region is called the Koch triangle. This region actually corresponds mostly to the superior isthmus.

The atrioventricular node is located in the anterior and superior angle of the triangle.

Underneath the endocardium of this region there can be found the artery of the atrioventricular node, coming from the crux cordis or from the right coronary groove.

The triangle has the following borders:

- Anteriorly and to the left, at the apex of the triangle, by the right fibrous triangle and the membranous septum. The fibrous triangle can be felt endocardially. It is crossed by the perforating part of the Hiss bundle.
- The left border is formed anteriorly by the tendon of Todaro (subendocardic and intramuscular) and posteriorly by the ostium of the coronary sinus.
- The right border is an imaginary line that continues anteriorly the right part of the ostium of the coronary sinus, up to the intersection with the insertion of the septal cusp.
- The anterior border is the insertion line of the septal cusp, up to the right fibrous trigone (Figs. 6.49).

In the area of the triangle, at the tip, there lies the atrioventricular node. More precisely, the node is located at the base of the right ventricle, bordered by the right fibrous triangle, contained partially in the connective-adipose lamina between the floor of the right atrium and the base of the right ventricle (at the tip of the pyramidal space).

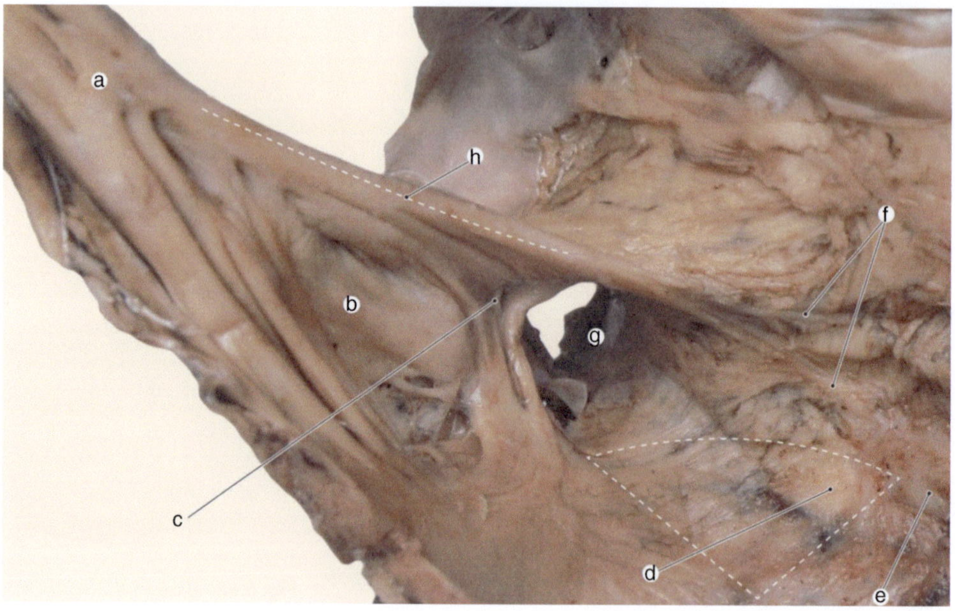

Fig. 6.49 The position of the atrioventricular node. Anterior view. *a* terminal crest whose inferior extremity splits, *b* subeustachian sinus, *c* subthebesian sinus, *d* atrioventricular node, *e* atrioventricular septum, *f* bifurcated Todaro tendon, *g* coronary sinus ostium, *h* eustachian edge

! The quick definition of the triangle can be made as follows: in the right atrium, the floor has a flat region located between the origin of the septal cusp, the ostium of the venous sinus and the base of the interatrial septum. The left and superior extremity of this region is the Koch triangle.

6.1.5.4 The Terminal Crest

The terminal crest is a muscular semicircular prominence that separates the atrial territory derived from the primitive atrium from the atrial territory derived from the venous sinus. On the outer surface it corresponds to a shallow groove called the sulcus terminalis. It derives from the fusion of the terminal fasciculus and the marginal fold (see embryology).

The terminal crest describes an almost circular course, beginning and ending in contact with the interatrial septum and it splits the right atrium embryologically, morphologically and functionally Figs. 6.12, 6.49, 6.50 and 6.51).

The terminal crest begins superiorly at the right of the opening of the superior vena cava (it is here in relative continuity with a sagitaltrabecula inside the right auriculus) (Fig. 6.9). It then descends on the anterior-lateral wall of the atrium. On this wall it gives two types of muscular trabeculae:

- one group of almost vertical ascending trabeculae, located in the upper part of the crest, difficult to spot and to demonstrate, that lie between the atrial crest and the atrial wall. These muscular cords are thin and they are usually continued by the subepicardic muscle fibers (Fig. 6.10).
- the second group of trabeculae consists of large, anteriorly-oblique elements, known as the pectinate muscles. Their branching pattern varies. The muscular fibers that form the pectinate muscles have their embryological origin in the primitive atrium (Figs. 6.2 and 6.3).

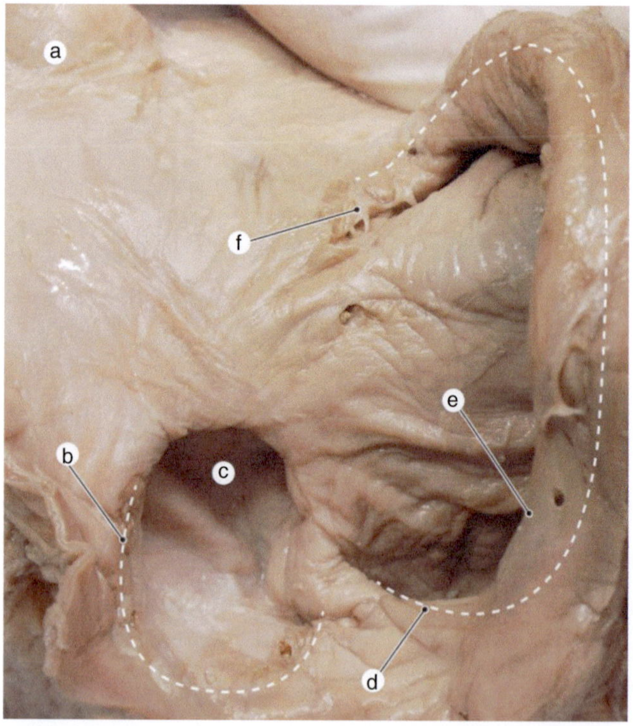

Fig. 6.50 Right atrium from the right and rear view. The atrial wall was folded over the terminal crest so the general disposition of the terminal crest can be highlighted. Valvular reminiscences (marked with *dotted lines*) demonstrate the initial disposition of the primitive sinus valves. *a* superior vena cava, *b* left valve reminiscence, *c* interatrial patent orifice, *d* right valve reminiscence, *e* inferior vena cava valve, *f* right valve reminiscence (named by some "superior vena cava valve")

The pectinate muscles also enter the right auriculus. The pectinate muscles sometimes attach on the sagital trabecula following a pattern that resembles the fibers of a palm-tree

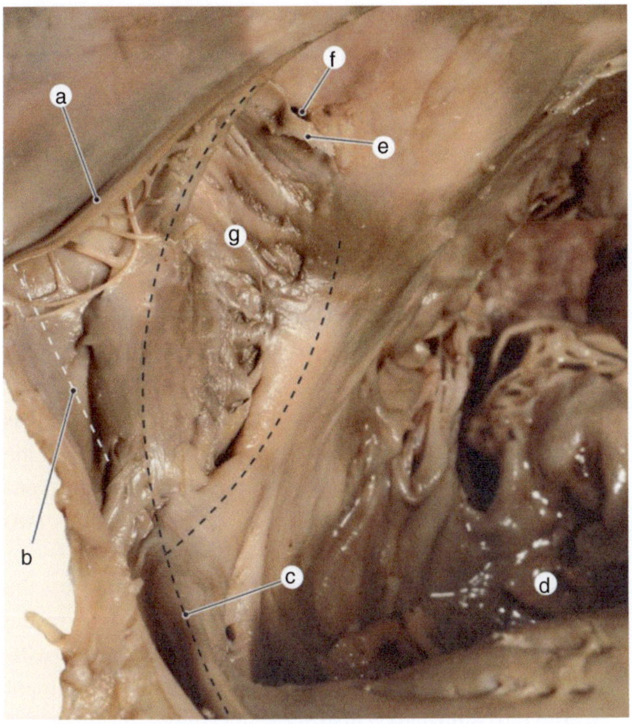

Fig. 6.51 Due to a deficiency of coalescence of the right valve, in an adult heart a rest of venous-marginal recess can be noticed. The existence of the superior bifurcation fascicle of the terminal crest explains the possibility of impulse conduction through the trabeculated part of the venous-tricuspid isthmus. View from the right and superior. *a* valve of the inferior vena cava, *b* venous-marginal recess with incomplete coalescence, *c* terminal crest which bifurcates inferiorly, *d* posterior cusp, *e* thebesian valve, *f* sinusal ostium, *g* subeustachian sinus

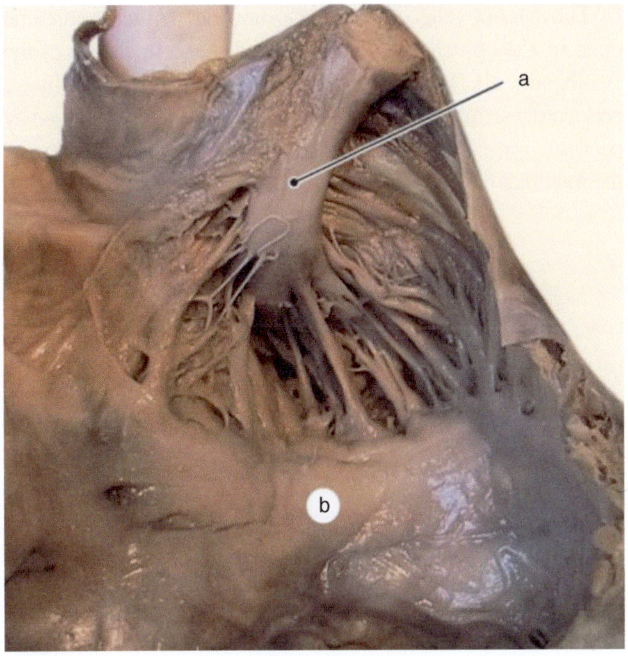

Fig. 6.52 Variant of distribution of the pectinate muscles in the right auricle. *a* sagittal trabeculae in the axis of the right auricle, *b* subauricular vestibule

leaf (Fig. 6.52). Other times, the distribution of the pectinate muscles is "palmed" (Fig. 6.6).

The atrial wall between the pectinate muscles is very thin, having a membranous aspect.

The behavior of the terminal crest towards the atrial floor is inconstant. It generally divides into two muscular fascicles, with a variable aspect (Figs. 6.49 and 6.51), called the posterior and anterior fascicles.

The posterior fascicle lines the valve of the inferior vena cava (Eustachio), forming together the eustachian border.

In intrauterine developement there is a cavomarginal recess[1] (proposed term) between the right valve of the embryonary venous sinus and the marginal fold.

This recess disappears through a coalescence process so that in the adult the Eustachian valve adheres to the terminal crest. Some rudimentary chordae may remain as imperfections of this coalescence (Fig. 6.51).

The anterior fascicle heads towards the septal cusp, some of its fibers diverging as a fan in the subendocardic layer of the floor of the atrium.

The muscle fibers of both fascicles reach the atrioventricular node.

There is a so-called "subeustachian" recess that generally has few muscular trabeculae. The atrial wall in this region is thin, membranous. Towards the left side of the subeustachian recess, in connection with the ostium of the coronary sinus there is a smaller recess, called the subthebesian recess (the sinus of Keith) (Fig. 6.49).

The right horn of the valve of the inferior vena cava is sometimes continued upwards by remnants of the right valve of the embryonary venous sinus. They reach the right side of the opening of the inferior vena cava as small membranes or tendinous chordae sometimes being excessively considered as proof of existence of a valve of the superior vena cava (Fig. 6.50).

6.1.5.5 The Subauricular Part of the Vestibule of the Right Atrium

The subauricular part of the vestibule is the segment of the vestibule located anteriorly and superiorly, between the base of the right auricle and the tricuspid ring. It is embryologically derived from the incorporation in the atrial wall of a part of the right atrioventricular junction (Fig. 2.80).

This part corresponds on the exterior to the right anterior segment of the coronary groove. The openings of some thebesian veins can be seen here.

[1]In many medical dictionaries, the terms infundibulum and conus are considered synonyms. This is due to a great variability of the existence of the infundibular territory. The infundibulum is sometimes very short and even absent while other times it has the appearance of a well-structured cylindrical segment (Figs. 4.8 and 4.35)

The anterior veins of the right atrium and ventricle sometime open in a deep venous channel located in the thickness of the vestibular wall. This channel has an entrance bordered by an endocardic semilunar fold (sometimes the entrance is covered by pectinate muscles). The length and diameter of the channel vary, the maximal dimensions being 2.6/0.6 cm (Figs. 6.53 and 6.54).

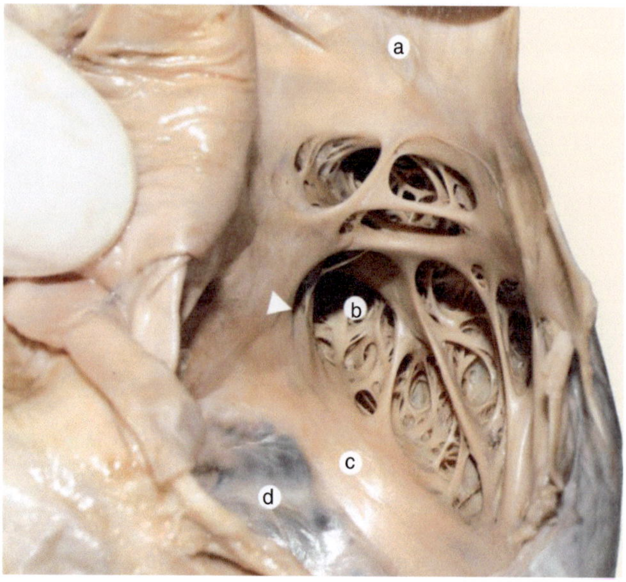

Fig. 6.53 Demonstration of the subaricular vestibule in the right atrium. The *arrowhead* indicates the drainage orifice of a deep venous canal. *a* superior vena cava, *b* right auricle, *c* subauricular vestibule, *d* anterior cusp

The aortic noncoronary sinus together with the fibrous center of the heart (the right fibrous triangle) lifts a prominence called the aortic torus in the right atrium.

An aneurysm of the aortic sinus (Valsalva) may burst in the right atrium (evolution favored by this rapport – Skandalakis) (Fig. 6.55).

6.1.5.6 Other Morphological Landmarks of the Cavity of the Right Atrium: The Atrioventricular Septum, Sinus Venarum, Crista Interveniens, Crista Dividens, Intercaval Tubercle

The commissure between the anterior and the septal cusps of the tricuspid valve (sometimes only the origin of the septal cusp) divides the membranous part of the interventricular septum (pars membranaceea septi) into two segments:

- the superior segment (inconstant) is represented by the membranous atrioventricular septum and belongs to the right atrium. It separates the right atrium from the vestibule of the aorta (the last part of the ejection compartment of the left ventricle) – also see embryology. Its surface is about 0.5 cm^2.
- the inferior segment belongs to the right ventricle and it forms the interventricular membranous septum. This septum is located exactly underneath the ring of the tricuspid opening, it is about 0.5–1 cm cm^2 in surface and it separates the right ventricle from the aortic vestibule (Figs. 6.56, 6.57, 6.58 and 6.59).

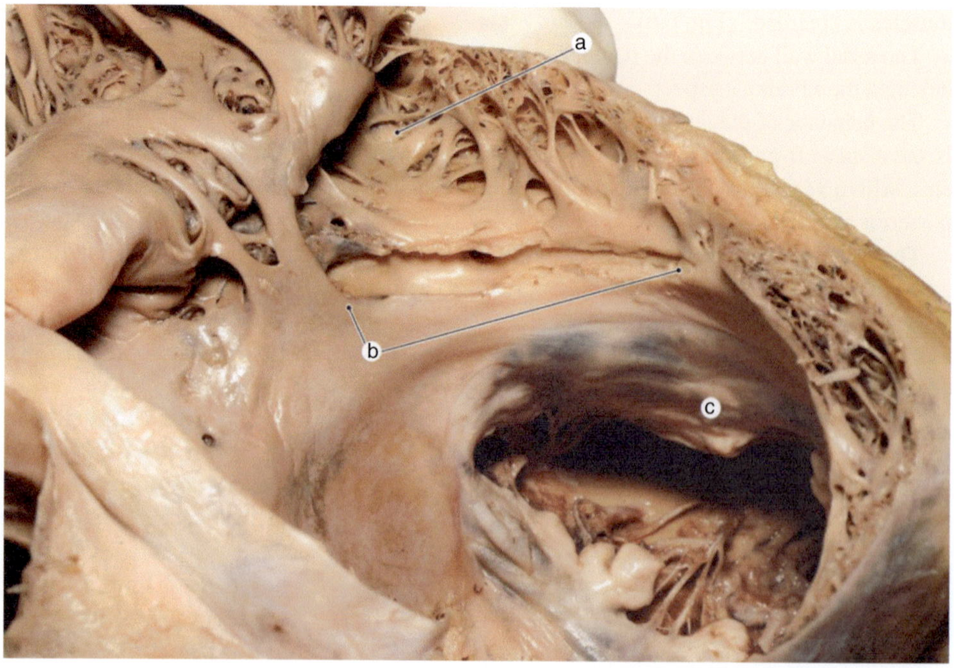

Fig. 6.54 Profound venous canal– stripped on its entire length. It can be observed in its lumen the drainage orifices of some anterior veins. *a* right auricle, *b* profound venous canal in the subauricular vestibule, *c* anterior cusp

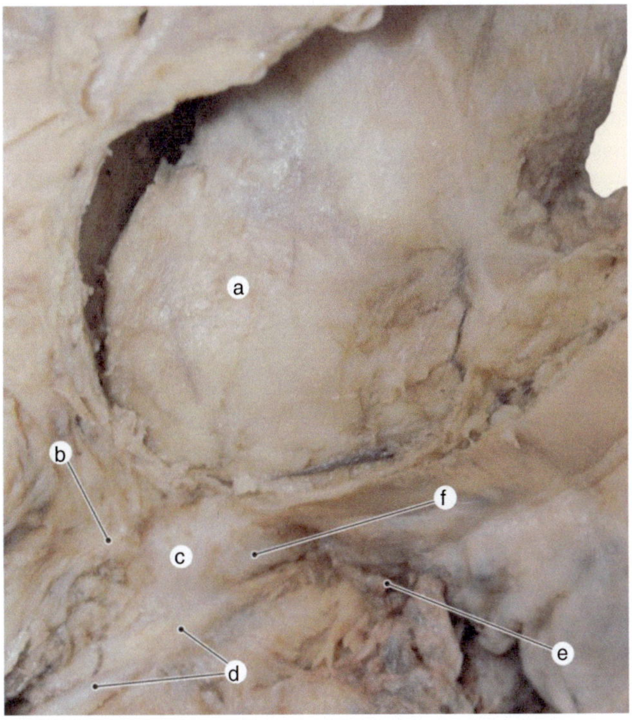

Fig. 6.55 The proeminence of the atrial wall (torus) determined by the compression of the noncoronarian aortic sinus was cropped to understand the intimacy of anatomical relation. View from the right and rear. *a* noncoronarian aortic sinus, *b* tendon of Todaro, *c* tendinous center, *d* atrioventricular node and its artery, *e* valvular commissure, *f* atrioventricular membranous septum

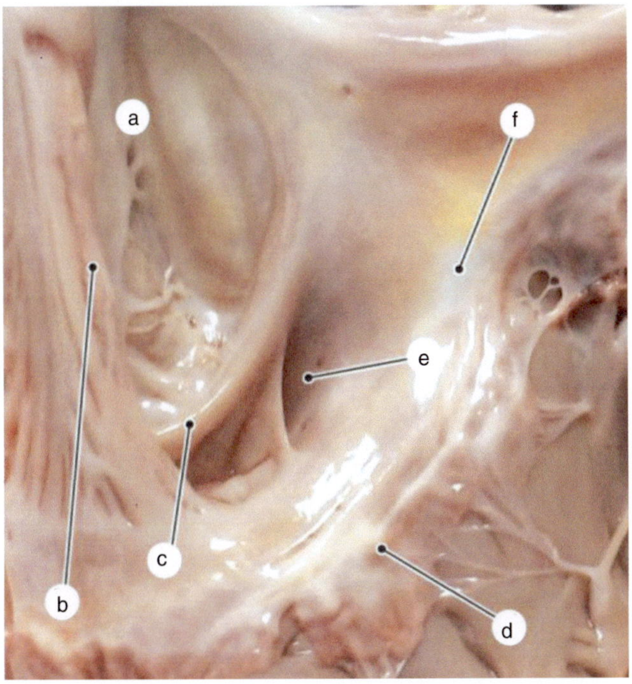

Fig. 6.56 Position of the atrioventricular septum. The heart showed was not preserved in formaldehyde. *a* fossa ovalis, *b* terminal crest, *c* eustachian edge, *d* septal cusp, *e* sinus ostium, *f* atrioventricular ostium

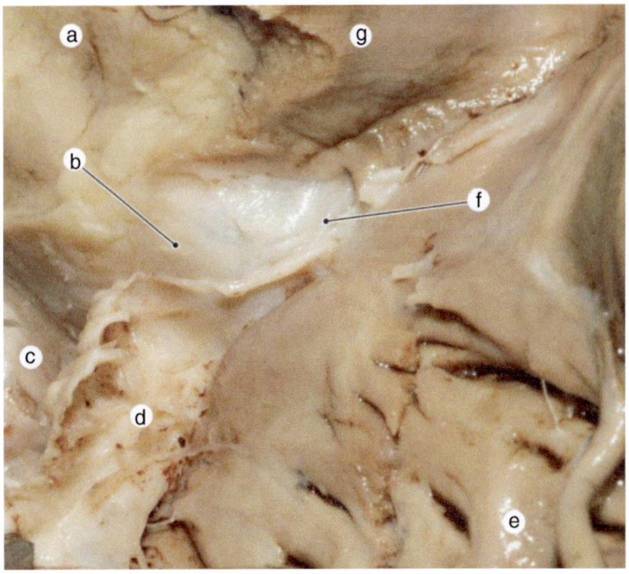

Fig. 6.57 Membranous septum, view from the right side of the heart. *a* aorta, *b* atrioventricular septum, *c* right atrium, *d* septal cusp, *e* right ventricle, *f* interventricular membranous septum, *g* supraventricular crest

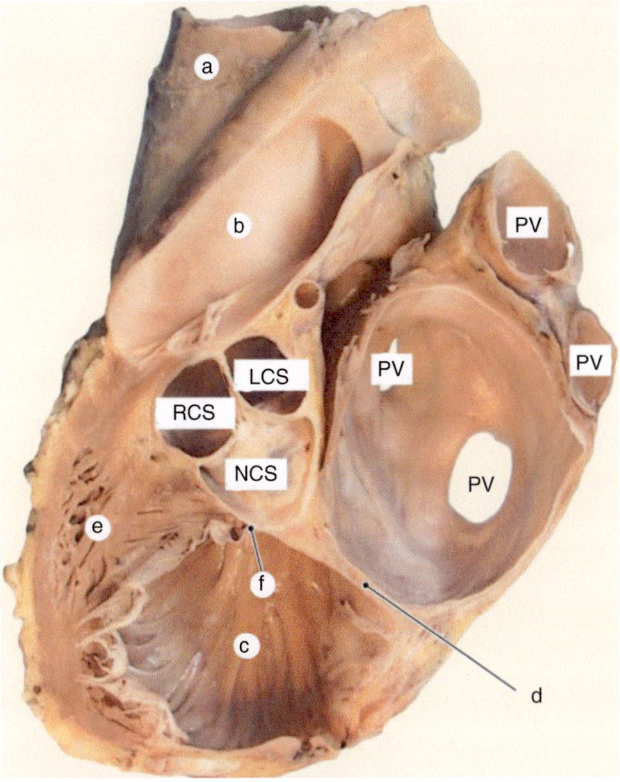

Fig. 6.58 Cross-section through the aortic valve. View from below. *LCS* left coronary sinus, *RCS* right coronary sinus, *NCS* non coronary sinus, *PV* pulmonary vein. The membranous septum separates the right atrium and right ventricle from the aortic vestibule. *a* aorta, *b* pulmonary trunk, *c* right atrium, *d* interatrial septum, *e* right ventricle, *f* membranous septum

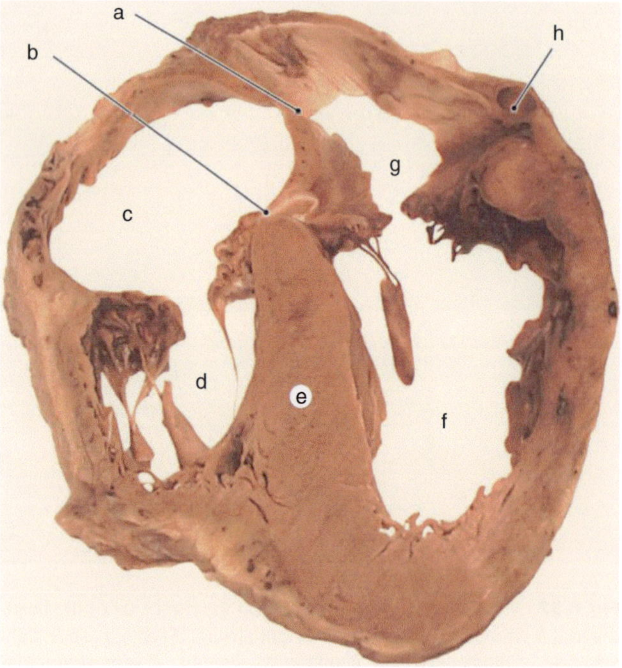

Fig. 6.59 Cross section, corresponding to the echocardiographic view of the four cavities. *a* interatrial septum, *b* atrivoventricular septum, *c* right atrium, *d* right ventricle, *e* interventricular septum, *f* left ventricle, *g* left atrium, *h* coronary sinus

The anterior wall of the right atrium corresponds to the right atrioventricular-tricuspid opening (Fig. 6.12).

Sinus venarum is the segment of the wall of the right atrium located between the openings of the two vena cava. It has a smooth appearance and contains the openings of a few thebesian veins (Fig. 6.11).

Crista interveniens and crista dividens are more likely embryological terms and they refer to the borders of the oval fossa. The upper segment of the border of the oval fossa is crista interveniens and its name resides in its location between the openings of the two vena cava. In intrauterine developement, we sometimes find at its level a prominent structure called the Lower intercaval tubercle (see embryology). The anterior segment of the border of the oval fossa is the crista dividens and it is actually the anterior border of the septum secundum. In intrauterine developement, the blood from the inferior vena cava is lead by the right valve of the primitive venous sinus towards the oval fossa. Some of this blood is deflected by the crista dividens towards the tricuspid opening (Fig. 2.34).

6.2 Internal Configuration of the Right Ventricle

By comparing the aspect of the two ventricles we notice that while the left ventricle has the shape of a cone with the tip downwards and through its size and symmetry it seems to be the main architectonic element in the structure of the heart, the right ventricle is somehow weaker, looks more asymmetrical and seems to surround the right and anterior part of the left ventricle.

We classically describe for the right ventricle an anterior wall, a posterior or posteroseptal wall and a septal wall.

For the clinical doctor, the french-derived terms "septal" and "mural" are also useful. These are mainly functional terms and they emphasize that the free "mural" wall is more mobile than the septal wall.

We can emphasize the particularities and the defining difficulties of the position of the ventricular walls by making a transversal cross-section in the distal third of the heart.:

- the septal wall is convex and it protrudes into the right ventricle.
- the right ventricle has an anterior and a posterior extension that overlap the left ventricle (Fig. 3.5).

The atrioventricular ring has an internal correspondent – a shallow atrioventricular groove (which can be palpated) that marks the atrioventricular limit.

The cavity of the right ventricle begins at this groove (see Sect. "The Right Atrioventricular Ring"), it descends close to the apex of the heart and it then continues anteriorly, superiorly and to the left with the cone of origin of the pulmonary artery. The terminal part of the ventricle continues the cone of the pulmonary artery and it is called the infundibulus of the pulmonary artery. It ends with the subvalvvar infundibular segment (the subvalvar infundibulus).

The Figs. 6.58, 6.59, 6.60, 6.61, 6.62, 6.63 and 6.64 present cardiac cross-sections in different planes realized for a better understanding of the relations between the chambers.

6.2.1 The Inflow and Outflow Compartments of the Right Ventricle

By following this general appearance, the cavity of the right ventricle is divided into an initial compartment for receiving the blood and a distal compartment for the evacuation of the ventricular blood (Figs. 6.65, 6.66 and 6.67).

The ventricular walls of the receiving compartment are covered by muscular trabeculae (muscle bundles forming a network that usually attach through both ends on the ventricular wall; some of them have a free center, unattached to the wall).

The theories in specialty literature regarding the role of these trabeculae do not converge, varying from the opinion that they slow the blood flow to the supposition that they increase the minute-volume. Starting from phylogenetic notions we

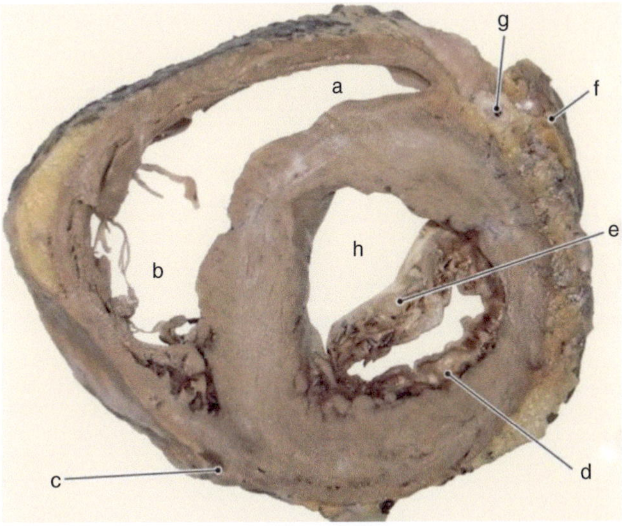

Fig. 6.60 Cross-section through the aortic vestibule. Inferior view. *a* infundibulum, *b* right ventricle, *c* posterior interventricular artery, *d* posterior mitral cusp, *e* anterior mitral cusp, *f* left auricle, *g* anterior interventricular artery, *h* aortic vestibule

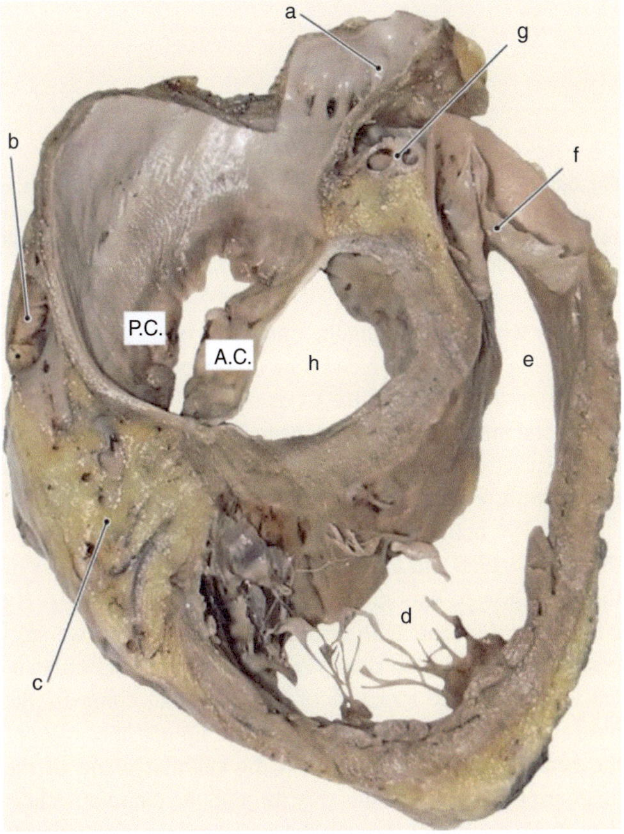

Fig. 6.61 Cross section at the level of the mitral valve. Superior view. Notice that the subvalvular infundibulum does not merge with the wall of the left ventricle. This type of arrangement allows the Ross surgical procedure. *AC* anterior cusp, *PC* posterior cusp. *a* left auricle, *b* coronary sinus, *c* cross of the heart, *d* right ventricle, *e* infundibulum, *f* pulmonary valve, *g* left coronary artery bifurcation, *h* aortic vestibule

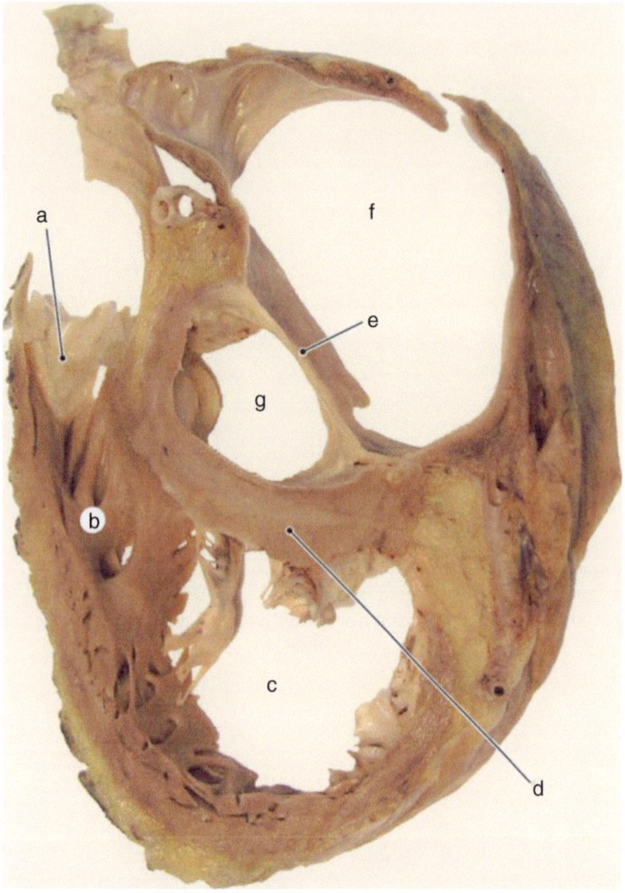

Fig. 6.62 Cross-section through the aortic vestibule, just below the aortic valve. Inferior view. *a* pulmonary valve, *b* infundibulum, *c* right ventricle, *d* interventricular septum, *e* mitral-aotric continuity, *f* left atrium, *g* aortic vestibule

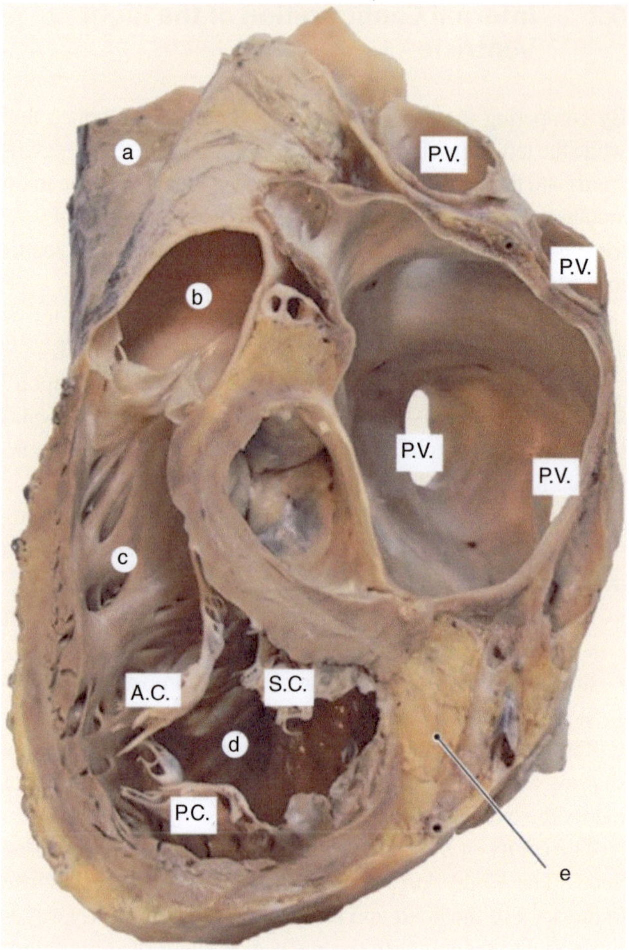

Fig. 6.63 Cross-section through the pulmonary infundibulum. Inferior view. There are noted the positions of the tricuspid cusps and the positions of the pulmonary veins. *a* aorta, *b* pulmonary trunk, *c* infundibulum, *d* right atrium, *e* pyramidal space

consider worth mentioning the initial role of these trabeculae in ensuring the laminar blood flow inside the single ventricle, preventing the mixing of the oxygenated with the deoxygenated blood in the three-chamber heart [3]. We mention the general disposition that seems to guide the blood flow on the mobile wall, leading it towards the ejection opening.

We also believe interesting the resemblance between these trabeculae and the disposition of the anti-wind bars of the Eiffel tower, bars that connect the structural pillars. By comparing the heart with an architectural element, we suggest that the evolution processes have involved the trabeculae in a resistance structure of the heart that connects the bases of the papillary muscles with the tip and the walls of the heart. The forces applied on the valvular plane of the heart are transmitted in this way through the tendinous chordae of the heart and through the papillary muscles towards the trabecular network to find both their support point and their origin in the working myocardium.

Returning to the right ventricle – the receiving compartment derives from the trabeculate part of the primitive bulb and it has:

- a septal wall, trabeculate, "at the entrance" (relatively immobile)
- a free – mural wall (mobile)
- an apical region

The last two segments are highly trabeculated (Fig. 6.68).

The evacuation compartment has relative smooth walls and its first part has a conic shape, giving its name the conus arteriosus (Fig. 6.67).

Embriologically this segment originates from the conal part of the primitive bulb and all the authors agree that its walls are smooth – this aspect increases the speed of the blood flow while leaving the ventricle.

The conus ends with the second part of the ejection compartment called the infundibulum of the pulmonary artery (infundibulum derives from the Latin word infundare – to clog, meaning the segment that ends at the pulmonary valve).

In many medical dictionaries, the terms infundibulum and conus are considered synonyms. This is due to a great variability of the existence of the infundibular territory. The infundibulum is sometimes very short and even absent while other times it has the appearance of a well-structured cylindrical segment (Figs. 4.8 and 4.35).

The subvalvar infundibulum (only the segment located inferior to the pulmonary valve) is formed after the muscular formation of the embryological conal septum (part of the spiral septum). The conal septum doesn't split like the rest of the spiral septum. It separates the aortic vestibule from the pulmonary one (Fig. 6.69).

As stated in the embryology chapter, the muscular transformation of the conal septum actually attaches the cone to the interventricular muscular septum.

The splitting of the spiral septum separates however, the subvalvar infundibulum from the aorta. This fact makes it possible to individualize the subvalvar infundibulum through surgical dissection and the achievement of the Ross procedure.

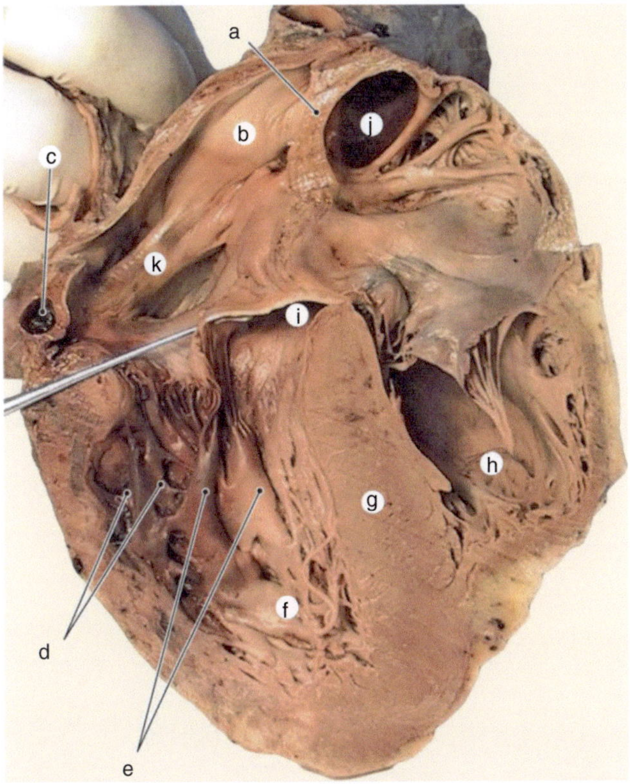

Fig. 6.64 Frontal cross-section through the four cavities. Posterior view. Note the unusual presence of a muscular trabeculae in the lumen of the left atrium, trabeculae know as comadin crest. *a* interatrial septum, *b* left atrium, *c* coronary sinus, *d* posterior papillary group, *e* anterior papillary group, *f* left ventricle, *g* interventricular septum, *h* right ventricle, *i* aortic vestibule, *j* right auricle, *k* comadin crest

6.2.2 The Muscular Interventricular Septum, the Conal Septum, the Membranous Interventricular Septum, the Septomarginal Trabecula the Supraventricular Crest

Here is how, after such a presentation, an inconsistency of anatomical terms appears. We shall explain how such a situation became possible.

In the development of the heart, the lumen of its exit pole is divided through the appearance of the spiral septum. This develops through the union of the endocardic crests (dextrodorsal and sinistroventral), forming the proximal part of the conal septum which continues in the distal part with the truncal septum – inside the lumen of the atrial trunk.

The conal septum will ensure the separation of the subvalvular (evacuation and vestibular) compartments of the aorta and pulmonary artery and will participate in the forming of the membranous interventricular septum. This septum is invisible from the ventricular lumen (Fig. 6.69).

The truncal septum will realize the distal separation of the intrapericardic part of the aorta from the pulmonary artery.

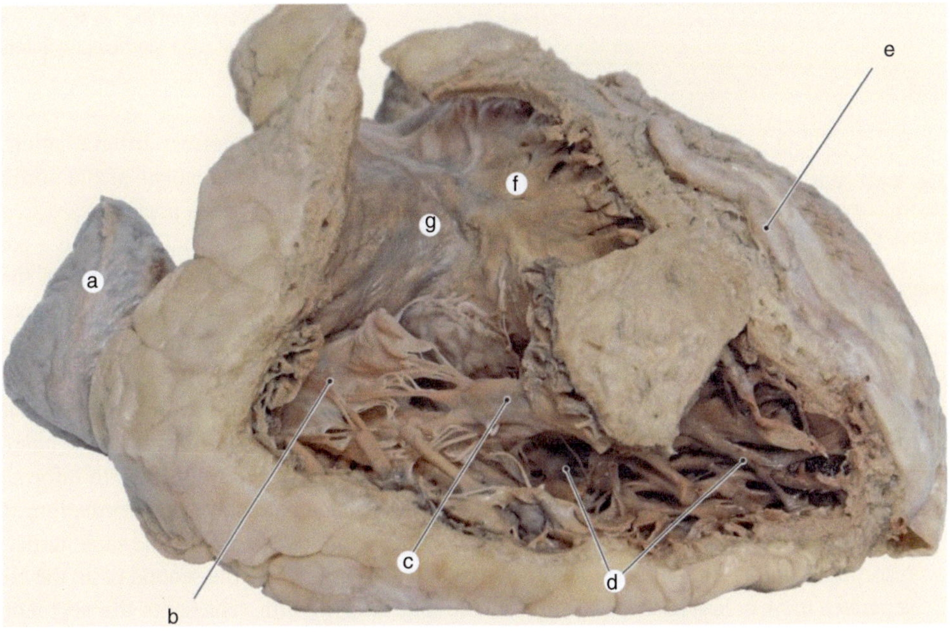

Fig. 6.65 View from the right side over the right ventricle. The receiving compartment is corresponding to the trabecular septum and the ejection compartment is corresponding to the pulmonary cone. *a* right auricle, *b* anterior cusp, *c* anterior papillary, *d* trabecular septum, *e* anterior interventricular artery, *f* pulmonary cone, *g* supraventricular crest

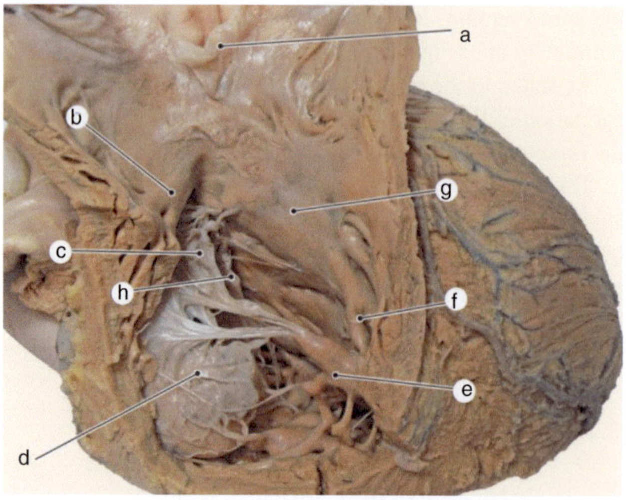

Fig. 6.66 Valvular apparatus and landmarks in the right ventricular cavity. *a* pulmonary valve, *b* supraventricular crest, *c* anterior cusp, *d* posterior cusp, *e* anterior papillary, *f* moderator band, *g* septal marginal trabecula, *h* Septal cusp

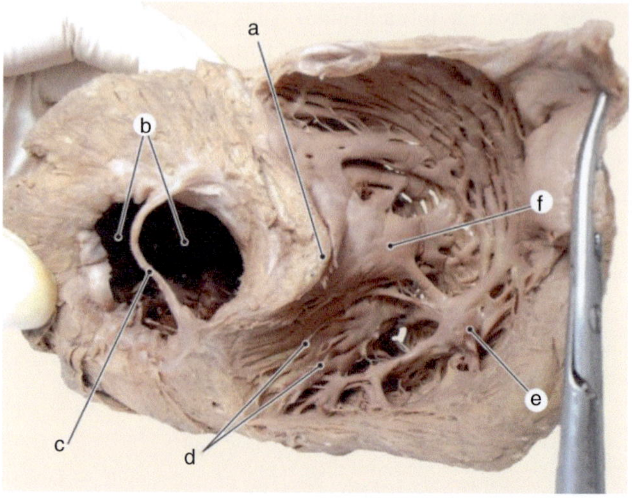

Fig. 6.68 Disposition of the trabeculae in the right ventricular cavity. *a* supraventricular crest, *b* mitral- aortic orifice, *c* mitral-aortic continuity, *d* parietal chordae without papillary muscles, *e* anterior papillary, *f* septomarginal trabecula

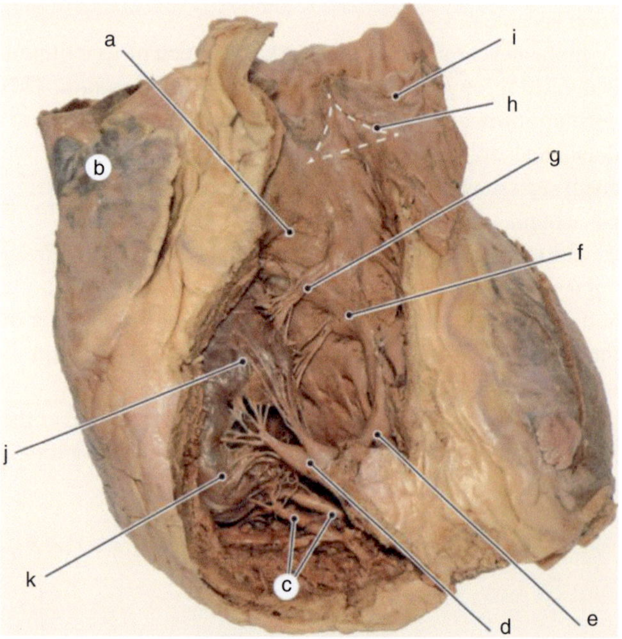

Fig. 6.67 Valvular apparatus and landmarks in the right ventricular cavity. *a* supraventricular crest. *b* right auricle, *c* posterior papillary group, *d* anterior papillary, *e* moderating strip, *f* septomarginal trabecula, *g* septal chordae, *h* subcomisural membranous space, *i* semilunar pulmonary valve, *j* anterior cusp, *k* posterior cusp

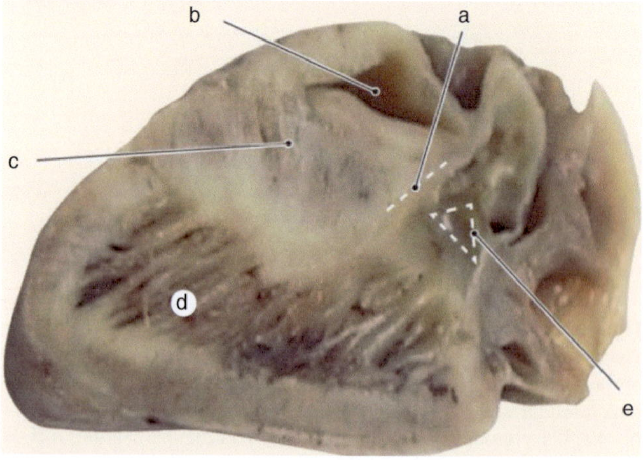

Fig. 6.69 Highlighting the conal septum in a fetal heart. Sagittal section. View from the left side. *a* conal septum area, *b* pulmonary trunk, *c* muscular interventricular septum, *d* left ventricle, *e* membranous septum area

We considered this interlude into the embryological development necessary to avoid the confusion generated by the term "conal".

The confusion can be made between:

- The conal septum as an embryological term (the inferior part of the spiral septum that separated the subvalvular regions of the two ventricles. According to its degree of resorption, the pulmonary subvalvar infundibulus can be separated more or less from the aortic vestibule (Fig. 6.95). Its correct differentiation makes the Ross procedure – the replacement of the aortic valve with its own pulmonary artery – possible).
- The conal septum as a part of the conus of the pulmonary artery – component of the ejection compartment that corresponds to the interventricular septum.

The inaccurate utilization of these anatomical terms by clinicians led to this confusion, imposing an ambiguous term in everyday practice. This situation is unfortunately frequent in the toponymy of the heart.

We would like to inform the clinicians that, with the globalization of information, they must carefully evaluate the meanings of the same terms in different medical cultures.

In the second case, the clinical conal interventricular septum represents the segment of the interventricular septum

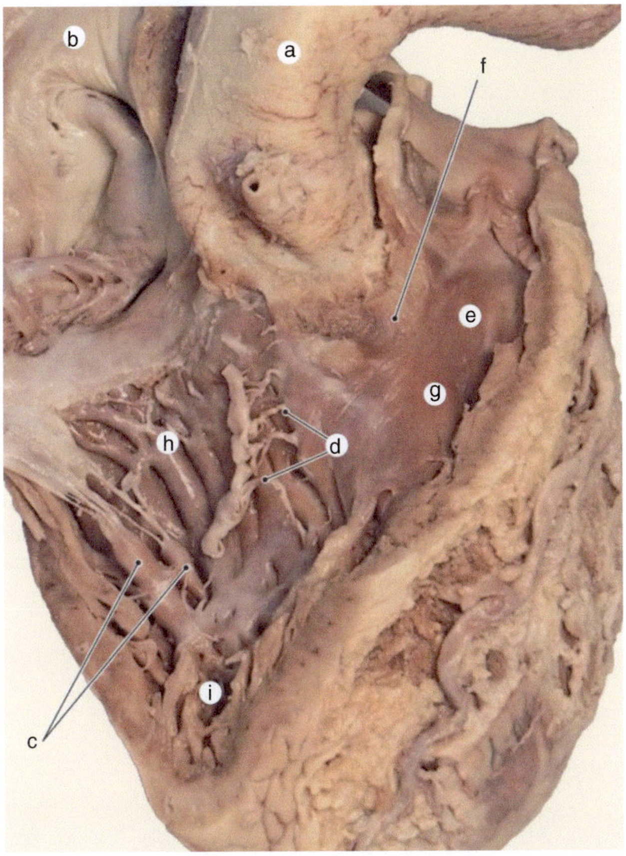

Fig. 6.70 Right ventricle after removing the mobile wall. There is no membranous septum. *a* aorta, *b* right atrium, *c* posterior papillary group, *d* septal chordae, *e* subvalvular infundibulum, *f* supraventricular crest- its base is corresponding to the embryological conal septum, *g* "clinical" conal septum, *h* the "entrance" part of the interventricular septum, *i* apical trabeculated part of the interventricular septum

that corresponds to the pulmonary conus (the ejection compartment). This conal septum has several parts (Fig. 6.68):

- the superior conal septum, represented by one or two septoparietal trabeculae (they connect the septum to the nonseptal wall)
- the inferior conal septum, represented by the septomarginal trabecula (it connects the septum to the acute margin)
- the supraventricular crest, represented by a prominent portion of the right ventricular wall that lines the vestibule of the aorta. This crest is bordered by the extensions of the septomarginal trabecula. The base of insertion of the crest on the interventricular septum corresponds to the embryological conal septum.

The topography of the interventricular septum contains some parts of the ejection compartment, besides the components of the clinical conal septum:

- the membranous interventricular septum (this is a segment of the pars membranaceea septi measuring about 0.5 cm^2 located immediately inferior to the commissure of the anterior and septal cusp) (Fig. 6.57). Sometimes the membranous septum does not exist (Fig. 6.70).
- the trabeculated part, also called "the inlet", to be differentiated from the conal trabeculae which represent "the exit" (Figs. 6.65 and 6.71).
- the trabeculated apical part.

This relatively complicated distribution of the components of the interventricular septum is necessary to be able to understand the location of various types of septal interventricular defects. There is actually one septal interventricular defect for each segment that forms the septum (see embryology).

The limit between the receiving and ejection compartments can be described as follows: the inferior border of the

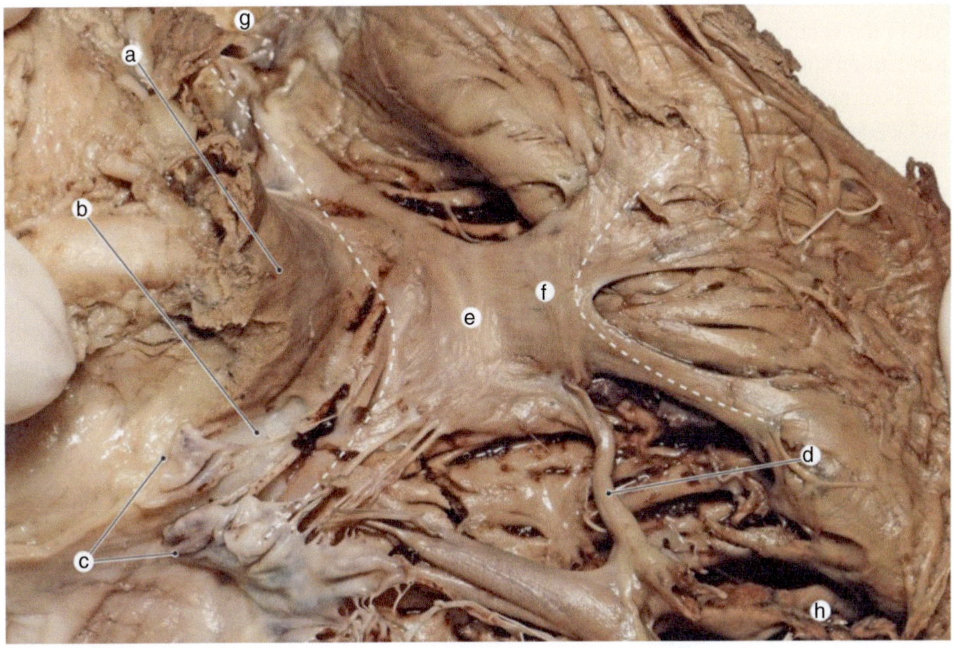

Fig. 6.71 Septomarginal trabecula has two branches (limbs) in the upper part, which include the supraventricular crest. Inferiorly it presents the moderating strip and two branches which strengthen the connection with the mobile wall. *a* supraventricular crest, *b* membranous septum, *c* anterior cusp and septal cusp do not fusion, *d* moderating strip, *e* septomarginal trabecula, *f* marginal fascicle, *g* pulmonary valve, *h* the apical trabecular part of the interventricular septum

anterior cusp, the anterior papillary muscle and the septomarginal trabecula (the septal band) (Figs. 6.66 and 6.67).

This trabecula leaves the septum in the distal part and bridges towards the base of the anterior papillary muscle, becoming the moderator band. In the thickness of the septomarginaltrabecula, on its inferior margin, within the myocardium lies the right branch of the bundle of Hiss (see the excitoconductor system).

! This branch can be located deeper or more superficial, in some extreme cases even intracavitary (normal situation in dolphins).

Regarding the role of the moderator band, we suggest its involvement in the homogeneity of the contraction of the two ventricles, like all the septoparietal trabeculae.

Proximally, the septomarginaltrabecula has an upper limb and a lower limb (Fig. 6.71). These extensions surround the supraventricular crest. The opposite extremity of the trabecula has:

- a fascicle that goes anteriorly and superiorly – the marginal fascicle.
- a posterior and inferior fascicle – the moderator band that reaches the base of the anterior papillary muscle.

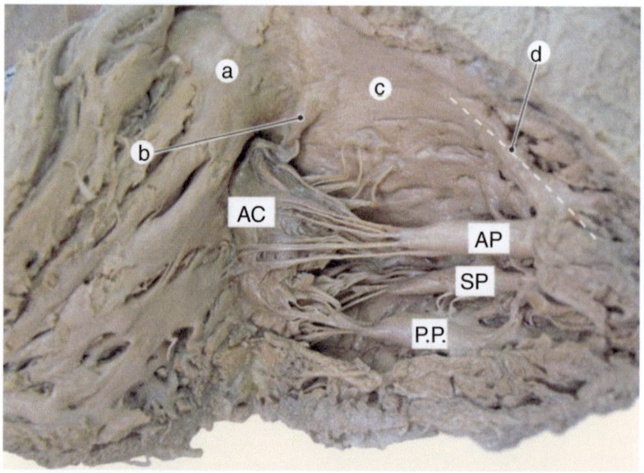

Fig. 6.72 Tricuspid valve apparatus. *AP* anterior papillary muscle, *PP* posterior papillary muscle, *SP* septal papillary muscle, *AC* anterior cusp. *a* supraventricular crest, *b* pyramidal papillary, *c* septomarginal trabecula, *d* moderating strip

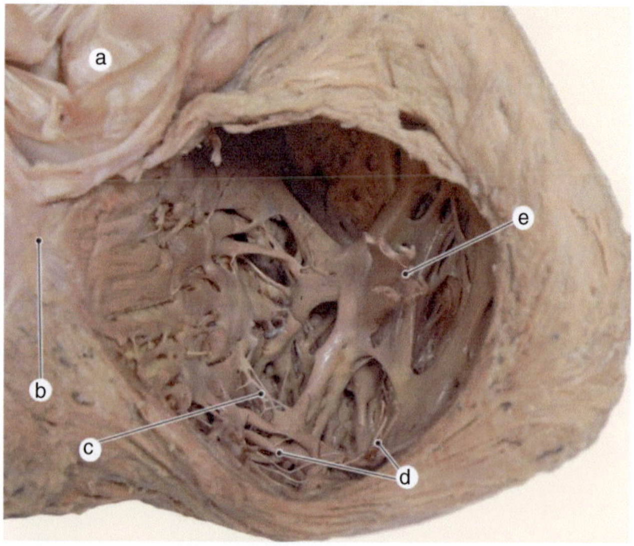

Fig. 6.73 Unique papillary muscle in the right ventricle. View from the top, after removing the right atrium. *a* aorta, *b* tendinous center, *c* false chordae, *d* chordae without papillary, *e* anterior papillary

6.2.3 The Right Atrioventricular Junction

6.2.3.1 The Valvular Apparatus of the Right Atrioventricular Opening

This apparatus is represented by the papillary muscles, the tendinous chordae and the cusps of the right atrioventricular (tricuspid) valve, attached on an "atrioventricular ring" which is a part of the structures of the fibrous skeleton.

The papillary muscles are relatively conic muscular prominences, unique or multiple, having the base fixed on one of the ventricular walls. Their tip provides origin to some formations suggestively called chordae tendineae.

Their opposite extremity is attached on the ventricular surface and on the borders of the atrioventricular cusps, acting as tendons that prevent the protrusion of the cusps inside the atrium during the ventricular systole (they are also called true tendinous chords due to their obvious function) (Fig. 6.72).

Inside the right ventricle, the papillary muscles show a great variability regarding the number, dimensions, position and disposition of the tendinous chords.

There is an anterior papillary muscle that classically corresponds to the anterior ventricular wall, easily recognizable because the moderator band ends at its base. This muscle can frequently be the only papillary muscle of the right ventricle (Fig. 6.73). In this situation, the papillary muscle is strengthened through muscular trabeculae towards all the ventricular walls, not only towards the anterior wall, as its name suggests. The muscle is often held in position through false chordae tendineae (named like this because they connect the muscle to the anterior and septal wall instead of the cusps). These false chords may contain elements of the excitoconductor system (Skandalakis) and are sometimes called pseudotendons.

The anterior papillary muscle actually acts as a distributer of the conduction system (arrived at its base through the moderator band) towards the ventricular network (Fig. 2.89).

There is a third kind of (false) tendinous chords inside the right ventricle, which are short, sometimes resembling connective bands and other times looking just like tendinous chords that stretch between the base of the cusps and the ventricular wall. They keep the cusps in position and prevent them from reflecting into the atriums (Figs. 6.74 and 6.75).

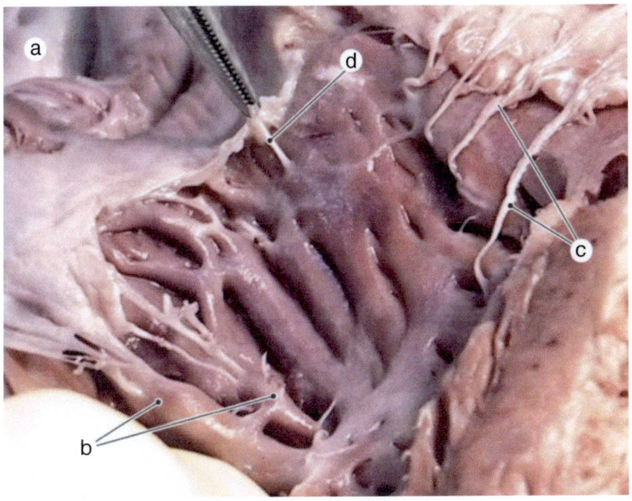

Fig. 6.74 Septal cusp of the tricuspid valve was resected near the base. We notice basal chordae tendineae which prevent the reflection of the cusp in the right atrium. *a* right atrium, *b* posterior papillary group, *c* chordae without papillary, inserted on the septal cusp, *d* basal chordae without papillary

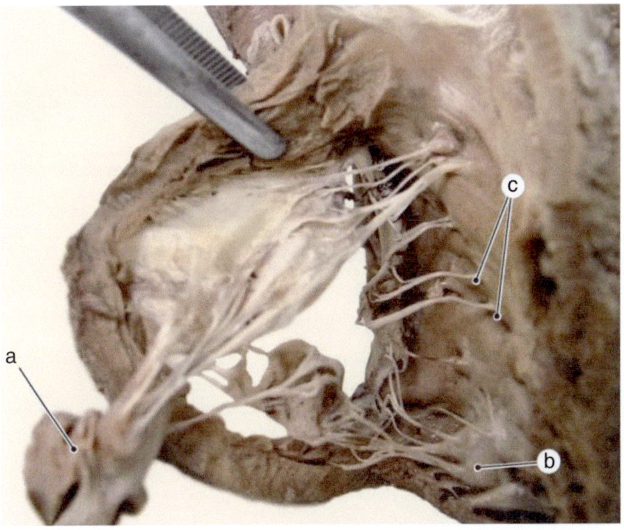

Fig. 6.76 The tendinous chords disposition in the right ventricle. Inferior view of the tricuspid valve. *a* anterior papillary muscle, *b* posterior papillary muscle, *c* tendinous chords without papillary muscle for the septal cusp

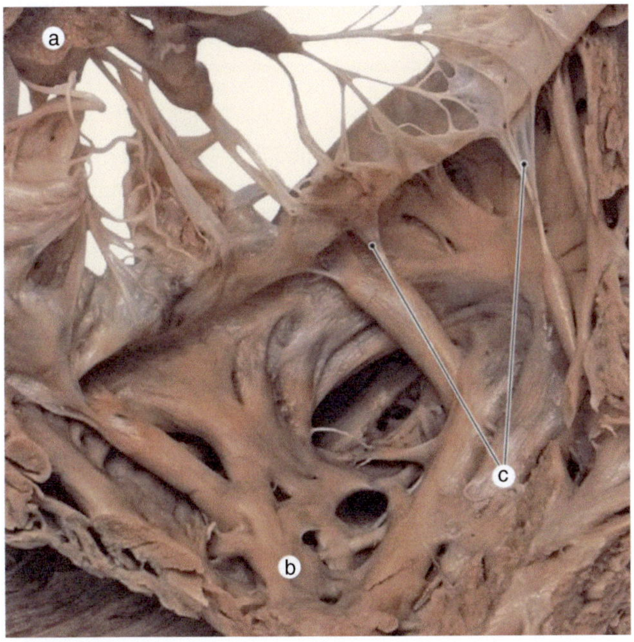

Fig. 6.75 Basal tendinous chords in the right ventricle with the same function as those from the previous image, but with another configuration. *a* posterior papillary muscle, *b* right ventricle, *c* tendinous chords without papillary muscle

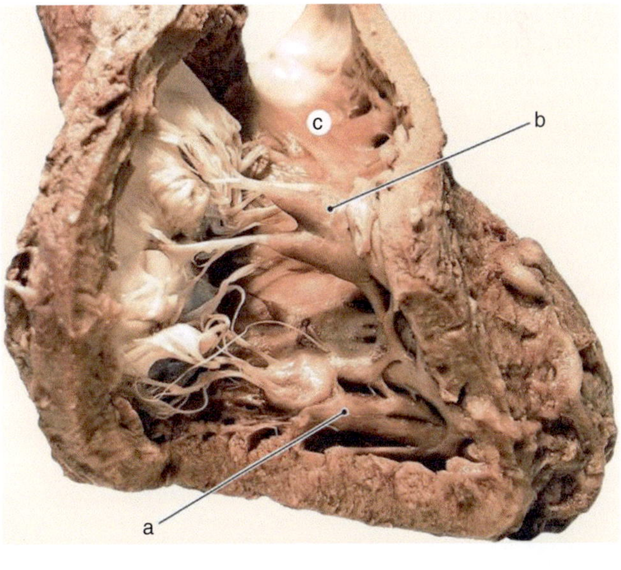

Fig. 6.77 Papillary muscles in the right ventricle. *a* posterior papillary muscle, *b* anterior papillary muscle, *c* subpulmonary infundibulum

There is classically described a single posterior papillary muscle which corresponds to the posteroseptal wall. In the cases when it truly exists, it is a thick muscle with a split tip (Fig. 6.76). We often see a posterior papillary group, formed by two or three papillary muscles, with their bases united or separated (Figs. 6.77 and 6.78). The absence of the posterior papillary muscle, with, instead, its corresponding tendinous chords attaching directly or through small conic prominences on the septal and posterior ventricular walls is also common.

There seldom is a well-individualized septal papillary muscle belonging to the septal wall. The corresponding tendinous chords most frequently attach directly onto the interventricular septum where the presence of one or two small conic prominences sometimes suggest the presence of some papillary muscles. When the first of these small muscular prominences is more voluminous, it is called the conal papillary muscle (Fig. 6.72).

In the anterosuperior part of the septal wall, between the tricuspid and pulmonary ostiums, the ventricular myocardium

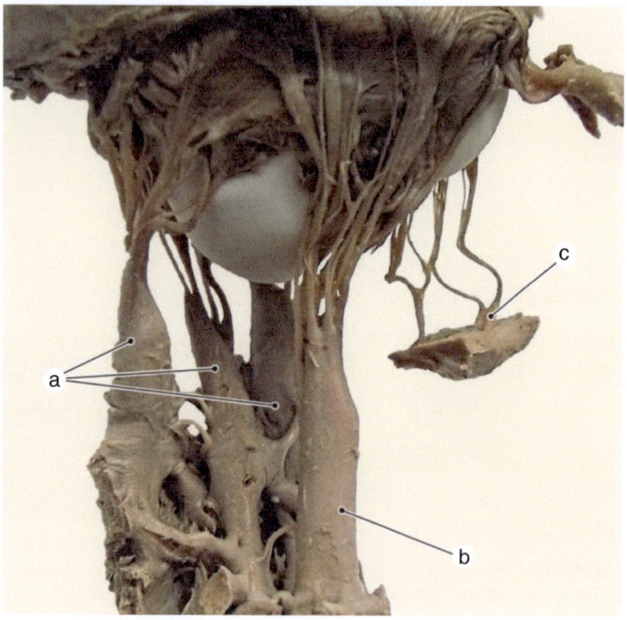

Fig. 6.78 Like in the left ventricle, in the right one the papillary muscles base is reinforced by muscular trabeculae, with eachother and also with the ventricular apex. *a* postero-septal papillary group, *b* anterior papillary muscle, *c* septal tendinous chords

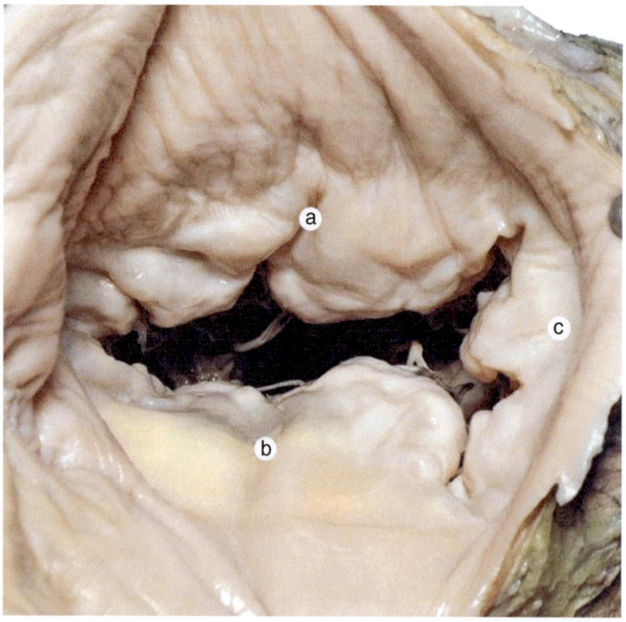

Fig. 6.79 Atrial view of the tricuspid valve – superior view. *a* anterior cusp, *b* septal cusp, *c* posterior cusp

that lines anteriorly the aortic vestibule protrudes inside the cavity of the right ventricle as the supraventricular crest.

The ensemble of all the described valvular components functions unitarily, insuring the unidirectional blood flow from the atrium towards the ventricle. The former anatomists wonderfully called the atrial appearance of the valve "vide supra" and the ventricular appearance of the valve "vide infra" (Figs. 6.77 and 6.79).

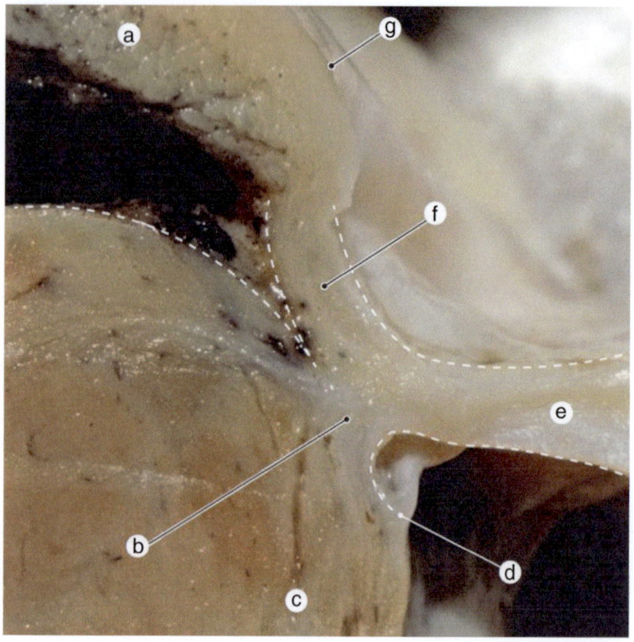

Fig. 6.80 The insertion apparatus of the cusp on the ventricular base. Sagittal section. View from the right. *a* atrial muscles, *b* subepi-subendocardial continuity, *c* ventricular wall, *d* inferior root, *e* cusp, *f* superior root, *g* atrial endocardium

The tricuspid opening has about 8–11 cm in circumference and classically allows the simultaneous introduction of the tip of three fingers.

6.2.3.2 The Right Atrioventricular Ring

The atrioventricular ring separates the right atrium from the right ventricle. Even though we would be tempted to think that the ring is oriented in a frontal plane, it actually is oriented in an oblique plane between the frontal plane and the sagital plane and it represents the anterior wall of the right atrium.

Structurally –we can say that the atrioventricular opening is classically formed from an atrioventricular ring on which the valvular cusps insert themselves. In reality, the link between the atria and the ventricles is complex and is realized through aatrioventricularjunctional area, having a heterogeneous structure, providing both electric and spatial separation and functional unity of the chambers of the heart at the same time.

The ring has a membranous structure and is located between the projection line of the superior and inferior roots of the cusps. It can be relatively compared with a membranous cylindrical segment, folded at the level of the cusps axis. In this strictly membranous structure the ring has the role of electrical insulator between the atrium and the ventricle (Fig. 6.80).

The inferior root of the cusps has an insertion that continues the ventricular endocardium at the base of the ventricular pyramid. Subepicardic muscle fibers are actually continued

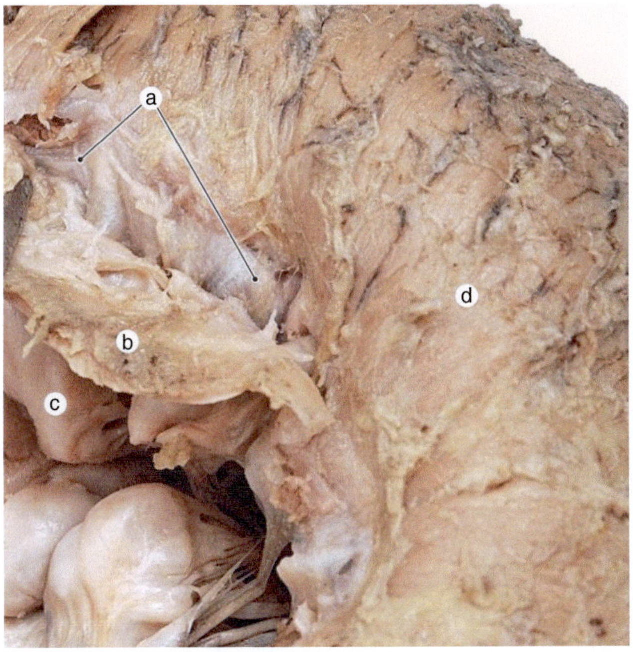

Fig. 6.81 The cleft between the cusps roots. *a* inferior root, *b* superior root, *c* ventricular base

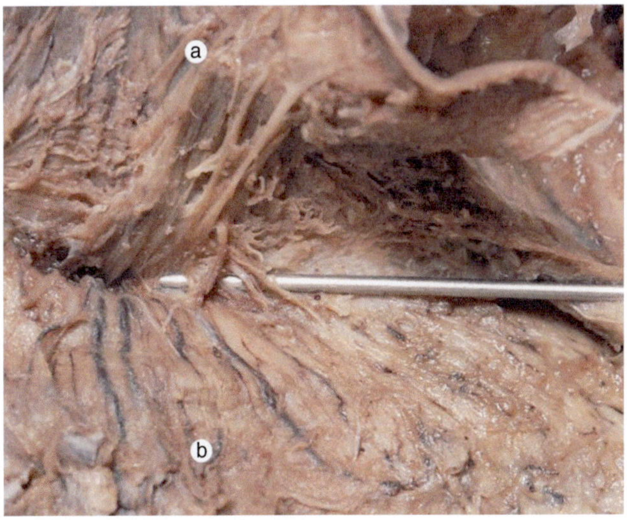

Fig. 6.82 Abnormal atrioventricular muscular fascicles at the heart cross. *a* atrium, *b* ventricle

with the subendocardic muscle fibers at the level of the insertion of this root, realizing the subepi-subendocardic continuity (marked by a fibrous condensation line).

This continuity represents an important support point for the muscle fibers that line the internal and external surfaces of the heart.

Connective fascicles that blend with the muscles at the base of the ventricle also begin at the level of the insertion of the root. This disposition supports the opinion according to which the region of the roots of the cusps is deeply involved in the dynamics of the myocardium.

After a short course, the upper root of the cusps is lined on the external side by the atrial muscular layer.

The segment between the inferior limit of the atrial muscles and the insertion of the inferior root is responsible for the electrical insulation between the atria and the ventricles (Fig. 6.81).

The described situation is reached in ontogenesis after important transformations and differentiations of the junctional mesenchyme (see embriology).

Aberrant mesenchymal fascicles differentiated into muscular tissue during ontogenesis may be aberrant conducting pathways between the atria and ventricles.

6.2.3.3 The Atrioventricular Fold and the Pyramidal Space

The atrioventricular junction resembles an atrioventricular fold. The tip of the folding angle represents the atrioventricular ring.

The atrioventricular folding is way more emphasized at the level of the tricuspid atrioventricular junction and the two components of the fold are better connected compared to the left side.

This detail is important in surgery, when the identification and resection of aberrant muscular fascicles located close to the valvular ring is required, fascicles that represent accessory transmission pathways in the WPW syndrome (Fig. 6.82).

The posterior segment of the right "atrioventricular fold" is called the pyramidal space. The blood vessels and nerves pass through this space towards the atrioventricular node, located at the tip of the space. The terminal part of the coronary sinus also passes through here in its way towards the atrial floor (Figs. 6.36 and 6.104).

The atrioventricular ring is indicated in an atrial view by a circular line where the atrial endocardium is continued by the cusps endocardium. This circular line, that actually shows the origin of the cusps, passes at the level of the interventricular septum over the membranous part of the septum, dividing it into the atrioventricular septum and the membranous interventricular septum (the area has been described at the right atrium).

Both the posterior right horn and the anterior right horn of the tendinous center sometimes extend with fascicles of fibrous connective tissue towards the atrioventricular ring. These fascicles are called filacoronaria (see the fibrous skeleton of the heart). Their connective tissue may become dense connective tissue or even partly transform into cartilage. These "fila" sometimes may deposit calcium. Fila coronaria do not describe a complete circular course in the atrioventricular ring, forming a fragmented contour (in the right part of the ring we have never found segments of the fila coronaria referred to in classical anatomy). We often found instead calcifications or

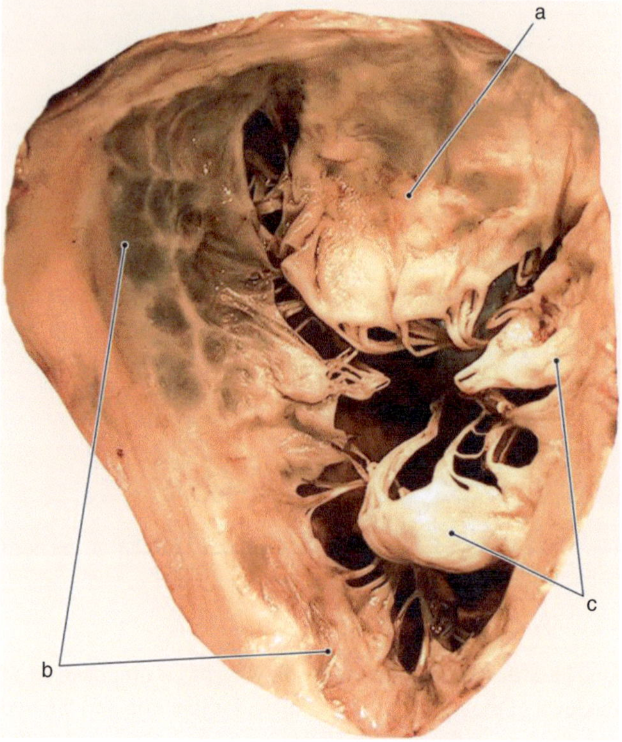

Fig. 6.83 Atrial view of the tricuspid valve. The septal cusp is in opposition with the other two. *a* anterior cusp, *b* septal cusp, *c* posterior cusp

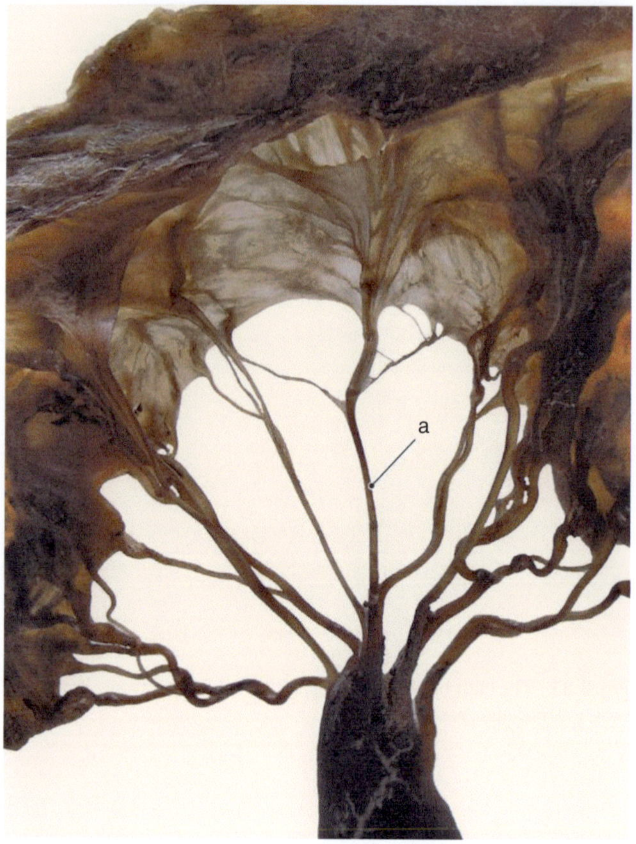

Fig. 6.84 Almost constantly in the commissural areas there is an axial tendinous chord which reaches the cusp base. *a* axial tendinous chord which reaches the basal area of the commissure

dense fibrous transformation of the horns of the tendinous center. We also must state that while the anterior fila coronaria of the tricuspid ring is a free-standing, well-defined structure, with a fibrocartilaginous aspect, the posterior fila coronaria is either the extension of the horn of the posterior triangle or appears as a more or less condensed connective fascicle, without an apparent connection with the triangle.

Fila coronaria provides attachment to the adjacent ventricular muscles giving resistance and elasticity to the ventricular base. They rarely enter the divergent fold represented by the two roots of the cusps.

Summarizing this, we may say that the right atrioventricular junction is represented by:

- the atrioventricular ring with the two divergent roots of the cusps and their different approach in atrial and ventricular junction;
- anterior and posterior fila coronaria;
- a segment of the membranous septum;
- the atrioventricular fold with its extension represented by the pyramidal space.

6.2.3.4 The Atrioventricular Cusps

The atrioventricular cusps are located as follows: anterior superior (in short, anterior), septal and inferior (the last one corresponds to the diaphragmatic surface also being called posterior cusp) (Fig. 6.83). The appearance and the number of the cusps is variable though. They may have one or more notches on the free margin, separating "valvular lobules". There usually is an anteroseptal commissure (dividing the membranous septum), an inferoseptal commissure and an anteroinferior commissure.

If we remove the cusps from the ring we realize that they form a continuous membranous veil. This continuity is marked by deeper notches that define the commissures and by shallower notches that separate the "valvular lobes". In other words, the commissures are rather continuation regions where the valvular veil is smaller than interruptions of this veil (Figs. 6.84, 6.85, 6.86 and 6.87).

A cusp contains: a base (basal area), a free, dense, harsh border and an intermediate translucent region between the two.

The tendinous cords are of several types according to their attachment point: cords for the free margin, for the translucent area for the basal area or for the commissural area (Fig. 6.88). There are also false chords that leave the posterior wall right below the origin of the cusp and attach on the basal part of the posterior cusp (Figs. 6.74 and 6.75). There are also false tendinous chords that connect the papillary muscles to the walls or very thin false chords that connect different parts of the ventricular wall.

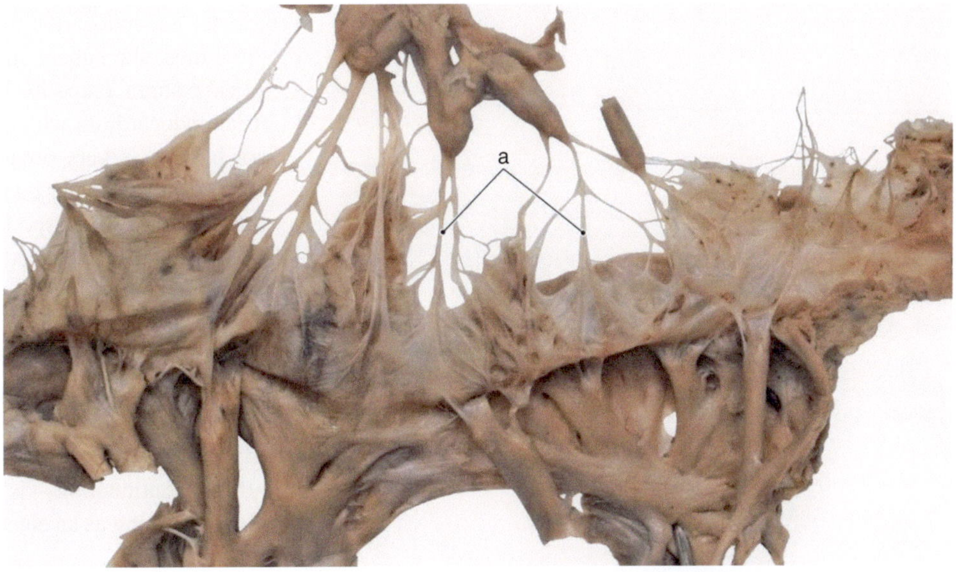

Fig. 6.85 The tricuspid valve unfolded. Ventricular view. *a* axial tendinous chord in commissural areas

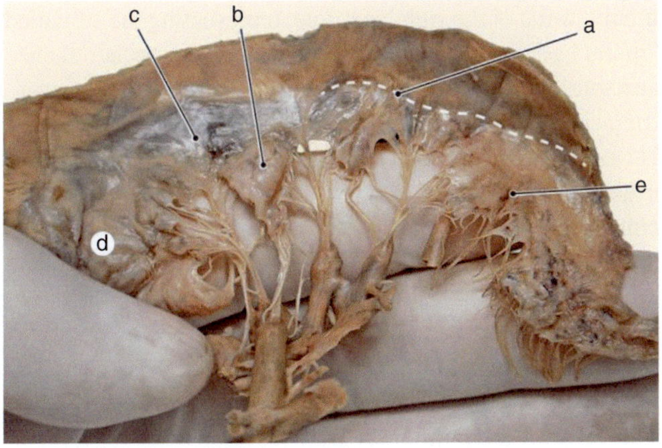

Fig. 6.86 The tricuspid valve unfolded. Atrial view. *a* atrioventricular border, *b* posterior cusp, *c* commissural area, *d* anterior cusp, *e* septal cusp

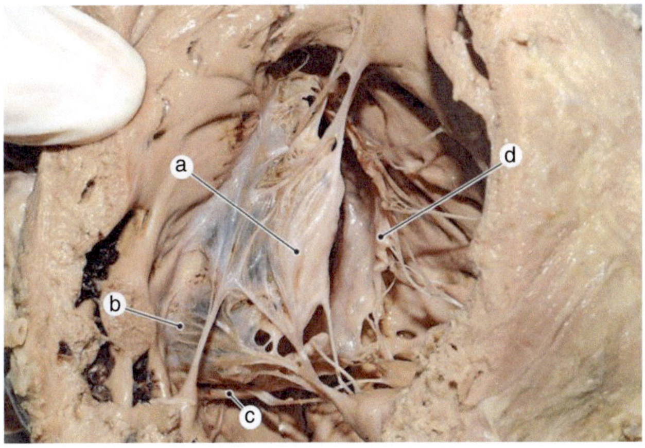

Fig. 6.88 Ventricular view of the tricuspid valve. Note the tendinous chords manner of insertion. *a* anterior cusp, *b* commissure, *c* posterior cusp, *d* septal cusp

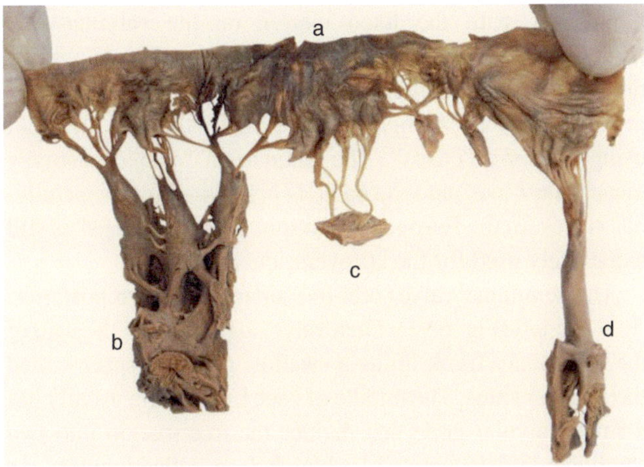

Fig. 6.87 The tricuspid valve unfolded. *a* the cusps form a continuous membrane veil, *b* postero-septal papillary muscle, *c* septal tendinous chords, *d* anterior papillary muscle

The tendinous chords from the anterior papillary usually spread towards the anterior and posterior cusps.

The tendinous chords from the posterior papillary usually spread towards the posterior and septal cusps.

The tendinous chords from the septum reach the septal and anterior cusps (the rule here is that a papillary muscle always sends tendinous chords towards two cusps).

The commissural areas usually have their own array of tendinous chords, being well-equipped in this way to prevent the rebound in this point. The Fig. 6.89 shows a stage in the development of the inferoseptal commissure.

We sometimes found hearts that showed a clear separation between the anterior and septal cusps at the commissure.

The rest of the valvular apparatus was perfectly normal, still the separation between the two cusps allowing rebound (Fig. 6.71).

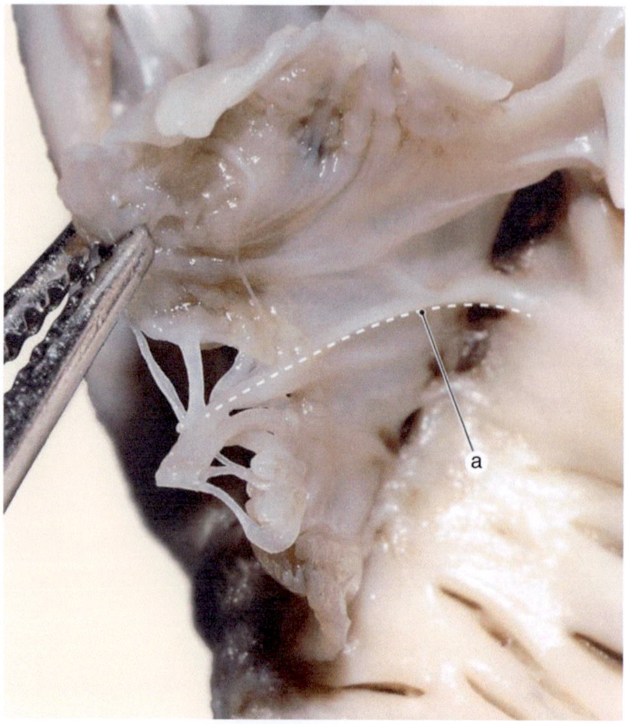

Fig. 6.89 Four months old fetal heart. Ventricular view. Differentiation of an axial tendinous chord. *a* axial tendinous chord in course of differentiation

For a better understanding of the notion of atrioventricular ring there are a few notes and remarks to make:

- the attachment base of the cusps consists of two laminas that diverge one superiorly and the other one inferiorly. The superior lamina is covered by atrial endocardium and the inferior lamina by the ventricular endocardium. These short laminas have a membranous aspect with a fibrous-connective structure.
- in the outer diverging angle between the laminas there is connective-fatty tissue, covered by epicardium, and the entire assembly, fila coronaria included, forms the atrioventricular junction.
- fila coronaria are usually located in the ventricular myocardium, providing support for its insertion.

The behavior of the atrial and ventricular epicardium, endocardium and myocardium in the vicinity of the ring is as follows:

- the epicardium doesn't strictly line the area of the ring. It descends from the atrium, leaps over the coronary groove, far from the base of the cusps. The coronary blood vessels travel in the space formed this way (that marks the coronary groove) in a connective-fatty environment.
- the endocardium leaves the ventricular wall and covers the inferior lamina of the base of the cusp at the level of the ventricular ring in vide infra (from the inferior view).

The place where it leaves the ventricular wall is a proper ventricular (inferior) root of the cusp. We can notice how the subepicardic ventricular muscle fibers are continued with the ventricular subendocardic muscle fibers at the level of this root (the muscular subepi-subendocardic continuity).

- in vide supra (superior view), the continuation of the atrial endocardium with the cusp endocardium (the superior lamina) is very obvious. We can palpate and sometimes see the circular contour of the atrioventricular ring at the base of the cusp. The atrial myocardium becomes thinner and disappears in the vicinity of the superior lamina of the base of the cusp.

The two laminas that represent the base of the cusps have no muscle fibers at all. This is how the myocardium is completely missing at the level of the atrioventricular ring.

The transmission of the electrical impulse – transmission based on the conductibility of the myocardium, therefore also on its continuation – is stopped this way, the atrioventricular ring acting as an electrical insulator between the atria and the ventricles.

If we look at the functional aspects of the valve, the anterior and posterior cusps are attached and solidary with the mobile walls of the right ventricle, representing the so-called "mural" part of the valve while the septal cusp is attached and solidary with the relatively immobile wall – the interventricular septum. This dichotomy of the valvular architecture is worth being taken into consideration both in physiological evaluations and mostly in surgical procedures (also see embryology).

6.2.4 The Pulmonary Valve (the Valve of the Pulmonary Trunk)

The valve of the pulmonary trunk separates the subvalvular ventricular infundibulum from the trunk of the pulmonary artery, preventing the return of blood into the ventricle (Fig. 6.67).

The valve is formed by three semilunar valves, attaching themselves with the fixed margin on the valvular ring (Fig. 6.90). If we remove the valves, it resembles an embattled fibrous condensation, just like the aortic ring.

Some authors wrongly name all the valves of the heart using the term "cusps". The Latin term "cuspid" actually means "nest like" and the name is best suited for the semilunar valves. In the European tradition, the term "cusps" is still extensively used for the atrioventricular valves.

The semilunar valves are: one anterior and two posterior: right and left (Fig. 6.91). Each valve, together with the wall of the pulmonary trunk limits a swallow nest-like space called the valvular sinus. The middle of each free margin usually has a small valvular node that divides the free margin into two semilunar translucent veil-looking halves, called lunules.

The semilunar valves are joined together at their extremities through commissures (Figs. 6.92 and 6.93).

Inferior to each commissure there is a triangular subcommissural space – right, left and posterior (Figs. 6.67 and 6.94).

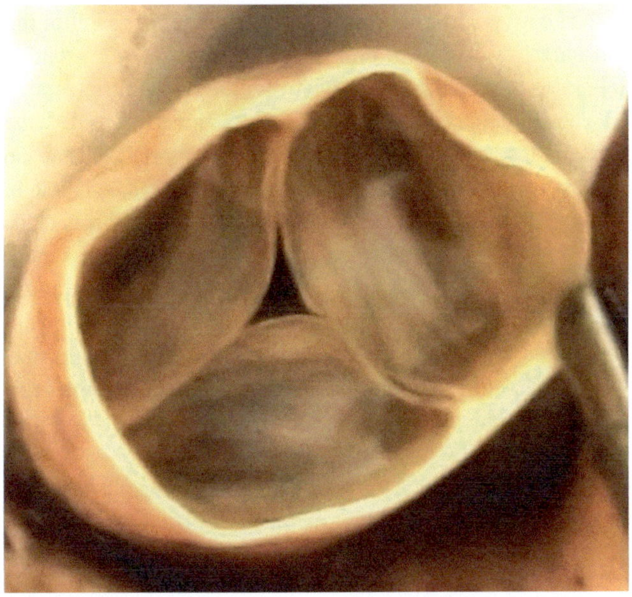

Fig. 6.90 Closed pulmonary valve due to demonstrative water filling. Superior view

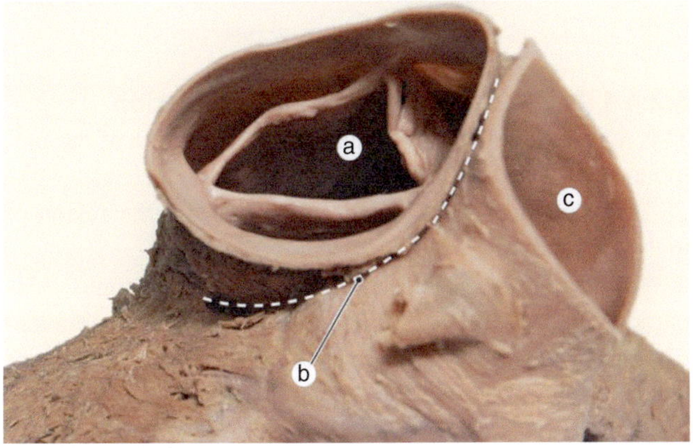

Fig. 6.91 Pulmonary valve. Superior view. Informative arrangement of the spiral septum. *a* pulmonary valve, *b* area of the former spiral septum, *c* aorta

These spaces are occupied by membranous- looking structures, containing a large amount of fibrous and elastic connective tissue. The pulmonary ring is attached to the infundibular myocardium through these structures (the connective-elastic fibers blend with the myocardic fibers).

The pulmonary valvular ring [4] (structure similar to the aortic ring) is connected posteriorly to the aortic valvular ring through short fascicles of dense connective tissue. This tissue forms a veritable "aortic-pulmonary symphysis" that unites the subcommissural space between the posterior pulmonary sinuses with the subcommissural space between the anterior aortic coronary sinuses. This aortico-pulmonary symphysis is called in many studies the infundibular tendon or the conal ligament. This structure is most likely to represent a remnance of the former spiral septum (Fig. 6.95).

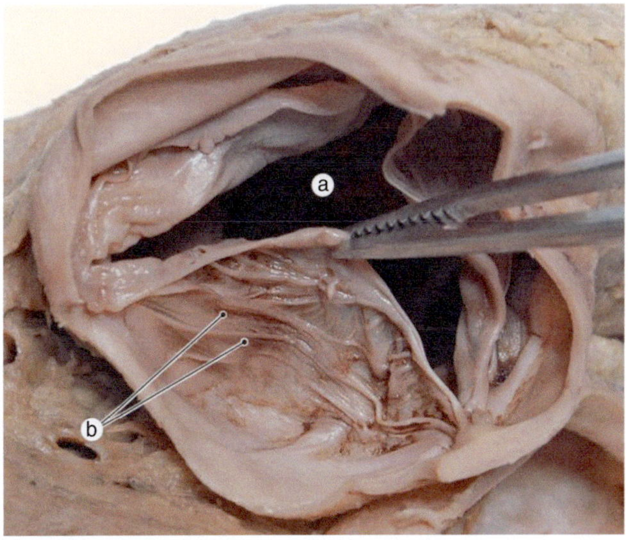

Fig. 6.92 Pulmonary trunk sinus with transversal bands. Postero-superior view. *a* pulmonary valve, *b* transversal fibrous bands inside the sinus

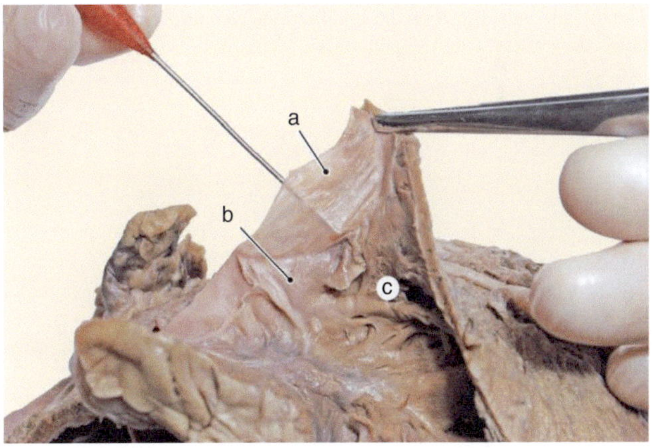

Fig. 6.93 Sino-infundibular junction. *a* semilunar valve, *b* subcommisural membranous trigone, *c* infundibulum

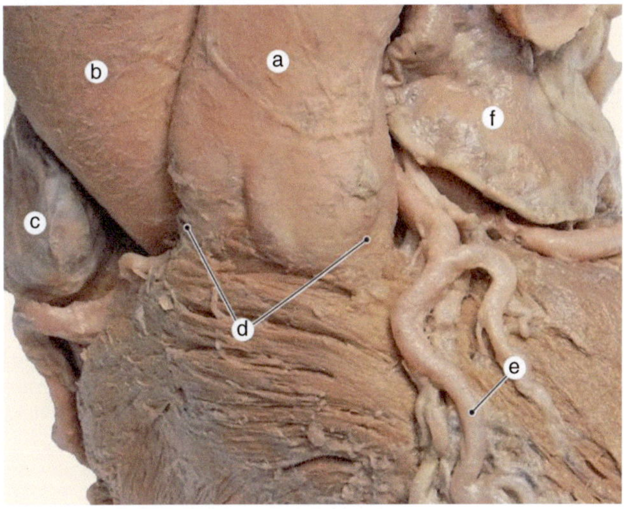

Fig. 6.94 The pulmonary "bulb" similar to the aortic bulb. *a* pulmonary trunk, *b* aorta, *c* right auricle, *d* pulmonary "bulb", *e* anterior interventricular artery, *f* left auricle

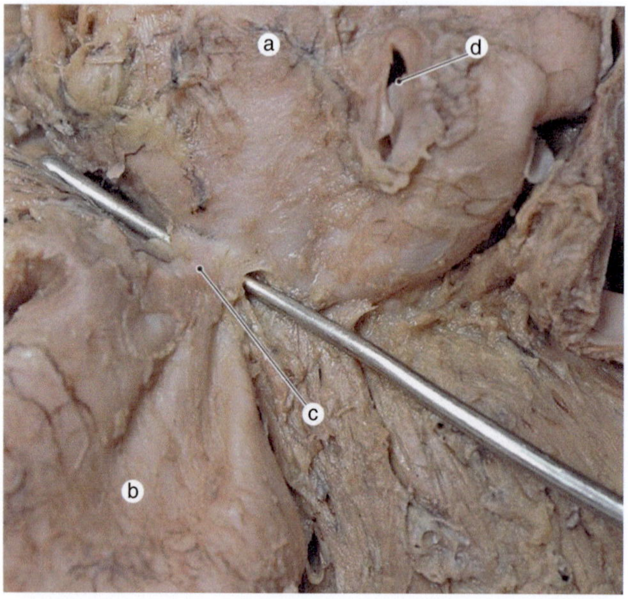

Fig. 6.95 Antero-superior view of the aorticopulmonary symphysis. The metalic indicator is on the conal septum (embryological). *a* aorta, *b* pulmonary artery, *c* aorticopulmonary "symphysis", *d* coronary artery

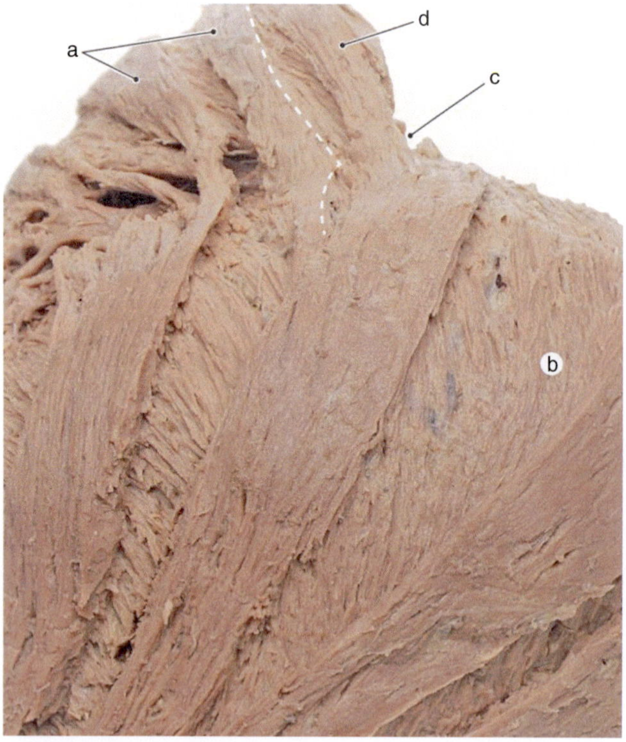

Fig. 6.96 Muscle fibers distribution on the left side of the ventriculo-pulmonary junction. *a* superficial fibers, *b* intermediate fibers, *c* ventriculo-pulmonary junction, *d* border of the infundibulum muscularisation

! The myocardium located just inferior is the result of the muscularization of the embryological conal septum and it separates the evacuation pathways of the two ventricles.

The pulmonary artery has a sinotubular junction just like the aorta, represented by the border between the sinusal wall and the pulmonary artery. The junction is weakly differentiated though.

On the other hand, the sinoinfundibular junction is characterized by the fact that the myocardium can ascend more onto the membranous subcommissural spaces than the aortic myocardium, and sometimes even on the sinusal wall. Individual variability is very important though. Otherwise, the attachment of the pulmonary valve has important similarities with the manner of attachment of the aortic valve (see the corresponding chapter).

In the pulmonary valve, the sinusal wall doesn't generally protrude towards the exterior as much as the aortic one. Still, we can sometimes observe here a "bulb-like" aspect (Fig. 6.94).

By comparing the sinusal wall of the aorta and pulmonary artery, we notice that the aortic wall is thicker. But surprisingly, the two vessels have a relatively equal number of elastic lamina in the sinusal wall. In both vessels, the number of elastic lamina and the thickness of the wall is higher in the tubular part than in the sinusal one.

6.2.4.1 The Ventricular-Pulmonary Junction

This notion refers to the way the area of the valve of the pulmonary trunk attaches on the wall of the left ventricle.

This area is embryologically derived from the fusion of the conus with the primitive ventricle (see).

This fusion is reached because the primitive conus folds partially over the primitive ventricle forming the supraventricular crest and the pulmonary infundibulus. The inferior border of the folded bulbar territory is the septomarginal trabecula (see embriology).

Through the resorption of the superior part of the spiral septum and the partial splitting of the conal septum results a cleavage space between the subvalvar infundibulus and the left ventricle, space that can be relatively easily dissected after the removal of the aorto-pulmonary symphysis. In this way the subvalvularinfundibulus and the pulmonary valve are separated from the aorta and the Ross procedure – the replacement of the aortic valve with its own pulmonary valve – becomes possible.

The principle is: the pulmonary conus is fused with the muscular interventricular septum, due to the muscularization of the conal septum, and the supravalvar infundibulus is disectable due to the dividing of the spiral septum.

One or two posterior conal arteries pass through this region and they have to be protected by the surgeon during the procedure (Fig. 6.98).

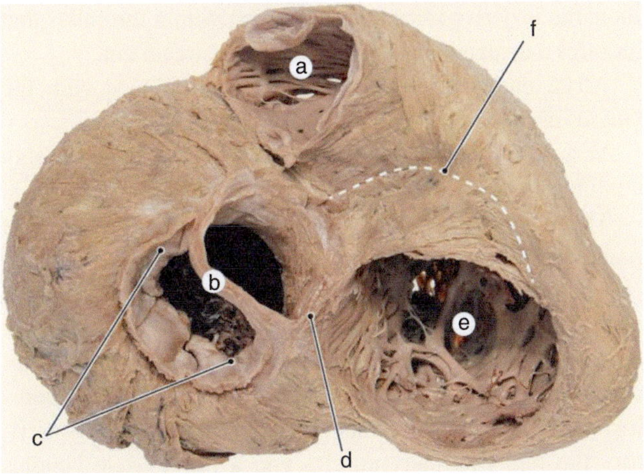

Fig. 6.97 The appearance of the ventricular pyramid base after the removal of the atria. The triorificial isthmus is limited laterally by the former superior bulboventricular sulcus. The mitral-aortic orifice becomes noticeable after the removal of the aorta and of the left atrium. *a* pulmonary ostium, *b* mitral-aortic ostium, *c* posterior mitral cusp, *d* bundle of Hiss, *e* tricuspid ostium, *f* the direction of the former superior bulboventricular sulcus marks the triorificial isthmus

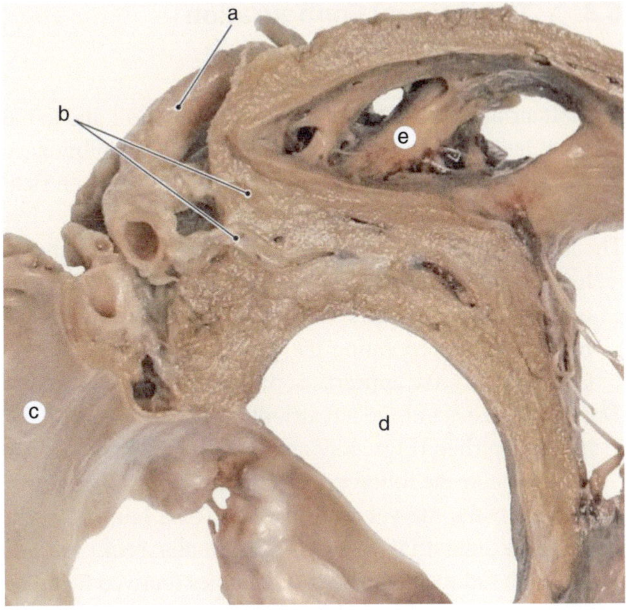

Fig. 6.98 Transversal section through the infundibulo-ventricular junction. Note the two posterior conal arterial branches. *a* anterior interventricular artery, *b* posterior conal arteries, *c* left auricle, *d* aortic vestibule, *e* subvalvulary pulmonary infundibulum

6.3 The Internal Configuration of the Left Atrium

The left atrium is a cavity which is partly posterior and to the left in relation to the right atrium. Here end the pulmonary veins, and the atrium communicates with the left ventricle through the bicuspid or mitral valvular opening.

The left atrium has an internal aspect marked by its embryological origin: mostly (the upper posterior-wall, located between the pulmonary veins ostia and around them) is formed by incorporating the primitive pulmonary vein. Consequently, the appearance of this wall will be smooth.

The interior aspect of the left atrium is poorer in details than the right atrium (Figs. 6.99 and 6.100).

Here we note the following specific structures: the pulmonary veins ostia, the valve of the oval fossa falx septi, the septum, the interatrial septum, the auricular neck, the left auricle with rudimentary pectinate muscles (derived from the primitive atrium), the ostium of the mitral valve and the vestibule of the mitral valve (it has a smooth aspect and comes from the atrioventricular junction).

Sometimes in the lumen of the left atrium a major prominent muscle can be found, which is stretched between the left auricle and the left upper pulmonary vein. It can be confused with a tumor or a thrombus. It Sometimes can appear as an imagistic breakthrough representing a variation of the structure of the left atrium called the cumadinic crest [5] (Fig. 6.64). Its name is derived from the confusion with a thrombus that requires a dispersion stabilizer (warfarin) treatment.

Atrial endocardium (in both atria) continues with the venous endothelium without a very clear border.

Very important, the atrial myocardium can variably continue around the terminal segment of the pulmonary veins.

This disposition is attributed to atrial electrophysiological pathology (fibrillation) (Figs. 6.101 and 6.102).

There are studies that report independent pulsations in the distal segment of the pulmonary veins [6] Only a small part of the left atrium derives from the primitive atrium . This part is represented by the left auricle together with a neighbouring territory. As a result, the left atrium presents in this territory the rare pectinate muscles and a few muscle bundles which penetrate the left auricle (Fig. 6.103).

The circular space located just above the mitral ring, is the mitral subauricular vestibule. As in the right part, the vestibule derives from the atrioventricular canal.

Sometimes, to the right of the ostia of the right pulmonary veins, the atrial wall has a vertical crease determined by the tangential direction of the pulmonary veins to the atrial wall. Although it is not easy to demonstrate, the left atrium has a tight inferior- posterior boundary with the wall of the coronary sinus when it enters into the dorsosinusal space. This boundary explains the possible existence of congenital atriosinusale communications (Figs. 8.56 and 6.104).

The left atrium is partially covered by the right atrium towards which it is positioned posteriorly and to the left. This is how we can explain why the left atrium is participating in the formation of the posterior wall of the transverse pericardial sinus. Another boundary of great clinical importance must be mentioned, namely the posterior boundary of the left

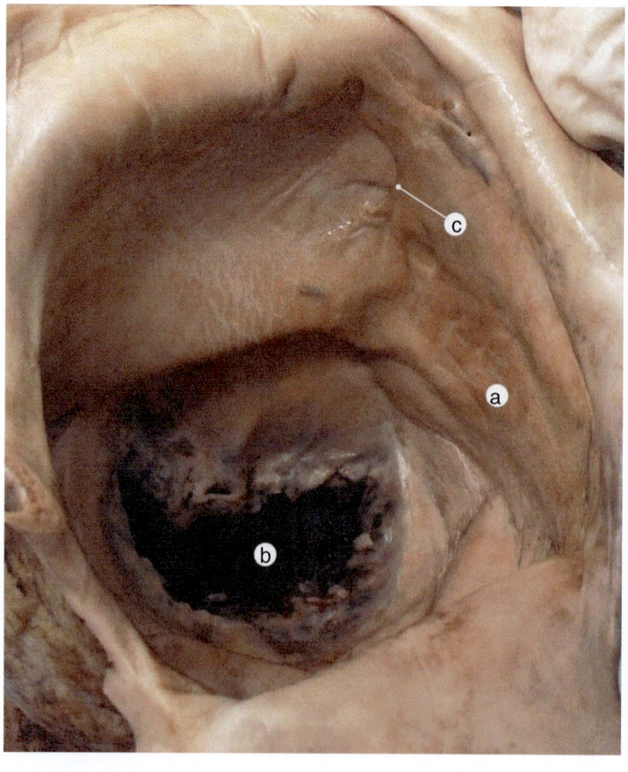

Fig. 6.99 he interior appearance of the left atrium. Postero-superior view. *a* mitral valve, *b* Interatrial septum, *c* falx septi

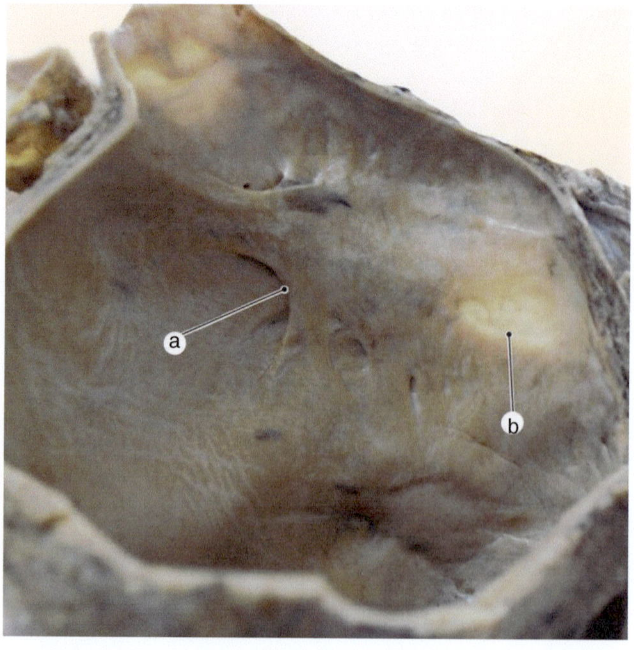

Fig. 6.100 Interatrial septum seen from the left atrium. *a* falx septi, *b* transillumination of the fossa ovalis

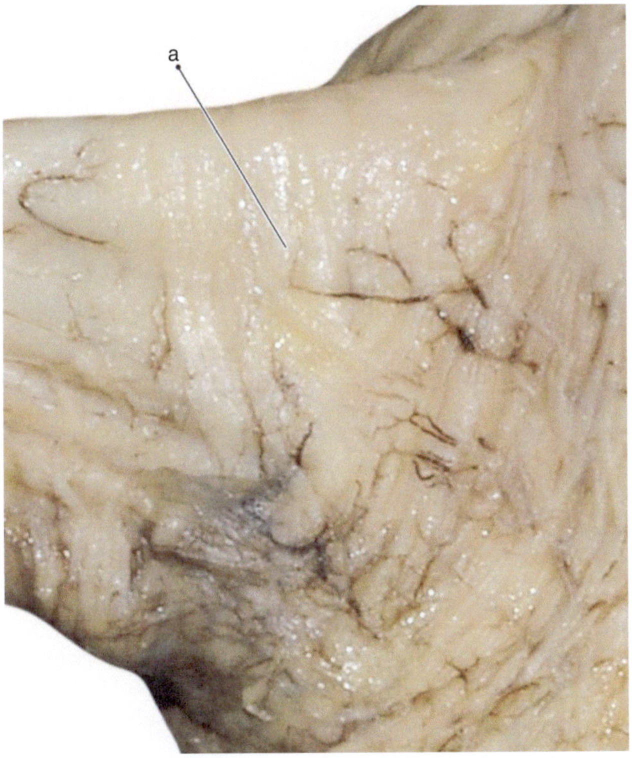

Fig. 6.101 Miocardisation of a pulmonary vein terminal part. Macroscopically, the peripulmonary muscular fibers are paler than the atrial ones (embryological trait). *a* the inferior left pulmonary vein with muscularised wall

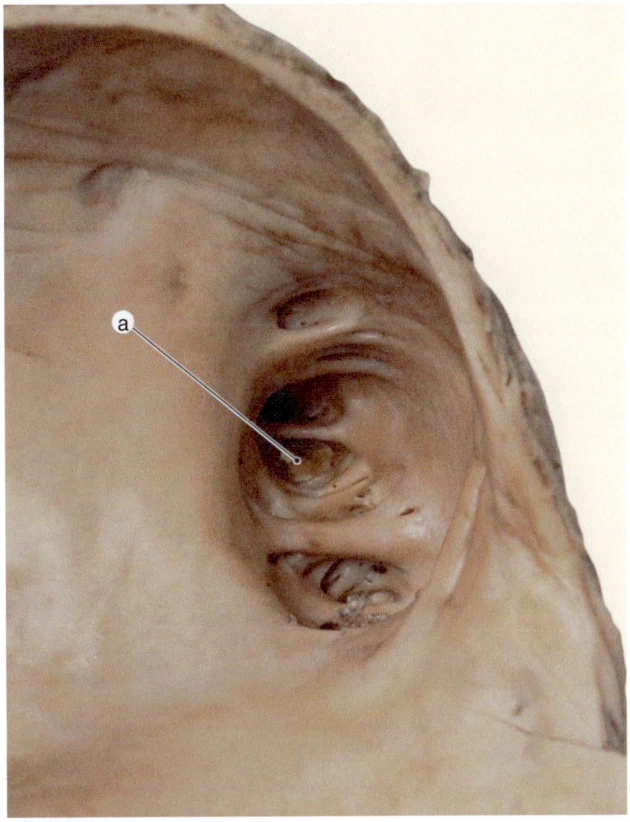

Fig. 6.103 The interior appearance of a small left auricle. *a* the left auricle with muscle trabeculae

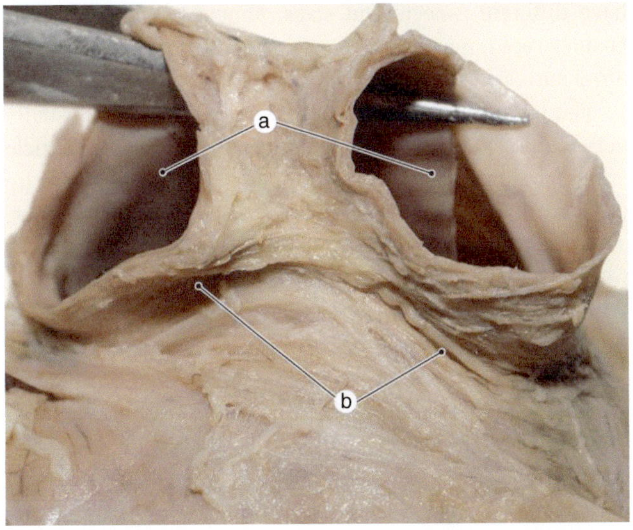

Fig. 6.102 Miocardisation of the pulmonary veins common opening. *a* left pulmonary veins, *b* circular muscle fibers around the common opening

atrium with the thoracic esophagus. The cavity of the left atrium has a globulous aspect, the interatrial septum representing the right and posterior part of the anterior atrial wall.

The exact anterior wall which corresponds with of the aorta is thin and can be easily ripped (unraveled) if it is excessively tractioned [6].

The anterior wall derives from the interatrial notch of the primitive atrium. As a result, the muscular blanket between the two atria is continuous, providing a right- left conduction pathway. (See the chapter about the structure of the atrial wall).

The interatrial septum is placed obliquely between the frontal and sagittal plan. On the septum there is an endocardic fold with a falciform (concave) aspect called the valve of the fossa ovale-falx septi. This "valve" has its concavity directed anteriorly and upwards. If we transilluminate septum we can notice that the falx septi is positioned in front of the oval fossa, which suggests the anterior oblique orientation of the interatrial aperture of communication in intrauterine period (Figs. 6.100 and 6.105).

On the posterior wall of the left atrium pulmonary veins commence through four ostia arranged into two pairs (Figs. 4.3 and 4.45). The ostia of the left veins are positioned superiorly to the orifices of the right pulmonary veins. Quite often the orifices from the same side may merge. Rarely the orifices from opposite sides can merge. As a consequence, the number of ostia sof the pulmonary veins in the left atrium is variable.

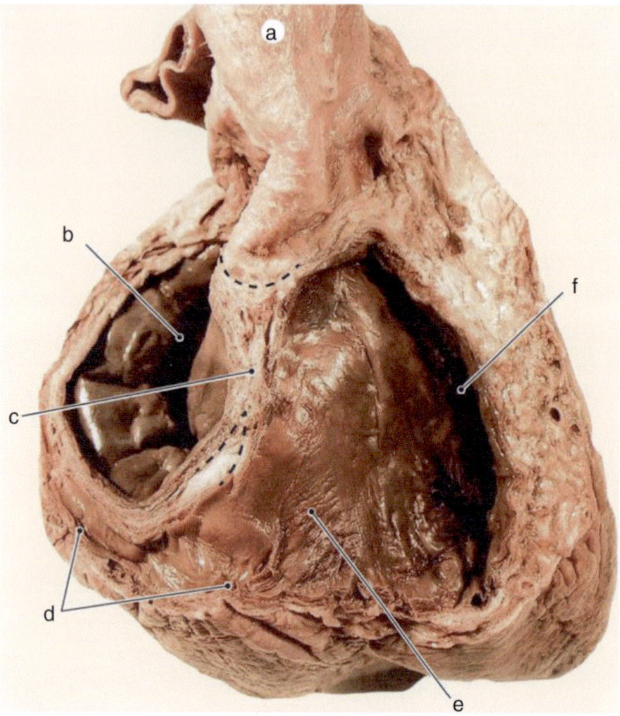

Fig. 6.104 The relation between the left atrium and the coronary sinus. The ventricular insertion base of the interatrial septum is marked with the dotted line. The coronary sinus appears as an extension of the right atrium. *a* aorta, *b* mitral ostium, *c* interatrial septum base, *d* the coronary sinus appears as an extension of the right atrium, *e* the right atrium floor corresponding to the pyramidal area, *f* tricuspid ostium

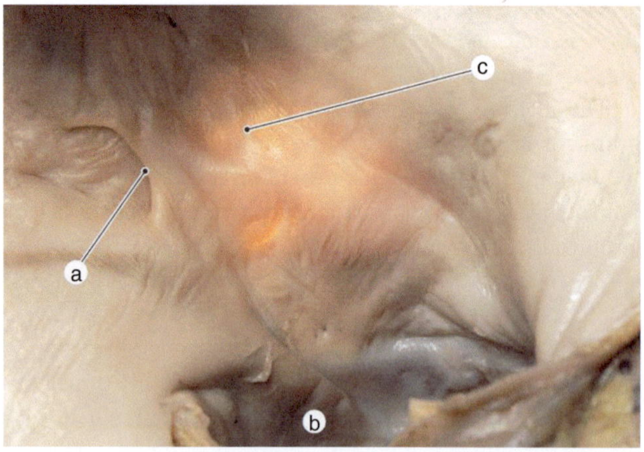

Fig. 6.105 Left side of the interatrial septum. The relation between falx septi and the fossa ovalis projection (transillumination). *a* falx septi, *b* mitral orifice, *c* fossa ovalis transillumination

According to Kato et al. [7], for the right side, besides the two pulmonaary veins, the superior and the inferior ones, the following variants can exist: a median pulmonary vein, two median pulmonary veins, a supreme pulmonary vein, a median pulmonary vein and a supreme pulmonary vein.

For the left side, besides the two pulmonary veins – the superior vein and the inferior vein – that open separately or

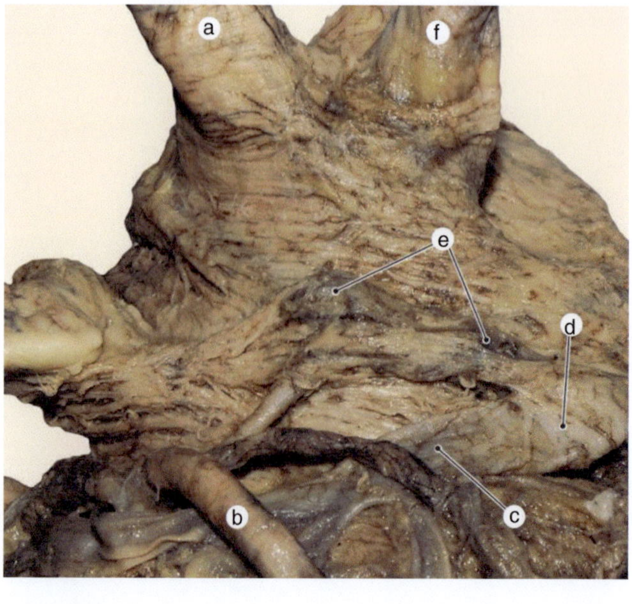

Fig. 6.106 The left pulmonary veins manner of drainage and their local anatomical relations. Left-side view. *a* muscularised superior left pulmonary vein, *b* circumflex artery, *c* great cardiac vein, *d* sinusal border, *e* oblique vein, *f* inferior left pulmonary vein

through a unique orifice the following variants exist: a short common trunk and a long common trunk (Figs. 6.102 and 6.106).

At the conjunction of the anterior wall with the lateral one we find the communication with the left atrial auricle.

The two atrial plural – auriculae the right and the left one have different aspects and sizes, almost typical. This fact ensures rapid, many times intuitive identification of the two atrial auricles.

The left atrial auricle is longer, narrower, having usually very embattled margins. The margins of the left atrial auricle are marked by deeper incisions. Sometimes the auricular tip can be bifid. The axis of the atrial auricle is often sinuous. The communication orifice with the left atrium is well-formed and sometimes the left atrial auricle has a distinct "neck"through which it inserts itself in the atrium. Intraluminally, a few rudimentary trabeculae can be observed. Pretty rarely, a trabecular pattern is developed. Surprisingly, the position of the left atrial auricle can be changed (varied) too. Its tip can reach the pulmonary infundibulum, next to the right atrial auricle. In some cases, the tip of the left atrial auricle can be situated behind the aorta. The right atrial auricle (as we have already shown) is shorter and larger, has smoother edges and a larger base of implantation. Its general aspect is cone-shaped and its tip is blunt. Its interior aspect is (as we have mentioned) heavilytrabeculated.

The basis of the left atrium is formed mostly by the left atrioventricular orifice – bicuspid or mitral. This will be described in the left ventricle. Unlike the right atrium, the mitral orifice is found on the basal wall, situated in antero-inferiorly to the left atrium.

6.4 The Internal Configuration of the Left Ventricle

6.4.1 General Considerations on the Left Ventricle Cavity

If we look at the heart with the eyes of an architect, the left ventricle seems structurally the main cavity of the heart: it has the thickest walls (8–12 mm), the most symmetrical form – cone-shaped with the apex pointing downwards, the trabeculae muscles are very well represented, connecting the bases of the papillary muscles both amongst themselves and with the ventricular walls. And functionally speaking, the left ventricle, which pushes blood into the systemic circulation, is the main pump.

Here are a few observations on the internal appearance of the left ventricle:

On the interventricular septum a part of the trabeculae situated in the direction of the blood flow (evacuation of the blood) are included (absorbed) variably in the septum. These trabeculae commence from the apex and end subendocardially in the root of the aorta.

- Such a disposition implies that the root of the aorta becomes solidary (through the septal trabecular system) with the dynami 133cs of the heart's apex and the septal wall is smoother, in order to facilitate ejection (Fig. 6.107).
- among the subendocardial muscle fibers of the aortic vestibule the left bundle branch of the bundle of Hiss descends, then divides into its own fascicles. Sometimes this branch or portions of it can be observed subendocardially (in dolphins for example, the left bundle branch and its fascicles travel intracavitary. When Purkinje described the fascicles of the excitoconductor tissue, he initially found them intracavitary and described them as gelatinous fibers) [8] (Fig. 6.108).
- the trabecular network at the apex of the heart is extremely well- represented as a connecting network on one hand between the bases of the papillary muscles and on the other hand, between the papillary muscles, the apex of the ventricle and its walls. Perhaps with the same function as in the right ventricle, these trabeculae transmit the pressures exerted by the mitral ring along the tendinous chordae and the papillary muscles towards the heart's apex and heart walls (Fig. 6.109).
- finally, a last observation is that the aortic ring and the mitral ring are interlocked via the aortic curtain and mitro-aortic continuity (it will be discussed later on).

In conclusion, these anatomical observations contribute to the explanation of one aspect of ventricular dynamics: during ventricular contraction both the transverse diameter of the ventricle (by contraction of the circular fibers of the myocardium) diminishes, as well as the longitudinal diameter (by lowering the plane of the heart valves, which also includes the two orifices).

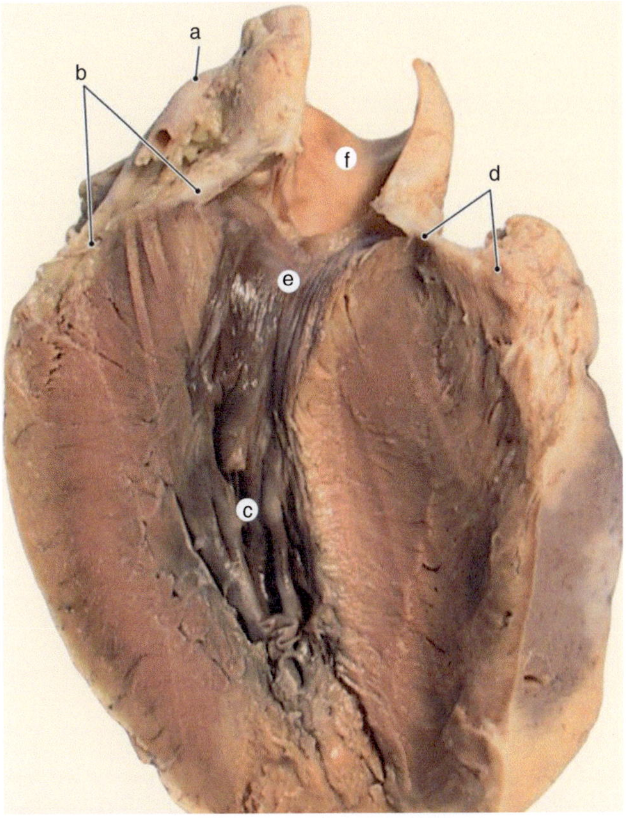

Fig. 6.107 Left side of the interventricular septum. The aortic root corresponding to the medium part of the septal base. *a* left coronary artery, *b* anterior part of the interventricular septum's base, *c* trabeculae embeded in the septum, *d* posterior part of the interventricular septum, *e* aortic vestibule, *f* aorta

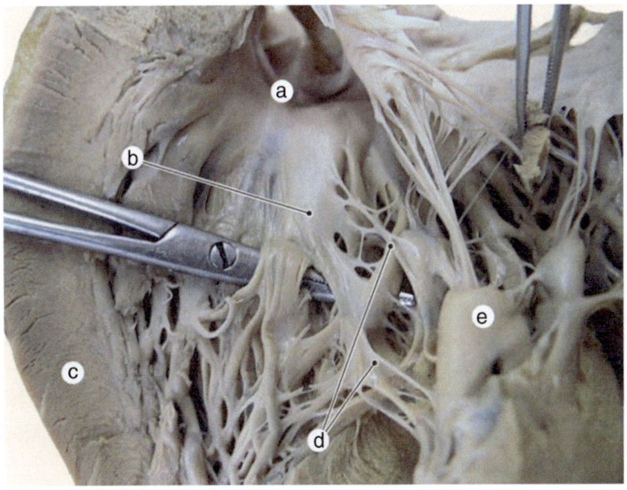

Fig. 6.108 The left branch from the bundle of Hiss descends under the vestibulary endocardium. *a* aortic vestibule, *b* left branch of the bundle of Hiss, *c* left ventricle, *d* purkinje fibers, *e* posterior papillary muscle

A transverse section of the heart at ventricular level will reveal that the right ventricle seems wrapped around the left ventricle (Fig. 6.60).

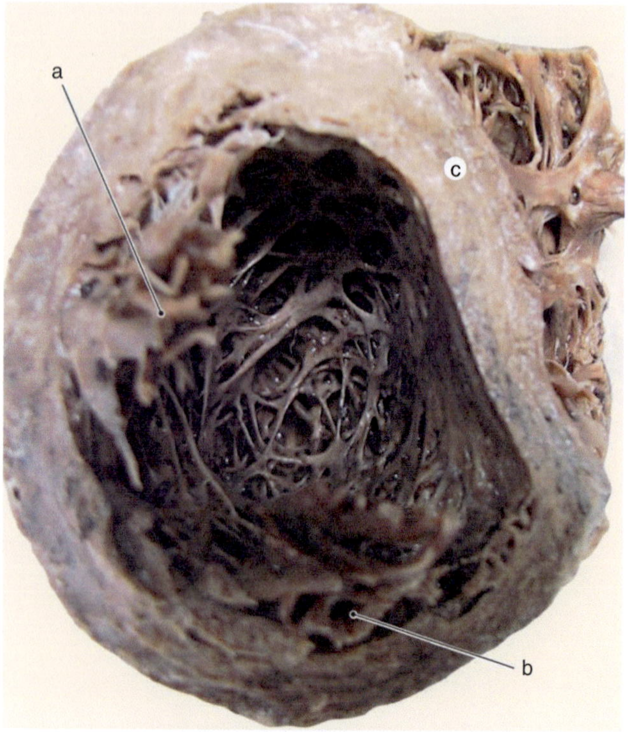

Fig. 6.109 The appearance of the trabecular network at the left ventricle apex. *a* anterior papillary muscle, *b* posterior papillary muscle, *c* interventricular septum

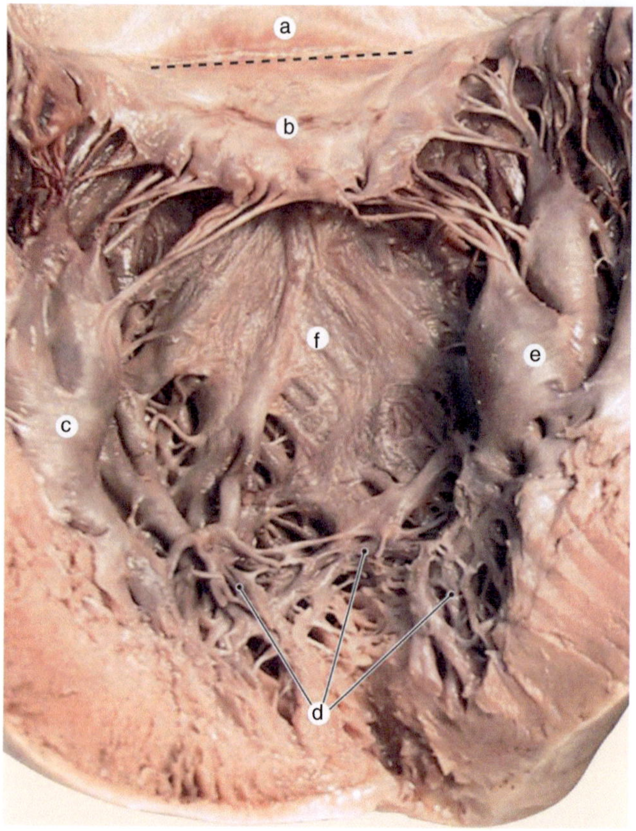

Fig. 6.110 Papillary muscles location inside the left ventricle. *a* mitral-aortic continuity, *b* anterior mitral cusp, *c* anterior papillary muscle, *d* aaical trabecular network which reinforces the papillary muscles bases, *e* posterior papillary muscle, *f* septum with embeded trabeculae

The left ventricle occupies a smaller area on the heart's sternocostal surface than the right ventricle, a larger area on the diaphragmatic surface than the right ventricle whereas the pulmonary surface of the heart (or the obtuse margin of the heart) is represented entirely by the left ventricle.

The classic statement used by for the specialists in anatomy is that in the ventricle there are two left papillary muscles – anterior and posterior. In reality, we are often talking about an anterior and posterior papillary group, the muscular cones of the papillary muscles being more or less connected at their base and branched towards the top.

Discussing the terms anterior and posterior when describing the papillary muscles, Anderson et al. [9] elegantly show that the classical descriptions were made with the heart opened on its obtuse aspect and with the apex pointing down. Reorienting the heart with its long axis to the left and inferiorly, we see that the anterior papillary group is in fact superior, mural and to the left, and the posterior papillary group is inferior, septal and to the right (Figs. 6.110 and 6.64).

The chordae tendineae which start from the tips of the papillary muscles insert fara on both cusps of the mitral orifice fara.

The atrioventricular cusps are arranged as followed: the anteromedial cusp (or short, the anterior cusp), is also clinically called the great mitral cusp. Due to its rapports with the root of the aorta the name "aortic cusp" is very suggestive (Fig. 6.111).

The second cusp is positioned posterolaterally and called, in short, the posterior cusp. Its dynamic solidarity with the ventricular non septal wall with the ventricular wall (not the ventricular septum) justifies the name fara mural cusp (Fig. 6.112). The free margin of the anterior cusp along with the area of the interventricular septum that opposes this margin delineates an orifice that divides the ventricular cavity into a lower reception compartment (with irregular walls due to the presence of the muscle trabeculae) and a superomedial ejection compartment (with walls relatively smooth).

In its terminal part, the ejection compartment changes direction upwards and to the right. This last portion of the ejection compartment, with an almost transversal floor (in respect to the bloodflow axis), located immediately below the aortic ring justifies its name as the aortic vestibule (Fig. 6.113).

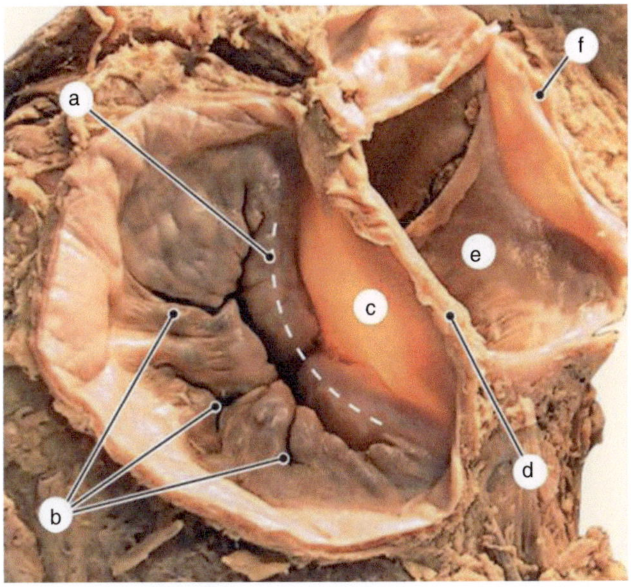

Fig. 6.111 Mitral cusps and their relation to the aortic vestibule. The notches divide the cuspidian lobules. *a* the apposition area, *b* notches in the posterior mitral cusp, *c* anterior mitral cusp, *d* mitro-aortic continuity, *e* aortic vestibule, *f* right coronary sinus

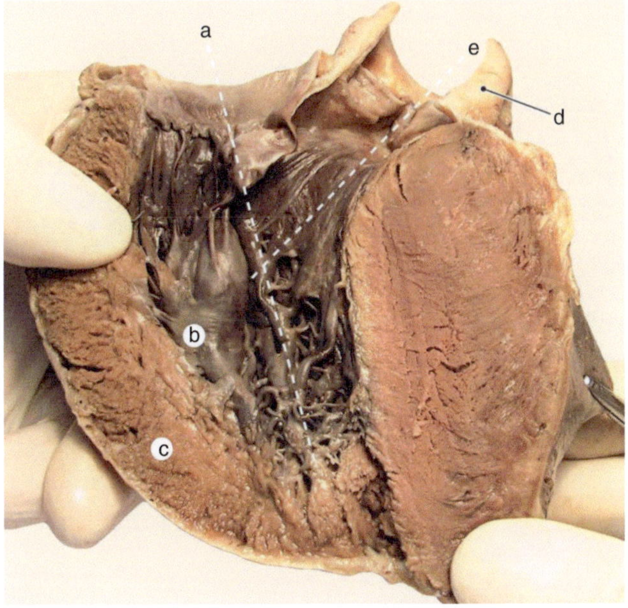

Fig. 6.113 The different orientations of the left ventricle compartments. View from the left side. *a* reception compartment axis, *b* anterior papillary muscle, *c* left ventricular wall, *d* aorta, *e* ejection compartment axis

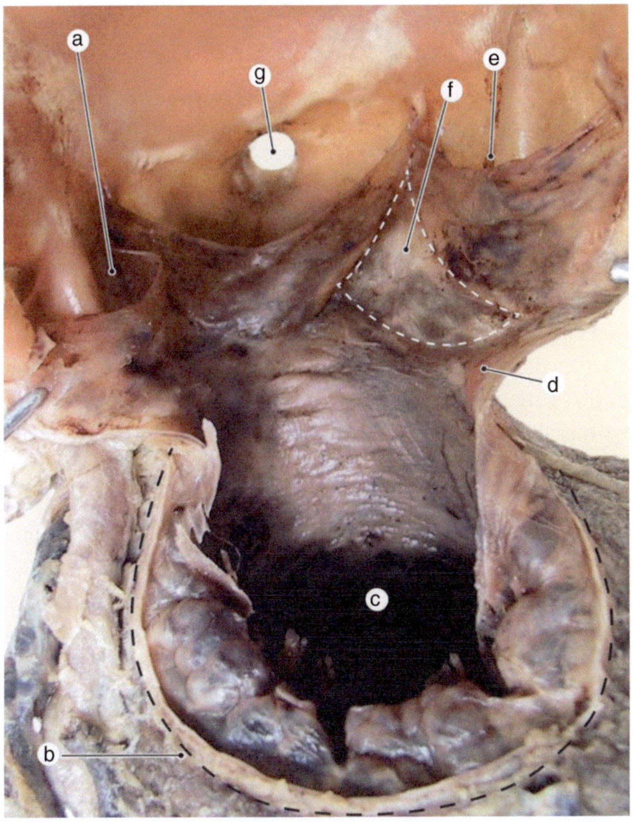

Fig. 6.112 The insertion of the posterior mitral cusp and the mitroaortic orifice after fara removal of the mitro-aortic continuity. *a* left coronary sinus, *b* the insertion of the posterior cusp on the mitral ring, *c* mitro-aortic orifice, *d* tendinous centre, *e* noncoronary sinus, *f* Henle trigone, *g* right coronary artery ostium

6.4.2 The Valvular Apparatus of the Left Atrioventricular Orifice

The left atrioventricular valve, bicuspid or mitral (mitral valvular complex) prevents the return of blood to the left atrium during the ventricular systole and consists of: the atrioventricular ring, the anterior and posterior cusps, the chordae tendineae and the anterior and posterior papillary muscles.

The mitral orifice has the circumference of 7–9 cm. Its shape resembles the "D" letter facing down and with the vertical segment of the letter to the mitro-aortic continuity (Fig. 6.114).

6.4.3 The Left Atrioventricular Ring

The atrioventricular ring correlates with a circular groove (which is palpable), where in superior view the atrial endocardium continues with the endocardium of the two cusps (Fig. 6.115).

The groove is the result of the "folding" of the endocardium of the atrioventricular canal which led to the formation of the left atrioventricular junction (see embriology). The segment of this fold situated in the angle between the aorta and the left atrium at the base of the aortic curtain, corresponds to the mitroaortic continuity (Figs. 6.116 and 6.113). In the depth of this circular fold, similar to the situation found in the tricuspid, the conjunctive from the cusp axis diverges into the coronary sulcus. The endocardium of the

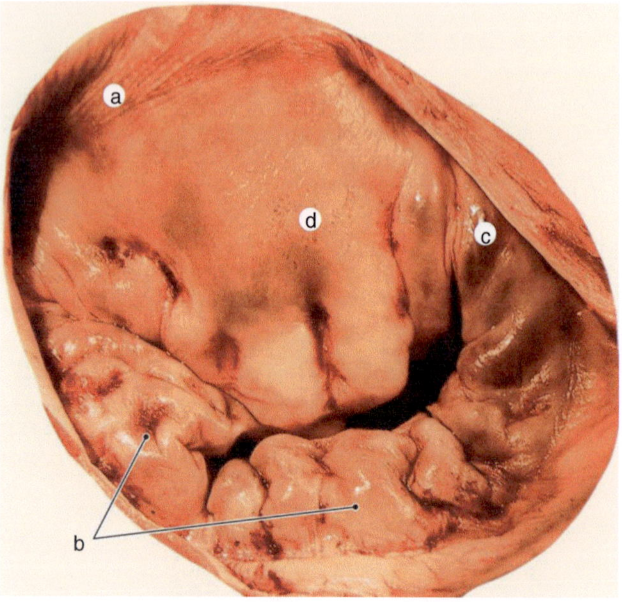

Fig. 6.114 Atrial view of the mitral valve. *a* mitral-aortic continuity, *b* valvular lobules, *c* commissure, *d* anterior mitral cusp

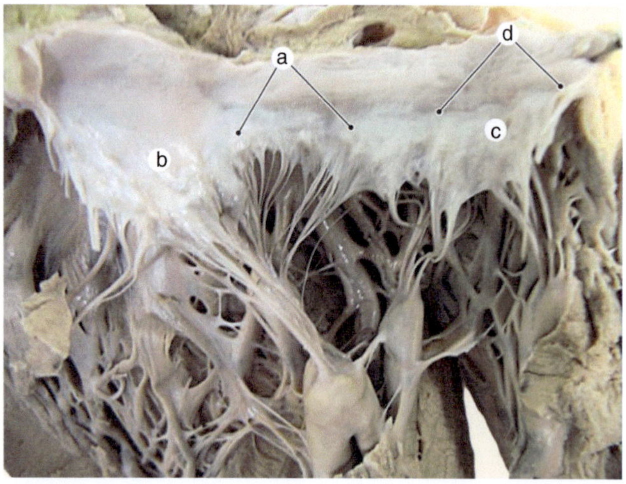

Fig. 6.115 Mitral valve unfolded. View from the left side. *a* velamentous commissural area, *b* anterior mitral cusp, *c* posterior mitral cusp, *d* circular atrioventricular sulcus

cusps coats the superior and inferior membranous blades which form the two roots of the cusps. After a very short path, the roots continue with the muscular walls. In this way, the roots of the cusps which are not muscled form a cylinder segment called the atrioventricular ring (Fig. 6.117). The mitral ring also has in its structure or in its neighbourhood the fila coronaria, and so on (see fibrous skeleton and tricuspid ring).

Deriving from the anterior horn of the fibrous triangle, we can sometimes find a short, anterior filacoronaria.

From the left horn of the fibrous triangle also derives a filacoronaria which penetrates the mitroaortic continuity

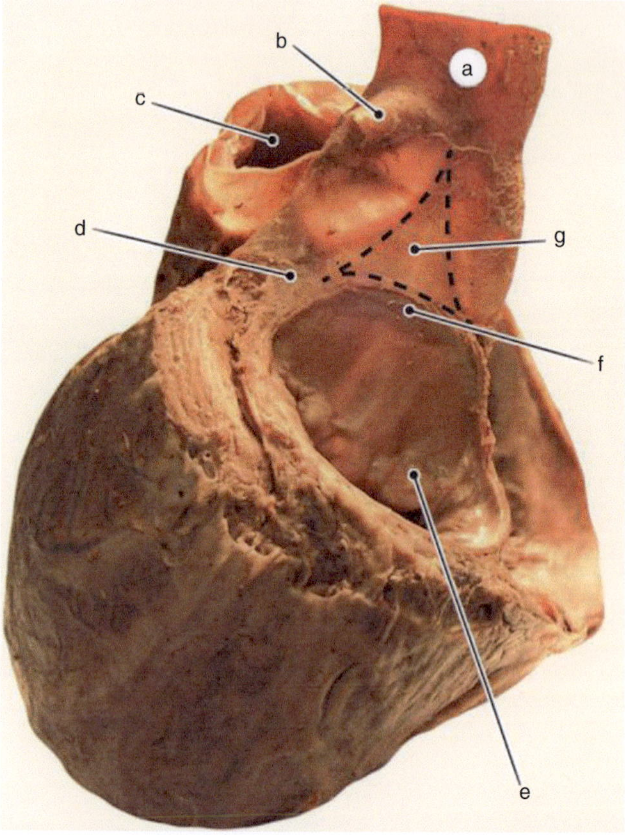

Fig. 6.116 The relation between the mitral valve and the aortic root. *a* aorta, *b* left coronary artery, *c* pulmonary valve, *d* left fibrous trigone, *e* anterior mitral cusp, *f* mitral-aortic continuity, *g* intervalvular septum – aortic curtain

and intertwines with the filacoronaria from the right horn of the triangle.

From the posterior horn of the tendinous triangle derives a left posterior filacoronaria towards the posterior half of the mitral ring. In this way, at the base of the aortic curtain, within the mitroaortic continuity, the mitral ring is well-defined and elastic.

As on the right side, the filacoronaria do not circumscribe the whole mitral ring (see images from fibrous skeleton).

For a better understanding of the concept of atrioventricular ring, we are going to repeat some observations which were also discussed at the tricuspid ring:

- the base of the cusps consists of two fibro-membranous roots which are divergent, one going upwards, the other downwards. The superior root is lined by the atrial endocardium and the inferior one by the ventricular endocardium (Fig. 6.117).
- After a very short path the two blades continue with the atrial and ventricular muscular walls.
- in the angle of divergence formed between the blades (with the appearance of a cylinder segment) there can be

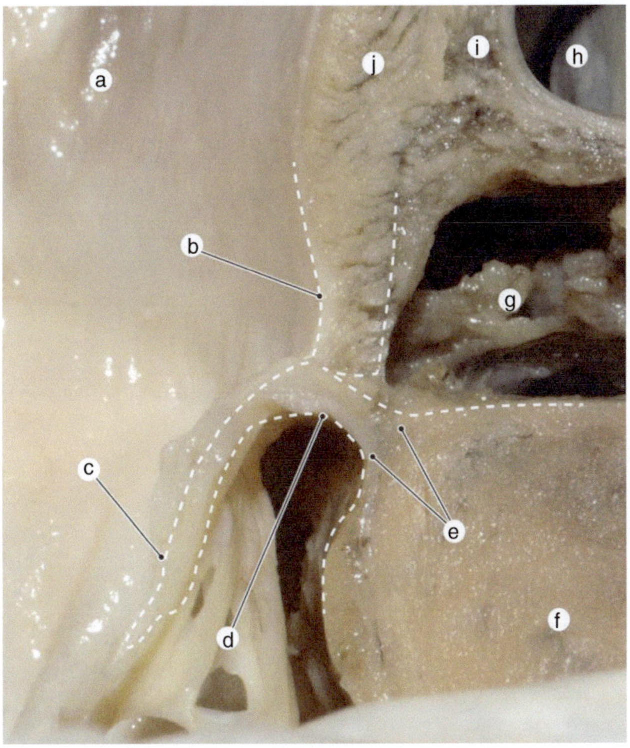

Fig. 6.117 Atrioventricular junction. *a* left atrium, *b* superior root, *c* posterior mitral cusp, *d* inferior root, *e* subepi-subendocardial continuity, *f* left ventricle wall, *g* coronary sinus, *h* right atrium, *i* interatrial septum, *j* left atrium muscular wall

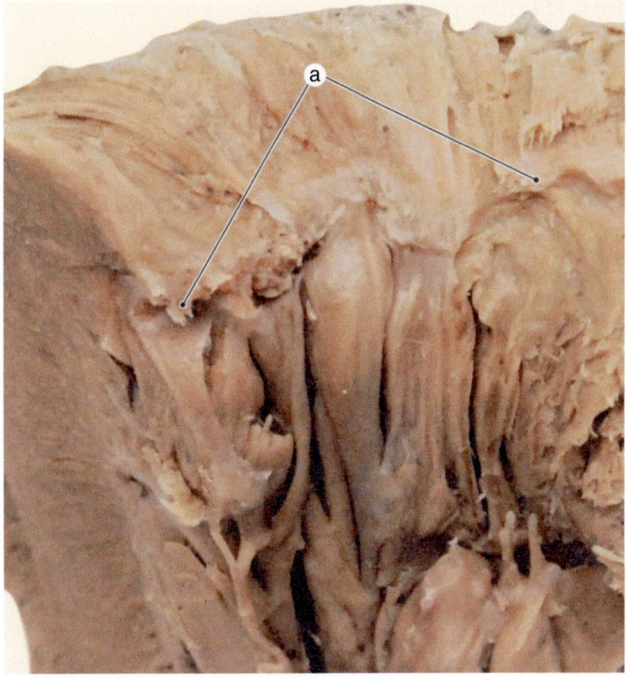

Fig. 6.118 The demonstration of the subepi-subendocardial continuity. At this level, the subepicardial muscle fibers and the subendocardial muscle fibers act in different directions as well as the roots of the atrioventricular cusps. *a* subepi-subendocardial continuity

found connective and fatty tissue, which along with the filacoronaria form the atrioventricular ring. This provides on one hand, atrioventricular electrical insulation and on the other hand, the mechanic connection between the atria and ventricles.

- the filacoronaria are found in the ventricular myocardium, in the middle of the myocardium, parallel with the margins of the atrioventricular rings, supporting the insertion of the myocardium and in the same time strengthening the complex area called the atrioventricular junction (see the fibrous skeleton).
- The behaviour of the epicardium, the endocardium and atrial and ventricular myocardium in the vecinity of the ring is as follows:
- the epicardium does not mold to the ring area. It descends from the atrium, skips the coronary sulcus, at a distance from the basis of the cusps. In the space thus formed (the coronary sulcus) pass the circumflex artery, the great vein, the oblique vein of the left atrium and the coronary sinus. All these course through a fatty and connective tissue environment.
- at the level of the atrioventricular ring, from the inferior view, the endocardium leaves the ventricular wall and coats the inferior root of the base of the cusp. The place where the endocardium leaves the ventricular wall, is an actual insertion for the ventricular root (the inferior root) of the cusp. At this level, we can observe how the subepicardic ventricular muscle fibers continue with the subendocardic ventricular muscle fibers (the subepi-subendocardic muscle continuity) (Fig. 6.118).
- from the superior view, the continuity of the atrial endocardium with that of the cusps (the superior blade) is very evident.

The place in which the endocardium of the superior root starts to coat the atrial muscle, can be considered the area of atrial insertion for the atrial (superior) root of the cusp (Figs. 6.119 and 6.120).

At the base of the cusp we can palpate and sometimes observe the circular outline of the atrioventricular ring. Between the atrial and ventricular insertions of the cusp, the two blades of the roots of the cusp create the aspect of a fibro-membranous cylinder segment coated by the endocardium and folded at the base of the cusp.

As we have shown in the case of the tricuspid valve at the level of the mitral valve in the vicinity of the atrioventricular ring, the transmitting of the electric impulse is interrupted. We mention that here also, remnant atrioventricular muscle

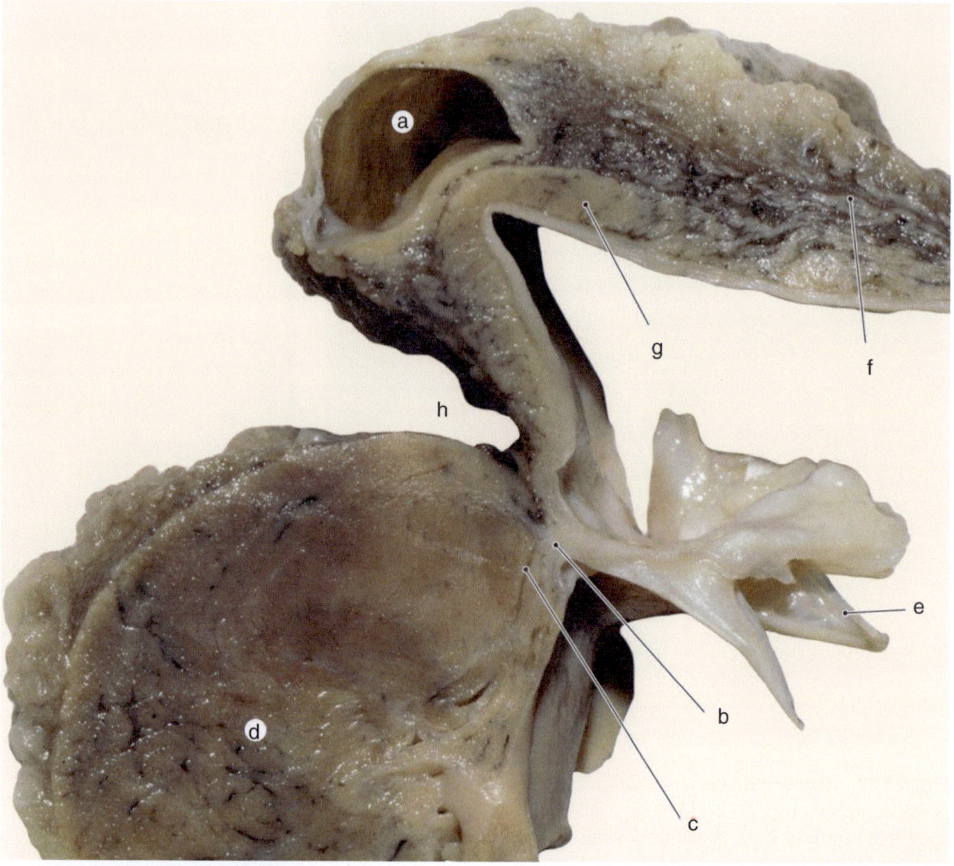

Fig. 6.119 Atrioventricular junction – general view. Note the atrioventricular fold. *a* coronary sinus, *b* Subepi-subendocardial continuity, *c* connective tissue trabeculae that fade away in the muscular thickness, *d* left ventricle, *e* posterior mitral valve, *f* subepicardial muscle fibers, *g* left atrium muscular wall, *h* atrioventricular fold

Fig. 6.120 Atrioventricular junction (in detail). *a* superior root, *b* posterior mitral cusp, *c* inferior root, *d* left ventricle, *e* connective tissue trabeculae that fade intramusculary, *f* subepi-subendocardial continuity, *g* left atrium muscular wall

bundles can be found, which may be involved in the inadequate transmission of the atrioventricular impulse. More often these muscle bundles can be found at the level of the crux cordis.

6.4.4 The Atrioventricular Cusps

The layout of the atrioventricular valves is very variable.

If we detach the cusps from the ring we can observe, as in the right ventricle, that they form a continuous membranous veil (Fig. 6.115). This continuity is marked by deep indentations that define commissures and by less deep indentations that separate the valvular lobules (Fig. 6.114).

In other words, the commissures are not areas of discontinuity, but actually of continuity, where the membranous veil is less spread.

From the superior view, the indentations extend by means of small grooves on the cusp, all the way up near the atrioventricular ring. These grooves are formed because the entire velamentous area of the cusps is greater than the surface of the atrioventricular ring. When the valve is open, within these grooves, the cusp folds. When the valve is closed, the surface between the grooves bulges towards the left atrium (Fig. 6.114).

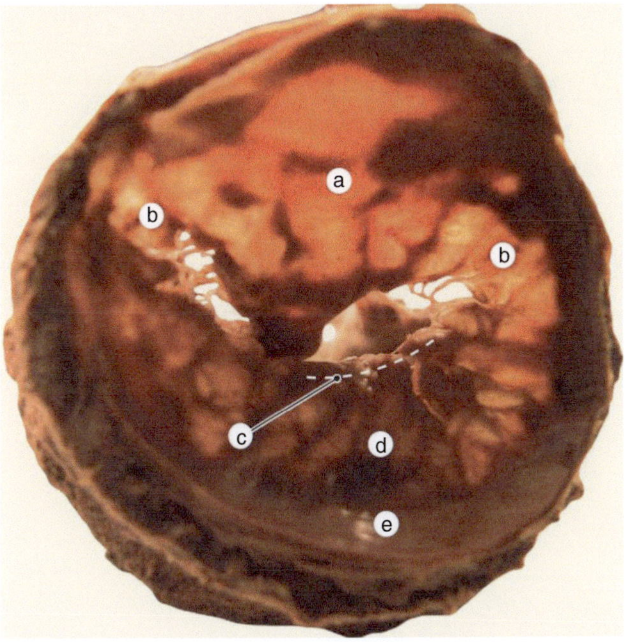

Fig. 6.121 The cusps topography. Superior view of the mitral valve. Transillumination. The apposition line of the cusps doesn't reach the fibrous ring. *a* anterior mitral cusp, *b* commissure, *c* rugged free edge, *d* intermediate area, *e* basal area

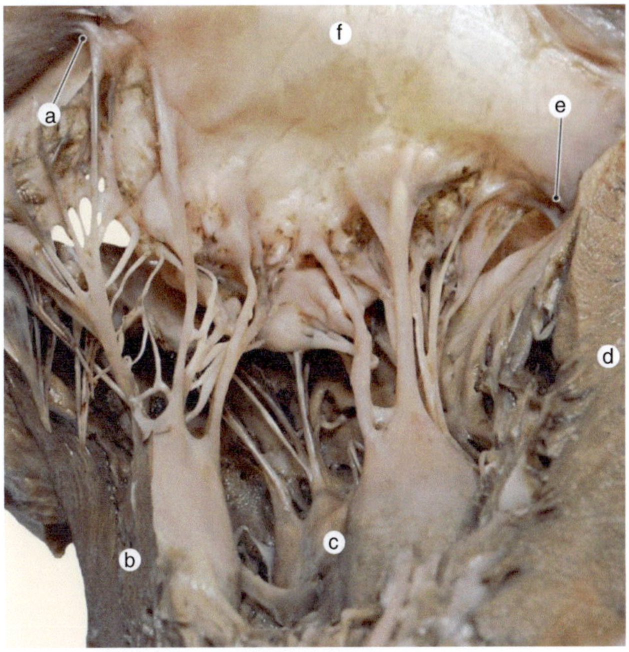

Fig. 6.122 Inferior and right-side view of the mitral valve. *a* posterior commissural area, *b* posterior papillary muscle, *c* anterior papillary muscle, *d* interventricular septum, *e* anterior commissural area, *f* anterior mitral cusp

We can observe an anterolateral commissural area and a posteromedial one (Figs. 6.114 and 6.121).

The anterior aortic cusp is wider, with small and inconsistent indentations. In Figs. 6.141, 6.153b and 8.56, we can observe variants of the lobulation of the anterior cusp.

The posterior-mural cusp is narrower and has two indentations which are almost constant and which subdivide it into three lobules (Figs. 6.111, 6.115).

Although the insertion of the aortic cusp occupies about one third of the atrioventricular ring, its size greatly increases towards the free margin, thus both cusps close relatively equal parts of the surface of the atrioventricular orifice [9].

Among the lobules, the central one has a greater tendancy to prolapse during ventricular systole.

A cusp can be described as having: a base (basal area), a free, floating, dense (rough) margin and between them an intermediary area, a translucent or "clear" area (Fig. 6.121).

The roughness of the cusp margins and also the grooves and indentations of the lobules facilitates a better closure (apposition) of the two cusps. The apposition line does not reach the fibrous ring. This shows the effectiveness of the commissural areas in the closure of the valves (these areas do not separate but bring the cusps together).

The tendinous chordae of the heart valves are of many types, depending on the area of insertion: chordae for the free margin, for the translucent area, for the basal area, for the commissural area and for the indentation area

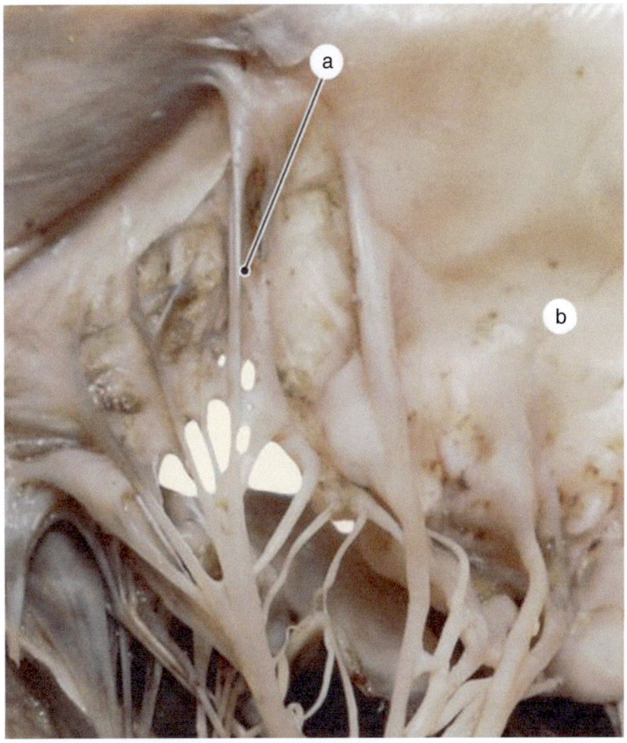

Fig. 6.123 Detail of the posterior commissure. *a* tendinous chord with ventricular insertion in the commissural axis, *b* anterior cusp

(Figs. 6.122, 6.123, 6.124, 6.125, 6.126, 6.127 and 6.128). There also exist false chordae which start from the ventricular walls and end in the ventricular walls. Sometimes the

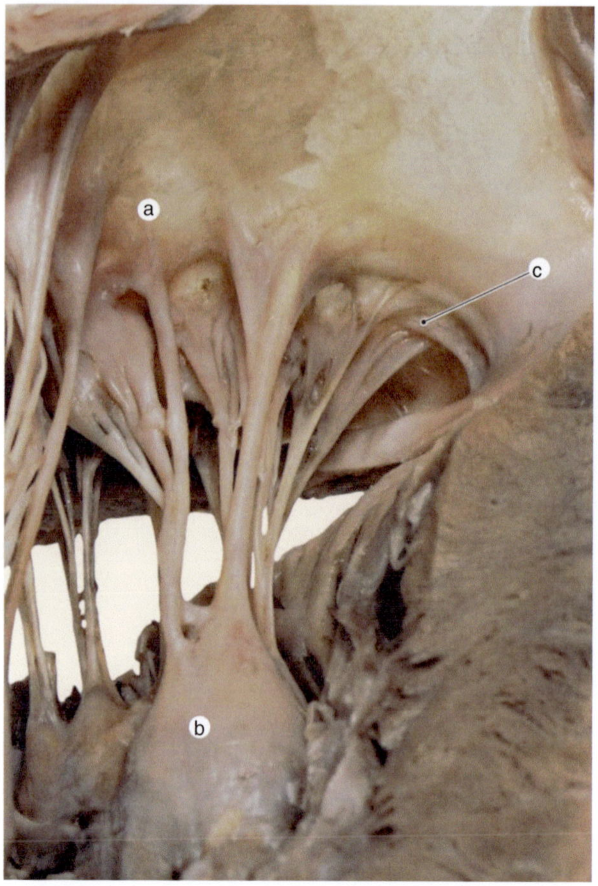

Fig. 6.124 Detail of anterior commissure. Inferior view. *a* anterior cusp, *b* anterior papillary muscle, *c* chordae tendineae with ventricular insertion in commissural axis

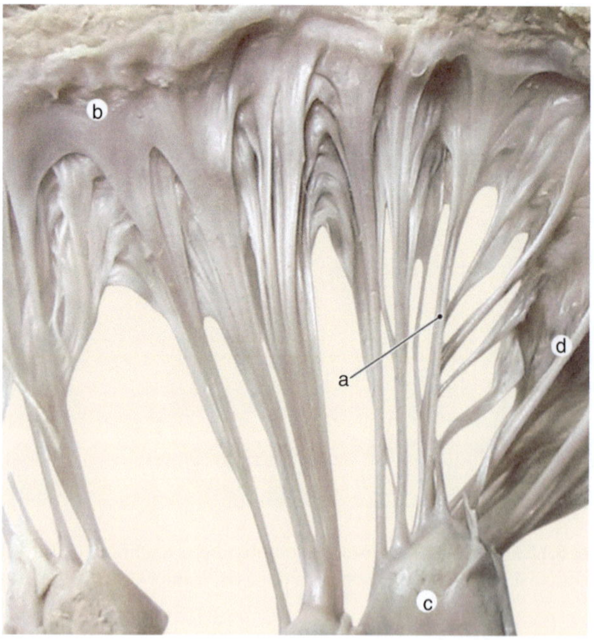

Fig. 6.125 The aspect of the chordae tendineae on the ventricular face of the mitral cusps. Structuralwise, the tendinous chords extremities form successive arches at the level of their cusp insertion. *a* chordae tendineae in the commissural axis, *b* posterior cusp, *c* posterior papillary muscle, *d* anterior cusp

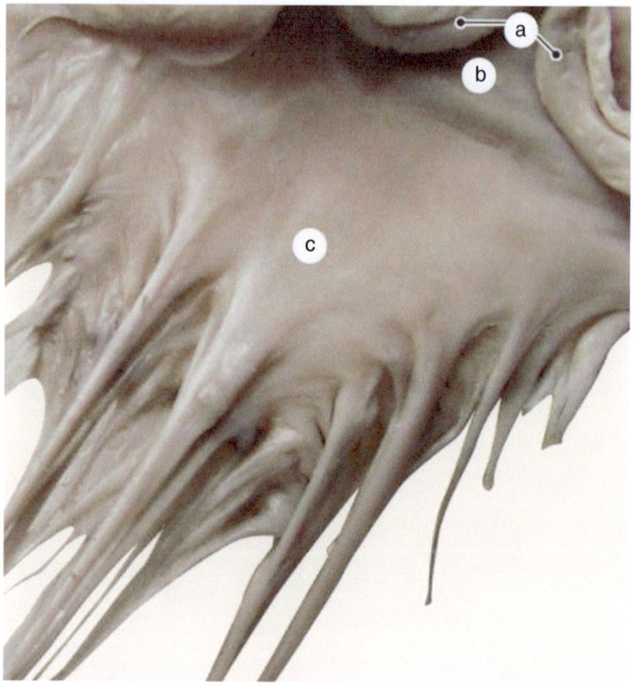

Fig. 6.126 Ventricular surface of the anterior mitral cusp. *a* aortic valvules, *b* aortic curtain, *c* anterior cusp of the mitral valve

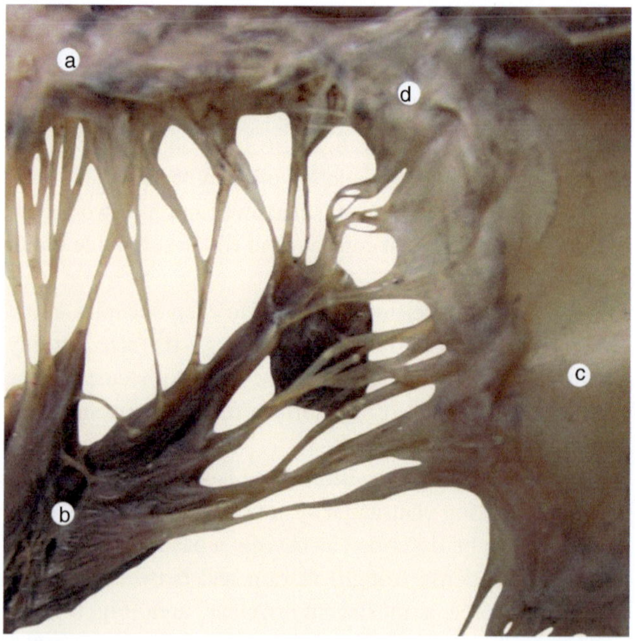

Fig. 6.127 Atrial view of the anterior mitral commissure. *a* posterior cusp, *b* anterior papillary muscle, *c* anterior cusp, *d* commissure

extremity chordae that start from the anterior papillary muscles and insert on the edges of the anterior cusp are thick and have a muscular aspect. Because of their sturdiness, they were suggestively also called "vainglorious tendinous chordae" [10] (strut chordae – engl.) (Fig. 6.129).

The tendinous chordae which leave a papillary muscle dominantly insert on the corresponding cusp, but they can also reach the opposite cusp.

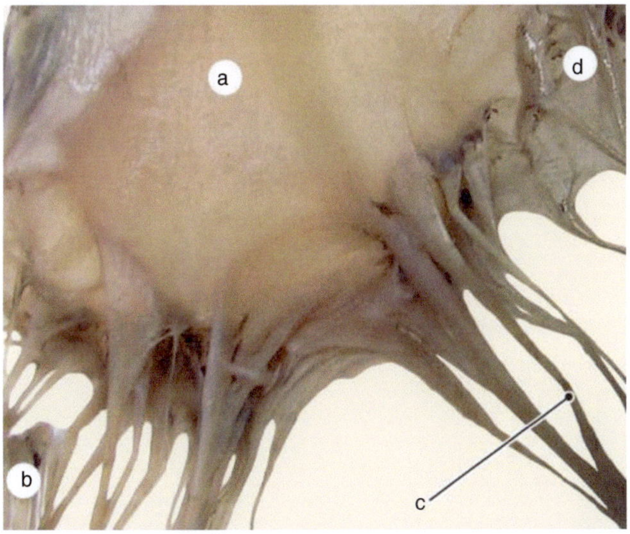

Fig. 6.128 The insertion of chordae tendineae on the anterior mitral cusp. Inferior view. *a* anterior cusp, *b* chordae of posterior papillary muscle, *c* chordae of anterior papillary muscle, *d* commissure

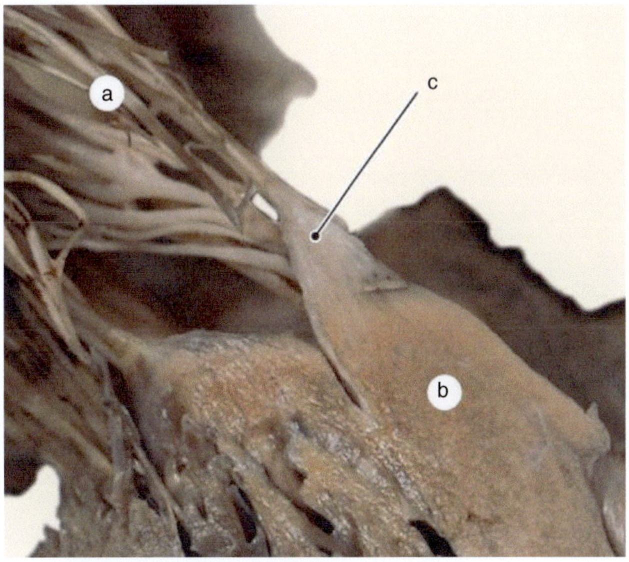

Fig. 6.130 Myotendinous junction. *a* chordae tendineae, *b* sagittal section of papillary muscle, *c*. junction area

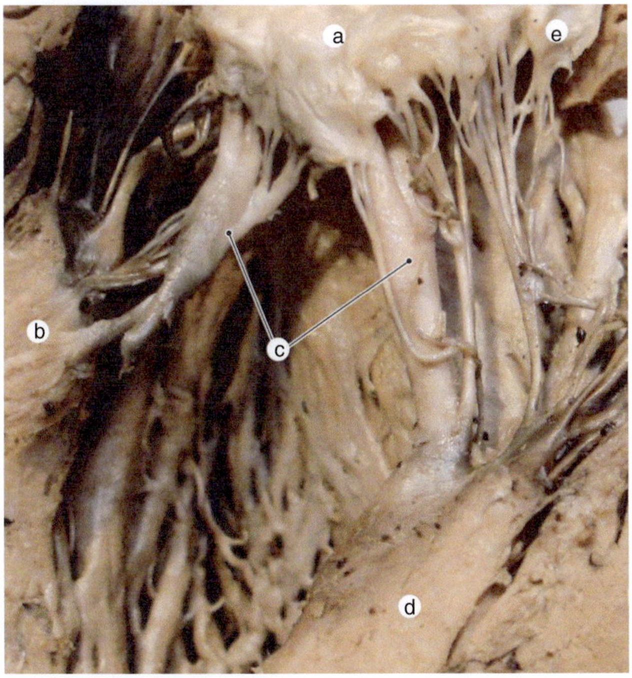

Fig. 6.129 Muscled mitral chords (strut chordae). *a* anterior cusp, *b* anterior papillary muscle, *c* strut chordae, *d* posterior papillary muscle, *e* commissure

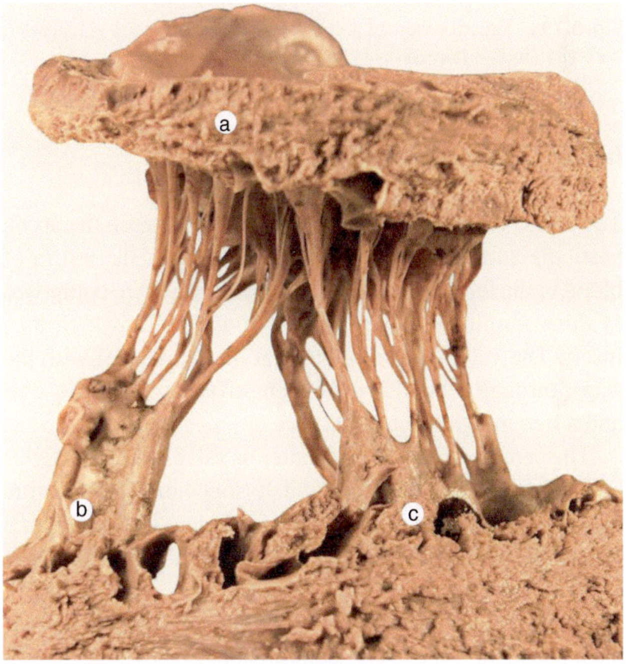

Fig. 6.131 Mitral valve (mitral parachute). General view from left side. *a* ventricular base of mitral valve, *b* anterior papillary muscle, *c* posterior papillary muscle

The papillary muscles, as we have observed, are rather represented by papillary groups:

- the anterior group (with its origin on the sternocostalwall)
- the posterior group (with its origin on the diaphragmatic wall).

Cusps are histologically composed of three structures: an internal layer of connective fibrous tissue and fibroblasts, a spongy middle layer composed of collagen bundles and a large quantity of proteoglycans (with a shock-absorbing function) and a superficial layer of endothelium and elastic fibers.

Normal cusps have NO vascularization. But blood vessels do invade inflamed cusps.

The tendinous chordae, as their name show, are fibrous bundles. But they can sometimes be muscularized. They are inserted on the tip of the papillary junction, where, in the junctional area, the connective tissue fibers penetrate between the myocytes (Figs. 6.130 and 6.131).

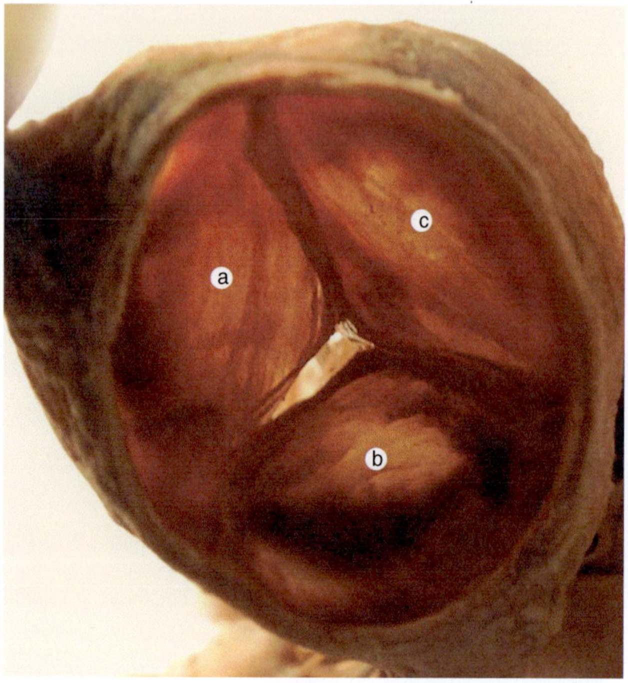

Fig. 6.132 Superior view of aortic valve. *a* right coronary sinus, *b* left coronary sinus, *c* non coronary sinus

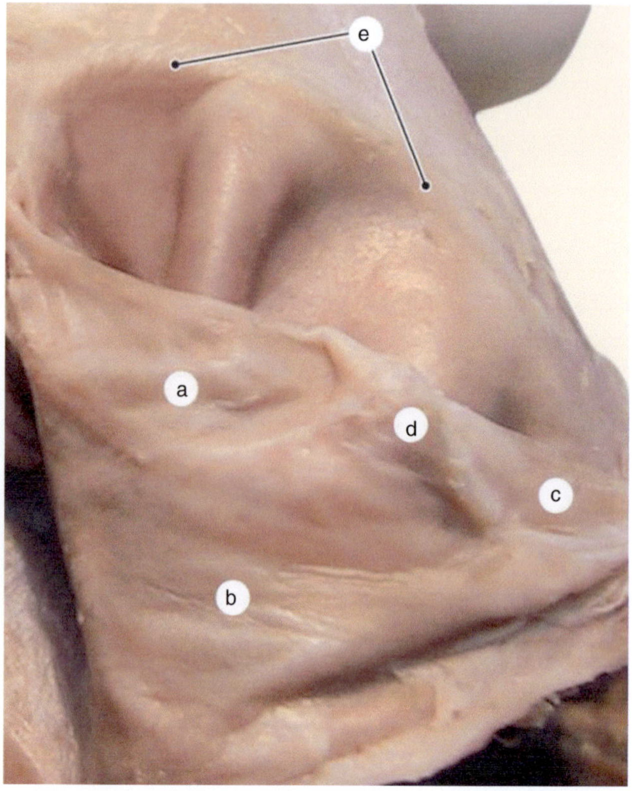

Fig. 6.133 Details on the ventricular surface of a aortic semilunar. *a* lunula, *b* aortic semilunar valve, *c* lunula, *d* nodule, *e* supravalvular ridge

6.4.5 The Aortic Valve

The aortic valve is found at the boundary between the aortic vestibule and the ascending aorta. It prevents the return of blood in the left ventricle. It is a complex structure composed of three semilunar valves and a fibrous ring on which they insert. The valvules have a base (at the same level with the ring), through which they fix themselves to the aortic wall and a free margin (Fig. 6.132).

The semilunar valves, two anterior valves (left and right) and a posterior one which delimitate, together with the aortic wall, the aortic sinuses (Valsalva). The most fortunate name for the aortic sinuses depends on the origin of the coronary arteries. Thus we have a right coronary sinus, a left coronary sinus and a non coronary posterior sinus. Just like the pulmonary valve, the valves have nodules and lunules (Figs. 6.133 and 6.134).

The configuration of the valves and of the valvular commissures is very variable. The interior aspect (the aortic surface) of the semilunar valve is not always smooth. Transverse fibrous bands, covered by the endocardium and centered by nodular structures or vertical bands can bulge into the sinusal space (Fig. 6.135).

The free margin of the valves can be quite often fenestrated, especially at the level of the lunules. At the level of the commissures, the free margins can have the following valvular behavior: either they unite and form a unique fascicle which inserts itself on the arterial wall, or they unite at the level of the arterial wall or they don't unite but insert separately on the arterial wall (Figs. 6.134 and 6.135).

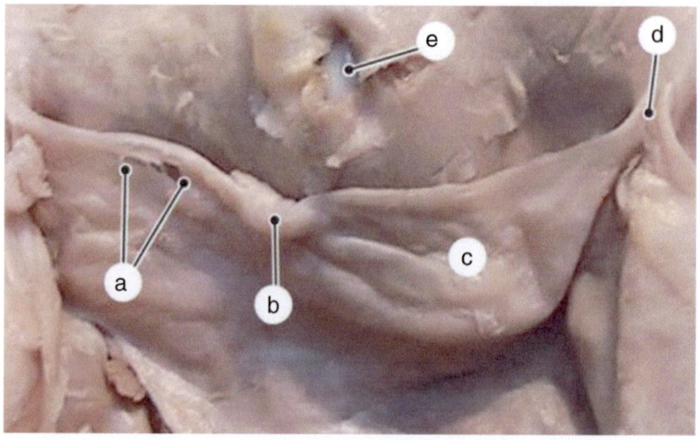

Fig. 6.134 Topography of a semilunar coronary sinus. Version of intervalvular commissure. *a* fenestrations, *b* nodule of semilunar valve, *c* lunula, *d* commissure, *e* ostium of the right coronary artery

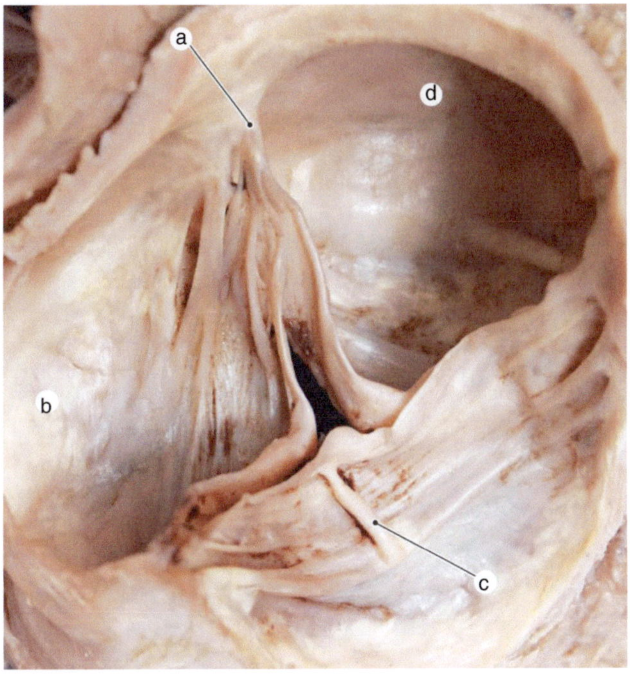

Fig. 6.135 Superior view of aortic sinuses where it can be observed vertical and transverse strips. Another version of intervalvar commissure is evident. *a* commissure, *b* left coronary sinus, *c* vertical strip, *d* right coronary sinus

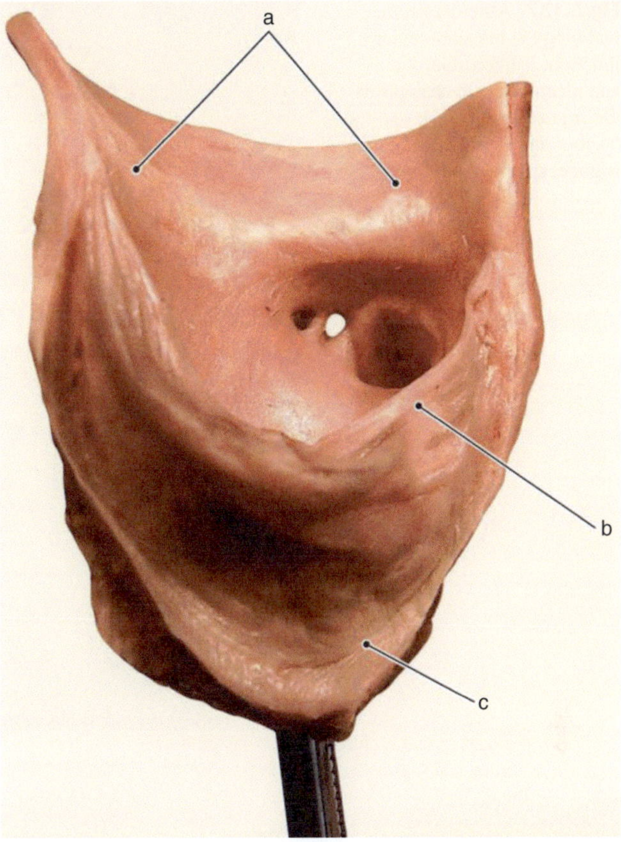

Fig. 6.136 Right coronary sinus with three arterial ostiums. *a* supravalvular ridge, *b* lunula, *c* insertion of semilunar valve on the aortic ring

If the free margin of the semilunar valve is shortened by disease, or if the sinotubular junction expands, the aortic valve becomes insufficient. If the free margin is longer than the valve can prolapse into the ventricle, thus becoming insufficient.

6.4.5.1 The Sinotubular Junction, Aortic Ring, Aortic Bulb

The upper limit of the sinuses is marked by a prominenceof the aortic wall called the supravalvular ridge. This ridge marks in fact the sinotubular junction (between the sinuses and the tubular part of the aorta) (Fig. 6.136).

With age, the sinotubular junction tends to dilate, causing a degree of insufficiency of the aortic valve.

During ventricular systole, the valvules mold the sinusal wall and the junction tends to behave like a threshold

which leads to a vortex flow. This explains the great frequency of the presence of atherosclerotic plaques in the perijunctional area (Fig. 6.137).

If we compare the structure and the dynamics of the aortic ring and the sinotubular junction, we note:

- the structure and contraction of the aortic ring extension is heterogeneous, thanks to the heterogenity of related structures;
- at the same time, the movement and expansion of the sinotubular junction is much more uniform;
- the root of the aorta suffers a degree of retrotorsion during the isovolumetric contraction of the left ventricle, similar and solidary with the rotation of the mitral ring;
- aortic root compliance decreases with age, affecting dynamics.

The ostia of the coronary arteries (the original orifices) can be found in the upper part of the sinuses, often under the supravalvular ridge but the position and number of these orifices can be variable (Figs. 6.136, 6.138 and 6.139). Practically the coronary ostia can open anywhere in the coronary sinus or in its vicinity.

The number of the ostia within a coronarian sinus varies between zero and three or four.

The right coronary artery emerges from the aorta relatively perpendicular to the aortic axis. Therefore the access of a catheter in the arterial lumen is relatively easy. The left coronary artery emerges

from the aorta anteriorly. As a result, access in the arterial lumen is more difficult.

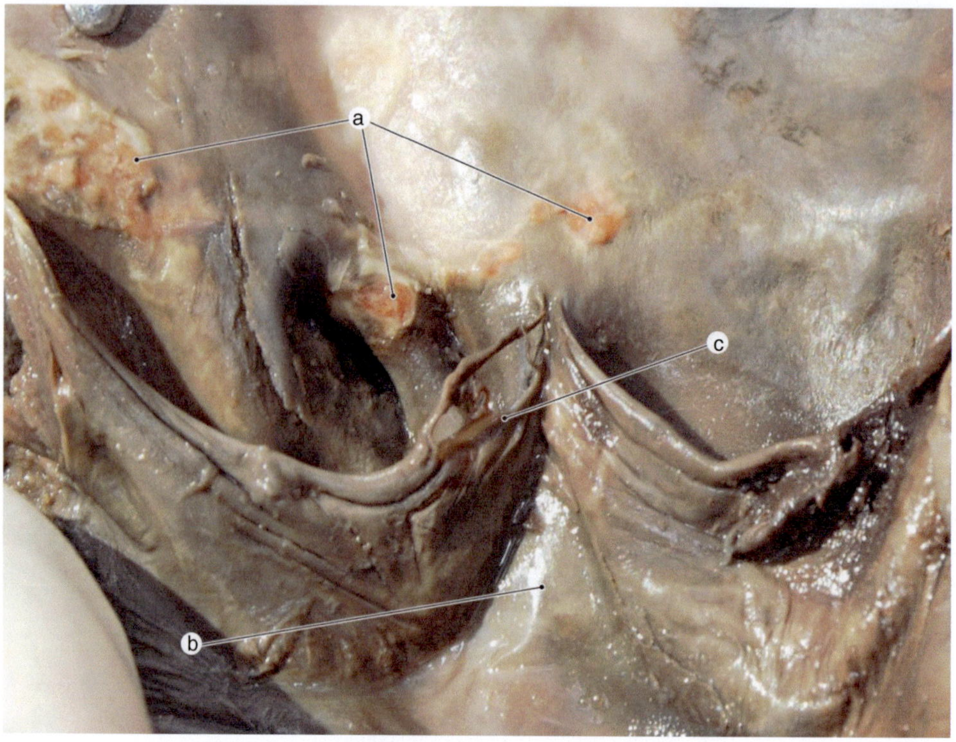

Fig. 6.137 Atherosclerotic pathology at the sinotubular junction. *a* atherosclerotic and ulceronecrotic changes on the supravalvular crest, *b* subcommissural membranous trigone, *c* fenestrated lunula

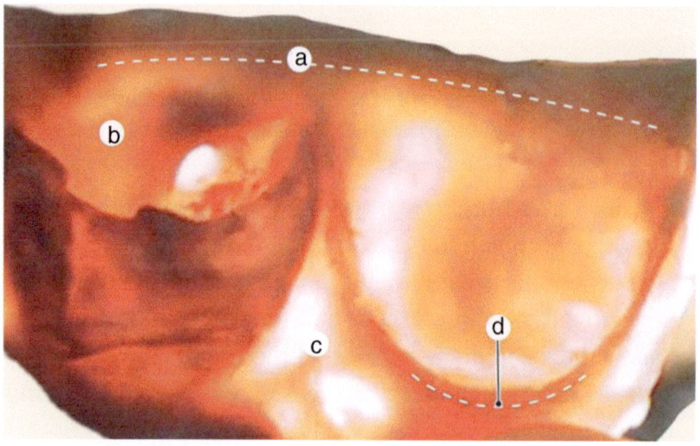

Fig. 6.138 Semilunar valvule of noncoronarian sinus was removed. *a* supravalvular ridge, *b* right coronary sinus, *c* Henle trigone, *d* aortic ring

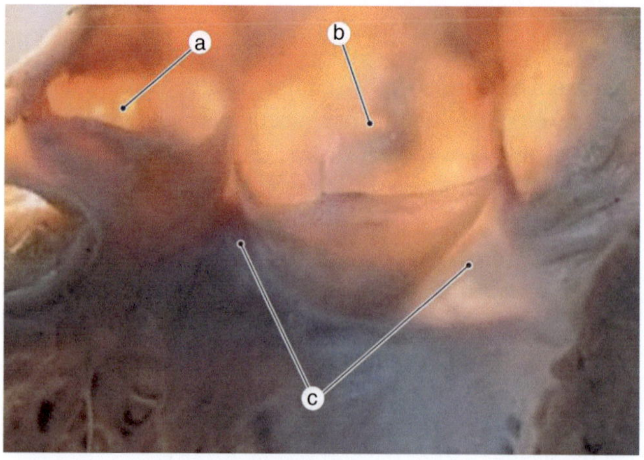

Fig. 6.139 Demonstration of the root of the aorta, of Henle spaces and coronary ostiums through transillumination. *a* left coronary ostium, *b* right coronary ostium, *c* Henle space

The aortic ring is a condensation of connective fibers in the aortic wall on which are inserted the fixed margins of each semilunar valve. It doesn't have the appearance of a circle but is composed of three segments of a circle, concave upwards and reunited at the level of some valvular commissures (the semilunar valves also come together to form a recess with an open angle facing downwards at the level of these commissures (Fig. 6.140). The rings shape is generally represented as sinous or crenelated. Very suggestive for the aortic ring is the comparison with a crown with three points, the points being represented by the commissures (Fig. 6.141).

Each aortic sinus bulges outwardly so that the origin of the aorta can be identified by the presence of the sinusal dilatations. The ensemble of these dilatations makes up the aortic bulb.

The bulb is located above the aortic ring and ends at the supravalvular ridge (Fig. 6.142).

Keep in mind!

The attachment of the base of the semilunar valves to the aortic wall is not a line but a surface bounded by the superior and inferior reflexion lines of arterial endothelium and endocardium. This surface may have a variable extension (Figs. 6.143 and 6.144).

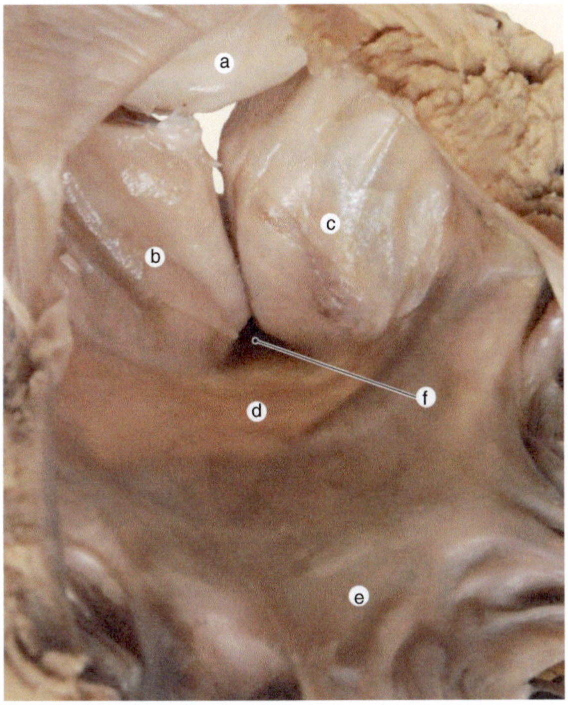

Fig. 6.140 Ventricular view of aortic valve with demonstration of the subcommissural recess. *a* right coronary sinus, *b* non- coronary sinus, *c* left coronary sinus, *d* aortic curtain, *e* anterior mitral cusp, *f* subcommissural recess

6.4.5.2 The Root of the Aorta

The aortic valve is found in a wider region, with intricate structures, which is appropriately named the aortic root. In literature the views are different on what forms the root of the aorta. If to these we also add the real difficulties of anatomic highlighting of the neighbouring structures we understand why the term "root of aorta" does not offer details.

For the beginning let us shape the notion of intraventricular septum ridge. We arrive at this structure if we cut away the interventricular septum from the heart and we can observe the ridge (the base) of the septum, it can be subdivided in three parts:

- the anterior third sustains the pulmonary infundibulum
- the middle third forms the floor of the aortic vestibule and gives way to the insertion of a part of the aortic root
- the posterior third supports to the right side a part of the floor from the right atrium (the cavotricuspidian isthmus) and to the left it supports the interatrial septum (Fig. 6.107).

After this preamble we further present the structures that make up the root of the aorta.

Under each aortic valvular commissure, there is a subcommissural membranous space (Henle'sintervalvular spaces) with a triangular form (Figs. 6.137 and 6.138).

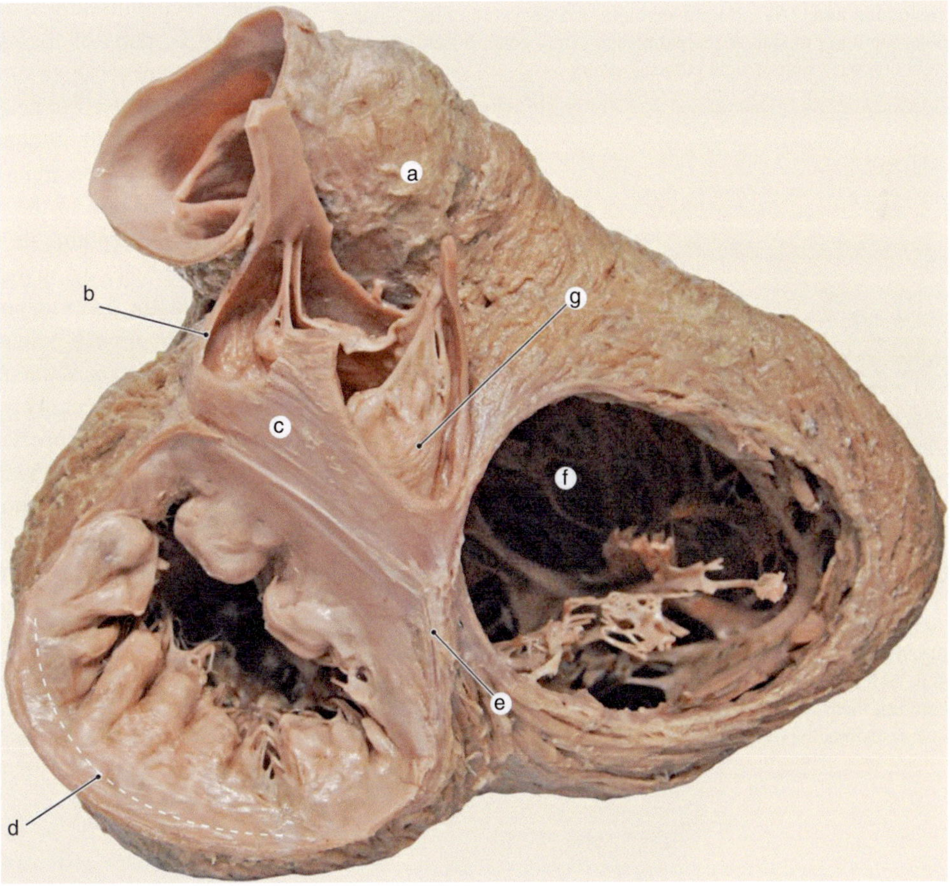

Fig. 6.141 Base of ventricular pyramid after removing the atria. Demonstration of aortic ring. *a* pulmonary infundibulum, *b* aortic ring, *c* aortic curtain, *d* posterior mitral cusp, *e* tendinous center, *f* right ventricle, *g* non-coronary sinus

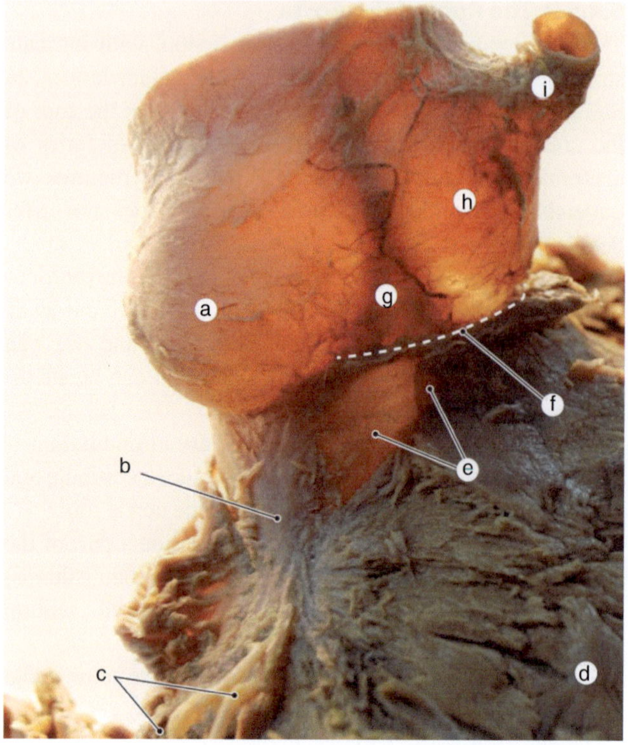

Fig. 6.142 Transillumination of aortic bulb. A part of left ventricular endocardium was kept to prove that membranous septum is composed of two layers. The tendinous centre is evident as an important resistance structure. *a* non- coronary sinus, *b* tendinous center, *c* arteries of atrio-ventricular node (AV), *d* right ventricle, *e* double wall of the membranous septum, *f* tendon of the pulmonary artery cone, *g* Henle space, *h* right coronary sinus, *i* right coronary artery

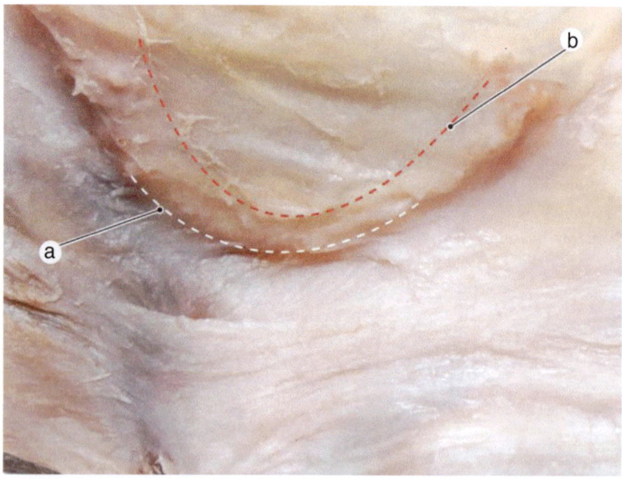

Fig. 6.143 Studying the insertion of a semilunar valve, the endocardial and endothelial reflection lines are noticeed, which comprise between them the condensation of aortic ring. *a* endocardial reflection line, *b* endothelial reflection line

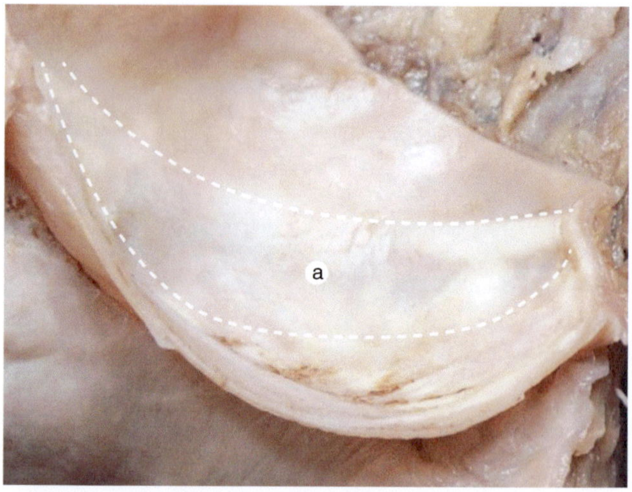

Fig. 6.144 After partial removal of a coronary sinus, its large base of insertion on the aortic wall is observed. Through endothelial transparency we can notice the fibrous condensation of the aortic ring. *a* true adherent surface to the aortic wall

These spaces achieve the "membranous anchorage" of the aorta to the left ventricle. Practically, the connective fibers in the base of these membranous segments attach themselves to the perimysium of the neighbouringmyocytes in the ventricular wall.

Keep in mind!

The subcommissural spaces are parts of the aortic vestibule, that is, parts of the ejection compartment of the left ventricle. There are three such spaces through which the aortic ring attaches itself to neighbouring structures:

Between the right coronary sinus and non coronary sinus there is the right subcommissural space (Fig. 6.142). It connects the aortic ring to the middle third of the ridge of the interventricular septum. Its connective fibers, after a short path, dissipate into the myocardial septum thickness. On the external side (the right side) of the subcommissuralspace there is, as we have already pointed out, the anteroseptal commissure (or the insertion of the septal cusp) of the tricuspid valve. This commissure generally divides the right Henle intervalvular space in a postero-superior region called the atrioventricular septum (separates the vestibule of the aorta from the right atrium) and an antero-inferior region called the membranous interventricular septum (separates the vestibule from the right ventricle). The tip of the Henle space remains outside the right heart. The base of this membranous septum is reached, subendocardially, by muscle fibers which continue the "absorbed" trabeculae in the septal wall of the left ventricle.

More important, however, is the fact that in relation to the membranous septum passes the common trunk of Hiss's

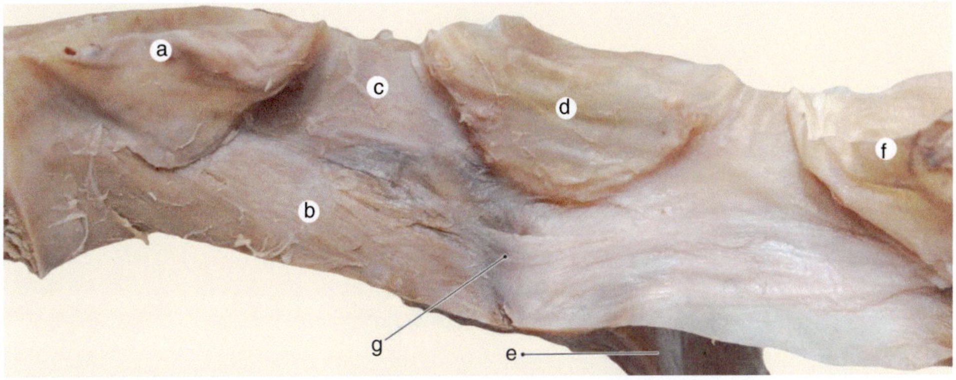

Fig. 6.145 Unfolded aortic valve. *a* right coronary sinus, *b* aortic vestibulum, *c* Henle space with membranous septum at its base, *d* non-coronary sinus, *e* interatria septum, *f* left coronary sinus, *g* fibrous condensation in the aortic vestibule corresponding to the tendinous centre

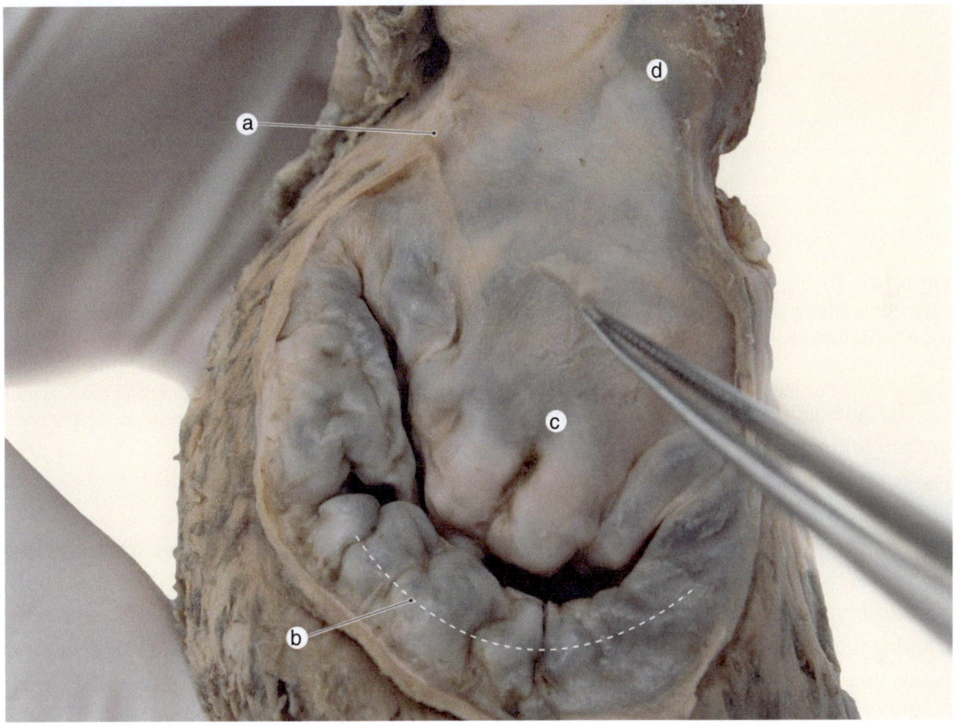

Fig. 6.146 The real continuity between the aortic curtain and anterior mitral cusp. The endocardium from the atrial surface of the cusp is caught in clip. *a* left fibrous trigone, *b* posterior mitral cusp, *c* anterior mitral cusp, *d* aortic curtain

fascicle which here divides into its two branches. Basically the perforating part of Hiss's fascicle crosses the right margin of the right fibrous triangle and enters as in a "cavum" in the space between the endocardium of the aortic vestible and the base of the membranous septum. After a short course it divides into its two branches (see the images of the excito-conductor tissue).

Between the right and left coronary sinus we find the anterior subcommissural space (Fig. 6.145). This membranous structure links the aortic ring to the ridge of the interverticular septum (derived from the muscle transformed primitive conal septum). On its external surface a fascicle of dense connective tissue (the aortico-pulmonary symphysis) links the aortic root to the pulmonary ring. This subcommissural space is often muscled in a great measure.

Between the left coronary sinus and the noncoronarian sinus, the left membranous subcommissural space is called the intervalvar septum- aortic curtain and it ends inferiorly, at themitro-aortic continuity, corresponding to the middle part of the base of the anterior mitral cusp. Basically, the aortic curtain is called the intervalvular septum because it unites the aortic ring with the mitral ring, stretching like a membranous wall between the two valves (Figs. 6.146, 6.147 and 6.148).

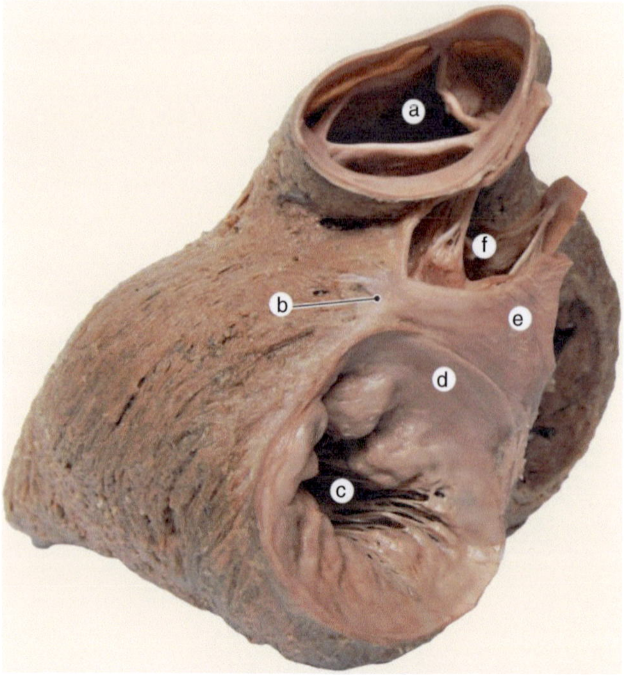

Fig. 6.147 Highlighting the aortic ring and the aortic curtain. *a* pulmonary valve, *b* left fibrous trigone, *c* mitral valve, *d* mitral-aortic continuity, *e* aortic curtain, *f* aortic valve

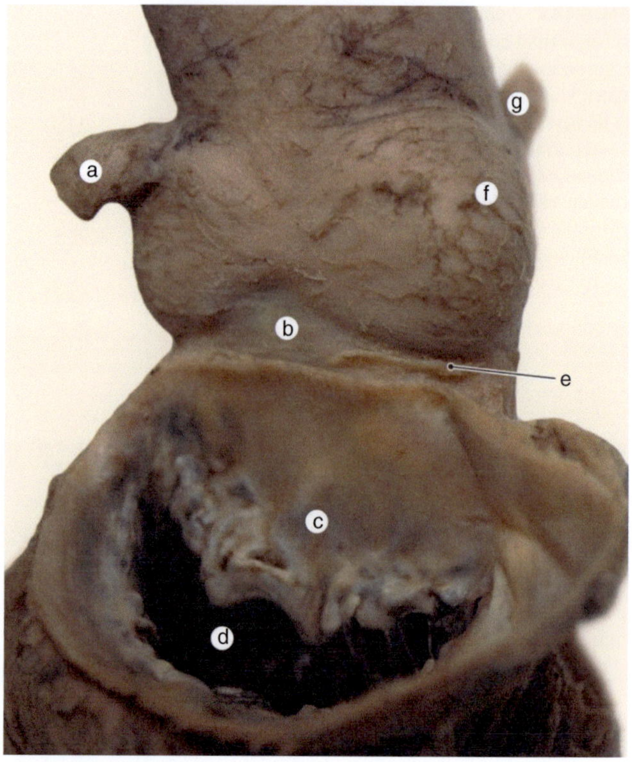

Fig. 6.148 Mitral-aortic continuity. *a* left coronary artery, *b* aortic curtain, *c* anterior mitral cusp, *d* mitral valve, *e* right fibrous trigone horn, *f* non-coronary sinus, *g* right coronary artery

The mitroaortic continuity is the place where the aortic curtain joins the left aortic wall. It contains the corresponding extentions of the two fibrous triangles. It serves as origin for the base of the aortic cusp of the mitral valve. During the embryonic period, between the origin of the aorta and the mitral ostia there is a narrow band of mesenchyme with a transversal disposition, which derives from the atrioventricular junction (Fig. 2.1). During the development of the heart, this mesenchyme suffers an epithelial transformation, is absorbed (included) in the aortic root and stretches between the mitroaortic continuity and a semicircular fibrous condensation which joins the most inferior segments of the aortic ring. I named this condensation "the primary ring" of the aorta (Fig. 6.149). The segment between the mitroaortic continuity and the primary ring reorientates vertically during the development of the heart, in the same plane with the aortic wall and becomes part of the root of the aorta – the inferior part of the intervalvular septum. Muscle remnants of the primary mesenchyme of this segment can modify the electrophysiology of the area. (Anderson predicts in his descriptions the existence of this "primary ring" [11], which he calls the "virtual ring", but is unable to individualize it.

The subcommissural membranous structures unite the aortic ring to the interventricular septum and mitral ring.

The aortic ring itself is bounded through short connective tracts, located in its most inferior parts (the maximum convexity of the sinuses), to the ridge of the interventricular septum. These tracts are quickly lost in the thickness of the myocardium, forming a part of the ventriculoaortic junction. Sometimes the connective tracts may suffer fibrocartilaginous transformations or accumulations of calcium. These short connective tracts, also known as "the third trigone", achieve "the fibrous anchoring of the aorta to left ventricle" (Fig. 6.150).

Heart specimens in which the most inferior part of the sinuses is muscularized, and the ventriculo-aortic junction ascends to the lower third of the sinus wall have been described [9].

We also mention that according to our observations, the maximum height that the ventriculoaortic junction can reach through myocardization is variable. This type of junction achieves "musculomembranous anchoring". It is different from the membranous anchoring, where the connective tissue fibers from the inferior part of the membranous segment interlace with muscle fibres, by the fact that, in this situation, the muscle fibres ascend onto the membrane, the muscularization having practically a membranous support (Figs. 6.147 and 6.149).

The aortic sinuses are additionally anchored to the working myocardium with the help of the two fibrous triangles which belong to the muscular skeleton of the heart:

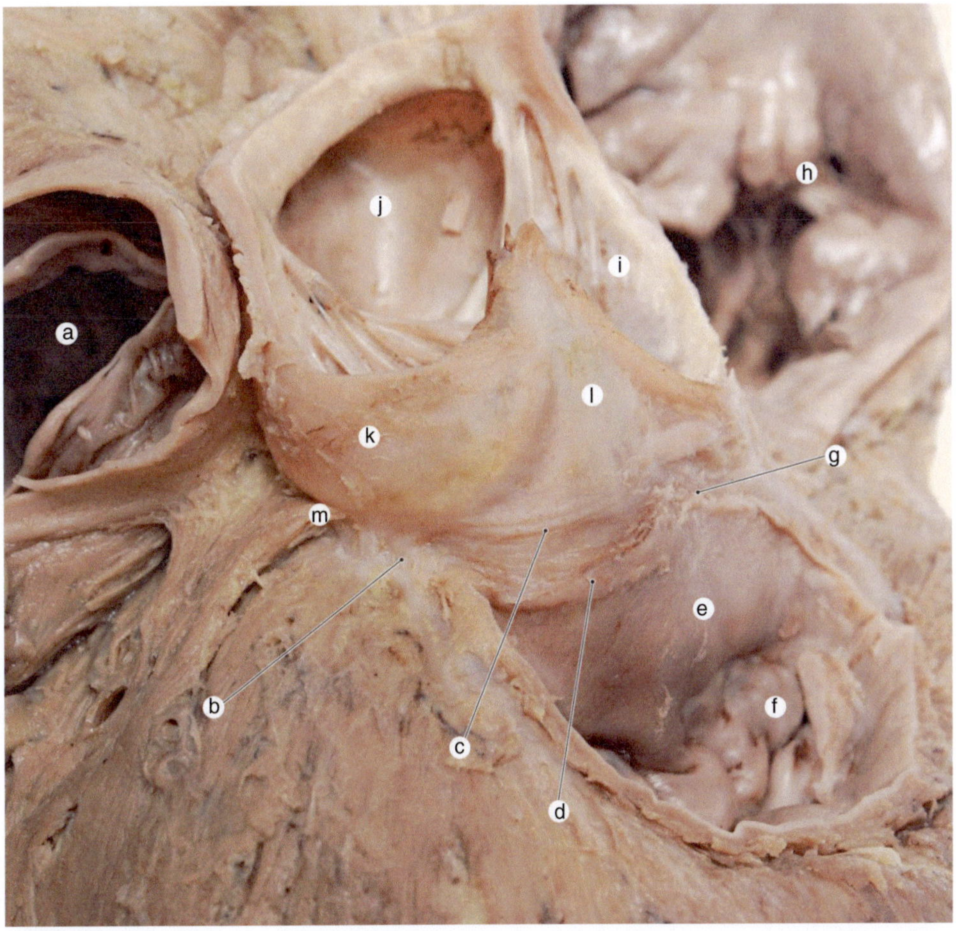

Fig. 6.149 Highlighting of primary ring and other aortic root components. *a* pulmonary valve, *b* left fibrous trigone, *c* primary ring, *d* continuity, *e* anterior mitral cusp, *f* mitral valve, *g* right fibrous trigone horn, *h* tricuspid valve, *i* coronary sinus, *j* right non-coronary sinus, *k* left coronary sinus, *l* aortic curtain, *m* "musculomembranous" anchoring of aorta

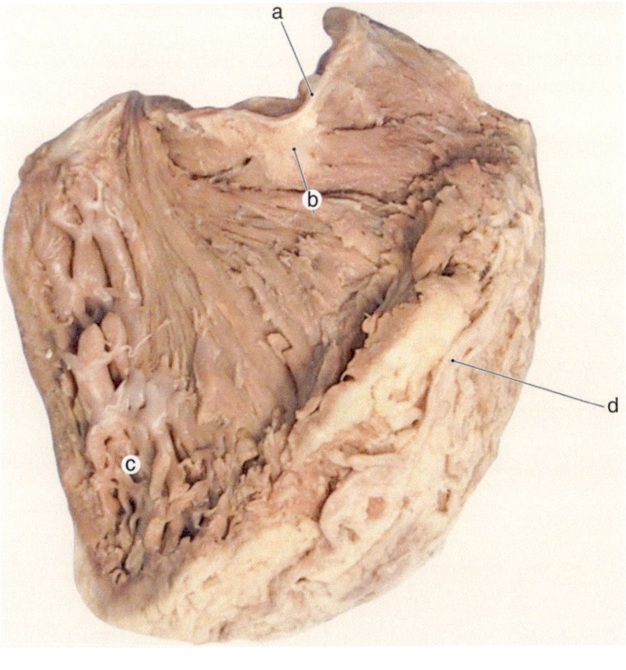

Fig. 6.150 Right side of interventricular septum dissected in order to highlight the changing direction of septal muscle fibers at different depths. *a* base of right coronary sinus, *b* fibrous anchoring – equivalent of the third trigone, *c* right ventricle, *d* anterior interventricular artery

the left coronary sinus is lined in its inferior part by the left fibrous trigone and with its help it attaches the aorta to the left ventrical and to the mitral ring. The non coronary sinus is molded by the right fibrous trigone on a much larger surface than the previous one. With its help, the aorta is simultaneously attached to the posterior third of the ridge of the interventricular septum, to the mitral ring and to the tricuspid ring. So we can state that in the same time, the right triangle separates the aortic valve from the mitral and tricuspidianvalves. The two trigones achieve "the skeletal anchoring of the aorta" (Figs. 6.141 and 6.149).

In conclusion, it is worth emphasizing that most of the components of the fibrous skeleton in fact surround the origine of the aorta and generically participate in the definition of the concept of the root of the aorta.

In other words, the root of the aorta is an integrative zone, which unites and facilitates the functionality of structures through which blood enters the heart, through which blood leaves the heart, and a large part of the fibrous skeleton.

- Summary: the root of the aorta represents the sum of the structures that achieve the following: membranous anchoring, fibrous anchoring, musculo-membranous anchoring and skeletal anchoring.

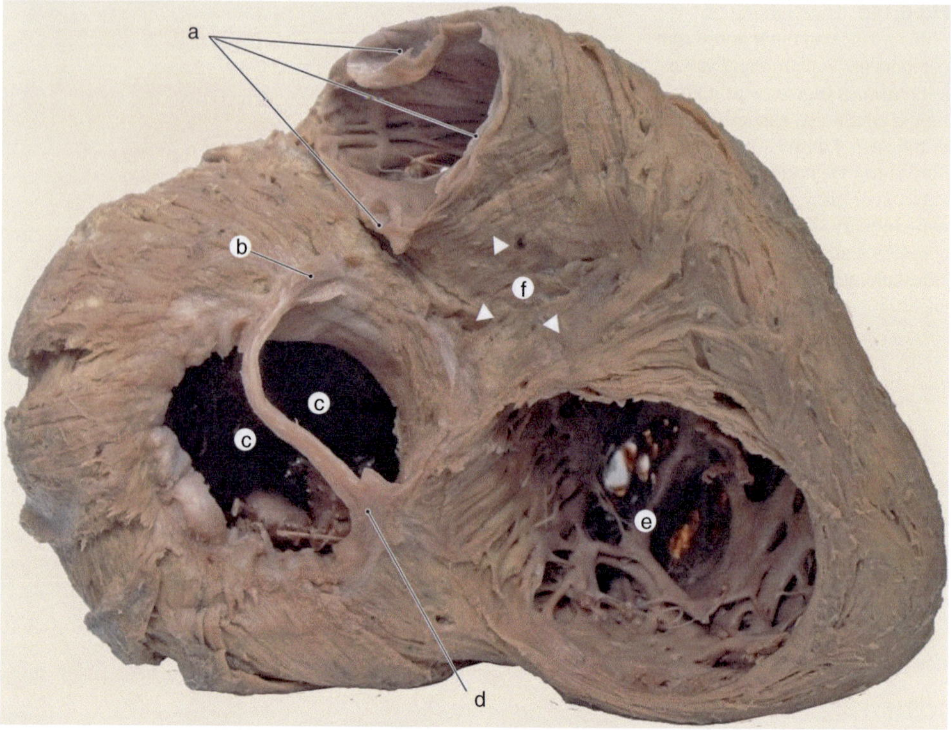

Fig. 6.151 Highlighting the mitral-aortic ostium and the triorifficial isthmus at the vase of the ventricular pyramid after atrial removal. *a* pulmonary semilunar valve, *b* left trigone, *c* mitral and aortic ostium, *d* right trigone floats in aortic vestibule, *e* right ventricle, *f* triorifficial isthmus (*arrowheads*)

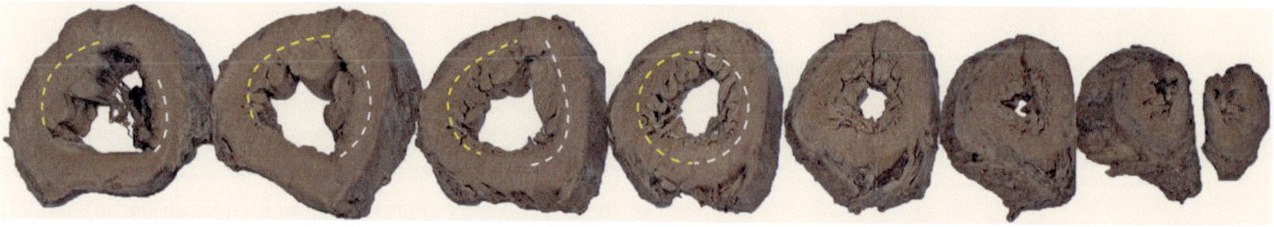

Fig. 6.152 Series of cross-section through the left ventricle, that demonstrate the relation between papillary muscles and ventricular trabeculae. The bases of the papillary muscles lose their individuality and fade into a trabecular network

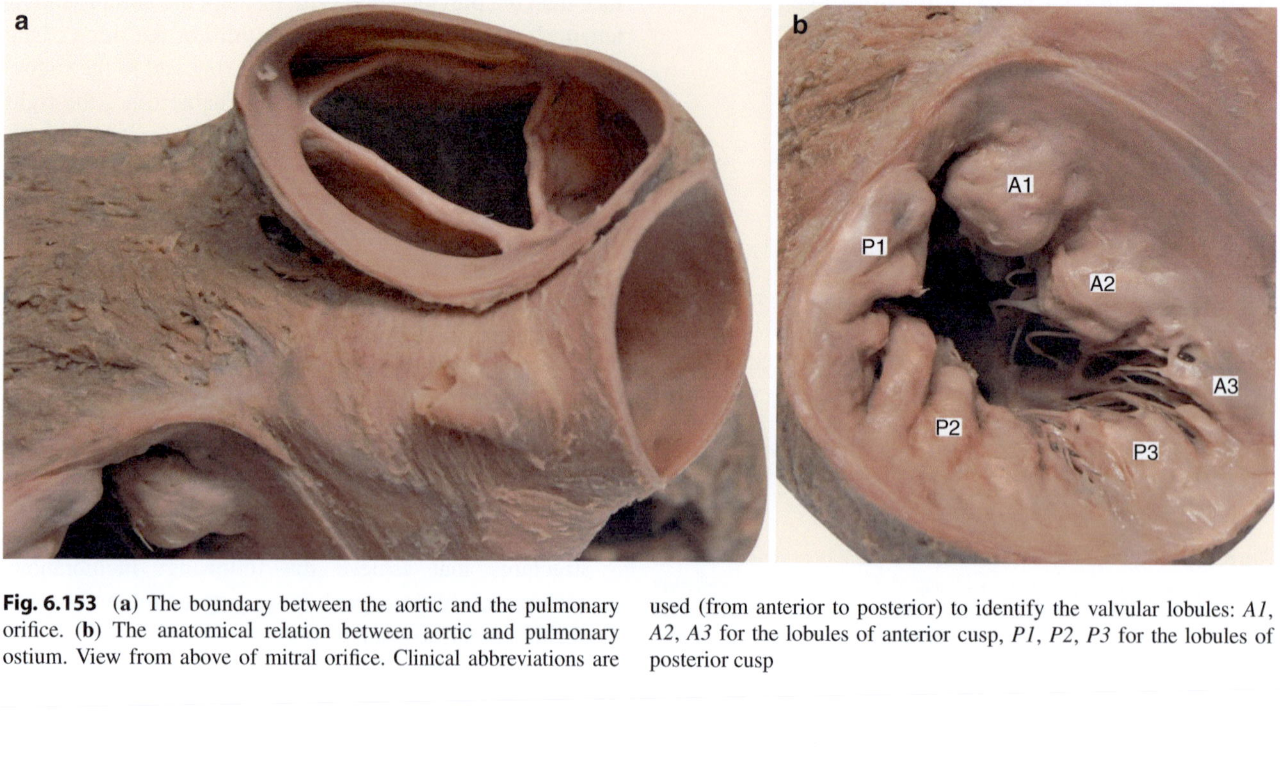

Fig. 6.153 (**a**) The boundary between the aortic and the pulmonary orifice. (**b**) The anatomical relation between aortic and pulmonary ostium. View from above of mitral orifice. Clinical abbreviations are used (from anterior to posterior) to identify the valvular lobules: *A1*, *A2*, *A3* for the lobules of anterior cusp, *P1*, *P2*, *P3* for the lobules of posterior cusp

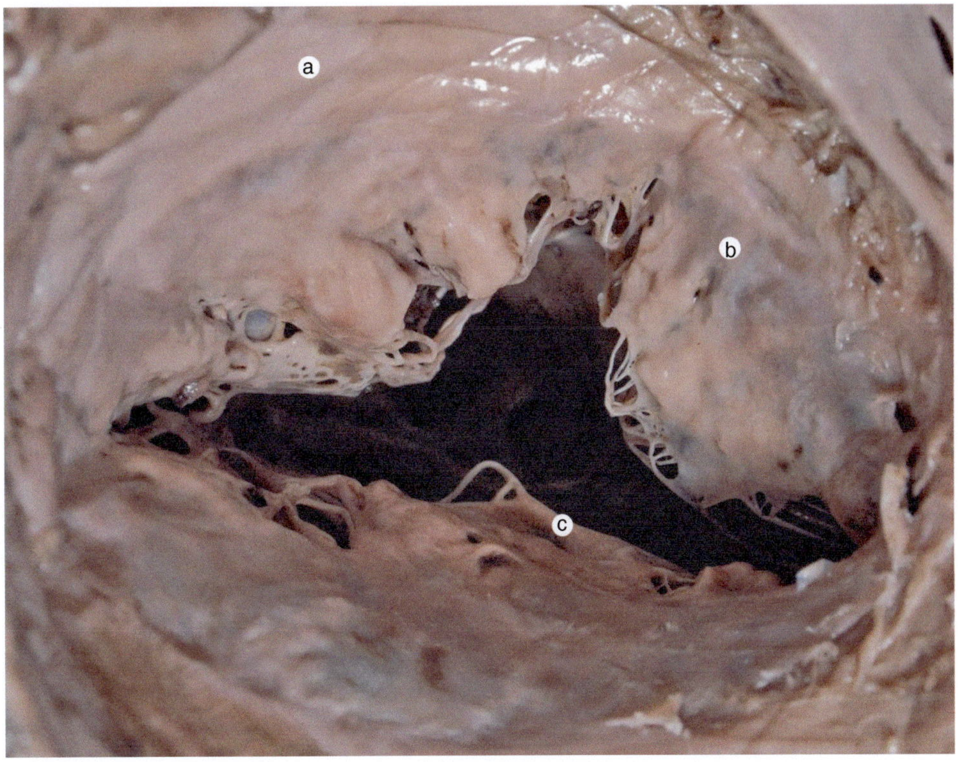

Fig. 6.154 View from above of tricuspid orifice. *a* anterior cusp, *b* posterior cusp, *c* septal cusp

- Also as a summary: the root of the aorta is made up of the following structures arranged consecutively and circularly, structures which are in contact with both the aortic ring and with the atrioventricular myocardium: the mitroaortic continuity, the insertion line of the atrial myocardium on the right triangle (when the atrioventricular septum is present), the tendon of the pulmonary cone, the aortico-pulmonary symphysis, the tendon of the sternocostal surface of the left ventricle (see fibrous skeleton), the left triangle. To these are added the fascicles from under the semilunar valves, the membranous subcommissural spaces, the aortic curtain, the mitroaortic continuity, the atrioventricular membranous septum and the interventricular septum.

6.4.5.3 Mitral-aortic Ostium

If we remove the atria and the aorta,we can notice that at the base of the left ventricle it exists a single mitral-aortic orifice, which is subdivided by the mitral-aortic continuity in the aortic ostium and the mitral ostium (Fig. 6.151).The right fibrous trigone is "floating" in the area of the mitral-aortic ostium, simultaneously separating and reuniting the mitral orifice, tricuspid orifice and the aortic orifice .The ostium does not represent only an individual anatomical element it has also a functional role in the heart dynamic, being for example entirely involved in the retro-torsional movement of the ventricular base. Mitral-ortic orifice formation results from the aortic protrusion into the superior endocardial cushion and partialy fusion of the same structures.

References

1. Inoue S, Becker AE, Riccardi R, Gaita F. Interruption of the inferior extension of the compact atrioventricular node underlies successful radio frequency ablation of atrioventricular nodal reentrant tachycardia. J Interv Card Electrophysiol. 1999;3:273–7.
2. Cabrera JA, Sanchez-Quintana D, Ho SY, Medina A, Wanguemert F, Gross E, Grillo J, Hernandez E, Anderson RH. Angiographic anatomy of the inferior right atrial isthmus in patients with and without history of common atrial flutter. Circulation. 1999;99:3017–23.
3. Necrasov OV, Dornescu GT. Anatomia comparată a vertebratelor. Bucureşti: Editura Didactică şi Pedagogică; 1971.
4. Hokken RB, Bartelings MM, Bogers JJC, Gittenberger-de Groot AC. Morphology of the pulmonary and aortic roots with regard to the pulmonary autograft procedure. J Thorac Cardiovasc Surg. 1997;113:453–61.
5. McKay T, Thomas L. 'Coumadin ridge' in the left atrium demonstrated on three dimensional transthoracic echocardiography. Eur J Echocardiogr. 2008;9(2):298–300.
6. Ernst G, Stollberger C, Abzieher F, et al. Morphology of the left atrial appendage. Anat Rec. 1995;242:553–61.
7. Kato R, Lickfett L, Meininger G, et al. Pulmonary vein – anatomy in patients undergoing catheter ablation of atrial fibrillation. Lessons learned by use of magnetic resonance imaging. Circulation. 2003;107(15):2004–10.
8. Silverman ME, Grove D, Upshaw CB. Why does the heart beat? The discovery of the electrical system of the heart. Circulation. 2006;113:2775–81.
9. Anderson RH, Razavi R, Taylor AM. Cardiac anatomy revisited. J Anat. 2004;205:159–77.
10. Muresian H, Diena M, Cerin G, Filipoiu F. The mitral valve: new insights into the clinical anatomy. Maedica. J Clin Med. 2006;1(4):5–12.
11. Anderson RH. Clinical anatomy of the aortic root. Heart. 2000;84:670–3.

7 The Structure of the Heart

This chapter presents aspects of the epicardium and endocardium, the microscopic anatomy and infrastructure of myocardium, the structure of myocardium regarding the atrial and ventricular territories, the fibrous frame of the heart and the excito-conductor system.

7.1 Epicardium and Endocardium

The *epicardium* is in fact the visceral layer of the serous pericardium. Histologically, it is a *mesothelium* (simple squamous epithelium, represented by a layer of flat cells, located on top of a basement membrane).

The *subepicardial space* contains connective adipose tissue (abundant subepicardic adipose deposits may form, especially along the coronary arteries). Precipitating of subepicardial fat can start during the intrauterine period, when small adipose lobules appear along the vessels. In the subepicardial space, nervous fibers can be found along with parasympathetic nervous ganglia, a vascular arterio-venous plexus, as well as lymphatic ganglia and vessels. The epicardium contains numerous free nervous endings (**pain receptors**).

The *endocardium* is the follow-up of *endothelium*, of the great vessels of the heart. The *subendocardial space* has a similar content to that of the subepicardial space. In addition, in this space, cells pertaining to the excito-conductor system are found, along with subendocardial muscular fibers and loose connective tissue. The atrio-ventricular valves are in fact, endocardial folds that cover both sides of a blade of connective fibrous tissue – *lamina fibrosa*. As the epicardium, the **endocardium is supplied by numerous sensitive fibers**.

! Lesions of the endocardium, but especially the epicardium, are responsible for cardiac pain, due to the profuse sensitive innervation of these structures.

7.2 Myocardium: Microscopic Infrastructure and Microanatomy

The term *myocardium* generally refers to the muscular part of the heart. The myocardium is in fact a generic term that describes a greater complexity of notions.

In the structure of the myocardium the following components can be found: proper cardiomyocytes ("working cardiomyocytes), excito-conductor myocytes, myoendocrine myocytes, the connective fibrous matrix (extracellular matrix), arteries, veins, capillaries, lymphatic vessels, nerves, interstitial cells (of Cajal). In order to be more accurate, the extracellular liquid and the migrated haematic cells must be taken under consideration. This extracellular contains mucopolysaccharides, which maintain the cellular adhesion but in the same time operate as a lubricant, allowing and favouring the gliding of structures.

7.2.1 Cardiac Myocyte: General Features and Microscopic Infrastructure

The strictly muscular component of the myocardium is represented by the *cardiac myocyte*. There are three types of cardiac myocytes: *proper cardiac myocyte* ("working" cardiomyocyte), *excito-conductor myocytes* and *myoendocrine cardiomyocyte*.

The proper cardiac myocyte is a striped muscular cardiac cell. The general aspect is relatively cylindrical and branched. Its diameter varies from 20 to 30 μm while the length is around 100–150 μm. It forms junctions with roughly 11 other adjacent myocytes and relates to a capillary (Figs. 7.1 and 7.2).

The cardiac myocyte is formed of a *sarcolemma* (cellular membrane), a *sarcoplasm* (cytoplasm) and usually *a single nucleus located in the center of the cell* (different from the

F.M. Filipoiu, *Atlas of Heart Anatomy and Development*,
DOI 10.1007/978-1-4471-5382-5_7, © Springer-Verlag London 2014

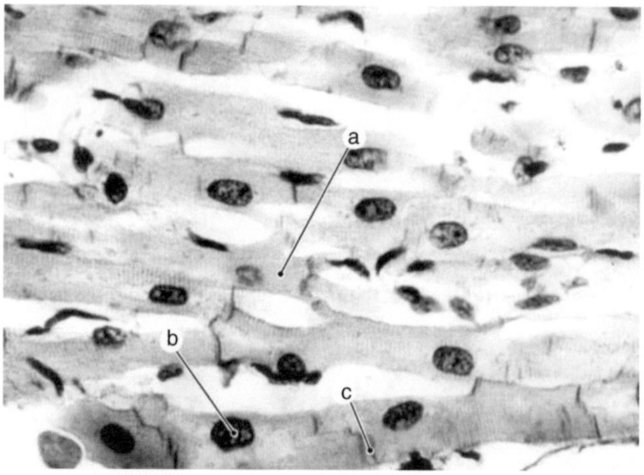

Fig. 7.1 Working myocardium. Electron microscopy (Professor's Nicolae Ionescu collection) *a* cardiomyocytes with ramifications, nucleus, *c* intercalary discs

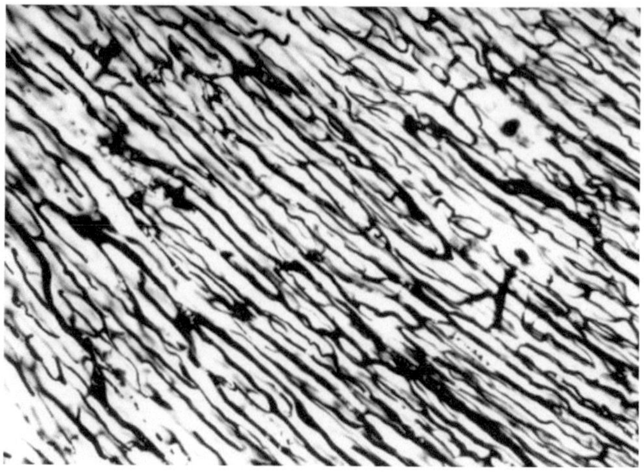

Fig. 7.2 Microscopic aspect of intra-myocardial vascular network after ink injection (Professor's Nicolae Ionescu collection)

skeletal muscular cells which have the nuclei situated at the periphery). As main differences of the cardiac myocyte from the striated skeletal muscular cell, the following should be noted: the absence of neuromuscular junctions, the increased number of mitochondrias and the presence of numerous glycogen granules in the cytoplasm.

The myocardium is a muscular tissue that **does not regenerate**. Its tolerance limit in acute ischemia is about 20 min.

The observation regarding its regenerating capacity has to be considered a postulate. Its validity may however become relative in time. For example, the presence of cardiac myocytes with two nuclei might be interpreted as a sign of regeneration (Fig. 7.7).

As it has already been described, one can observe that, from an anatomic point of view**, the myocardium is not a cellular syncytium** (a syncytium is a cytoplasmatic mass with many nuclei, and no intercellular limits), because the myocyte has a clear individuality. Classically, the *myocardium is considered a functional syncytium* [1].

This notion is not appropriate due to the fact that the cardiac myocytes are connected by junctions, in which the speed of the electric impulse is modified (even if favorable). Microscopically, the nature of conducting the electric impulse is discontinuing, which proves that in reality the myocardium is not a functional syncytium.

However the notion of functional syncytium is still used to express that when a cell is excited, all the cells in the network will suffer the effect.

The structural components of the proper cardiac myocyte ("working" cardiomyocyte) are next to being discussed.

Basement Membrane

The *basement membrane* is a laminar structure which can be observed with the aid of an electron microscope. It covers at the exterior, the cardiac myocyte. It is formed mainly of type IV collagen, proteoglycans and glycoproteins (laminine and fibronectine). It participates in the cellular interchange, but it also interacts with the extracellular matrix, *forming an insertion point for the extracellular collagen*. In this way, the *basement membrane depends on the intercellular cohesion*.

The basement membrane is considered a border structure between the components of the extracellular matrix and the components of the myocyte.

Sarcolemma

The *sarcolemma* is the actual cellular membrane, bonded to the internal aspect of the basement membrane. Like any other cellular membrane, it has two lipid layers and contains proteins called *integrines*. These proteins connect the transmembrane collagen from the extracellular matrix to the intracellular cytoskeleton. As their name implies, the integrines play a major role in transforming the cellular contraction into an ejection force.

The sarcolemma is involved in the process of forming the intercalated discs and the "T" tubules.

The *Intercalary discs* (Fig. 7.3) are specialized junctions between myocytes. Their role is to confer endurance, assuring the mechanic cohesion of the myocytes, but they also interfere in conducting the electric impulse. Following electron microscope examination, the junctions are: desmosomes, zonula adherens and gap junctions (communicating junctions).

The *desmosomes* obtain cellular adhesion with intermediate filaments of desmin.

Zonula adherens determines the mechanic adhesion of the cells. The zonules are link zones between the extremities of the actine filaments pertaining to two adjacent myocytes.

The *gap jonctions* [2] are the equivalent of electric synapses and allow the electric link between myocytes. The gap

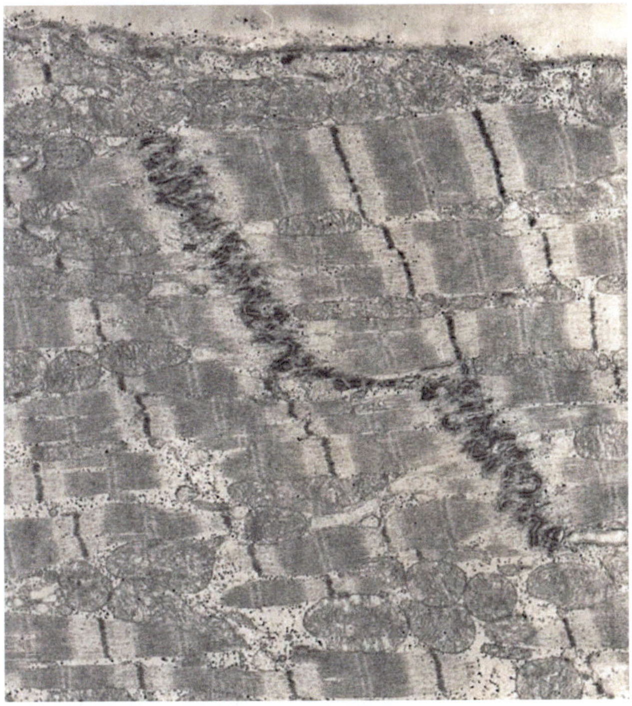

Fig. 7.3 Cardiomyocyte infrastructure. Electron microscopy. Intercalary disc (Professor's Nicolae Ionescu collection)

junctions contain proteins called conexines, formed from units named conexons.

The *"T" tubules* are involved in the excitation – contraction coupling.

The sarcolemma presents on its surface a protein called *dystrophin*, found in all the types of myocytes in the organism. Its role is to accomplish the adhesion of actine filaments to the laminin of the basement membrane. The synthesis of this protein is affected in a genetic X-linked disease with a recessive transmission, called the Duchenne progressive myopathy. This disease leads to a slow degeneration of the muscular fibers and death around the age of 20.

Sarcoplasm

The *sarcoplasm* has a striped aspect, due to the sequence of segments called sarcomeres. Following electron microscope examination, a sarcomere is bounded by two Z membranes (dark vertical bands). On each side of the Z membrane a clear band is located (the zone where the actine filaments attach on to the Z membrane; it is an isotropic zone in polarised light microscopy). Between two clear bands one can find a dark band (anisotropic zone in polarised light microscopy). At this level, the *thin myofilaments* (actine, tropomyosin and the troponin complex: troponin T, I and C) overlap, connect and interact with the *thick filaments* (myosin).

The M band (which is narrow) is located in the center of the dark band and it is limited on each side by two thin and lighter (in electron microscopic examination) bands, called the H bands.

There are two types of actine: F actine (filamentous) and G actine (globular). The long polymers of F actine result from G actine segments assembling.

Myosin can be decomposed enzymatic. Thus, under the action of trypsin, myosin can be fractionized into light mero-myosin, and heavy mero-myosin. Another enzyme – papain, may fractionize myosin in two sub-fragments, S1 and S2.

The sarcomeres align end to end and form myofibrils. These are grouped in packs just like electric wires in a multifillar cable.

Myofibrils align parallel to the longitudinal axis of the cardiac myocyte and stretch from one end of the cell to the other.

In a transversal section of a sarcomere, the myo-filaments are arranged as a hexagon, following a recurrent pattern, determined by the way the *myosin bridges* are fixating on actine myo-filaments [3].

From this pattern results the ability of a myocyte to contract only in the direction of the longitudinal axis. Alterations of the short axis are passive or elastic.

The contraction is initiated by the income of calcium in the sarcoplasmic reticulum. Thus, determines the interaction myosin-actin, the hydrolysis of ATP and the energy release with the *alteration in the angle of myosin bridges*. The modification in this angle leads to the overlapping of the myosin microfilaments with the actine ones and therefore to the *shortening of the sarcomere*.

The packs of myofibrils (structured in sarcomeres formed of myo-filaments) constitute a *cardiac myocyte*. The cardiac myocyte presents a basement membrane and a sarcolemma. Packs of cardiac myocytes, conjoined by collagen bundles of the extracellular matrix, form a *muscular fiber* covered by endomysium. The endomysium covers each cell and connects the muscular cells with the capillaries. Several muscular fibers form a *muscular bundle* covered by perimysium. Several bundles form a lamella, covered by epimysium. In areas where the striped structure is not obvious, several bundles form trabeculae, a papillary muscle or a larger bundle, covered by epimysium.

The epimysium (of the lamellae) merges inside the heart (covering the cavities), but it also fuses externally (it covers the subepicardic region of the heart and it connects the lamellae).

Cytoskeleton

The *cytoskeleton* connects the adjacent sarcomeres at the level of the Z membranes. Structurally, it is composed of microtubules and intermediate filaments of desmine, with the thickness of about 10 nm. Titine (conectin) is another protein of the cytoskeleton with role in maintaining the alignment of the sarcomere and preventing an over-stretch and elastic rebound. Titine connects the M bands with the Z membranes [4]. The cytoskeleton also contains alfa actinin,

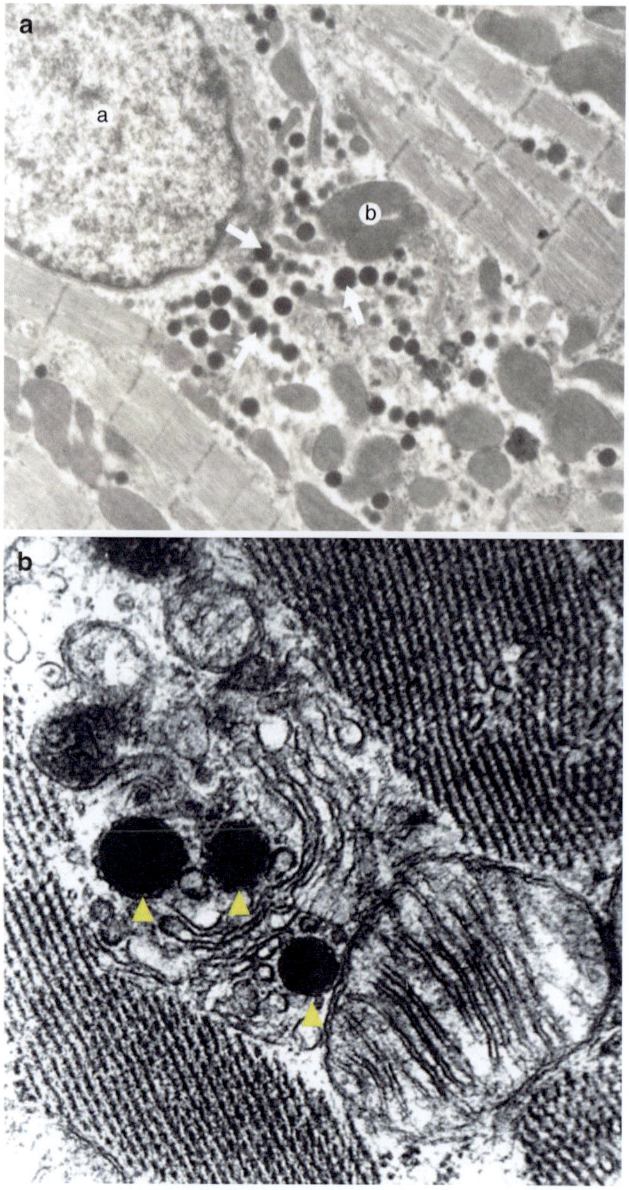

Fig. 7.4 (**a**) Cardiomyocytic infrastructure. In the cardiomyocytic cytoplasm, near the nucleus, the *arrowheads* indicate vesicles containing natriuretic peptide. Electron microscopy (Professor's Nicolae Ionescu collection) *a* nucleus, *b* mitochondria. (**b**) Vesicles containing natriuretic peptide near the rough endoplasmic reticulum. Electron microscopy (Professor's Nicolae Ionescu collection)

tubulin and talin. *The presence of proteins of the cytoskeleton integrates the extracellular matrix and also influences the mechanic performance of the cardiac myocyte.*

! Atrial cardiac myocytes contain in the sarcoplasm vesicles that stock *atrial natriuretic peptide* (Figs. 7.4 and 7.5).

The proteins of the cardiac-myocyte can be identified by imunohistochemical analysis.

Nucleus

The nucleus is unique, round or oval, central and it usually presents one nucleolus (Fig. 7.6). At times (rarely) one cell can have two nuclei (Fig. 7.7). The nucleus is surrounded by a *clear area* in which some cellular organelles accumulate.

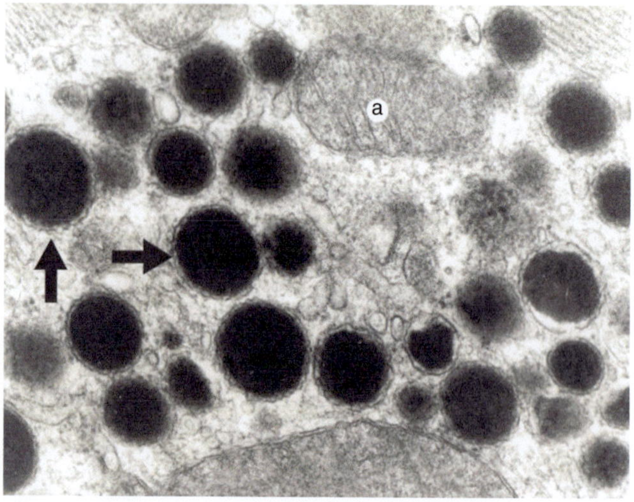

Fig. 7.5 Detail of vesicles containing natriuretic peptide. Electron microscopy (Professor's Nicolae Ionescu collection) *a* mitochondria

7.2.2 Extracellular Matrix: Definition, Components, Structure

7.2.2.1 The Definition and General Features of Extracellular Matrix

Inside the myocardium, the determined functional contractile part, named *parenchyma*, is represented by three types of cardiac myocytes (proper cardiac myocytes, excito conductor myocytes, secretory myocytes). The structure which supports and connects them, named *stroma,* is represented by the extracellular matrix (it is not a parenchymal cellular component) (Figs. 7.7, 7.8 and 7.9).

The extracellular matrix, also called the fibrous matrix, is composed of fibrous connective tissue, vessels, nerves, lymph vessels, migrated haematic cells and Cajal's interstitial cells.

The cells of the fibrous matrix constitute 60 % of the entire number of cells of the heart.

Adjacently to its mechanic role to confer the shape of the organ, the resistance to contortion, the resistance to elongation, support, alignment and connection of myocytes, an important role of the extracellular matrix is to *intercede the transfer of forces resulted during the contraction and to convert them into ejection systolic force.*

The re-elongation (drawback to initial length) of myocytes during the diastole is also partially determined by the extracellular fibrous matrix [5].

The extracellular matrix can be partially defined as the reunion of the three fascial connective structures of the myocardium – endomisium, perimisium, epimisium.

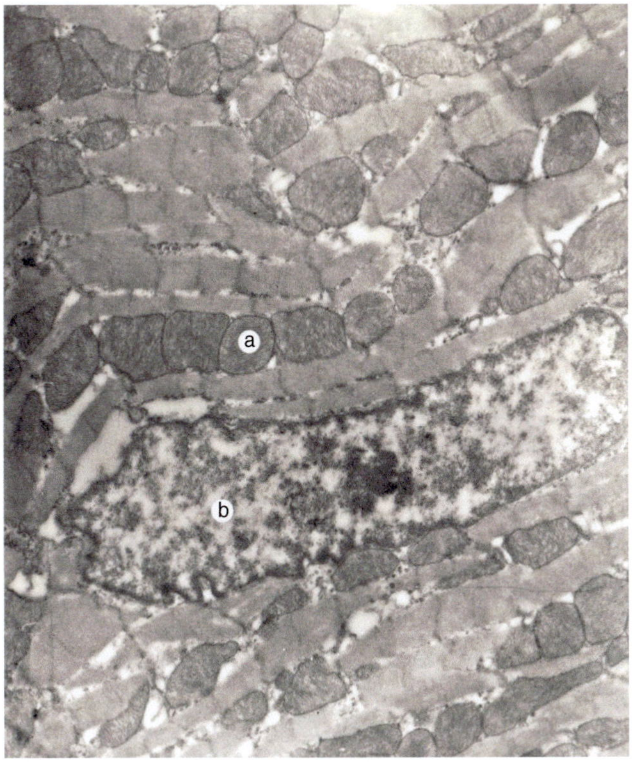

Fig. 7.6 Cardiomyocyte. Mithochondial chains between the myofiber bundles near the nucleus, proof of intense energy generating activity. Electron microscopy (Professor's Nicolae Ionescu collection) *a* mitochondria, *b* nucleus

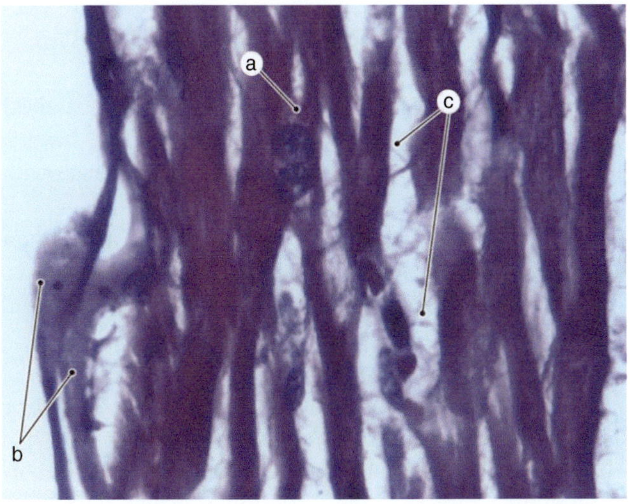

Fig. 7.7 Working myocardium. Optical microscopy. The image captures two extremely rare to objectify facts: a binuclear muscular fiber and, especially, the presence of some intramyocardial neurons in direct junction with muscular fibers. *a* binuclear muscular fiber, *b* neurons in direct junction with muscular fibers, *c* extracellular matrix

Endomisium binds the myocytytes and connects them with the nutritive vessels. Some authors consider that the cuspids and the tendinous cords are exterior structures of the extracellular matrix [6].

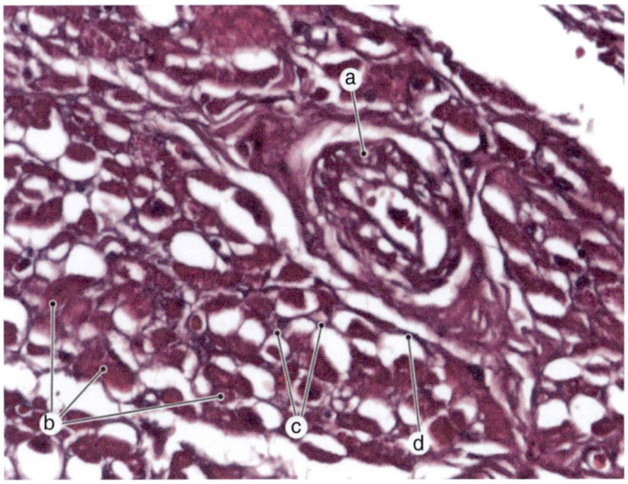

Fig. 7.8 Atrial myocardium. Highlighting some components of the extracellular matrix. *a* Arteriole, *b* myocytes, *c* fibroblasts, *d* epimisium

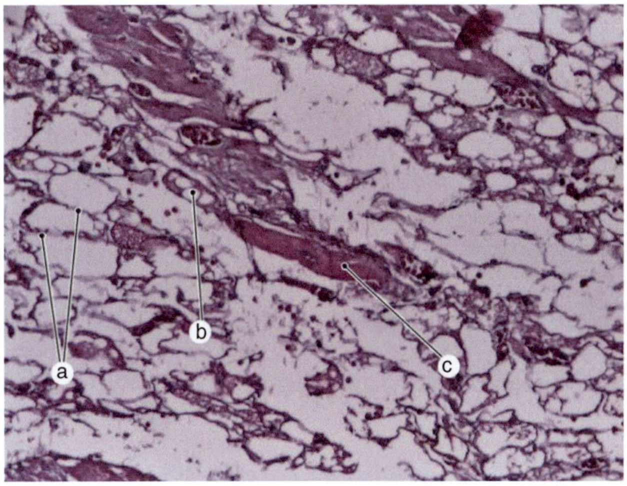

Fig. 7.9 Subepicardial necrosis in the atrial teritory allows us to observe an unaffected cardiomyocyte and episium sheets remaining after the myocyte dies. *a* epimisium, *b* myocyte necrosis allows episium visibility, *c* cardiomyocyte with ramifications

Fibroblasts (which can develop into fibrocysts), miofibroblasts (a phenotypic variety of fibroblasts), connective fibers (collagen, reticular and elastic fibers) and intercellular substance form the fibrous connective tissue of the extracellular matrix.

7.2.2.2 The Types of Connective Cells of the Extracellular Matrix

The following section reviews the types of connective cells of the extracellular matrix.

Fibroblasts [7] can develop into fibrocytes. These cells produce *vinmentine* – a protean intermediate filament, which is also found in other cells, such as the smooth muscle, endothelial cells or lymphocytes. These cells have the capacity of tissue movement because they can extend cytoplasmatic prolongations called *lamelipodes.*

Miofibroblasts are a phenotypic variety of fibroblasts. They produce actinic filaments which have contractile properties. It is a paradox that although these cells are genetically fibroblasts, the phenotype appears to be of a myocyte.

Tissular macrophages (histiocytes) have the capacity of tissue movement and phagocytosis. They are involved in the local immune mechanisms.

7.2.2.3 The Group of Migrated Haematic Cells of the Extracellular Matrix

The passage of the blood cells is accomplished by diapedesis. These cells and the endothelial cells display on their membrane specific proteins – *selectins,* which determine the adhesion of leukocytes to the wall of vessels.

The cells of this group are:

- mast cells contain numerous deposits of heparin and histamin
- plasmocytes are antibody-secreting cells
- monocytes can develop into macrophages
- lymphocytes are involved in the specific immune mechanisms
- eosinophil cells have the capacity of phagocytosis

7.2.2.4 The Types of Fibers of the Connective Tissue of the Extracellular Matrix

- *The collagen fibers* – they have a protean structure, resulting from the junction of smaller segments, called tropocollagen. The protean structure is abundant in glycine (30 %), prolyne, hidroxyprolyne, lysine and hidroxy-lysine.
- *The reticular fibers* have a protean structure, which is mainly made of type III collagen that anchors on basement membranes.
- *The elastic fibers* are compound of glyco-proteins, with a high concentration of glycine and prolyne.

7.2.2.5 Basement Membrane

It is a structure of the extracellular matrix, compounded of type IV collagen fibers displayed in a network-like architecture, located on the external aspect of the sarcolemma. It is involved in maintaining the cellular cohesion, while in the same time it is an anti-diffusion barrier for glucose and oxygen.

The elements which build-up the basement membrane are: type IV collagen, fibrillin [8], laminine and fibronectine. Among these components, the non-collagen glyco-proteins, laminine and fibronectine play an important role in the cellular adhesion and interaction.

7.2.2.6 The Intercellular Substance and Its Components

The intercellular substance (amorphous) is assembled from the following:

- *Proteoglycans.* They are heavy weight substances, characterized by the presence of a protean axis on which lateral chains of sulfated glycosaminoglycans, anchor. Proteoglycans are linked to hyaluronic acids.

  The proteoglycans associated to the basement membrane are: heparan sulfate proteoglycans and syndecan.

  The proteoglycans associated to the intercellular substance are: chondroitin sulfate, heparan sulfate, dermatan sulfate.
- *Glycosaminoglycans* are polymers of disaccharide acids, which contain amine sucrose.
- *Glyco-proteins for cellular adhesion*
- *Fibronectine* is a dimeric glyco-protein which can be fibrillar (in the extracellular matrix) or soluble (in the plasma). It may form connections with the proteoglycans, integrines and collagen.
- *Laminine* is a glycoprotein, of the basement membrane. It may link with proteoglycans, integrines and entactines.

7.2.2.7 The Cellular Receptors of the Extracellular Matrix and the Metalloproteinases

The cellular receptors of the matrix are:

- *Integrine* is in fact, a group of trans-membrane proteins, formed of alfa and beta units. They link to the cellular adhesion molecules of the matrix, as well as to the ones of the cytoskeleton.
- *Syndecans* are a subtype of trans-membrane proteoglycans. The protean core of these proteins perforates the sarcolemma. The external extremity connects with heparan sulfate. The internal extremity (cytoplasmatic) connects with the cytoskeleton.

The matrix metalloproteinases [9]

This is a family of **enzymes which degrades (reshapes) the proteins of the extracellular matrix. They have a specific bonding situs for zinc**. They are at balance with inhibitors of metalloproteinases.

Examples of matrix metalloproteinases: *stromelysin* which degrades laminine, fibronectine and proteoglycans. The *collagenase* degrades the type I and type III collagen. The *gelatinase* degrades elastine and type IV collagen.

7.2.2.8 The Types of Collagen of the Extracellular Matrix

The type I and type III collagen are the main types of collagen in the structure of the extracellular matrix. The resistance to elongation of the type I collagen is approximate equal to that of steel. As a repercussion, having remarkable mechanic properties, the matrix is considered to be a determinant factor in maintaining the shape and diastolic rigidity [10,11].

Eighty-five percent of the total collagen of the extracellular matrix is represented by fibrillar type I collagen [12]. This is synthesized by fibroblasts and myo-fibroblasts. The rest of the percentage is filled by fibrillar type III and type V collagen and type IV and type VI collagen, of the basement membrane.

Collagen is a protein with a slow turnover, of about 80–120 days. This slow turnover in a healthy heart is replaced with a very fast turnover in certain pathological situations, when aggregation of collagen leads to *fibrosis*. These pathologic conditions lead to a new type of phenotypic fibroblast called, myo-fibroblast, which is fibrogenic.

! In morphologic terms, aggregations of collagen may be *reactive interstitial fibrosis* (the perimisium component enlarges) or a *repair fibrosis – replacement* fibrosis (appearance of scars which replaces the dead cells).

A fact to be taken into consideration is that because apoptosis ("cellular suicide") is not being accompanied by inflammation, it is not followed by fibrosis.

It is now well known that not only lesions of the contractile system may lead to heart failure, but also lesions of the extracellular matrix!

7.2.2.9 Examples of Pathological Situations in Which the Extracellular Matrix Is Incriminated

The role of the extracellular matrix and its importance can very well be underlined, presenting a few pathological conditions in which lesions of the matrix have important repercussions [13].

- **Fibrosis with massive growth in type I and type II collagen**

  At a certain expansion level of fibrosis, the rigidity of myocardium increases and may lead to diastolic heart failure - heart failure with preserved ejection rate. This condition is frequent in patients with concentric cardiac hypertrophy which accompanies arterial hypertension.

- **Alteration of fibrillar collagen**

  If the collagen is highly and massively degraded, as for example in idiopathic dilated cardiomyopathy, the destruction of fibrillar collagen leads to excessive gliding of muscular fibers which determines rarefaction of myocardium and dilated ventricles. The heart becomes globular and systolic heart failure appears, with decreased ejection rate.

Monitoring of the serologic markers linked to synthesis and degradation of collagen may be an important part of a follow up strategy in the evolution of these diseases.

We would like to underline the fact that, in the myocardic mass, besides the possibility of variation in parameters of the extracellular matrix, *the structure and the aspect of the cardiomyocyte are themselves dynamic.*

Like the extracellular matrix, the dimensions of the muscular cells may also vary under the influence of physiologic or pathologic stimuli (increase defines myocyte hypertrophy).

7.2.3 The Structure of the Myocardium of the Atrium. The Continuous Atrium Theory

The logic of the embryologic evolution from the two atria – structures which develop from a *unique cavity* – must be found in the distribution of the main muscular bundles pertaining to these cavities.

In other words, on one hand the atria must be reunited through muscular bundles which form **a continuous atrium** (do not forget that the muscular fiber is the sub-layer of conduction of the nervous impulse). On the other hand, given the complex embryogenesis, atrial muscles have a distribution that may vary. Due to the ontogenetic complexity, a **breakage of the continuous atrium appears.**

Normal connections between muscles of the right and left atrium are highly important, due to the fact that they allow the transfer of the physiologic electric impulse on a normal pathway from the right atrium towards the left one.

Abnormal connections represent the sub-layer of pathologic electro-physiologic manifestations.

The wall of the primitive atrium is composed of an endocardic layer, with a membranous aspect, which will develop into myocardium.

The continuous atrium *initially is altered and becomes non homogenous due to a few elements responsible for generating heterogeneity of the adult atrial wall:*

- embedment of segments of the atrio-ventricular junctions into the wall of atrium
- embedment of extensions of the endocardial cushions into the wall of atrium
- embedment of extracardial cellular populations into the wall of atrium
- embedment of the venous sinus into the wall of right atrium
- embedment of the primitive pulmonary vein into the wall of left atrium
- the development of septa and different venous ostia.

The physiologic heterogeneity of the atrial architecture has as a main effect - abruption of the continuous atrium and therefore avoids a circular pathway of an electric impulse and a possible re-entry mechanism!

The wall of left atrium is generally thicker than the wall of right atrium, which reaches laminar *dimension and aspect in the interpectinate spaces.*

In fact, the *disposal of the atrial muscular bundles* follows a few patterns:

- Circular, internal and external muscular bundles are present at the base of the atria, in the vestibular territory. The external bundles connect with the ones on the opposite side, while the internal bundles connect with the septal muscles.

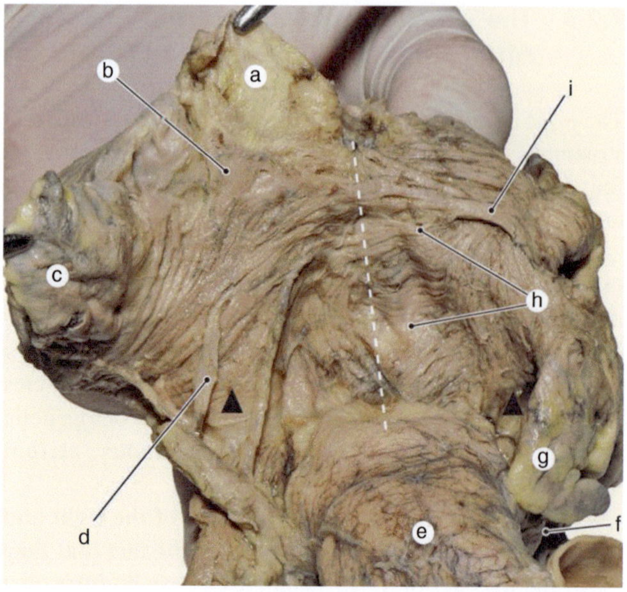

Fig. 7.10 Distribution of muscle fascicles from the anterior-superior face of atria. *Dotted line* indicates the interatrial boundary. *Arrows* show vestibular bundles. *a* superior vena cava, *b* area of sinoatrial node, *c* right auricle, *d* sinoatrial node artery, *e* aorta, *f* left coronary artery, *g* left auricle, *h* interatrial notch fascicle, *i* Bachmann fascicle

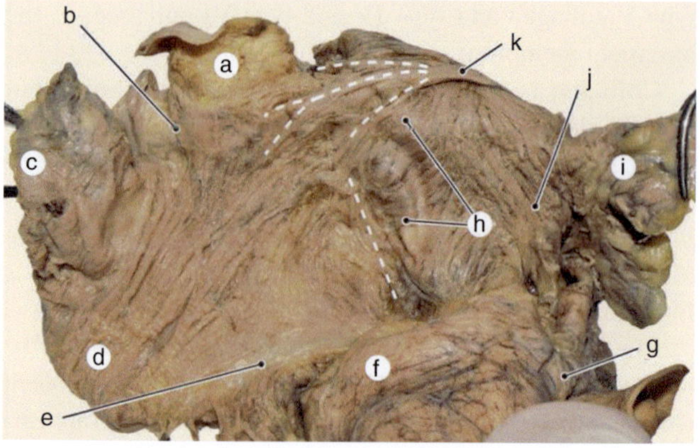

Fig. 7.11 Detail of previous image, with highlighting of the roots of the Bachmann fascicle. *a* superior vena cava, *b* area of sinoatrial node, *c* right auricle, *d* Anterior vestibular fascicle, *e* atrial-ventricular junction, *f* aorta, *g* left coronary artery, *h* interatrial notch fascicle, *i* left auricle, *j* Anterior vestibular fascicle, *k* Bachmann fascicle with its three originary roots: atrial, one anterior and one posterior to the vena cava

- Around all venous ostia detour bundles are present, on each side of the ostium, which emerge from a main bundle with a route towards the ostia. These bundles fuse with circular bundles at the base of the atria.
- The base of the auricles is surrounded following the same pattern by two detour bundles, which afterwards unite.
- Muscular interatrial bundles are also present.
- In each atrium one can find intraatrial bundles.

7.2.3.1 The Muscular Bundles of The Right Atrium

In the structure of the right atrium, several bundles have been described:

The vestibular muscles of the right atrium are represented by two *circular vestibular bundles, one internal and one external.* These bundles surround a large area of the base of the atrium.

- *The internal circular vestibular bundle* is better structured anteriorly, while posteriorly, it fades in the atrial wall of the atrio-ventricular crease, at the level of the terminal crest.
- *The external circular vestibular bundle* of the right atrium is the right continuity, below the right auricle, of Bachmann's interatrial bundle (look forward) (Figs. 7.10 and 7.11). It is less structured than it, and after it reaches the acute margin, due to the crimped atrio-ventricular junction, it becomes profound and fades posteriorly in the vestibule of the atrium, at the limit with the terminal crest. This bundle is continued by a "delicate" superficial branch called **the external bundle of right atrium** (Figs. 4.36 and 6.10).

The external bundle is not always well structured, but when it exists, it consists of *thin muscular fibers which connect the epicardium with the pectinate muscles.* A part of these fibers form subepicardic loops (in the subepicardic space, they connect the deep bundles). The external bundle of the right atrium ends at the level of the terminal groove. At times, it may continue towards the posterior with the intercavum bundle (non-constant) which lays between the terminal groove and the interatrial groove of Waterstone. *The intercavum bundle may be an accessory route of interatrial transmission* (Figs. 7.12 and 7.13).

Both the intercavum and the external bundles are frequently under-developed and cannot be individualized.

- *The pectinate muscles* emerge from the *terminal crest* and fade into the vestibule, almost right-angled on the internal circular bundle. There is a group of pectinate muscles with an opposite direction (however see the cavity of right atrium).
- *The muscular bundle of the terminal crest* divides towards inferior, at the level of the cavo-tricuspide isthmus into two bundles:
  - The inferior bundle fades into the floor of atrium; its fibers reach the triangle of Koch.
  - The superior bundle fades into the structure of the Eustachian margin (it is a variable structure). Its fibers may reach the triangle of Koch.
- *The (semi)circular bundle of fossa ovalis* is also known as the *greater limbic bundle.* It connects with other septal bundles (Fig. 6.25).
- *As far as the interatrial septum* is concerned, it must be noted that the superior and posterior part of septum secundum is in fact a crease of the atrial wall. As consequence, it is but logic that the superficial bundles continue their pathway in the thickness of the interatrial septum (to

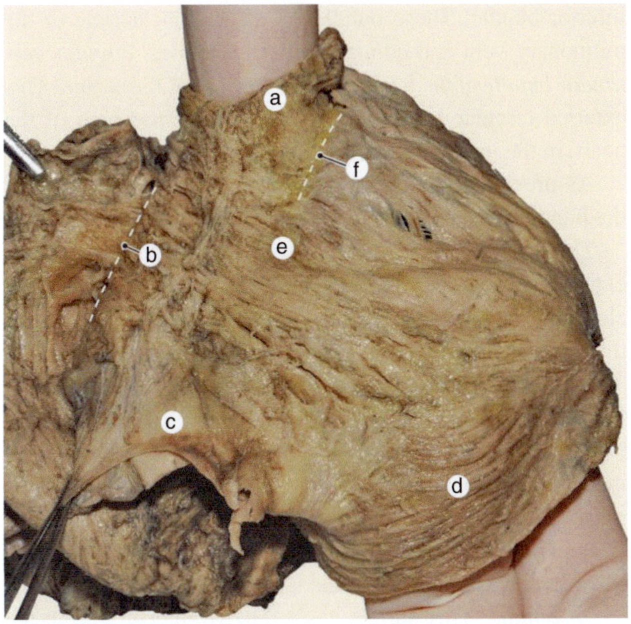

Fig. 7.12 Heart with a very well represented intervenous fascicle. Posterior view. *a* superior vena cava, *b* interatrial sulcus, *c* inferior vena cava, *d* vestibular fascicle, *e* intervenous fascicle, *f* terminal sulcus

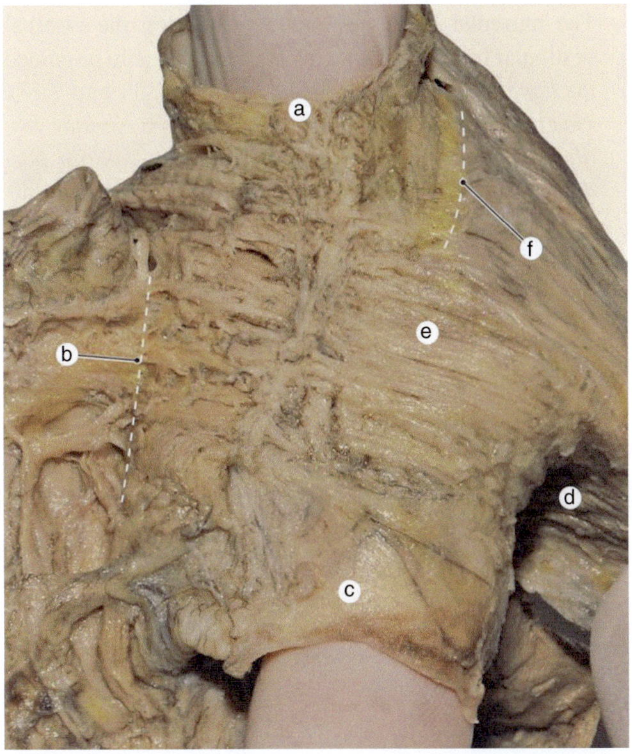

Fig. 7.13 Detail of previous image. Notice the existence of a thin vertical fascicle, which seems to bypass the intervenous fascicle fibers. *a* superior vena cava, *b* interatrial sulcus, *c* inferior vena cava, *d* external circular vestibular fascicle, *e* intervenous fascicle, *f* terminal sulcus

follow the configuration of the crease and connect with the opposite side).

- *The bundles of the dorsosinusal space* have been discussed in the dedicated chapter.

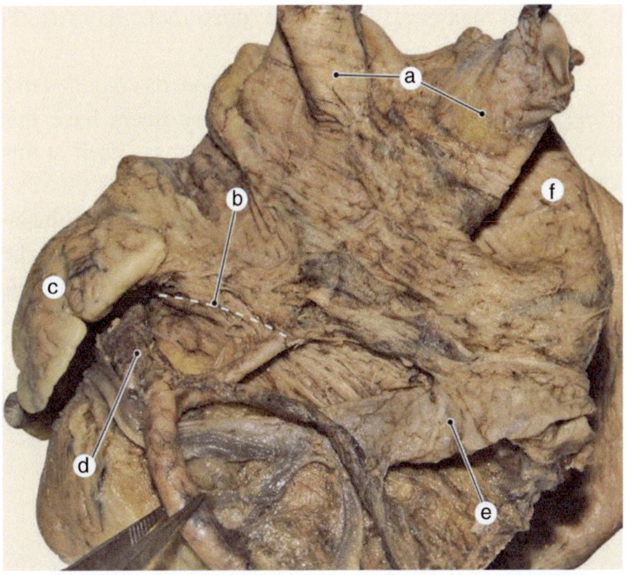

Fig. 7.14 Postero-lateral segment of the vestibular fascicle seen from the pulmonary surface of the left atrium. *a* left pulmonary veins, *b* vestibular fascicle, c left auricle, *d* Circumflex artery, *e* limit of coronary sinus, *f* inter-pulmonary fascicle

7.2.3.2 The Muscular Bundles of Left Atrium

- **In the structure of the left atrium,** one can find: *the septal-atrial bundle*, which emerges from the anterior and inferior part of the septum and fades into the anterior wall of the atrium, corresponding to the aorto-mitral continuity (on which it also partially inserts). It is possible that this muscular bundle develops from the left extension of the superior endocardial cushion (Fig. 2.9).
- The opposite of the previous is *a muscular bundle that consolidates the base of the interatrial septum on the left side* (developed from the extensions of the inferior endocardial cushion) (Fig. 2.16).
- *The external circular vestibular bundle of the left atrium surrounds the base of the left atrium* and it fades posterior, near the interatrial groove. In fact, all the other bundles of the left atrium fuse in with this one (look forward) (Figs. 7.14 and 7.15).
- *The inter-pulmonary bundle descends* in the space between the right and left ostia of the pulmonary veins and it ends in the angle between the coronary sinus and the interatrial groove, where they may o may not fuse with the external circular vestibular bundle (Figs. 4.39 and 7.15).
- *The interatrial bundle of Bachmann* is considered the main interatrial transmission pathway [14]. **It is formed on the trajectory line of reflection of pericardium on the atria** (Fig. 7.16).

It may very well be observed anterior and to the left of the orifice of superior vena cava (Figs. 7.10, 7.17 and 7.18).

It has a transversal disposal, crossing over like a bridge to the other side of the atria. *The right extremity* originates in two *roots* (*superior and inferior*), on each side of the orifice of superior vena cava. Sometimes, three roots may fuse in order to form this extremity.

At the limit between the atria, fibers from this bundle have a deep trajectory into the septum. These fibers have this direction because the atrial wall tends to crease itself at this level in order to form the limb of the fossa ovalis.

In its trajectory towards left, the bundle of Bachmann crosses the interatrial border and fades either at the base of the left auricule or at the level of the orifice of left superior pulmonary vein. In each situation, it divides into a superior and inferior bundle. These bundles circle the left auricle or the pulmonary vein and connect with the *external circular vestibular bundle of the left atrium,* at the base of the atrium. This external circular bundle fades posterior, at the base of the heart, in the inferior part of the interatrial groove or near it.

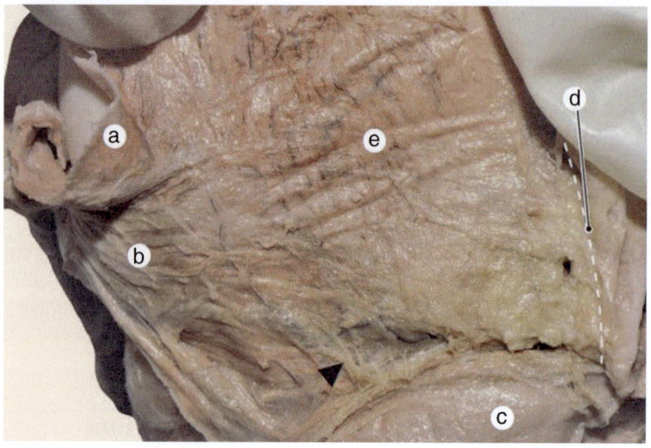

Fig. 7.15 Posterior aspect of the left atrium. Inter-pulmonary and vestibular fascicles end near the inter-atrial sulcus. Thin muscular periinusal fibers continue with the vestibular ones (*arrow*). *a* inferior left pulmonary vein, *b* vestibular fascicle, *c* venous sinus, *d* inter-atrial sulcus, *e* inter-pulmonary fascicle

As previously discussed, *in its trajectory towards right,* the bundle of Bachmann originates in two roots.

The inferior root continues not only the pathway of the external circular vestibular bundle of the right atrium but also a group of muscular fibers that originate in a region near the sinoatrial node. *It is possible that along this pathway the electric impulse generated in the sinoatrial node reaches the left atrium.*

The superior root continues the pathway of the inter-cave muscular bundle (Fig. 7.11).

- As previously demonstrated, around fossa ovalis, in the thickness of the limb, one can find a very well structured muscular bundle, called *the limbic (semicircular) muscular bundle*. This bundle has a relative interruption in the posterior and inferior region fossa ovalis.
- At the base of the atria, anterior, on the trajectory of the former interatrial notch of the primitive atrium, there is a fine layer of muscular fibers that connects the two atria. The muscular layer continues towards left the external vestibular bundle of the right atrium and it could be named *the bundle of the interatrial notch* (Figs. 7.11 and 7.17). *This bundle unites towards inferior with the circular vestibular bundle of the left atrium, while its superior part descends as the inter-pulmonary bundle.* Having this

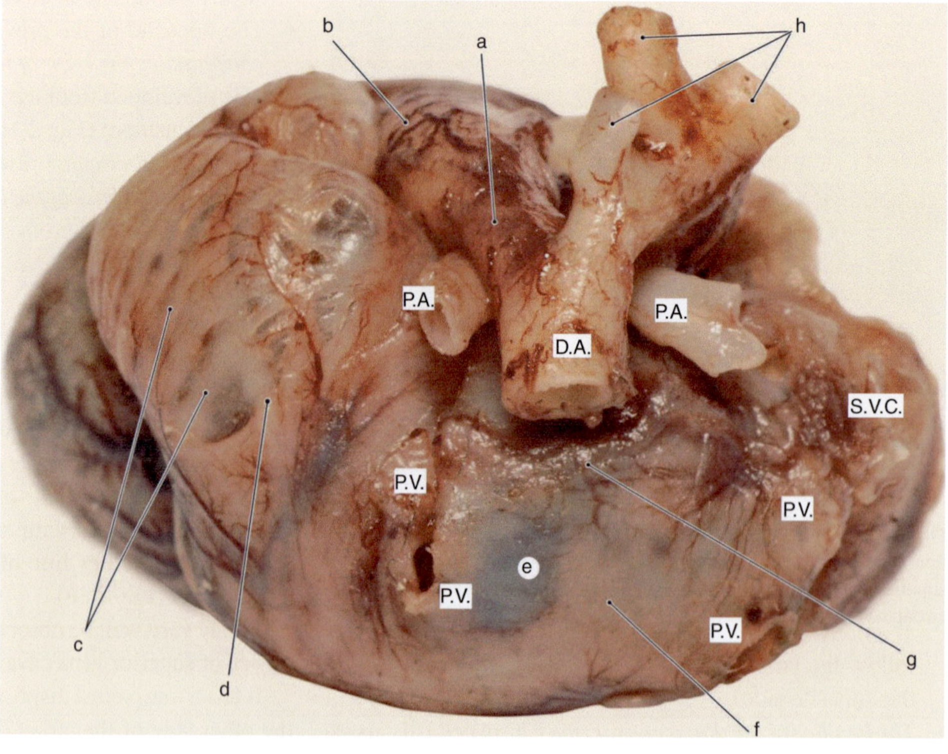

Fig. 7.16 Fetal heart – 5 months old. Posterior view. Myocardic formation process of the atrial walls is captured in evolution. Notice the left auricle muscularisation pattern in circular strips. The image captures remarkably the anatomical relation between the arterial canal, descending aorta (*DA*) and the pulmonary arteries (*PA*). *a* arterial canal, *b* pulmonary trunk, *c* left auricle muscularisation pattern in circular strips, *d* sagittal muscularisation strip, *e* low muscularisation area, *f* inter-pulmonary fascicle, *g* forming area of the Bachmann fascicle, *h* branches from aortic arch, *PV* pulmonary veins

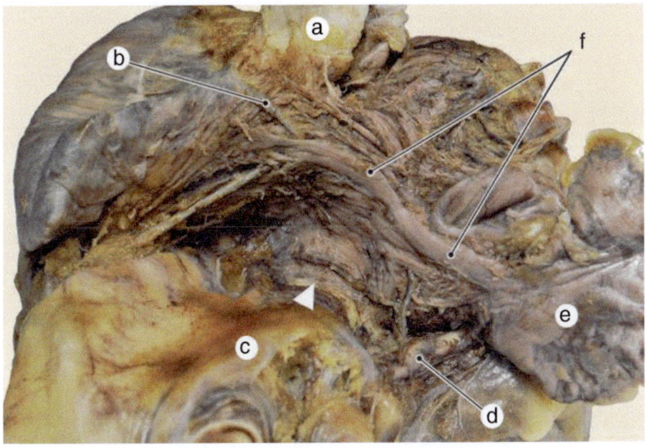

Fig. 7.17 Bachmann fascicle ends divergent at the base of the left auricle. Its root forms a myocardic bridge over the sinoatrial node artery. Inter-atrial notch fascicle (*arrow*). *a* superior vena cava, *b* sinoatrial node artery, *c* aorta, *d* left coronary artery, *e* left auricle, *f* Bachmann fascicle

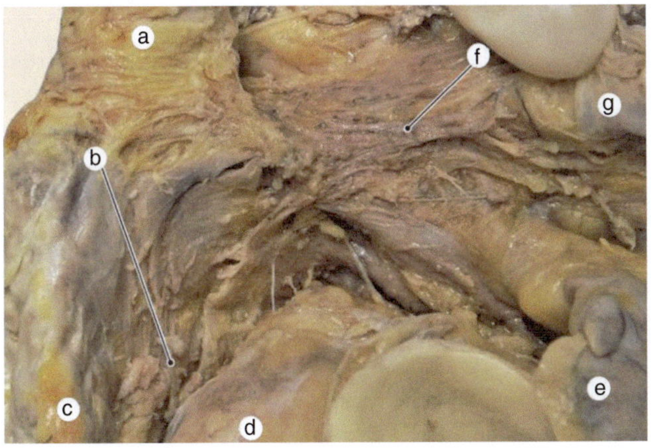

Fig. 7.18 Variant of Bachmann fascicle that ends near the ostium of left superior pulmonary vein. *a* superior vena cava, *b* artery of sinoatrial node, *c* right auricle, *d* aorta, *e* left auricle, *f* Bachmann fascicle, *g LPV* left pulmonary vein

conformation, we consider that **this bundle must also be remarked as an interatrial transmission pathway!**

7.2.3.3 The Conveyance of Electric Impulse Through the Muscular Continuous Atrium

For an assembly preview, we will shortly discuss the possible trajectories of the electric impulse generated in the sinoatrial node towards the two atria, **following the muscular continuous atrium**.

There are two areas from which the nervous impulse can depart towards the walls of atria, due to the fact that the excito-conductor system extends into the terminal groove:

1. **The superior area of the terminal groove** – the inferior root of the bundle of Bachmann and then the main bundle, with two possibilities:
   (a) profound, towards the interatrial septum (and possibly towards the atrioventricular node)
   (b) towards the left atrium, *through the peri-venous bundles and the peri-auricular bundles*, which fuse with the *external circular bundle of the left atrium.* This bundle fades near the interatrial groove.

   In the space between the ostia of the pulmonary veins, the muscular bundles fuse and form a thin layer (which is sometimes incomplete) of muscular fibers, which might be named *pulmonary inter-venous bundle* (Fig. 7.15). As already discussed, this bundle continues the bundle of the interatrial notch.

   The eventual muscular inbreaking of the terminal part of the pulmonary veins, forms a peri-venous circular muscular route that might alter the local electrophysiology.

   In the left auricle, the main circular bundles are merged into a *sagital bundle* that allows physiological transmission but inhibits the re-entry mechanism (Figs. 2.52 and 7.16).
2. **The median and inferior area of the terminal groove** may represent another zone from which the electric impulse generated in the sinoatrial node is launched on the following trajectory: pectinate muscles – vestibular bundles of the right atrium – bundle of the interatrial notch – external circular bundle of the left atrium (or sometimes inter-pulmonary bundle) – posterior interatrial groove.

! As discussed, the area represented by the sinus venosus and located between the terminal and interatrial grooves, interrupts the muscular continuous atrium. Sometimes at this level, one can find the inter-cave bundle which may vary or alter the atrial electrophysiology.

7.2.3.4 The Variability of Embryologic Myocardic Inbreaking of Atrium Walls – Anisotropic Substratum of Electrophysiology

Due to the complexity of the development of the atrial wall, we consider that the best way to present the atrial myocardium is to relate to its embryologic evolution and the process of muscular inbreaking.

The muscular inbreaking of atria follows a membranous (endocardic) pattern (Fig. 7.19), on multiple variable ways, regarding the territory involved:

- The mesenchymal extensions of the endocardial cushions (Figs. 2.4 and 2.9) will form cardio-myocytes. This group is represented by territories derived from the fusion of endocardial cushions, as well as those derived from their extensions: base of the interatrial septum, the territory derived from the former intermediate septum, the anterior region of septum secundum and the anterior and medial parts of the left and right atrial vestibule.

- The extra-cardiac mesoderm which invades the membranous part of the septum primum, through the vestibular spine, determines myocardic inbreaking, rendering to the formation of the muscular part of the interatrial septum, mainly the floor of the fossa ovalis (Fig. 2.20).
- Regarding the formation and presence of the vessels (conditioned mostly by the evolution of the cells of the proepycardic organ) -the myocardic inbreaking begins either in the territories around the venous ostia, or in the auricles, in mostly circular patterns (Fig. 2.52, 2.54 and 7.16). The bundle of Bachmann develops on the reflection line of pericardium on the atrial wall.
- The myocardic inbreak of segments derived from atrioventricular junctions, which are encircled in the atrial vestibule (Fig. 2.80). **The remnant bundles derived from the mesenchyme of these regions may suffer a process of muscular inbreak and may represent abnormal pathways of transmission between atria and ventricles** (Fig. 6.82).
- The myocardic inbreak of the coronary sinus is obviously part of the same process which takes place near by, at the level of the left atrial wall. One can observe that the same vessel supplies simultaneously the adjacent regions of right and left atria, as well as the wall of the sinus venosus (Fig. 7.20).

This process underlines the fact that the coronary sinus is an extension of the right atrium and **explains the possibility that remnant muscular bundles may represent abnormal transmission pathways between the two atria, around or through the wall of the sinus venosus.**

Normally, due to the involution of the left cornus of the primitive sinus venosus, the muscles of the coronary sinus should have devolved and lost their connection with the right atrium.

- The embedment of the right cornus of the sinus venosus in the atrial wall is followed by a heterogeneity increase of the atrial architecture, due to the development of the eustachian margin, the terminal crest, dorsosinusal space and eustachian and thebessian valve.

Electro-physiologically, the embedment of sinus venosus into the wall of atrium and *the variability of the myocardic inbreak of structures* represent major events which lead to an increased anisotropism of the wall of atrium.

After the myocardic inbreak process has begun in these specific areas, the inbreak zone increases due to local proliferation and these zones tend to fuse, in order to form the atrial muscular layer. Incomplete myocardic inbreak areas may still be sometimes visible in adults (Fig. 7.20).

7.2.4 Myoendocrine Cardiomyocyte – The Heart as an Endocrine Organ

In mammals, the atrial myocyte contains in its cytoplasma a great number of electron-opaque granules [15], with a diameter of 0.3–0.4 μm, associated with structures of the Golgi Complex (Figs. 7.4 and 7.5). Ever since 1956 it has been known that the majority of human atrial myocytes contained the so-called atrial specific granules. Soon a conclusion was reached that these granules result from a secretory function. This is how morphological studies led to a radical change of the image of the heart, which is currently seen not only as a simple central pump but also as an endocrine organ with crucial regulatory functions in the vascular and even the renal system. Cardiomyocytes have four fundamental properties: excitability, conductibility, contraction and secretion. It seems reasonable to conclude that all these functions are inter-linked [16].

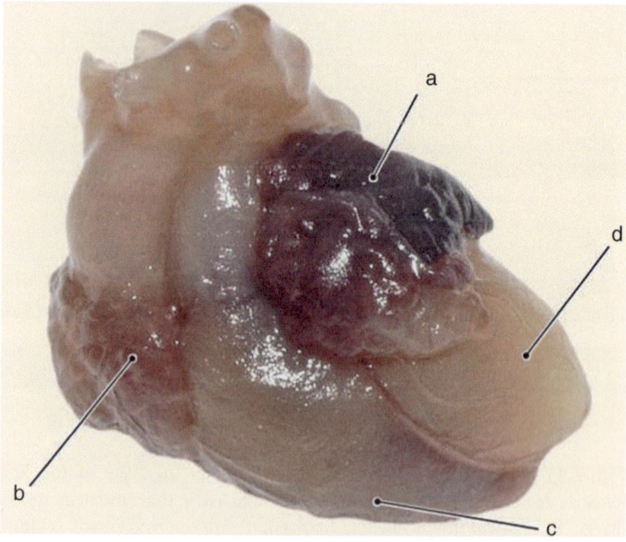

Fig. 7.19 9 weeks old heart. The atrial walls still have a membranous aspect. *a* left atrium, *b* right auricle, *c* left ventricle

As far as secretion is concerned, we can say that there is a group of substances found to be secreted by cardiomyocytes, both the atrial and the ventricular. These substances are *peptidic hormones which reveal a structural equivalence but have a distinct genetic determinism*. These substances are:

- Atrial Natriuretic Peptide (ANP)
- Brain Natriuretic Peptide (BNP or GC-B). It is called this way because it was initially discovered in pig brains
- Natriuretic Peptide Type C (CNP).

These substances are secreted both by the atrial and the ventricular myocytes. ANP is secreted particularly by the atrial and BNP by the ventricular myocytes. CNP is present in a variety of tissues (paracrine hormone).

The main actions of these substances are: to decrease peripheral vascular resistance, to decrease central venous pressure, to increase natriuresis and diuresis.

BNP is co-secreted together with a terminal fragment of amino acid, biologically inactive, called NT-pro BNP. The period for the division of BNP is longer than that of ANP, and NT-pro BNP has the longest period of division. This fact makes NT-pro BNP to be preferable for blood diagnostic

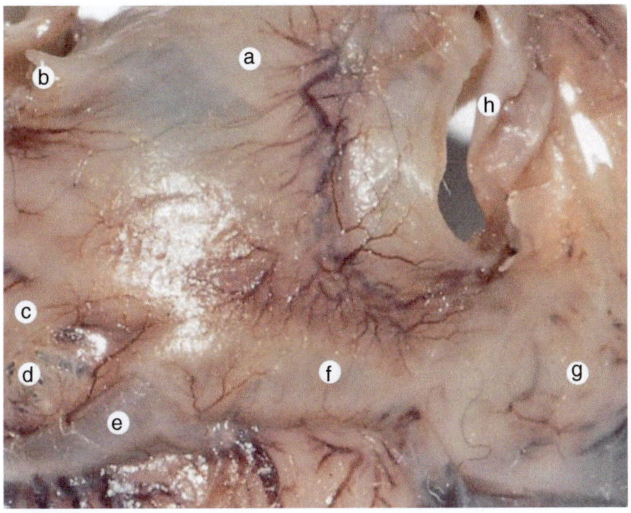

Fig. 7.20 5 months old fetal heart. Posterior view of the cross region of the heart. Detail. The local muscle formation process of the two atria and the sinusal wall is unitary and continuous. The process depends on vascular presence. *a* intrapulmonary fascicle, *b* left inferior pulmonary vein, *c* vestibular fascicle, *d* loss of compacting of the atrial wall, *e* great vein, *f* muscle formation of the sinusal wall, *g* right atrium, *h* inferior vena cava

tests. Blood levels of BNP and NT-pro BNP are used to diagnose acute cardiac insufficiency.

7.2.5 Architecture of the Myocardium-General Considerations. The Theory of "Shutters"

Every concept of microstructure that has been presented represents the basis for the next stage, that of describing the macroscopic structure of the ventricular myocardium. Although it may seem surprising, at the moment, there is no description of the architecture of the myocardium which is sufficiently well-reasoned, thorough and general in order to be unanimously accepted. This is due to the difficulty of the subject as well as to the fact that until now only minimal concepts have been necessary for clinical needs. These minimal concepts can be summed up as follows:

The atrial myocardium is thinner than the ventricular one. It consists of superficial muscle fibers and deep muscle fibers. Superficial fibers make up a system of ansae which bind the two atria. Deep muscle fibers are specific to each atrium.

As far as the organization of the ventricular myocardium is concerned it is generally accepted that there is a superficial layer that passes from one ventricle to the other and which at the top of the heart twists and goes deeper, forming the vortex cordis. There is also a middle muscular layer in each ventricle, well represented particularly in the left ventricle. There is as well a deep muscular layer specific for each ventricle. This classification cannot by far exhaust the topic of the myocardium architecture.

Once the technical opportunities to explore the heart increased, it was discovered that the current anatomical data do not provide a theoretical framework that should be sufficient for the technical capacities of morphofunctional exploration. This fact re-launched the race to solve "the problem of the myocardium structure".

As it often happens in research, numerous opinions were put forward, which, surprisingly, were quite often divergent. These opinions vary from the theory of the myocardium structured as a helical band to mathematical models where the fiber orientation is governed by strict formulas.

Beyond some exaggeration, we consider that each study has brought up a specific point of view, so a data basis has been built which helps us come closer to forming a universally valid conclusion. In what follows we will present, with arguments, the results of our observations regarding the myocardium structure.

In the anatomical description we will proceed from the premise that a structural theory is correct if there is a correspondence between organizational and functional details.

7.2.6 The Architecture of the Ventricular Myocardium

First we will go over the summary of the microstructural organization: Packs of myofibrils (structured as sarcomeres consisting of myofilaments) make up a cardiomyocyte. The aspect of the cardiomyocyte is essentially longitudinal, branched and anastomosed. This aspect can be found as a pattern at different organizational levels. The cardiomyocyte has a basal and sarcolemmic membrane. The cardiomyocyte packs, bound by collagen fascicles and varied proteins of the extracellular matrix make up a muscular fiber, surrounded by a connective tissue sheath called endomysium. The endomysium covers every cell as well as the fiber itself and binds muscle cells at the capillary wall. More muscle fibers make up a bundle, surrounded by the perimysium. More bundles make up a muscle lamella [17], surrounded by the epimysium. In the areas where the strand structure is not obvious, more bundles make up a trabeculation, a papillary muscle or a larger bundle, surrounded by the epimysium.

Practically, the epimysium (of the lamellae) fuses both at the interior of the heart (lining cavities subendocardially) and at the exterior (lining the heart subepicardially and binding lamellae).Fibers, bundles and lamellae are essentially branched and anastomosed. The acceptance of the lamellar arrangement is important and (for some) obvious in the myoarchitecture of the left ventricle. In comparison with the long axis of the left ventricle (originating in the primitive ventricle) the muscle lamellae are flat, superposed and circular, the

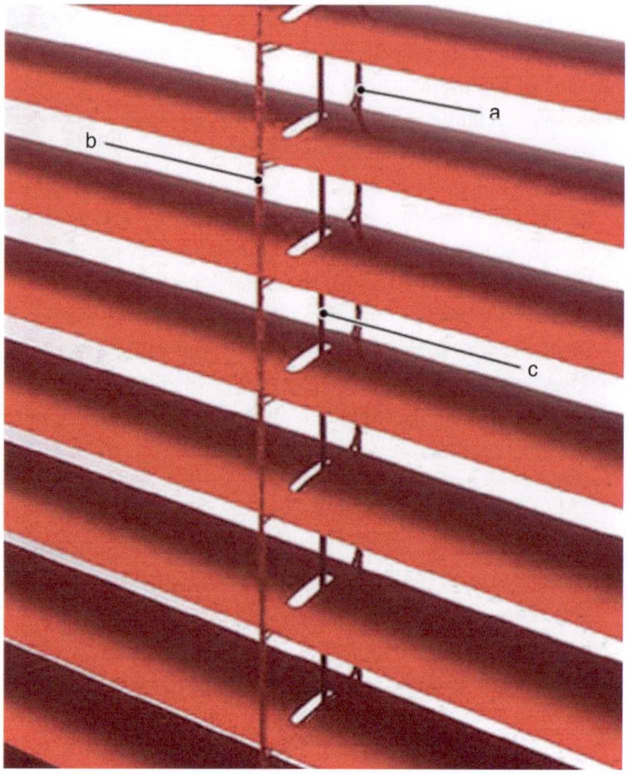

Fig. 7.21 Blind-like structure formation. See the position of the cohesion lines that allow the system to work like a unit. *a* external cohesion line, *b* internal cohesion line, *c* central cohesion line

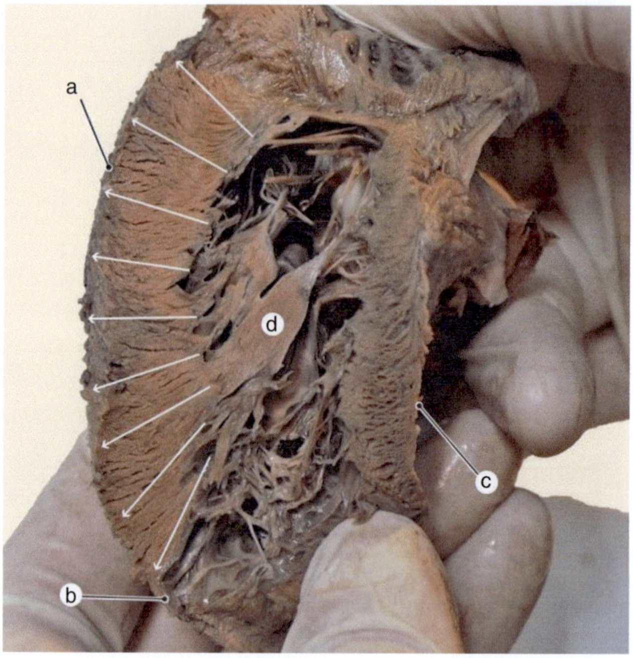

Fig. 7.22 Paramedian sagittal section through the left ventricle. The *arrows* show radial arrangement of the lamellae in the ventricular wall structure. The subepi-subendocardic superposition from the apex allows ventricular wall extension. *a* pulmonary side of the left ventricle, *b* epi-endocardic superposition at the ventricular apex, *c* diaphragmatic side of the left ventricle, *d* posterior papillary group

most suggestive comparison being that of a horizontal blind (Fig. 7.21). Consequently, we will call this type of organization "the theory of shutters".

Towards the top and the basis of the ventricle, the lamellae slant, and towards the ventricular center they are almost horizontal. They are not perfectly horizontal because the outer edges have a divergent tendency. We say that the lamellae are oriented relatively radially towards the surface of the heart. The inter-lamellar anastomoses play the role of the cohesion threads from the structure of a shutter. These threads are arranged in three columns: the central (near the middle of the lamella), the interior and the exterior column- a position similar to that of the cohesion threads from the structure of a shutter (Figs. 7.22, 7.23, 7.24, 7.25, 7.26, 7.28, 7.29 and 7.30). Similarly to the functional principle of the shutter, the central column ensures, first of all, co-axiality, while the inner and outer columns modify the inclination angle of the lamellae. This is possible due to the progressive excitation of the myocardium starting from the apex toward the basis and from the interior towards the exterior. During the systole the lamellae become horizontal, thus explaining the thickening of the wall in systole. The horizontalization of the lamellae concentrates myocyte forces, offering the maximum of expulsion power. During the diastole the lamellae become slanted, explaining the thinning of the ventricular wall. This type of behaviour of the lamellar structure should not be understood as an isolated behaviour, but, on the contrary, as integrated in the generality of a coherent parietal contraction, which is multisectorial and multiaxial! The lamellae have a luminal region, a central and a superficial one (towards the epicardium). The fibers and muscular bundles from the luminal region, forced by the blood flow to re-orientate during ontogeny, do not keep the lamellar arrangement, they are cut off from the lamellae and arranged in the direction of the blood flow. These fibers still keep the anastomoses with the fibers and the bundles from the neighbouring lamellae. They change into trabeculations oriented in the direction of the flow forces. In the classic description they correspond to the deep myocardial layer. The trabeculations contain bundles from more neighbouring lamellae (Fig. 7.34). The fibers and the bundles from the superficial region, under the influence of intrapericardial pressure (in phylogeny and ontogeny) gradually lose the lamellar arrangement, preserving however the anastomoses with the neighbouring fibers and bundles as well as with the original lamellae. These fibers will make up the superficial layer. Their orientation (as well as the orientation of the other layers) is mostly the result of the folding and reorganization of the heart tube (Figs. 7.35 and 7.36).

The fibers from the central region of the ventricular wall make up characteristic lamellae, anastomosed by the three types of interlamellar columns. They form the middle layer

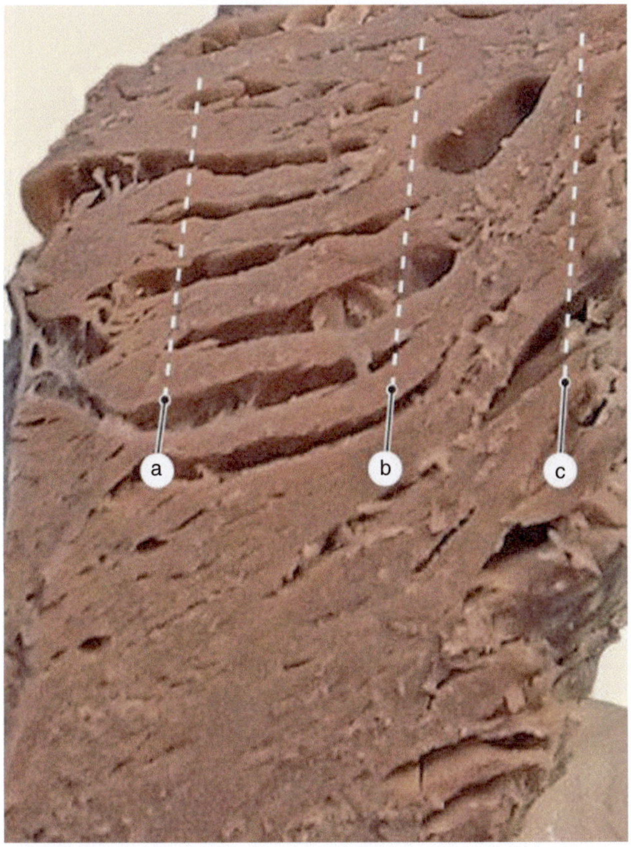

Fig. 7.23 Inter-lamellar muscular anastomoses are arranged like cohesion lines from the structure of a horizontal blind system. Between lamellae are three cohesion areas arranged from top to bottom in the depth of the ventricular wall. *a* internal cohesion area, *b* central cohesion area, *c* external cohesion area

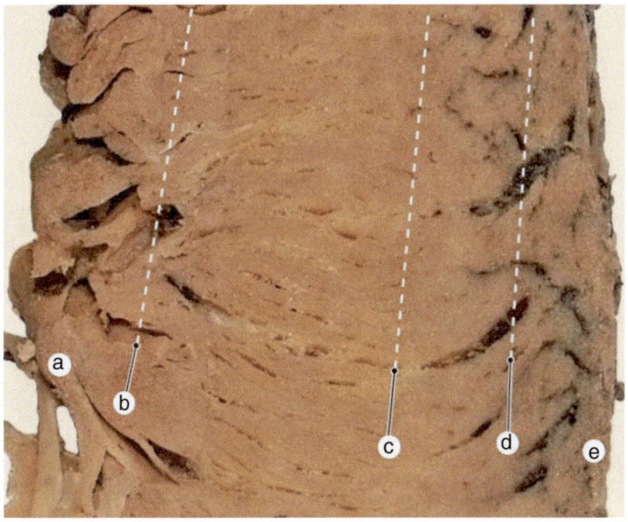

Fig. 7.24 Arrangement of the most important sights of inter-lamellar cohesion in the middle third of the left ventricular wall, on the pulmonary face. *a* trabeculae with origin in different lamellae, *b* internal cohesion area, *c* central cohesion area, *d* external cohesion area, *e* diaphragmatic face of the left ventricle

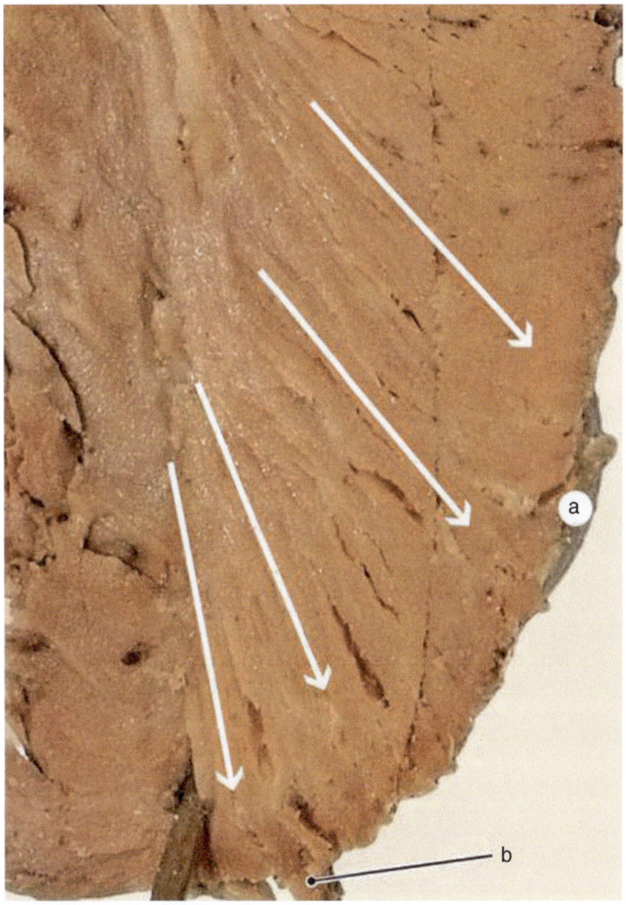

Fig. 7.25 Sagittal section through the wall of the left ventricle, on the pulmonary side. Approaching the apex the lamellae orientation (*arrows*) in the ventricular wall becomes oblique, until in the apex area the lamellae are almost vertical. *a* diaphragmatic side of the left ventricle, *b* apex

in the classic description. There is no uniformity in the size and orientation of these lamellae. Clearly, the lamellae do not reach (and there is no need to do so) the subendocardium or subepicardium. Their arrangement is not perfectly regulated and uniform in the whole ventricular wall, but they certainly exist. The columns are not perfectly sketched, rigorous, yet the interlamellar anastomoses between the envisaged areas certainly exist and the described structures perform their function, in all probability, according to the metaphor and the principle of the shutter. Thus structured, the myocardium really forms three layers, without a strict delimitation between them, the orientation of the fibers progressively changing, from the superficial towards the deep layer. Due to the progressive change in the direction of the fibers, the wall of the heart is compact and resistant. There are areas, however, near the apex of the heart and in the vicinity of interventricular grooves, where this superposition of differently oriented layers is not perfect. Thus the danger of the decompaction of myocardial structure appears (Fig. 7.37), leading to the superposition of the epicardium and the endocardium. The possibility of decompaction is

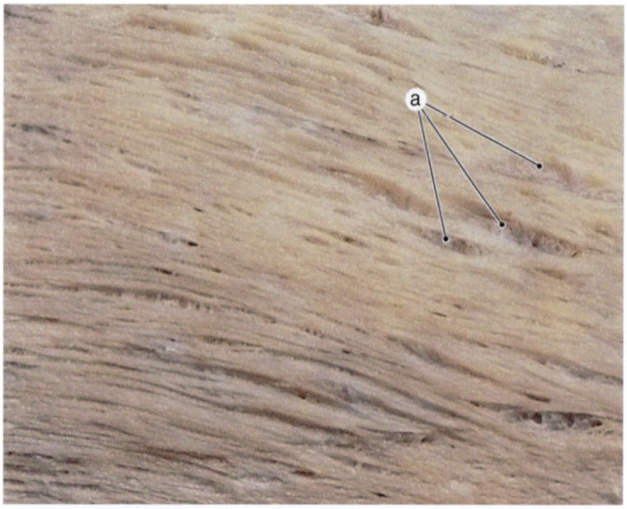

Fig. 7.26 Tangential section in the wall of the left ventricle on the diaphragmatic surface. The lamellar structure of the wall and extra-cellular matrix are obvious. *a* extra-cellular matrix

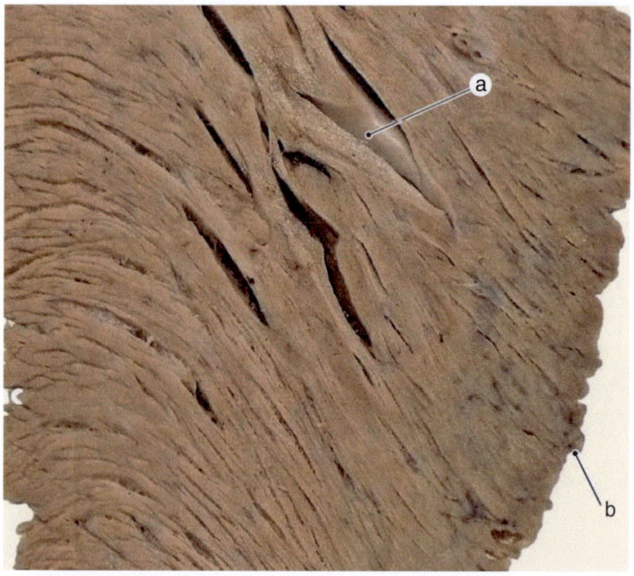

Fig. 7.28 Sagittal section in the wall of the left ventricle the diaphragmatic surface in the inferior third. The lamellar structure is evident. The muscular trabeculae have origin in the nearby lamellae. *a* trabecula with origin in different lamellae, *b* diaphragmatic side

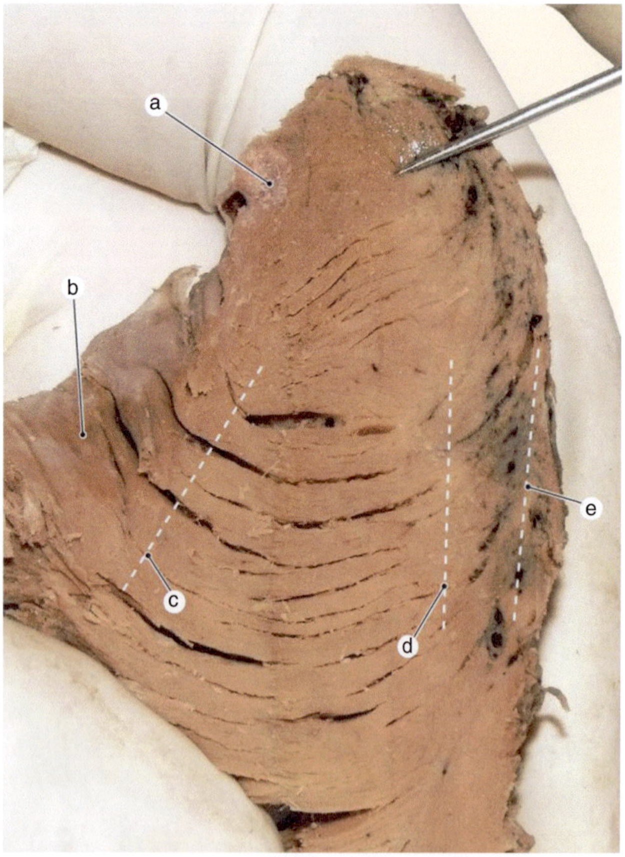

Fig. 7.27 Sagittal section in the wall of the left ventricle, on the diaphragmatic surface, near the ventricular base. The top of the needle is placed above a lamellar system of the ventricular base, that assures the semi-sphincter behavior of the left ventricular base. *a* mitral fila coronaria, *b* aortic vestibule, *c* internal cohesion area

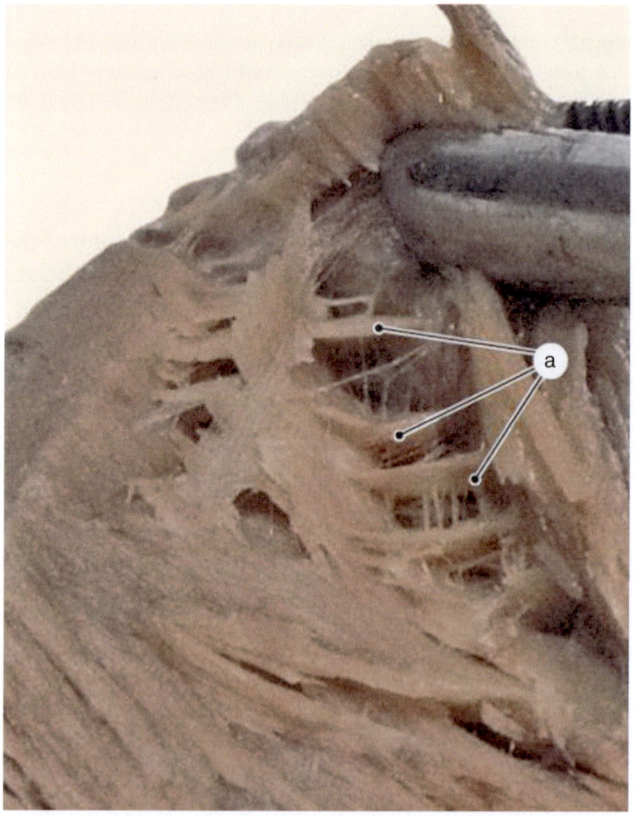

Fig. 7.29 Besides the most important areas of cohesionm, the lamellae are interconnected on their entire length through small inter-lamellar fascicles. *a* uniting inter-lamellar fascicles and extra-cellular matrix

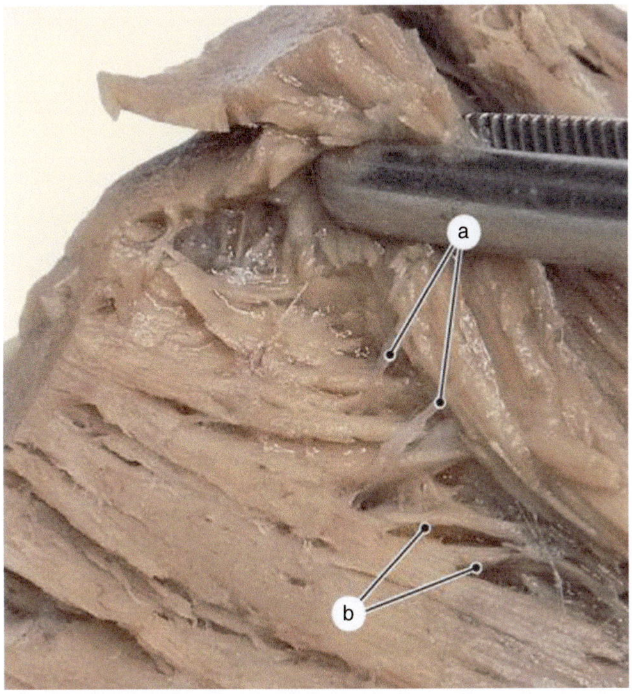

Fig. 7.30 Connecting inter-lamellar fascicles. *a* extra-cellular matrix, *b* uniting inter-lamellar fascicles

raised in dilated hearts with probably an altered extracellular matrix. In conclusion, the structure of the ventricular myocardium is simultaneously lamellar and stratified. The structural unities (fibers, bundles, lamellae) are branched and anastomosed, which creates structural interdependency and functional unity. There are certainly three layers: the superficial layer with predominantly slanted fibers towards the long axis. The middle layer has predominantly circular fibers, perpendicular on the long axis. The deep, trabecular layer has a reversed obliqueness towards the superficial layer. The transitions between the three layers are progressive. There are no cleavage planes or strict delimitations at the borders between layers.

In a nutshell, the direction of myocardial fibers varies progressively in the bulk of the ventricular wall, towards the longitudinal axis, from the surface to the depth thus: slantwise- circular-slantwise. The character of "clockwise or anticlockwise" movement can be determined by watching a clock set on the apex of the heart, with the central axis corresponding to the long axis of the heart and the screen towards the observer (Fig. 7.55).

The orientation of superficial slanted fibers is clockwise (if we look from the apex of the heart). Thus it becomes clear why their contraction participates in the torsion movement- an anticlockwise movement (Fig. 7.32). The orientation of the middle fibers is circular. Thus it is clear why their contraction reduces the transverse diameter (Figs. 7.31, 7.32, 7.33 and 7.39).

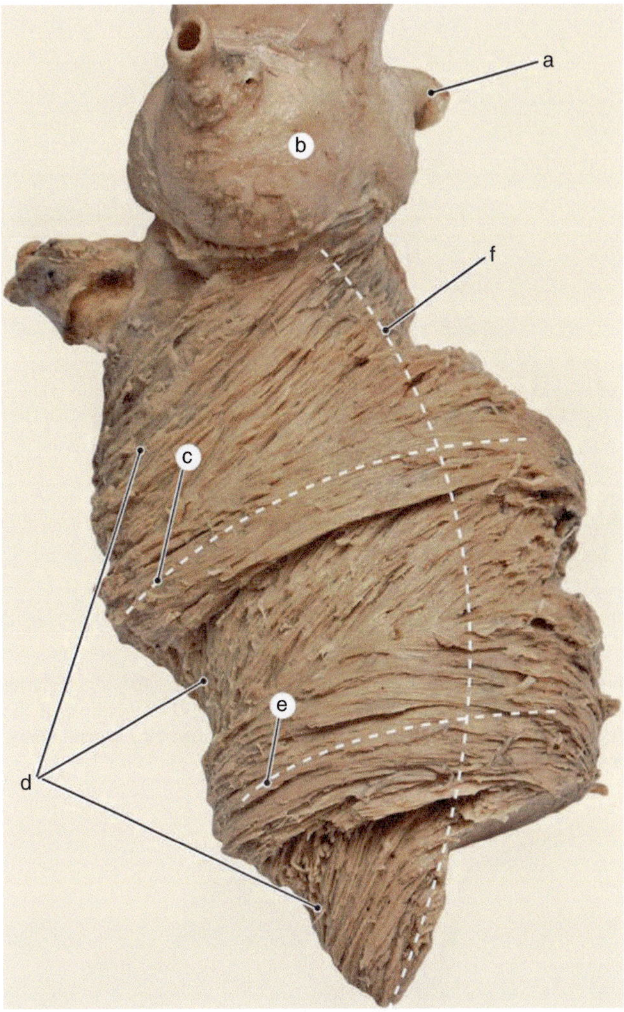

Fig. 7.31 Dissection of the left ventricular wall with the outlining of the direction of the fibers in the central and deep area. The *vertical pointed line* corresponds to the direction of the superficial fibers on the pulmonary surface. *a* left coronary artery, *b* aorta, *c* direction of the central fibers, *d* direction of the deep fibers, *e* direction of the central fibers, *f* direction of the superficial fibers on the pulmonary surface

The orientation of deep slanted fibers is anticlockwise. Thus it is clear why their contraction participates in the retrotorsion movement- a clockwise movement (Fig. 7.34). The superficial layer, because of its obliqueness, achieves through its contraction the shortening of the longitudinal axis and the anticlockwise torsion.

The Figs. 7.35, 7.36, 7.37 and 7.38 show the orientation of superficial fibers in the different areas of the heart.

The middle layer achieves the major reduction of the transverse diameter. The deep layer has two elements: Parietal trabeculations (located in relation to the wall) (Fig. 7.34) represent the visible part of the deep layer, connected to the lamellar structure by a transition area, with muscle fibers which gradually become spiralled anticlockwise. These parietal trabeculations are oriented spirally anticlockwise and are implied in longitudinal shortening and

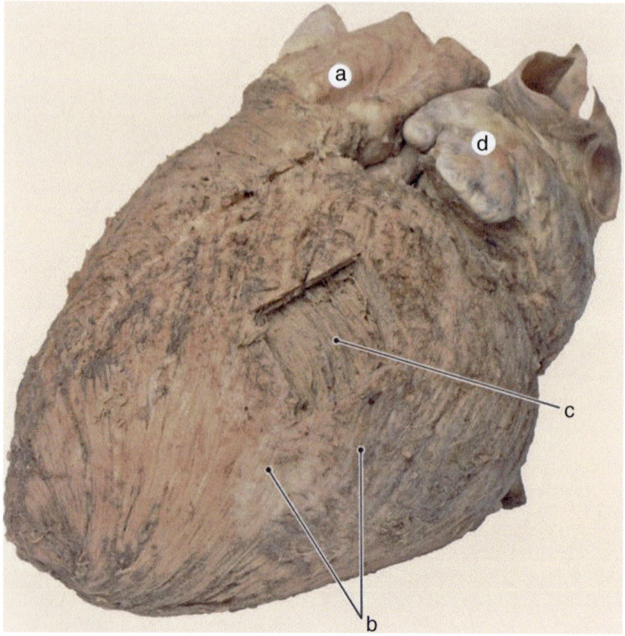

Fig. 7.32 "Window" in the left ventricular wall, for highlighting superficial and central fibers. *a* pulmonary trunk, *b* direction of the superficial fibers on the pulmonary side, *c* direction of the central fibers, *d* left auricle

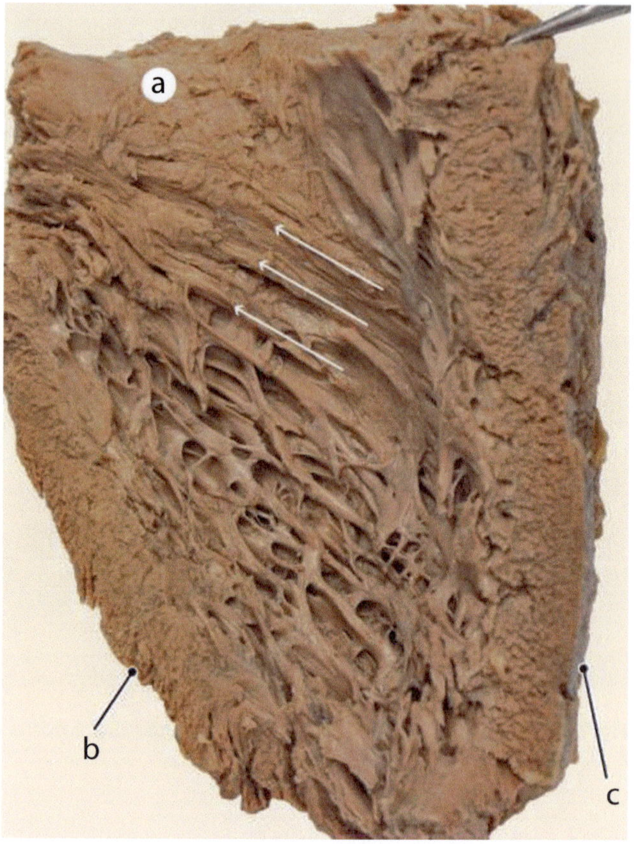

Fig. 7.34 Sagittal section of the left ventricle, seen from the left side. The *arrows* show the direction of the parietal trabeculae. The luminal trabeculae were resected before. *a* aortic vestibulae, *b* anterior side, *c* diaphragmatic surface

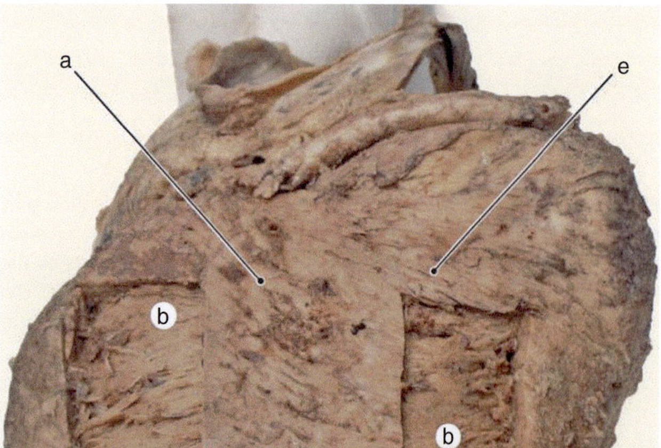

Fig. 7.33 "Windows" on the diaphragmatic surface for outlining central fibers of the two ventricles. *a* direction of superficial fibers, *b* direction of central fibers, *c* diaphragmatic surface of the left ventricle, *d* diaphragmatic surface of the right ventricle, *e* direction of the superficial fibers

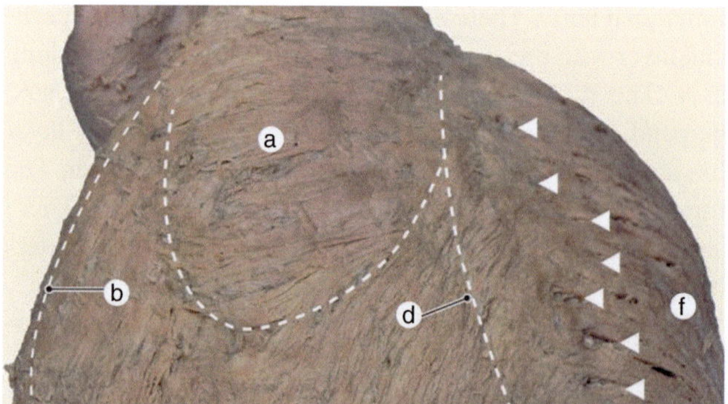

Fig. 7.35 Careful dissection in order to make visible the superficial fibers permits identifying change of their direction. The *pointed lines* show bulbo-ventricular grooves and delineation of the cone of the pulmonary artery. The *arrows* mark the areas in which the septal arteries reach ventricular wall depth, at the left of the anterior inter-ventricular groove. *a* the cone of the pulmonary artery – area of the primitive bulb, *b* direction of the superior bulbo-ventricular superior line, *c* right ventricle, *d* inferior bulbo-ventricular groove, *e* incisura of the heart apex, *f* left ventricle

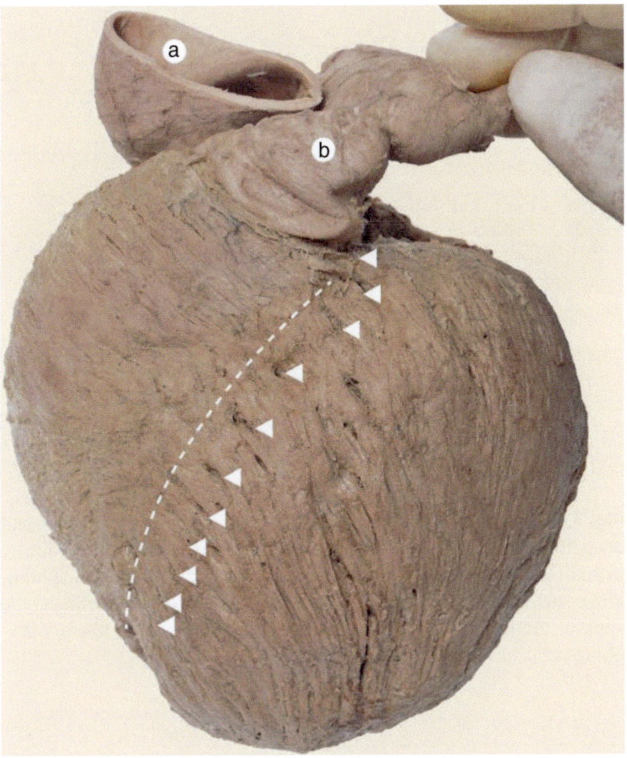

Fig. 7.36 The *arrowheads* mark the origins of the septal arteries and the direction of the anterior inter-ventricular artery. The *pointed line* shows the anterior inter-ventricular groove. The unbinding between the direction of the groove and the artery is evident. *a* aorta, *b* pulmonary trunk

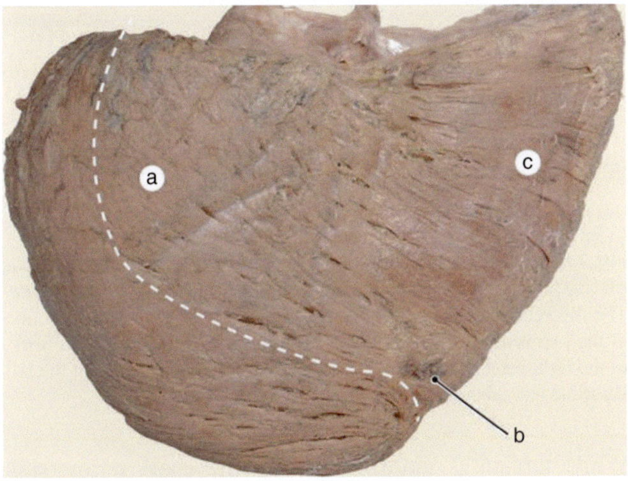

Fig. 7.37 The *pointed line* shows the direction of the superficial fibers on the diaphragmatic surface of the left ventricle. *a* diaphragmatic surface of the left ventricle, *b* parietal decompacting of the apex of the left ventricle, *c* diaphragmatic surface of the right ventricle

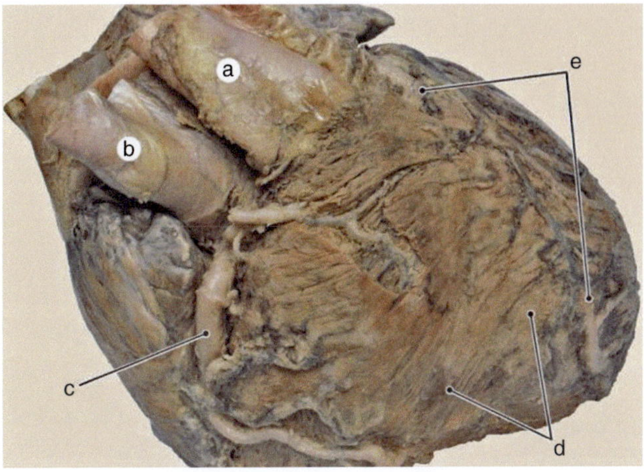

Fig. 7.38 Direction of the superficial fibers in the right ventricle. Great myocardial pons over the anterior inter-ventricular artery. *a* pulmonary trunk, *b* aorta, *c* right coronary artery, *d* direction of the superficial fibers on the right ventricle, *e* anterior inter-ventricular artery covered by myocardial pons

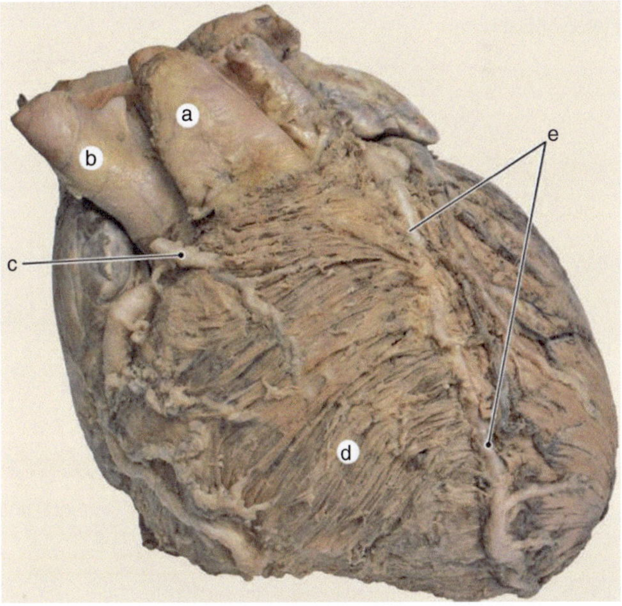

Fig. 7.39 Same heart from the last picture. Superficial fibers and myocardial pons were resected. *a* pulmonary trunk, *b* aorta, *c* artery of the pulmonary cone, *d* central circular fibers, *e* anterior inter-ventricular artery after removing the myocardial pons. Observe the greater diameter of the artery pre and post pons

clockwise retrotorsion. Luminal trabeculations (Figs. 6.109 and 6.110), relatively independent of the parietal lamellar structure. In the apical region they form a network involved in the binding of the walls and the cohesion of the contraction. On one hand, this network concentrates little by little in longitudinal trabecular columns (parallel with the long ventricular axis) which continues in the papillary muscles. Some of these columns (absorbed in the septum) reach subendocardially the vestibule of the aorta. On the other hand, the trabecular network joins together the bases of the papillary muscles. This way the cardiac apex is dynamically coherent with the basal plane (the apex comes close to the basal plane in systole and the longitudinal ventricular diameter shortens). The septoparietal trabeculations of the

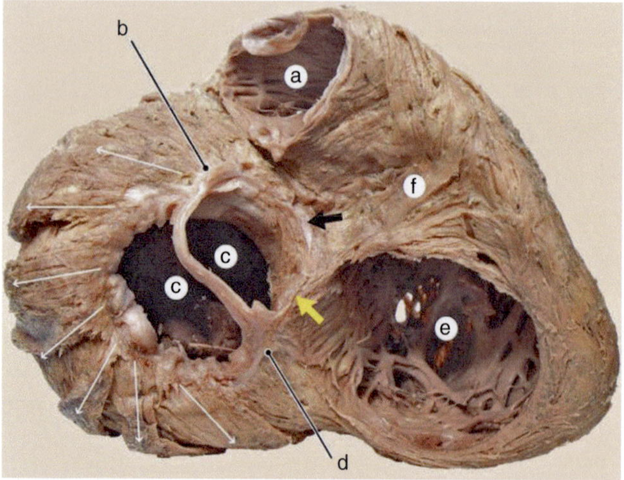

Fig. 7.40 The atria and greater arteries have been removed. The mitral-aortic orifice is visible, divided by the mitral-aortic continuation. *White arrows* show the orientation of the superficial fibers at the base of the left ventricle. The *yellow arrow* shows the Hiss fascicle and the *black arrow* shows the base of the right coronary sinus. *a* infundibulum, *b* the left trigone, *c* mitral-aortic orifice, *d* right trigone, *e* right ventricle, *f* three orifice istmus

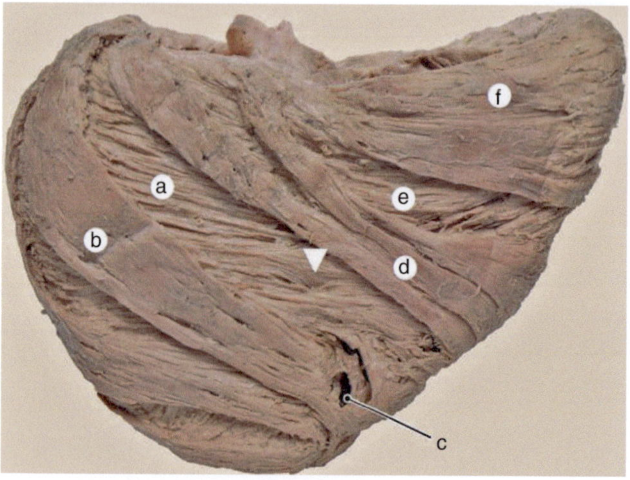

Fig. 7.42 Difference of orientation between the superficial fibers and deep fibers on the diaphragmatic surface. The *arrow* shows the splitting to right and left of the septal trabeculae. *a* central fibers, *b* diaphragmatic surface of the left ventricle, *c* area of parietal decompacting at the apex of the right ventricle, *d* superficial fibers, *e* central fibers, *f* diaphragmatic surface of the left ventricle

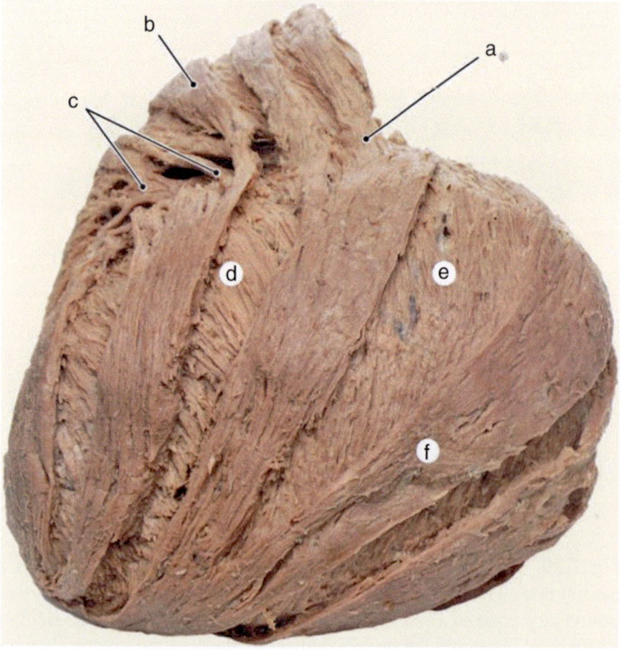

Fig. 7.41 Dissection for highlighting the progressive change of direction of the muscular fibers. The intermediate layer is found between the superficial and central layers. *a* ventricular-infundibular junction, *b* infundibulum, *c* septal-parietal trabeculae, *d* circular middle layer, *e* intermediate layer, *f* direction of the superficial fibers

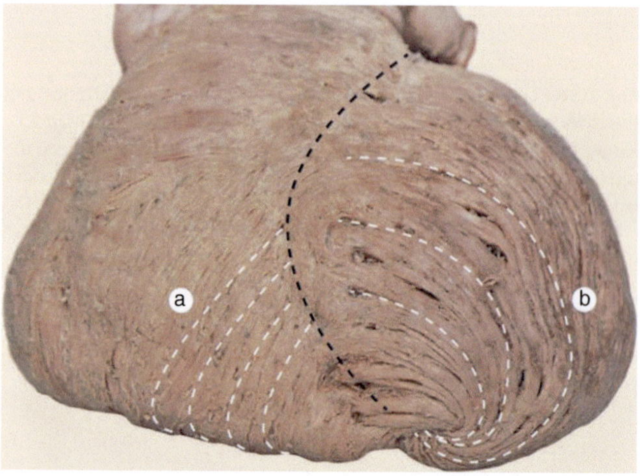

Fig. 7.43 Different direction of the superficial fibers for the two ventricles. The inter-ventricular groove is marked by the *black pointed line*. The dissection is very suggestive for the different ways of contraction of the two ventricles. *a* "hood-like" disposition of the superficial fibers in the right ventricle wall, *b* direction of the superficial fibers of the left ventricle that create the vortex

right ventricle are involved in interventricular binding, the homogenization of the contraction and also in the torsion determined by the superficial fibers (Fig. 6.68).

The transitional muscle fibers between the layers achieve the homogenization of the contraction. The retrotorsion. While torsion is more obvious at the apex, retrotorsion is more obvious at the ventricular basis. The coupling of torsion and retrotorsion engage the heart in a general movement of "wringing". If torsion is mostly due to the vertical distribution of superficial fibers at the apex of the heart, retrotorsion is generally due to the slanted arrangement of the superficial fibers around the mitral ring (mitral aortic) and it is defined as a circular clockwise movement of the ventricular basis (in fact of the mitral aortic orifice) (Figs. 7.40, 7.41 and 7.42). The recoil is a return to the situation before the systole. It is mostly an elastic phenomenon, produced by the

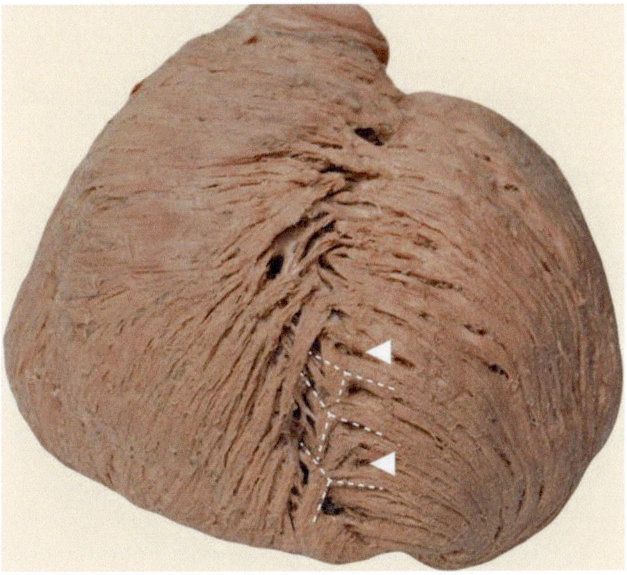

Fig. 7.44 The muscular trabeculae on the right side of the interventricular septum split at their anterior pole in a right fascicle and a left fascicle. These fascicles take part in creating the inter-ventricular walls. The trabeculae splittings superpose from top to bottom and create the anterior inter-ventricular groove. The left splitting fascicles superpose and mark entry spaces for the septal arteries

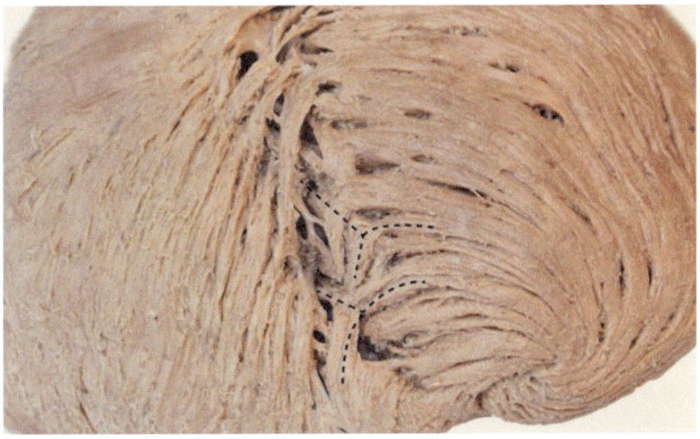

Fig. 7.45 Splitting of the septal trabeculae. Detail

tensional charge of the muscle fibers and the extracellular matrix. In fact, during both stages of contraction, the matrix is charged with elastic tensions bringing forward the recoil. In connection with this arrangement it must be specified that the ventricular myocardium is not a homogeneous territory, and its architecture is marked by the way in which the ontogenetic evolution of the heart tube and the septating of the heart takes place. There are a few areas where, originating from the basic structural principle, specific myocardial architectural solutions appear. These areas are: the interventricular grooves, the base of the ventricular pyramid, the cardiac apex, the ventricular-infundibular junction, the root of the aorta. These will be presented separately.

7.2.6.1 The Arrangement of Muscle Fibers at the Level of the Anterior Interventricular Sulcus

The groove can be found at the surface of the heart, on the sternocostal surface, as a longitudinal depression which descends from the left of the pulmonary ostium to the notch of the cardiac apex. This notch separates more or less obviously the apexes of the two ventricles (Figs. 7.43 and 7.53). The anterior interventricular vessels run down through the groove or frequently to its left. The anterior interventricular artery divides into septal branches to the left of the groove (Fig. 7.36). The classic description says that superficial fibers cross like a bridge at the level of the groove over the interventricular border. This statement was underlined by the observations on the coronary-myocardial bridges, observations which suggested that the anterior interventricular artery was in fact engaged between the middle and the superficial layer. We have been the prisoners of this opinion for a very long time. Minute repeated dissections, performed according to different methods have shown that in fact:- Septoparietal trabeculations from the cavity of the left ventricle (Fig. 6.68) bifurcate at their anterior extremity in a right and left fascicle. This bifurcation is responsible for the existence of the anterior interventricular sulcus at the level of the divergence angle (Figs. 7.44, 7.45, 7.46, 7.47, 7.48, 7.49 and 7.50). The angle of this bifurcation is filled with and covered by a thin mass of muscle fibers which link the two ventricles. This mass of muscle fibers is involved in the making of the myocardial bridges. In the inferior third of the anterior interventricular sulcus this lamella is missing or it is quite reduced. The observation should be correlated with

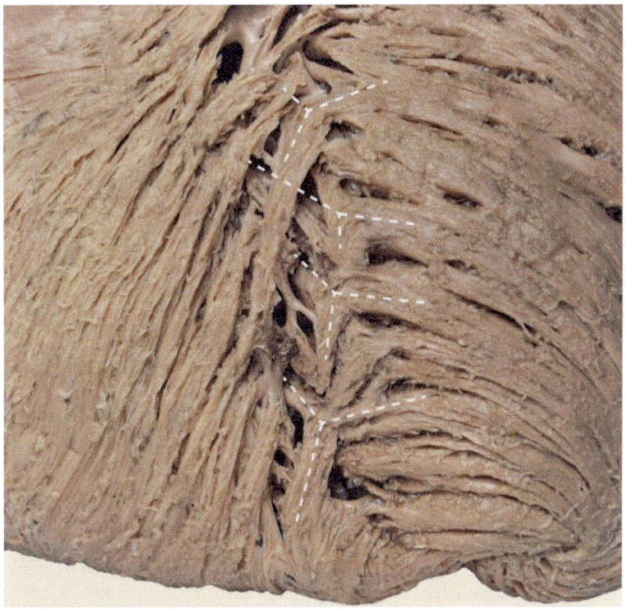

Fig. 7.46 Splitting of the septal trabeculae in the apex area

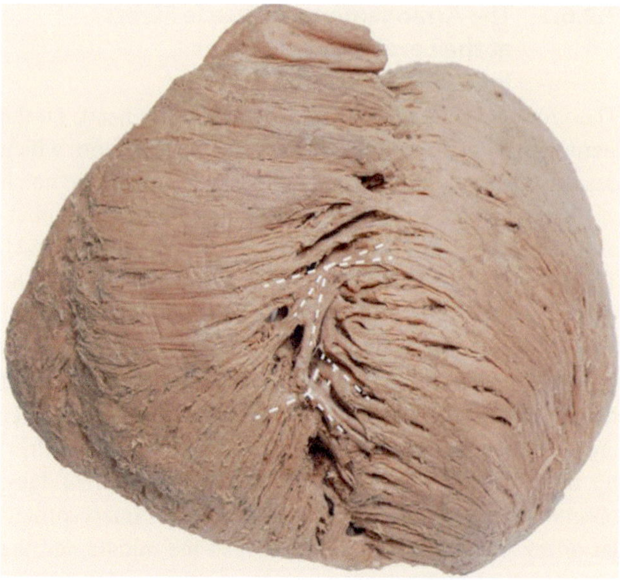

Fig. 7.47 Splitting of the septo-marginal trabeculae

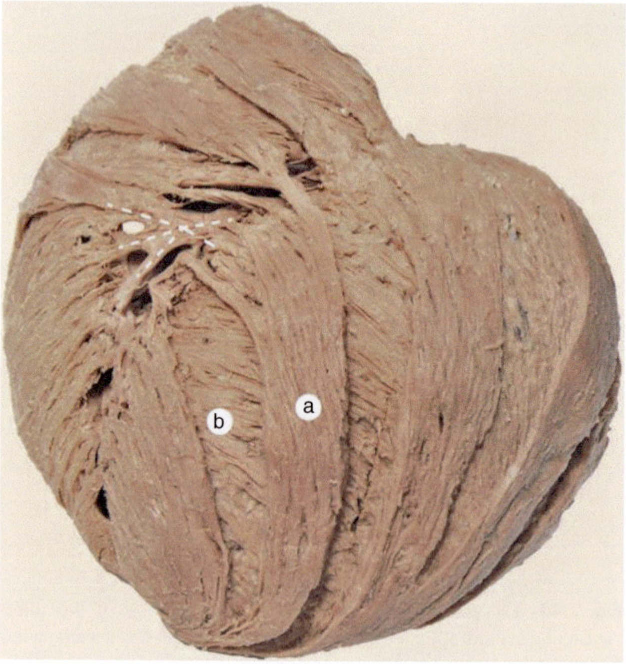

Fig. 7.49 The split trabeculae continue in the superficial layer as well as in the middle one. *a* superficial layer, *b* middle layer

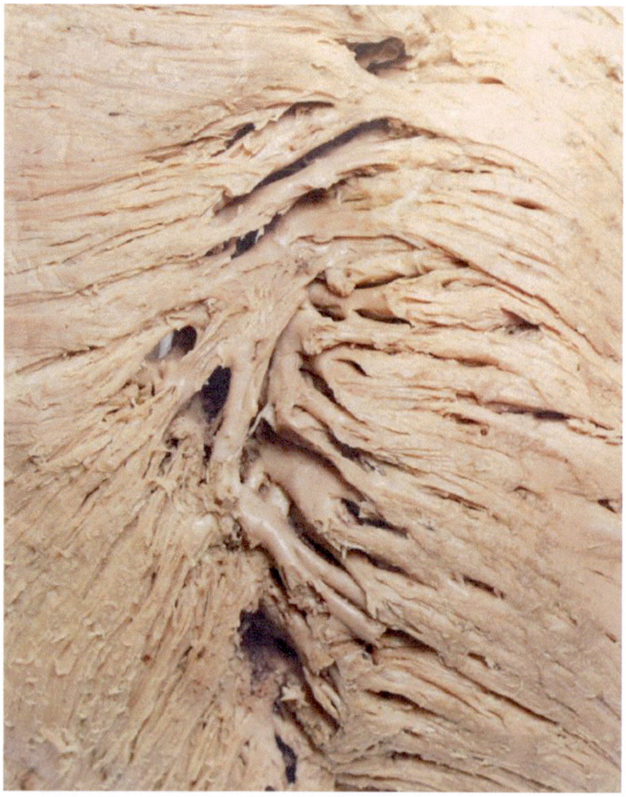

Fig. 7.48 Splitting of the septo-marginal trabeculae. Detail

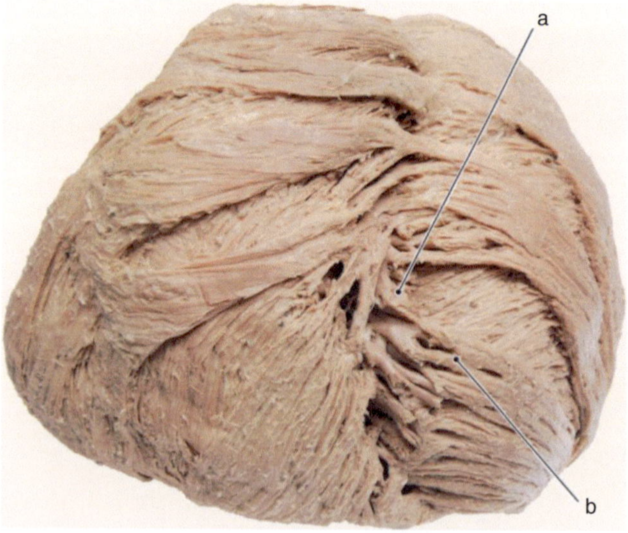

Fig. 7.50 The split trabeculae continue in the superficial layer as well as in the middle layer. *a* trabeculae that continue in the middle layer, *b* trabeculae that continue in the superficial layer

the decreasing number of the myocardial bridges towards the cardiac apex. The anterior trabecular extremities and their bifurcation bundles are superposed and make up a network that makes the interventricular limit compact.

The superposition of the bundles on the left side forms a network and through its orifices pass the septal perforating arteries. The engaging orifices are well- defined and besides the arteries they contain extensions of the extracellular matrix.

Practically it is possible that these perforating arteries would pass through the anterior extension of the left ventricle lumen. The line resulting from the reunion of the origins of these arteries actually marks the anterior limit of the right ventricle.- The bundles on the left side are continued in the bulk of the left ventricle wall, mostly in the bulk of the superficial layer and more deeply in the lamellar structure of the middle layer.- The superposition of the bundles on the right side is continued in the same manner in the bulk of the right ventricular wall, forming the most part of it.- The anterior interventricular sulcus appears in this theory as a vectorial balance area between divergent forces right-left. This is a dynamic balance, accomplished according to every moment of the contraction. The integrity and efficiency of bundles on one side are indispensable to the efficient contraction of the bundles on the other side. The loss of the yielding seat represented by the interventricular sulcus will have a general effect on the organ. We can now understand why septal infarction globally affects the pump capacity of the heart. Although ontogenetically and phylogenetically the interventricular septum has a separating role, from an architectural point of view it is built as an integral part of the structure of the left ventricle. In other words, the left ventricle has the harmonious architecture of an ovoid only if the interventricular septum belongs to it conceptually and structurally. On both ventricular surfaces the septum is covered by trabeculations, whose orientation is parallel to the local sanguine direction. At the center of the septal myocardial mass the myocardial structure is quasi-lamellar. The septal trabeculations are gradually bound to the lamellar edges towards the lumen of the left ventricle by anastomotic transitional bundles.

7.2.6.2 The Arrangement of Muscle Fibers at the Level of the Posterior Interventricular Sulcus

The groove can be found at the surface of the heart, on its diaphragmatic surface, as a longitudinal fossa which descends from the crux cordis to the notch of the cardiac apex. It is less visible than the anterior groove and contains the posterior interventricular vessels (Figs. 7.37, 7.42 and 7.51). The trabeculations that can be found in the right ventricle on the septum near the groove have essentially the same behaviour as those described above, i.e. they bifurcate in left and right bundles that are superposed. This behaviour is less evident than in the anterior region and it is present especially in the inferior two thirds of the interventricular sulcus. In the superior third of the groove, next to the crux cordis, the muscle fibers that fill the bifurcation space are better represented than in the anterior region. They probably originate in the muscularisation of the inferior endocardial cushion.- The difference of architecture between the inferior two thirds and the superior third of the posterior interventricular sulcus can derive from the embryological differences (the inferior two thirds originate in the inferior limbus of the muscular interventricular septum and the superior third in the inferior endocardial cushion and probably in the primitive ventricle).

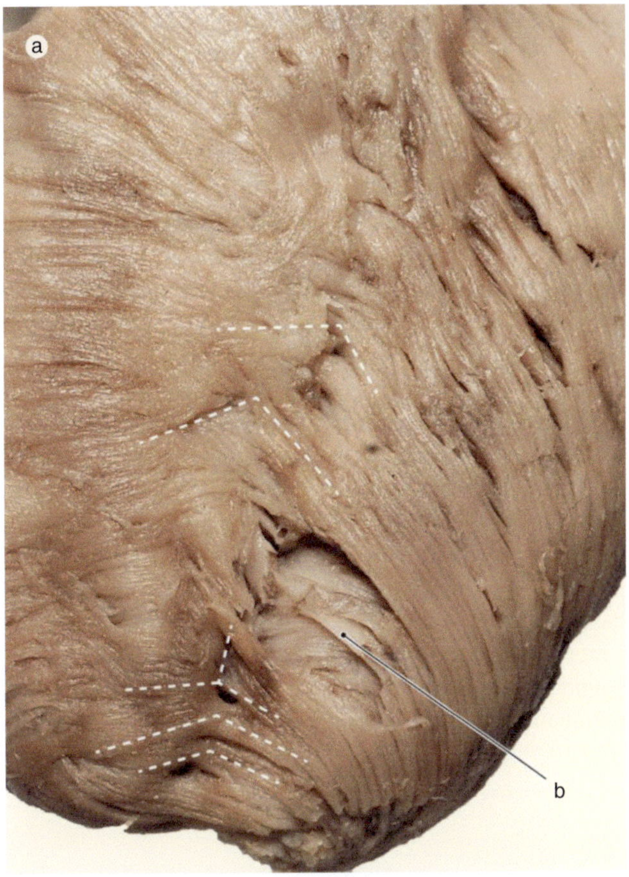

Fig. 7.51 Septal trabeculae from the right ventricle also split at the level of the posterior inter-ventricular groove. *a* diaphragmatic side of the left ventricle, *b* middle circular fibers in the right ventricle. The *pointed lines* show the splitting fascicles

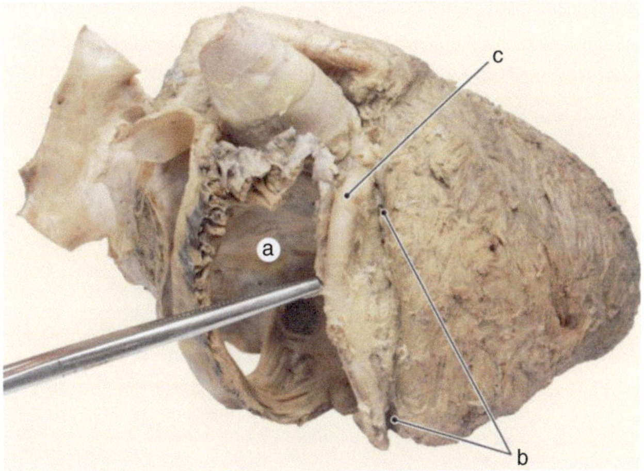

Fig. 7.52 The atrio-ventricular fold is deeper in it's right side than in it's left side. The maximum of expanding of this fold is in it's posterior side, that represents in fact the piramidal space. *a* right atrium, *b* atrio-ventricular fold that continues in the posterior with the piramidal space, *c* right coronary

7.2.6.3 The Mitro- Aortic and Tricuspid Orifices and the Arrangement of the Muscle Fibers at the Base Level of the Ventricles

There are practically two orifices at the base of the ventricles in the myocardial wall: the mitro- aortic and the tricuspid. The base of the ventricular pyramid together with these orifices and the atrioventricular rings is called the basal plane. In principle, at the level of these orifices a transition is made between the superficial, subepicardial myocardial fibers and the luminal, subendocardial myocardial fibers. Between the mitro- aortic and the tricuspid orifices, corresponding to the middle area of the interventricular septum crest there is a subepicardial-subendocardial transition. We say 'in principle' because the tendinous center and the membranous center mark the boundary between two subendocardial muscular territories. These fibrous structures bind the two mitral aortic and tricuspid orifices. The mitral aortic orifice is the orifice that results if we take out the aorta and left atrium from the base of the left ventricle (Fig. 7.40). The 'in situ' preservation of the mitral aortic continuity evidently marks the boundary between the aorta and the pulmonary artery. The mitral aortic orifice has thick, well represented margins, and at the ventricular root of the cusps the arrangement of superficial fibers is continued by the direction of subendocardial fibers. This way the base of the left ventricle is caught as if in a hammock by the subepicardial-subendocardial continuity and on one hand pulled towards the cardiac apex, while on the other hand, engaged in retrotorsion. The strong bundles of superficial muscle fibers anchor the two fibrous trigones, pulling them divergently and thus keeping the aortic orifice open during the ventricular systole. If we look at the arrangement and orientation of the subepicardial fibers at the level of this orifice (a slanted direction towards the posterior surrounding the circumference), we notice that by contracting, these fibers achieve the clockwise rotation of the mitral aortic orifice (looking from the cardiac apex), accomplishing the retrotorsion of the ventricular base (Fig. 7.40). The circular lamellar middle layer is well represented at the ventricular base (Fig. 7.27). Its contraction during systole should close the aortic orifice, yet this does not happen principally because of the involvement of the fibrous skeleton.

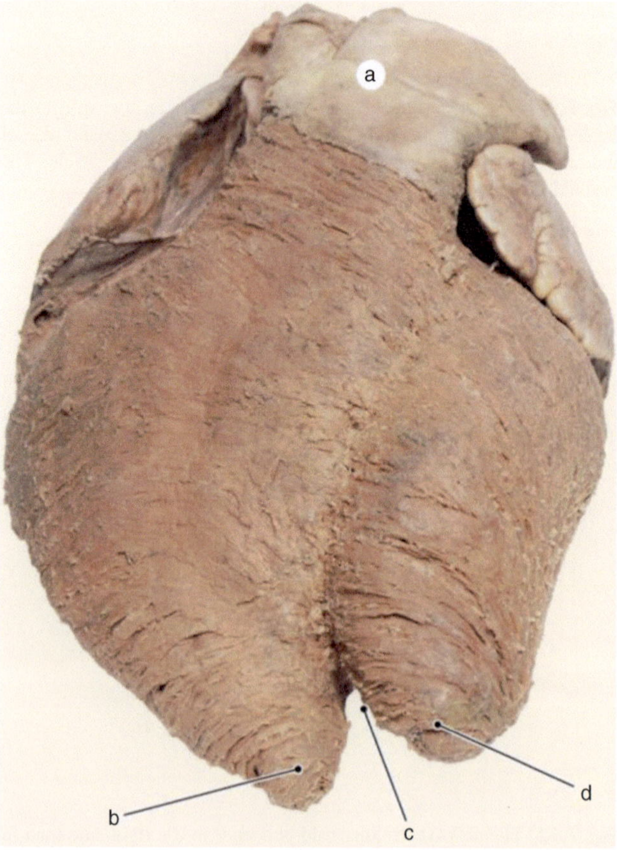

Fig. 7.53 The bifidus aspect of the heart is given by the deepening of the apex notch. The two apices are independent. *a* pulmonary trunk, *b* right ventricular apex, *c* apex notch, *d* left ventricular apex

The diameter of the aorta is maintained constant through a number of mechanisms: The three fibrous trigones (2 + 1) at the base of the aorta are well anchored through myocardial fibers which pull them divergently. The septal segment of the aortic vestibule has a reduced mobility due to the fact that at the level of its crest there is a quasi-continuity of the subendocardial fibers from both ventricles. These fibers are inserted on the tendinous center and the membranous septum and envelop as in a hammock the superior part of the septum, prohibiting the septal crest a sphincter-like dynamic. The superficial fibers of the mitral aortic orifice have a radial divergent orientation. They pull the ventricular root of the cusps, preserving the contour of the orifice. The most mobile part of the mitral aortic orifice is the mural segment which has a quasi-sphincter-like behaviour (we have shown the existence of a circular bundle of the ventricular base in Fig. 6.113). The tricuspid orifice is quite different from the mitral aortic one.

Its margins are a lot thinner at the level of the mural leaflet, where the margin is made up from a veritable marginal bundle (Fig. 7.40). This bundle consists of superficial muscular bundles contiguous with subendocardial ones. If in the left ventricle the subepicardial-subendocardial continuity is more superficial (regarding its position in the atrioventricular fold) and close to the internal margin of the mitral orifice, in the right ventricle the continuity can be found deeper in the atrioventricular fold, towards the ventricular lumen, on the internal surface of the mural segment of the tricuspid orifice (Figs. 7.40 and 7.52). The subepicardial fibers are not slanted as in the mitral aortic orifice, but almost parallel with the margin of the tricuspid orifice. These fibers take the tendinous center as a steady position, they surround the tricuspid orifice, the infundibulum and the ventricular wall and they end at the anterior interventricular sulcus. Consequently,

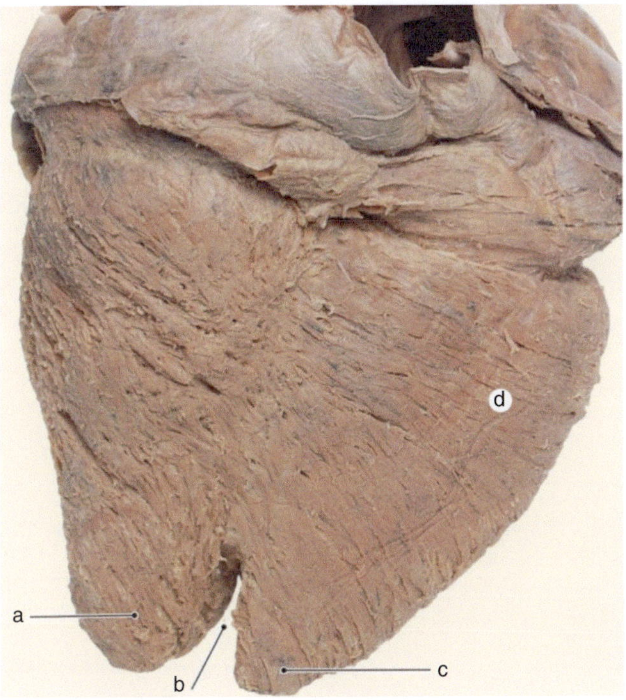

Fig. 7.54 The bifidus aspect is also present on the diaphragmatic side. *a* left ventricular apex, *b* apex notch, *c* right ventricular apex, *d* diaphragmatic side of the right ventricle

the contraction of these fibers mobilizes the free- mural segment of the tricuspid orifice and the ventricular sternocostal wall, joining them on the septal segment.

7.2.6.4 The Apex of the Heart

The classic conception regarding the apex of the heart is the following: the apex of the heart is represented by the apex of the left ventricle. Here the superficial fibers twist and penetrate the deep layer, forming the vortex cordis. From the apex towards the right, the margin of the heart separates the sternocostal surface from the diaphragmatic one. To the right of the apex on the margin of the heart there is the cardiac notch. This short presentation does not take into account the fact that there are two ventricles, with two apexes, separated in reality by an interventricular septum. The depth of the notch of the cardiac apex can be variable. The existence of hearts with extreme depths of this notch leads to the aspect of bifid cardiac apex (Figs. 7.53 and 7.54). Only after noticing such cases we understand what is obvious, namely the fact that each ventricle has its apex. This trivial detail becomes important in the context where we can ecographically measure the torsion movement of the apex of the heart (with strict reference to the apex of the left ventricle). The measurement of the torsion movement according to different parameters can be correlated with the degree of efficiency of the myocardial contraction, counting as a global indicator. In this context, the apical architecture becomes important. The left fascicles of the septomarginal trabeculations in the right

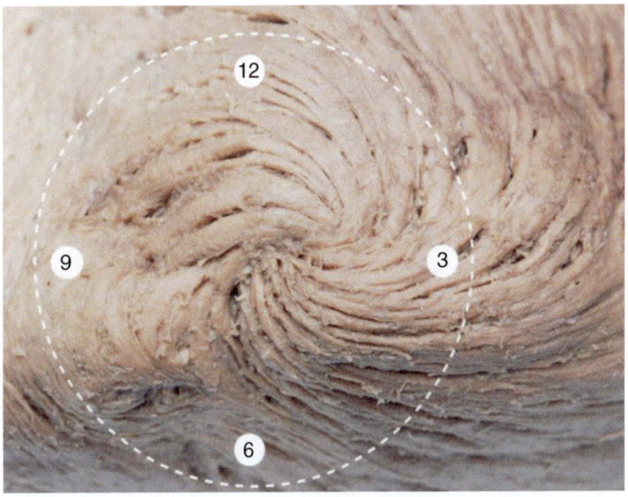

Fig. 7.55 Over the apical vortex of the left ventricle a clock frame is superposed. This way we can understand better the notion of clockwise and anticlockwise movement referring to the direction of the ventricular fibers contraction

ventricle make up a large part of the superficial fibers on the sternocostal face of the left ventricle (Fig. 7.50). These descend obliquely and have the tendency to spiral down clockwise near the ventricular apex. The totality of the muscle fibers with a spiralled arrangement from the cardiac apex is called the vortex cordis (Fig. 7.55). A quasi-complete rotation around the left ventricle is only accomplished by the fibers originating in the basal areas. These superficial fibers have their origin in the vicinity of the free (mural) part of the mitral ring. At the apex of the left ventricle, the superficial fibers form a vortex and then obviously penetrate the depth of the wall. The radius of the spiral decreases as the fibers approach the central long axis and the ventricular apex becomes narrow. At the level of this axis the perimysium of the muscle fibers merges and forms a dense, slightly protruding, quasi-nodular structure, with a diameter of around 3–4 mm. Due to the axial positioning and condensation as well as to the spiralled structure, we propose that this slight prominence should be called a modiolus (central spiralled axis) (Figs. 7.56 and 7.58). Less obvious is what happens with the subepicardial fibers after they penetrate in depth.

Thorough dissections have shown that part of the vortex fibers end at the level of the modiolus, whereas the great majority continues in the luminal trabecular network, in the mass of trabeculations (Figs. 7.57 and 7.58). Because of this myocardial architecture, the traction forces exerted by the superficial fibers are conveyed to the trabecular network and they set it in tension. The trabecular network becomes a yielding seat for the papillary muscles, their contraction becoming necessary to the support of the tendinous cords and implicitly of the cusps during the ventricular systole.

The whole ventricular wall and not only the superficial fibers (the vortex) participate in the structuring of the apex.

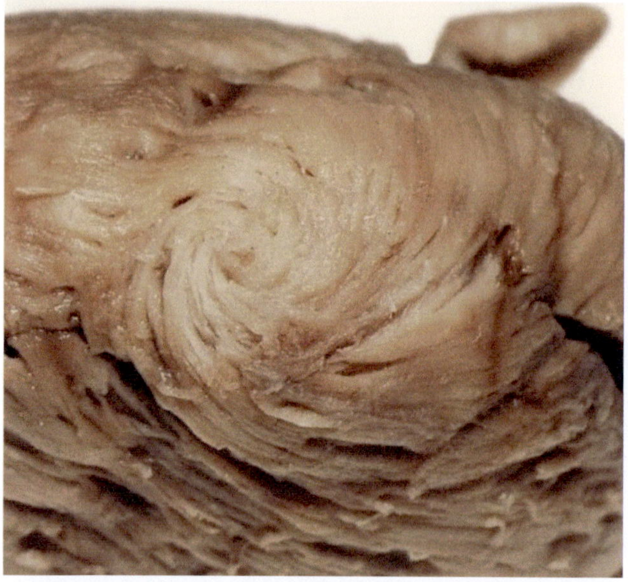

Fig. 7.56 Detailed image of the modiolus: compact muscular centre of the vortex

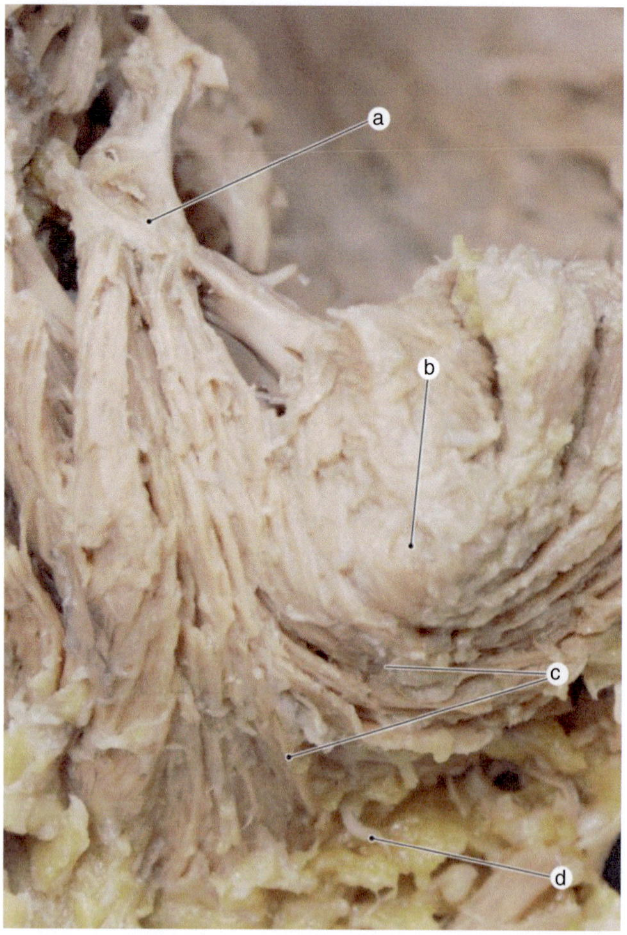

Fig. 7.57 Superficial fibers located just under the subepicardial fat, continue at the apex of the heart in the thickness of luminal trabeculae. The axis of the vortex is represented by a muscular fascicle with a modiolus aspect. *a* luminal trabeculae, *b* modiolus, *c* subepicardial fibers, *d* subepicardial fat

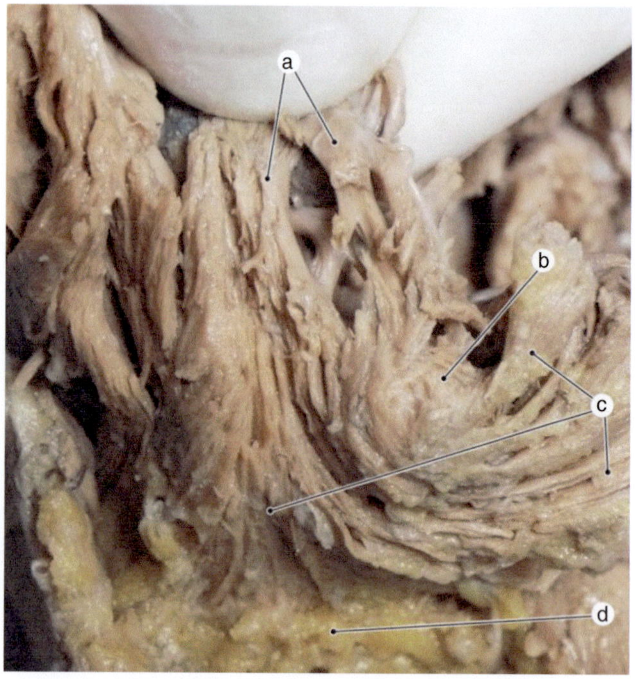

Fig. 7.58 The modiolus has a slightly umbilical aspect. *a* luminal trabeculae, *b* modiolus, *c* subepicardial fibers, *d* subepicardial fat

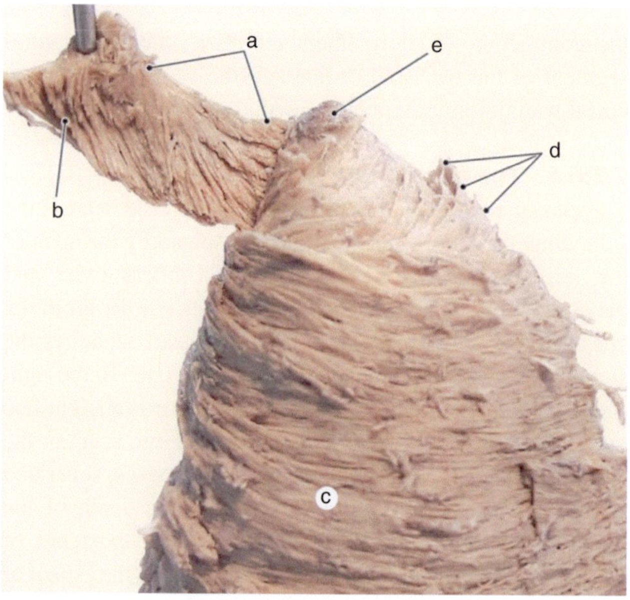

Fig. 7.59 Muscular lamellae and their fibers insert at the level of the apex on a terminal fascicle. *a* terminal fascicle, *b* narrow lamellae, *c* left ventricle – circular fibers, *d* narrow lamella, *e* modiolus

As they come close to the apex, the lamellae from the depth of the ventricular wall slant (the shutter is closed). Around the modiolus the myocardial lamellae can be joined in a terminal bundle (Fig. 7.59). We have seen that at the base of the ventricles the continuity between the superficial and the deep fibers is achieved at the level of the inferior roots of the cusps.

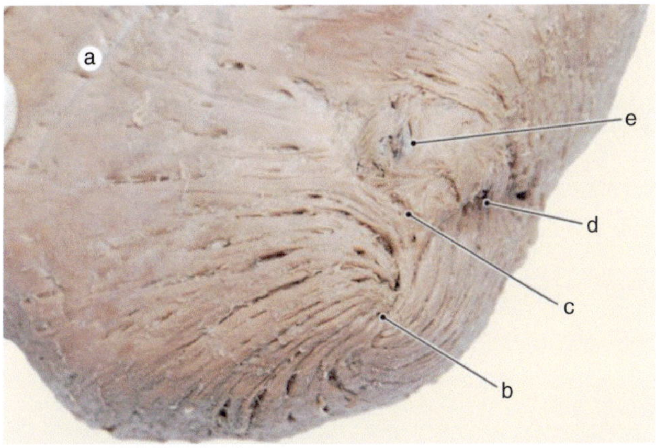

Fig. 7.60 The two ventricular apices are reunited by muscular fascicles. Notice the decompacting area of the ventricular wall at the apex of the right ventricle. As a remaining of the disorganization of the muscular fiber network, an epi-endocardial superposition occurs. *a* diaphragmatic surface of the left ventricle, *b* vortex, *c* apex of the right ventricle, *d* anterior inter-ventricular sulcus, *e* parietal decompacting

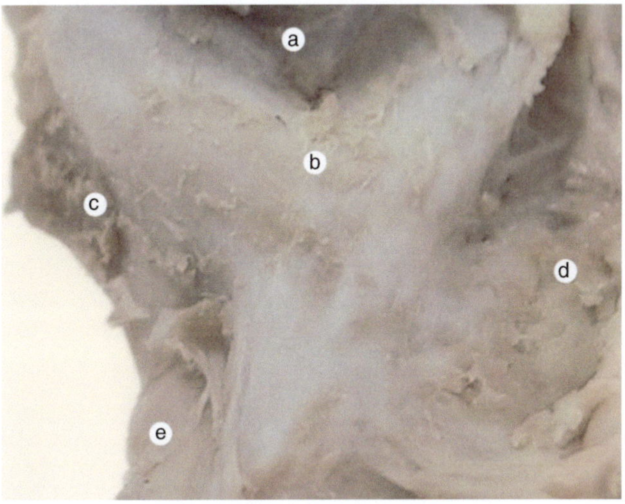

Fig. 7.61 In pigs, the tendinous center has a cartilaginous aspect and is very well defined. *a* aorta, *b* tendinous center, *c* left atrium, *d* right ventricle, *e* left ventricle

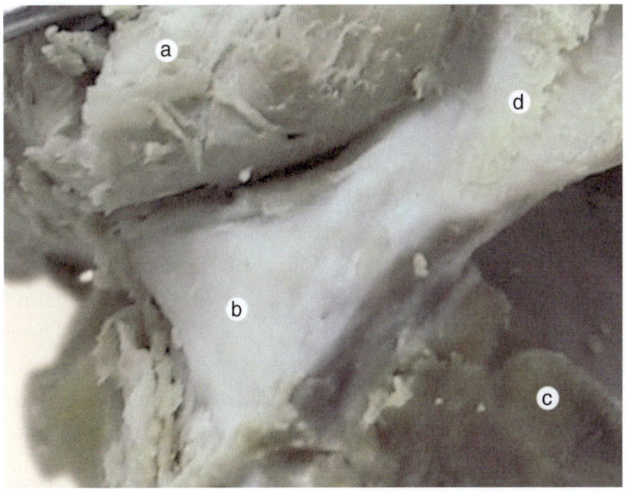

Fig. 7.62 Also the left fibrous trigone is cartilaginous in pigs. *a* aorta, *b* left trigone, *c* left ventricle, *d* continuity

At the apex of the heart the subepicardial-subendocardial continuity is clearly marked only at the center of the vortex, at the level of the modiolus. The rest of vortical subepicardial fibers penetrate without apparent delimitation, the mass of luminal trabeculations (Fig. 7.58).

The cardiac vortex is in fact a vortex of the left ventricle!

The superficial fibers that structure it do not belong only to the sternocostal surface, but also to the pulmonary and inferior diaphragmatic surfaces of the heart. These fibers originate in the inferior root of the mitral cusps (Figs. 7.40, 7.41 and 7.42) on the mural leaflet of the mitral ring. Due to this arrangement, they accomplish both the apex torsion and the retrotorsion (the backward torsion from the apex) of the mitral orifice and possibly of the mitral aortic. In conclusion, the superficial fibers are in fact the extension, in the ventricular walls, of the septal trabeculations from the right ventricle. This way the septal trabeculations of the right ventricle are of service to both ventricles! Returning to the left ventricle, these superficial fibers are in fact subepicardial-subendocardial continuities at the base of the left ventricle and the apex cordis, within the vortex. Their spiralled arrangement comprises like a glove the ventricular surface and achieves the opposite rotation movements of the ventricular base and apex. The movement begins at the apex, is anticlockwise and is known as torsion. Torsion is followed by a reverse, less pronounced rotation of the ventricular base, known as retrotorsion. The parietal trabeculations in the left ventricle have a spiralled tract in a reversed direction towards the superficial fibers. Their contraction can be a logical participant in the two rotation movements.

The described morphofunctional ensemble is also involved in: a general movement of wringing of the left ventricle and the setting in tension of the trabecular network, thus offering a yielding seat for the contraction of papillary muscles and the efficient activation of cusps during the systole. This setting in tension is associated with the shortening of the ventricle on the long axis and the coming close of the basal plane and the apex. The existence of the subepicardial-subendocardial continuities explains the participation of superficial fibers in the shortening of the long axis.

The rotation movements, after reaching maximum amplitude, are followed by recoil. As we have previously shown, this is mainly elastic and dependent on the extracellular matrix. The fact that the ventricular superficial fibers stem from the bifurcation of septal trabeculations into right and left bundles creates an interdependence of the dynamics of the two ventricles, including at the level of the apexes. The lowest septal trabeculation bifurcates. The left bundle ends

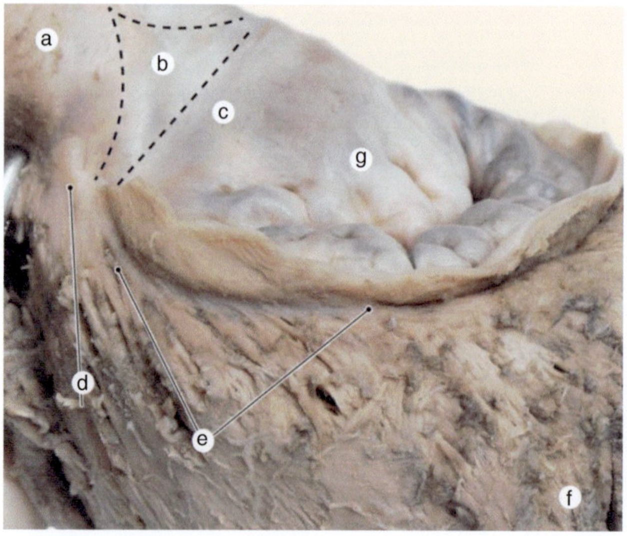

Fig. 7.63 Highlighting the left fibrous trigone and it's anatomical relations. Fila coronaria extends the mass of the trigone. *a* aorta, *b* aortic curtain, *c* continuity, *d* left trigone, *e* fila coronaria, *f* left ventricle, *g* anterior mitral cusp

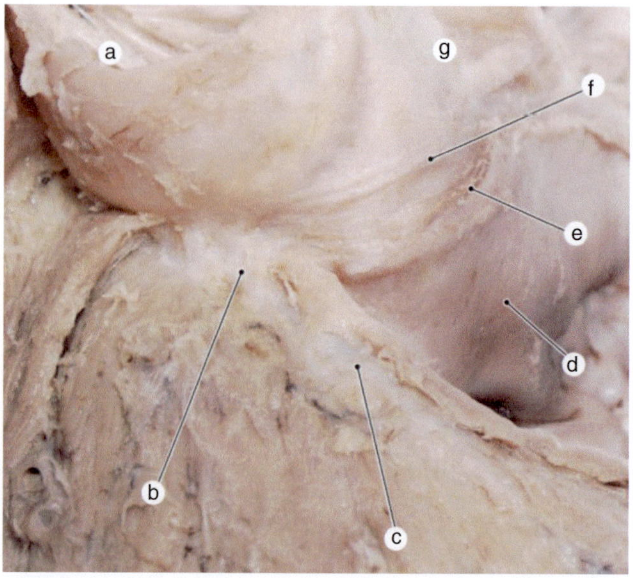

Fig. 7.64 After removing the left atrium, the mitral-aortic continuity and the fibrous condensing that defines the primary aortic ring are revealed. *a* left coronary sinus, *b* left trigone, *c* fila coronaria, *d* anterior mitral cusp, *e* mitral-aortic continuity, *f* primary aortic ring, *g* aortic curtain

in the vortex, while the right bundle frames the apex of the right ventricle and then reaches the diaphragmatic surface of the left ventricle.

Practically this bifurcation delimitates the inferior limit of the right ventricular apex. All the other right bundles of the septal trabeculations make up the wall of the right ventricle, which delimitates like a hood the inferior part (originating in the primitive ventricle) of the right ventricle cavity. These bundles end at the posterior interventricular sulcus (where they become bifurcation bundles on the right side of the posterior extremity of the septal trabeculations). The apex of the right ventricle is formed through the superposition and the interweaving of the right slanted bundles of the last septal trabeculations. This arrangement can be capable of decompaction (Fig. 7.60). From a bio-mechanical point of view, the anterior interventricular sulcus represents a vectorial boundary between the two ventricles. At its level, the traction direction of the superficial fibers of the two ventricles is divergent. If the divergence line of the traction vectors remains relatively steady, constituting a support area, the reverse contraction of the superficial fibers of the two ventricles leads to the adherence of the mobile walls to the septum. For the left ventricle, this is achieved through wringing and torsion. For the right ventricle there is no vortex structure. Here the "hood-like" orientation of the superficial fibers contained between the interventricular grooves makes possible the juxtaposition of the mobile wall and the septum (Fig. 7.43)! The anterior interventricular sulcus does not represent a certain morphological boundary between the two ventricles, especially in its inferior third. To its left, we can still find the anterior extension of the right ventricle. The certain boundary is in the place in which the left bifurcation branches of the septal trabeculations attach to the left ventricular wall. The variability of reports between the two ventricular apexes is enormous. Sometimes these can be situated almost at the same level. In most cases, however, the apex of the right ventricle is situated slightly higher than that of the left ventricle. The notch of the cardiac apex has different degrees of depth, ranging from some barely perceptible dimensions to depths that completely separate the ventricular apexes, leading to the aspect of bifid cardiac apex.

7.3 The Fibrous Skeleton of the Heart

7.3.1 General Observations on the Concept of Fibrous Skeleton

The fibrous skeleton of the heart is an ensemble of structures which have in common a great quantity of fibrous connective tissue. Representing a dense and non-contractile territory, these structures are resistant enough to offer support or insertion to varied myocardial formations. Parts of this system are defined as membranous or cartilaginous. A number of these structures can undergo sclerous and cartilaginous changes or, in extremis, calcium deposits may give them a "bony" appearance. The fibrous skeleton comprises: the atrioventricular rings, the aortic and pulmonary arterial rings, the subcommissural spaces situated below these rings, the aortic curtain, the mitral aortic continuity, the infravalvar fibrous fascicles, the interventricular and atrioventricular membranous septum, the tendon of Todaro, the tendon of the arterial horn, the left and right fibrous trigones and fila coronaria. To these we should add (in our opinion) the fibrous insertion lines of the atrial myocardium on the tendinous center and of a part of the superficial myocardium of the left ventricle on the anterior subcommissural space. The scientific treaties assign a number of roles to the fibrous skeleton. Gray's Anatomy [18] says, for example, that the fibrous skeleton:-"….ensures electric discontinuity between the atria and ventricles;- represents an insertion territory for the ventricular myocardium;- maintains the position of the heart in the interior of the pericardium;- represents a stable but deformable basis for the fixing of the cardiac valves." In our opinion, these extremely analytical statements exclude the synthetic, general view: the fibrous skeleton, apart from being some simple supporting scaffolding, is an integrating ensemble for the cardiac anatomy, which participates in the maintenance of the functional unity of the heart. It is likely that its involvement in the physiology of the heart is even greater, making a contribution to the maintaining of the general shape of the organ, the orifices and to the modulation of intramyocardial elastic forces. So that the contraction may be efficient, the forces exerted on the fibrous skeleton have to find, in the end, an extra-cardiac yielding seat. These forces are transferred from the tendinous center through the interatrial septum and aortic wall to the big mediastinal vessels that are well-fixed and offer sufficient support. Last but not least, the role of electric insulator of the fibrous skeleton structures has to be emphasized, with two special references: the atrioventricular rings prevent the passage of the electric impulse from the atria to the ventricles; the tendinous center isolates the atrioventricular node from the ventricular myocardium. In classic studies the following are not specified about the fibrous skeleton: the fact that the tendinous center is also the insertion place for some septal atrial muscle fibers. The fact that the commissures of the mitral valve are attached to both trigones. So far we have presented, by describing the orifices of the heart, many of the formations of the fibrous skeleton. We will continue with the following, in order to review all the component structures of this ensemble. The left and right fibrous trigones are masses of fibrous connective tissue that surround the root of the aorta. In other mammals- and the most suggestive example is the pig- the fibrous trigones are in fact cartilaginous, extremely well-formed and structured like trigones (Figs. 7.61 and 7.62). In man, their aspect is variable, having different degrees of structuring and outline. They can undergo sclerous, cartilaginous or quasi-osseous modifications. Sometimes the fibrous tracts which bind the base of the right coronary sinus to the crest of the interventricular septum are well-structured, thus capable of being considered the equivalent of the third trigone.

7.3.2 The Left Fibrous Trigone

The left (or anterior) fibrous trigone surrounds the base of the left coronary sinus at the exterior of the aorta. When it is well-structured it has a right anterior horn that reaches towards the aortic pulmonary symphysis, a posterior horn that penetrates the mitral aortic continuity and a left anterior horn which continues (and identifies) with the fila coronaria in the anterior part of the mitral ring (Figs. 7.63 and 7.64). The left fibrous trigone offers insertion for all types of myocardial fibers of the left ventricle in its vicinity (superficial and deep), for the base of the left coronary sinus, the mitral aortic continuity and the mitral anterior commissure (Fig. 6.124).

The position of the trigones at the base of the ventricular mass. Both trigones are component elements of the root of the aorta. They participate in the formation of the aorta vestibule wall and bind the aortic ring with the mitral aortic orifice. Using a metaphor, we can say that both trigones "float in the aortic vestibule", that is, only their base is bounded by the ventricular base. If we make a section through the mitral cusps at the level of their inferior roots, we get a projection line of the inferior root along the mitral orifice. The line begins at the left trigone, surrounds the mitral orifice, reaches the right trigone and closes at the level of the mitral aortic continuity. In contrast to the right trigone, which is situated on the internal margin of the mitral aortic orifice, the left trigone lies closer to the external margin of this orifice. Consequently, this line is more superficial towards the area of the anterior trigone and the corresponding fila coronaria. The line is less superficial towards the posterior, near the posterior commissure. In other words the cavity of the left ventricle passes beyond the superior margin of the ventricular base towards the anterior, which does not happen towards the posterior! From this orientation the different aspect of the mitral commissures emerges: The anterior commissure, with a more closed insertion angle is bound to the anterior trigone by semicircular endocardial folds. The tendinous cords do not reach this trigone (Fig. 6.124). The posterior commissure, with a more open and visible insertion angle is bound to the posterior trigone both by semicircular endocardial folds and basal tendinous cords that reach the trigone (Fig. 6.123). The left fibrous trigone mediates the subepicardial-subendocardial continuity of some muscle fibers from the left ventricle.

7.3.3 The Right Fibrous Trigone and the Atrioventricular and Interventricular Membranous Septum

The right fibrous trigone (the central fibrous body of the heart or the tendinous center) clings to the base of the non-coronary aortic sinus and the crest of the interventricular muscular septum. It is larger than the left one, better outlined, and has a surface of about 1 square cm and a thickness of about 3 mm. The height to which the trigone clings to the non-coronary sinus is variable (Fig. 7.65). The trigones are joined by the bases of the aortic sinus and the aortic ring, through connective tracts that are so well represented so that their decollating is very difficult, even impossible.

The right trigone offers insertion to:-the base of the non-coronary aortic sinus- the posterior mitral commissure- the mitral aortic continuity-the tricuspid ring- the ventricular myocardium from the central mass of the interventricular septum- some septal subendocardial muscle fibers, belonging both to the right and the left ventricle; in this way the right trigone mediates a subepicardial-subendocardial continuity.-some atrial muscle fibers, mainly belonging to the interatrial septum, to the neighbouring parts of the two atrial walls and also to the bottom of the right atrium- the tendon of Todaro. The junction between the right atrium and the right ventricle in the area of the septal commissure of the tricuspid atrioventricular cusps is a critical and difficult to distinguish area. The difficulty to discern it resides in the fact that ontogenetically this is the area where the fusion of the right endocardial cushion with the dextro-dorsal crest of the arterial trunk took place, and the structures emerging from this fusion are not clearly individualized. According to the degree of fusion, there is sometimes an atrioventricular septum, resembling a superior extension of the interventricular membranous septum, an extension that separates like a unique wall the right atrium from the vestibule of the aorta. The tricuspid ring fuses with the membranous septum and with an extension of the right fibrous trigone. Practically, in this situation the following are inserted on the subcommissural membranous septum: the atrial and ventricular myocardium from the area of atrioventricular junction; the right atrioventricular ring. The insertion of the atrial and ventricular myocardium is done following a line which delineates at the bottom the triangular outline of the right subcommissural space, and the insertion of the atrioventricular ring in front of the septal commissure is done following a line situated lower and perpendicular on the previous one. The

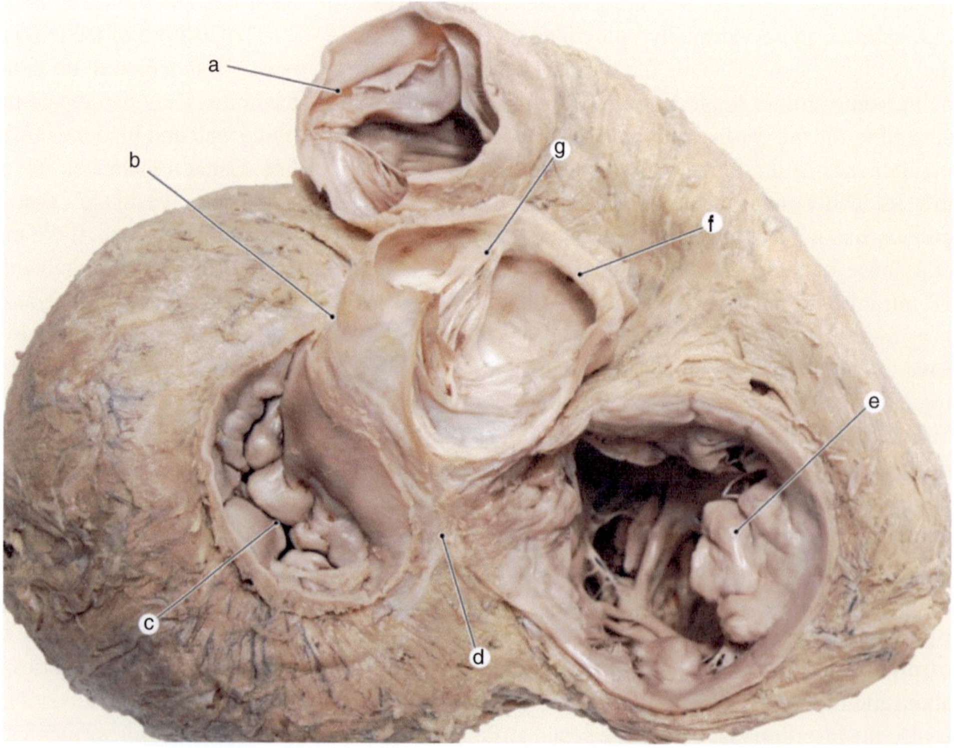

Fig. 7.65 The base of the ventricular pyramid after removing the atria. The roots of the great arteries have been kept. The non-coronary sinus was removed in order to highlight a segment of the aortic ring. The tendinous center connects the three orifices. *a* pulmonary valve, *b* left trigone, *c* mitral valve, *d* tendinous center, *e* tricuspid valve, *f* supravalvular crest, *g* aortic valve

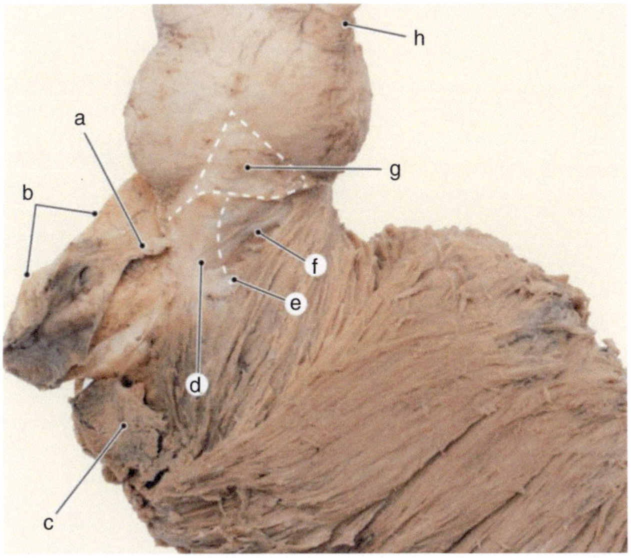

Fig. 7.66 Topography of the root of the aorta. The right atrium and ventricle were resected. The *dotted lines* delineate the regional membranous structures. Notice their continuity. *a* tendon of Todaro, *b* left atrium, *c* circular fascicle at the base of the left ventricle, *d* atrio-ventricular membranous septum, *e* the limit of the atrio-ventricular ring, *f* inter-ventricular membranous septum, *g* membranous Henle trigone, *h* right coronary artery

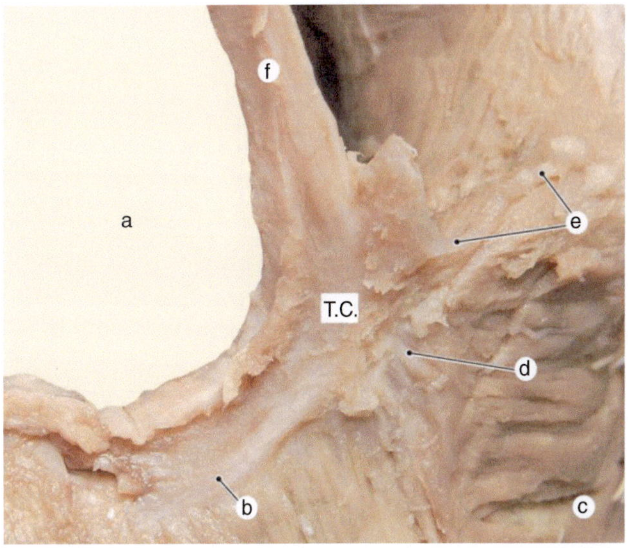

Fig. 7.67 Tendinous center (*TC*) "floating" in the vestibulum of the aorta. Posterior view. *a* left ventricle, *b* left posterior fila coronaria, *c* right ventricle, *d* fibrous insertions of the ventricular myocytes, *e* Hiss fascicle

whole plane of the tricuspid ring is perpendicular on the plane of the subcommissural trigone from the root of the aorta (Fig. 7.66). In this way, the right subcommissural space is divided into three segments:

The superior segment, with a triangular shape, is the classic (Henle) right subcommissural space (Figs. 7.117 and 7.118).

The anteroinferior segment is the interventricular membranous septum.

The posteroinferior segment is the atrioventricular membranous septum.

These two septae are inserted at the bottom on the crest of the interventricular muscular septum, strengthening the root of the aorta. They separate the two cavities from the vestibule of the aorta.

The existence and length of the inferior segments is variable. Sometimes both are lacking. Frequently, the interventricular septum is lacking. When there is no atrioventricular septum, the wall of the aortic vestibule is tied to the fusion between the tricuspid ring and the right fibrous trigone. Consequently, instead of a real atrioventricular septum represented by a single membranous wall, there is a pseudo-septum (a sandwich-like structure) resulting from the superposition of the aortic and the atrial vestibular walls. Although we have previously shown, we wish to underline the central position of the right trigone between the two valvular atrioventricular and aortic rings. The non-coronary aortic sinus together with the right trigone gives birth to a protuberance of the right atrium wall in the atrial cavity called torus aorticus (the aortic mound). When it is well-structured, the right trigone has a posterior horn that extends on the posterior third of the crest of the interventricular septum. From the apex of this horn, a fila coronaria goes and penetrates the posterior part of the mitral ring.

Sometimes the posterior horn doubles and sends a right extension that forms the fila coronaria for the posterior part of the tricuspid ring. The left anterior horn penetrates the mitral aortic continuity (we described it at the mitral ring). The left anterior horn clings to the superior limit of the membranous septum and continues with the tendon of the arterial cone (it will be described later) (Figs. 7.67 and 7.68) From the level of the tendinous center leaves another fila coronaria to the anterior part of the tricuspid ring. This fila is variable and difficult to be identified macroscopically because it lies in the myocardial mass and in general has to be dissected. When it exists, it is very long and well-structured. It can have a cartilaginous aspect (Fig. 7.69). "The atrioventricular bundle passes across the posterior trigone, goes down the posterior margin of the membranous septum and, on reaching the interventricular muscular septum, divides into its branches "(Gray's Anatomy). Our observations (concordant with a lot of data from specialized literature) show that the atrioventricular bundle perforates the right margin of the tendinous center (Fig. 7.69). We also note that in order to fulfill its function of electric insulator the surface of the tendinous center is increased by small fibrous tendons which insert the neighbouring myocardium. Near the posterior horn on right trigone, subendocardially, on the bottom of the right atrium, at the junction with the interatrial septum, one can sometimes feel a small protuberance called the tendon of Todaro. This tendon will be described separately.

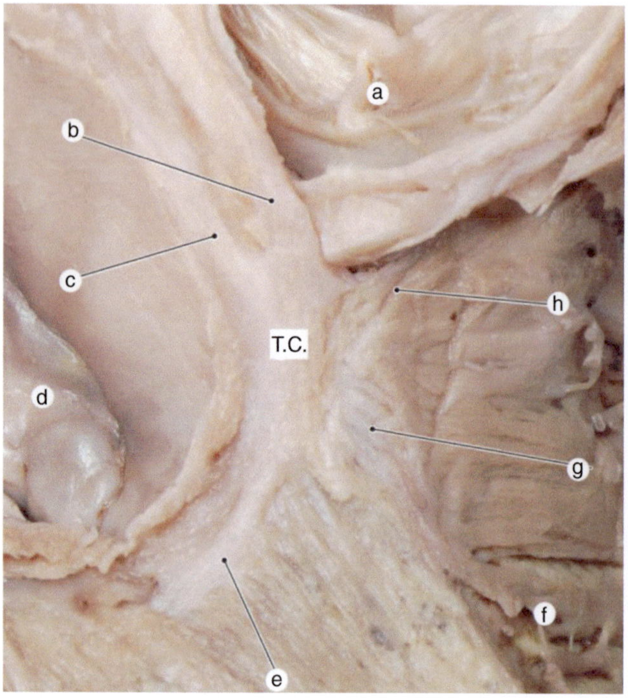

Fig. 7.68 Tendinous center (*T.C.*) posterior view. The aortic wall was removed at the level of the noncoronary sinus. Tendinous center unites the three neighbouring orifices and connects them to the crest of the muscular interventricular septum. *a* aortic noncoronarian sinus, *b* extension into the aortic ring, *c* mitral-aortic continuity, *d* anterior mitral cusp, *e* left posterior fila coronaria, *f* right ventricle, *g* fibrous insertions of the ventricular myocardiocytes, *h* right fila coronaria

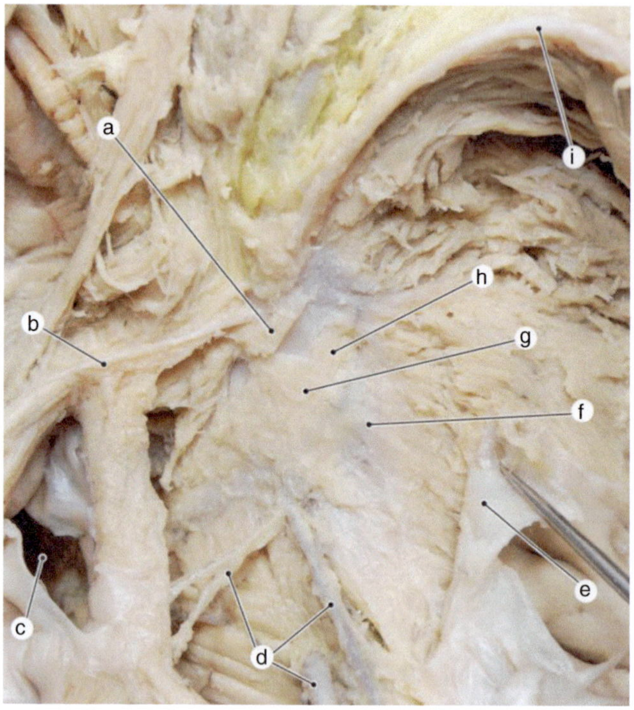

Fig. 7.69 The atrioventricular node is electrically isolated from the ventricular myocardiocytes through the surface of the tendinous center, enlarged by the fibrous insertions. Observe the posterior extensions of the node and the perforating segment of the bundle of Hiss. *a* atrial floor resected, *b* tendon of Todaro, *c* coronarian venous sinus, *d* node vessels, *e* septal cusp, *f* fibrous insertions of the ventricular myocytes that enlarge the isolation of the node, *g* atrioventricular node, *h* perforating segment of the bundle of Hiss, *i* anterior right fila coronaria

We will only note that it is inserted near the center of the posterior trigone. The basal plane of the heart is an approximate term, more physiologically than anatomically adequate, and it refers to the fact that the planes of the right and left atrioventricular orifices descend simultaneously toward the apex of the heart in systole, while the posterior walls of the atria stay fixed in the venous pedicles. In this way the intraatrial negative pressure increases and implicitly, the aspiration force of venous blood in the atria. The atrioventricular orifices seem to be functionally situated on a single plane- the basal plane- although anatomically they are not obviously co-planar. Truer to fact is the anatomical reference which considers both the mitral aortic and the tricuspid orifices as component elements of the basal plane. These orifices lie in closer planes than those of the atrioventricular orifices.

Strictly anatomically the atrioventricular orifices mark the limit between the atria and the ventricles. Their orientation is difficult to describe, because they have simultaneous orientations in different planes.

In relation to the vertical line of the frontal plane, in diastole the tricuspid orifice is slightly slanted towards the anterior, while the mitral is slanted more towards the posterior. If we extend the planes where the two orifices lie, these intersect at the bottom, forming a dihedral angle, open anterolaterally and to the left. The right trigone mediates the subepicardial-subendocardial continuity of myocardial fibers belonging to both ventricles. The two trigones are pulled in different directions by the superficial muscle fibers which are inserted at their level. Consequently, the aortic orifice remains open in the ventricular systole.

The position of the trigones at the base of the ventricular mass. Both trigones are constituents of the root of the aorta (Fig. 7.70). They participate in the delimitation of the aortic vestibule and bind the aortic ring to the mitral aortic orifice (Figs. 6.150 and 6.151). Through its central mass and its extensions, the tendinous center separates, yet at the same time unites and binds the aortic, mitral and tricuspid orifices. The trigones can be found at the base of the ventricular pyramid. In regard to the thickness of the ventricular wall, the right trigone is closer to the endocardium, while the left one is closer to the epicardium. Therefore, compared to the internal outline of the muscular wall, the outline of the mitral ring is external and moved to the anterior. The tendinous center offers support as electric insulator both to the atrioventricular node and to the Hiss fascicle which perforates it.

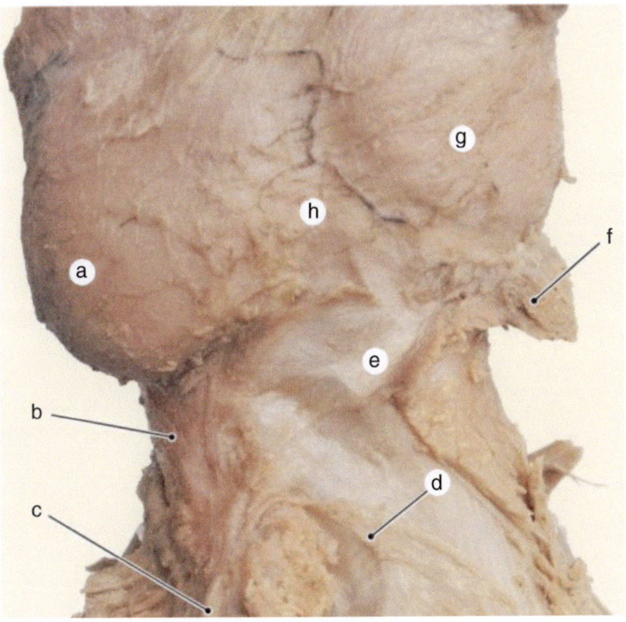

Fig. 7.70 The aortic root was extracted from the ventricular base together with the aortic vestibule endocardium. View from the right side. A fragment of the left branch of the bundle of Hiss that continues its perforating segment, situated above the muscular interventricular septum crest, can be observed subendocardial. *a* noncoronarian aortic sinus, *b* tendinous center, *c* atrioventricular node artery, *d* fragment of left branch of the bundle of Hiss under the left ventricular endocardium, *e* membranous septum, *f* right ventricle, *g* right coronary sinus, *h* trigone of Henle

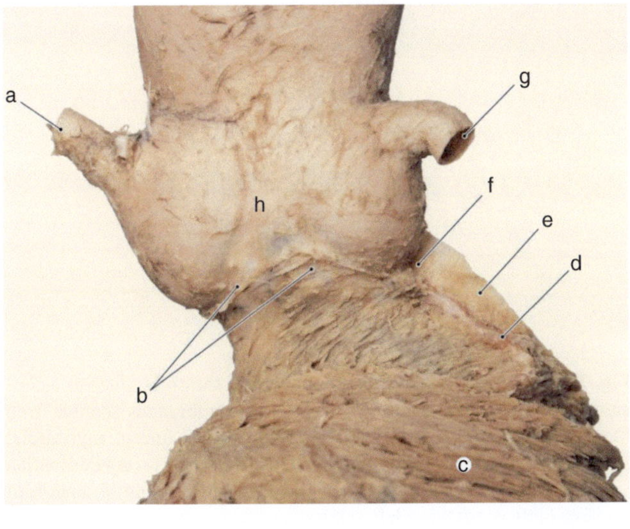

Fig. 7.71 Anterior view of the aortic root after the superficial and middle muscular fibers of the left ventricle were removed. The myocardial line of insertion follows the pulmonary cone tendon and continues with the left trigone, confirming the continuity of fiber links between the two trigones, both to the right and to the left. *a* right coronary artery, *b* line of myocardial insertion on the aortic root (the right side being the pulmonary cone tendon), *c* left ventricle, *d* fila coronaria, *e* left atrium, *f* left trigone, *h* left coronary artery, *i* Henle trigone

7.3.4 Fila coronaria

The Latin translation of fila coronaria is "circular thread". This name is very suggestive: fibrocartilaginous structures with a filiform aspect (diameter 0.5–1.5 mm) and variable length (0.5–3 cm) which surround segments of the mitral and tricuspid orifices. In the rest of the circumference of these orifices small discontinuous fragments of similar structures can be found. The presence, aspect and dimensions of the fila coronaria are extremely variable. The fila coronaria provides support for insertion to the myocardium from the ventricular base and sometimes mediates subepicardial-subendocardial continuities.

According to our experience there are two kinds of fila coronaria:

- some are superficial, easily to identify and are in fact the narrow elongated extensions of the horns of the two trigones;
- others are profound, difficult to illustrate, do not gradually become narrow, are inserted on the trigones and have a uniform cylindrical shape on their whole length. This is the case of the tricuspid anterior fila and of the mitral posterior fila. We have made an inventory of the following locations for the fila coronaria: anterior mitral, posterior mitral, posterior tricuspid (for superficial fila) (Figs. 7.63, 7.65, 7.71 and 7.72) anterior tricuspid and posterior mitral (for deep fila) (Figs. 7.73 and 7.74).

7.3.5 The Tendon of Todaro

The Tendon of Todaro is an extremely controversial structure regarding both its ontogenesis and its anatomical description. Furthermore, its very existence is sometimes contested.

We can safely state that we have identified this tendon (in various development stages) in all dissected hearts.

The most frequent aspect in which this tendon is usually found is that of a fibrous connective bundle, well organized and cylindrical in shape. Its diameter is variable (1–2 mm) and its length varies between 1 and 3 cm (Fig. 7.98).

The tendon is accompanied by subendocardial connective tissue and muscle fibers which are a continuation of the left commissure of the coronary sinus ostium. These fibers give the tendon consistency and have the same insertion area, on the right fibrous trigone.

From the point of insertion in the center of the right trigone, the tendon passes posteriorly to the dorsosinusal region, behind the coronary sinus ostium, at which point its structure loses its individuality in progressively thinner fibrous tracts. The tendon passes intramuscularly, 1–3 mm below the endocardium, on the floor of the right atrium, at the junction with

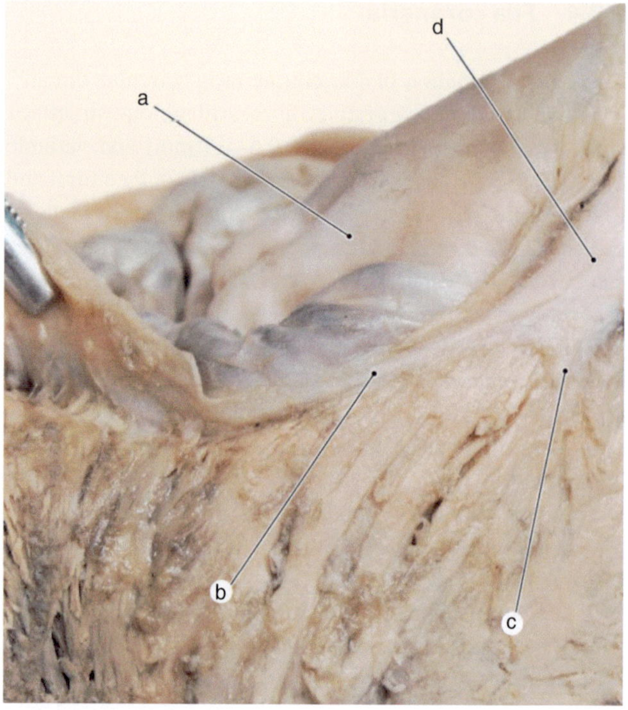

Fig. 7.72 Left posterior fila coronaria continues the tendinous center. *a* anterior mitral cusp, *b* Left posterior fila coronaria, *c* right posterior fila coronaria, *d* tendinous center

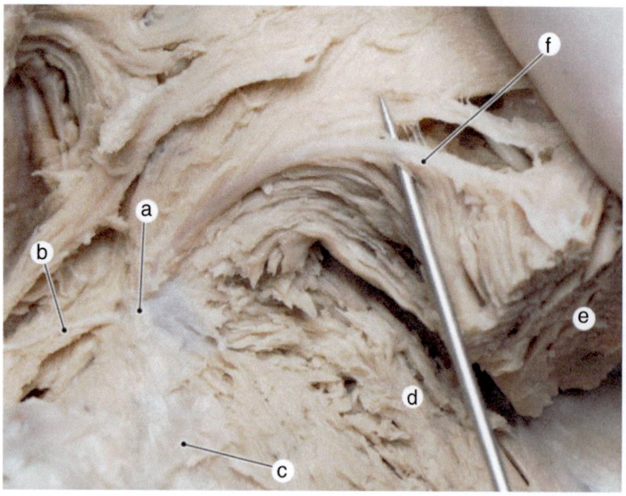

Fig. 7.73 Anterior tricuspid fila originates on the tendinous center, near the insertion of the Todaro tendon. It has an intramuscular course. *a* tendinous center, *b* tendon of Todaro, *c* root of the septal cusp, *d* right ventricle- septum, *e* right ventricle (sterno-costal wall), *f* anterior tricuspid fila coronaria

the interatrial septum. It is in this place that a small prominence on the tendon can be palpated, 3–4 mm long and 1–2 mm wide. This prominence is more noticeable if the tendon suffers a fibrocartilaginous transformation.

Sometimes the presence of the tendon is marked by a trabecula which is a continuation of the inferior horn of the limbus of fossa ovalis or a continuation of the tip of the

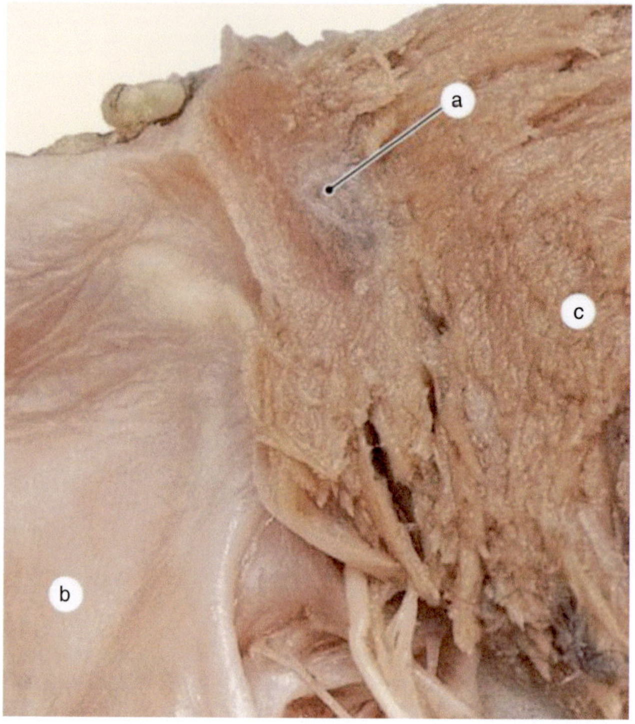

Fig. 7.74 Posterior mitral fila coronaria has a deep intramuscular course. *a* posterior mitral fila coronaria, *b* anterior mitral cusp, *c* left ventricle

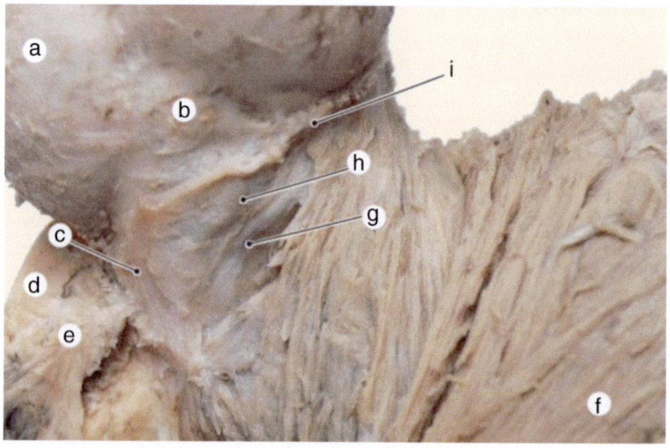

Fig. 7.75 Pulmonary cone tendon continues the right anterior extension of the tendinous center, separates the membranous septum from the Henle trigone and continues with the fibrous line of myocardial insertion, reaching the aortic-pulmonary "symphysis". *a* noncoronarian sinus, *b* Henle trigone, *c* tendinous center, *d* left atrium, *e* tendon of Todaro, *f* left ventricle, *g* left ventricular endocardium, *h* membranous septum, *i* pulmonary cone tendon

Eustachian valve, and which will take (by extension) the name of the tendon of Todaro.

Although the possibility of identifying it through inspection and palpation is variable, the tendon of Todaro is famous for its contribution to the delimitation of the Koch triangle (see right atrium).

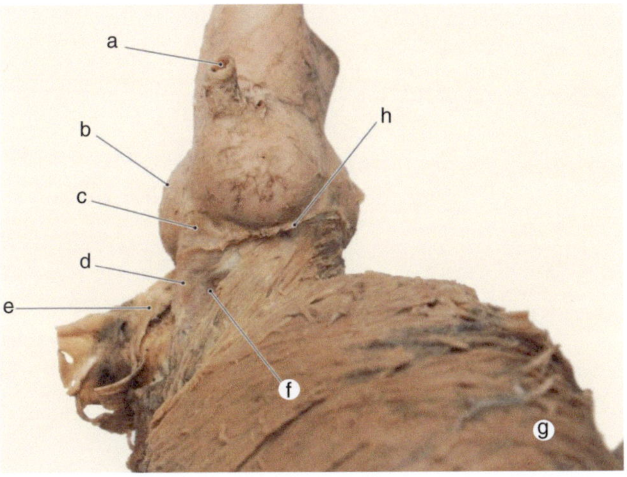

Fig. 7.76 Comparing with the previous picture, the pulmonary cone tendon is observed towards its anterior segment. Superficial and middle muscle fibers were resected. *a* right coronary artery, *b* noncoronarian sinus, *c* Henle trigone, *d* tendinous center, *e* tendon of Todaro, *f* endocardium of the left ventricle, *g* left ventricle, *h* pulmonary cone tendon

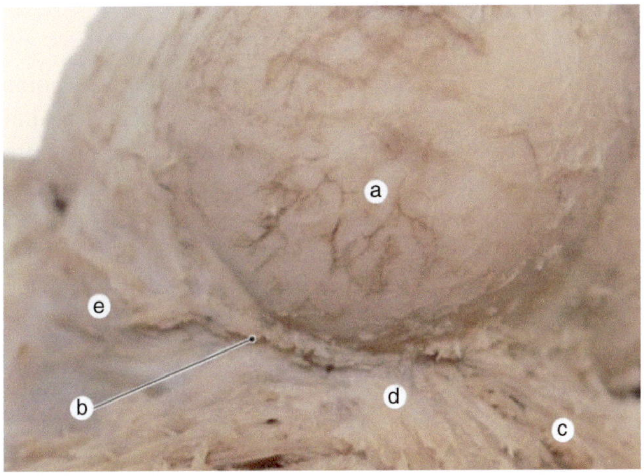

Fig. 7.77 The pulmonary cone tendon passes under the base of the right coronary sinus. *a* right coronary sinus, *b* pulmonary cone tendon, *c* left ventricle, *d* area of the third trigone, *e* superior right horn of the tendinous center

7.3.6 The Tendon of the Conus Arteriosus

The superficial myocardial fibers of the **tri-orificial isthmus** (see page 179) are inserted around the aortic root. The line of insertion is practically formed by small fascicles of fibrous connective tissue. After slicing the junction between the myocardial fibers and these fascicles we can visualize the projection of this line of insertion, which can be compared to a true tendon of the conus arteriosus.

The initial argument which probably led to the assignment of this name was the fact that the local muscular fibers apparently belong to the conus arteriosus. As we have mentioned before, in the chapter referring to the structure of the heart,

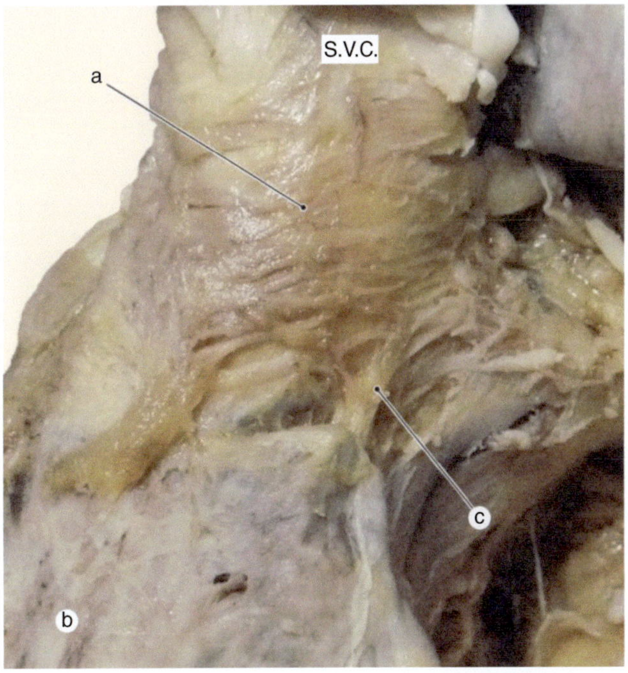

Fig. 7.78 Anterior view of the terminal segment of the superior vena cava (*SVC*). Notice the muscularization of the venous wall with pale myocardial fibres, with an embryological aspect. *a* muscularization of the superior vena cava, *b* right atrium, *c* cavoauricular notch, with a fibrous fascicle in the vecinity

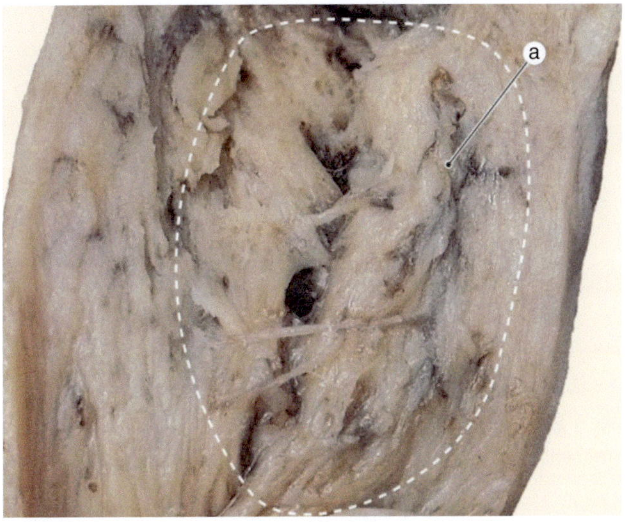

Fig. 7.79 The superior part of the terminal sulcus was resected parallel with the course of the sinoatrial node artery. The *dotted line* suggests the stretching of the compact area of the sinoatrial node. *a* sinoatrial nodal artery

these fibers seem to belong to the conus only in appearance, but in reality they belong to the **tri-orificial isthmus** – a part of the primitive ventricle.

The tendon arises from the right superior horn of the **central fibrous body**, passes over the right subcomissural membranous space and ends in the anterior

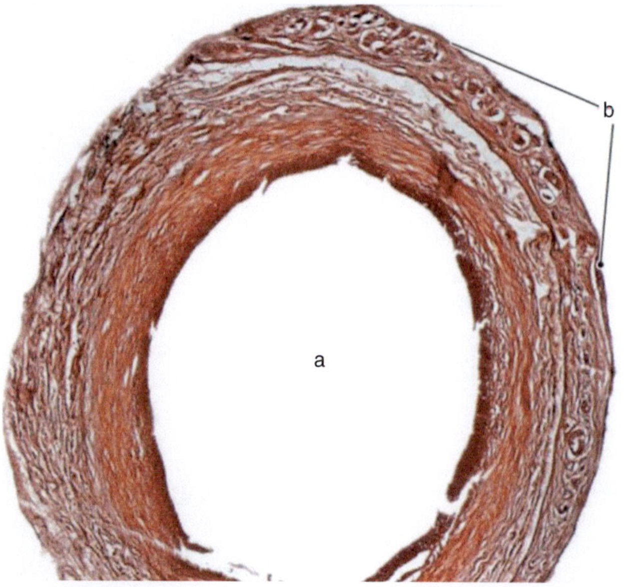

Fig. 7.80 Microscopic study of the node from the previous image, in its superior region. The obvious presence of the connective sheath (with an isolation role) suggests the existence of implicit specialized areas of pulse output from the node. *a* sinoatrial node artery, *b* sinoatrial node with connective sheath and myocytes disposed in "nests"

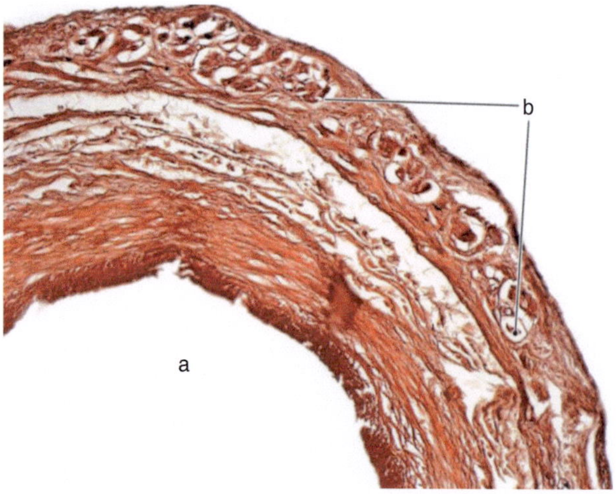

Fig. 7.81 Detail of the previous image. *a* sinoatrial node artery, *b* sinoatrial node with connective sheath and myocytes disposed in "nests"

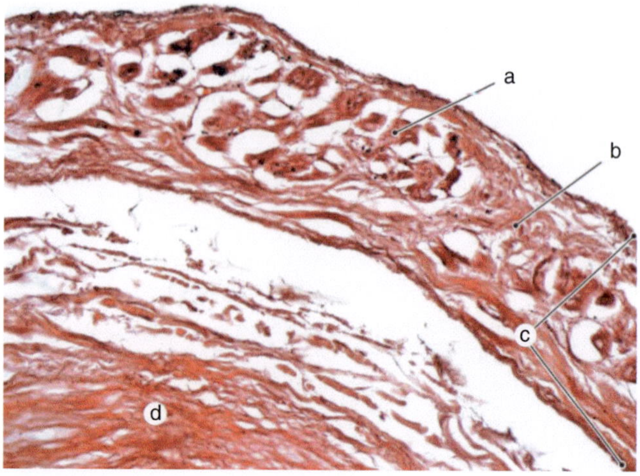

Fig. 7.82 Detail of the sinoatrial node structure. Notice the great amount of connective fibers that isolate the myocytes "nests" with irregular fibers. In an eventual inflammation of the area, the connective tissue can develop exuberant, suffocating the conduction system cells. The white spaces around the conductive myocytes appear due to post mortem retraction. *a* irregular fibers myocites, *b* connective tissue, *c* connective sheath, *d* node artery wall

subcomissural membranous space. At this point, it joins the tendon of insertion of some superficial myocardial fibers belonging to the left ventricle. The latter structure is not mentioned in specialized literature, but it could be named *the tendon of the sternocostal surface of the left ventricle* (Fig. 7.71).

In the above-mentioned disposition the tendon marks the limit up to which the right ventricle myocardium ascends along the aortic root (Figs. 7.75, 7.76, 7.77 and 7.71).

Some are of the opinion that the bundle of connective fibrous tissue that joins together the pulmonary ring and the aortic ring (Fig. 6.95) should be named the tendon of the conus arteriosus. In this case there is no longer a connection with the central fibrous body, which is usually found in classical descriptions.

We consider (as we have previously shown) that the term *aortopulmonary symphysis* is more appropriate for this fibrous structure that connects the two rings.

7.4 The Excitoconductive System

The excito-conductive system of the heart consists of modified cardiomyocytes grouped in nodes and bundles which *generate and conduct* electric stimuli to the substance of the heart.

These modified muscular cardiac cells are also called cardionector cells or *P*-type cardiomyocytes (*P* for pacemaker). From a histological point of view they are smaller compared to the cardiac contractile **myocytes** (5–10 μm), have a single nucleus and their myofibrils are arranged irregularly, which results in less visible striations.

Immunohistochemistry and electron microscopy studies demonstrate the existence of at least two types of P cells in the sinoatrial node, commonly known as "spindle-shaped" and "spider-shaped"[19].

Light microscopy samples show that the elements of the excitoconductive system are grouped in clusters and are surrounded by a fine capsule of connective tissue. The connective tissue provides electrical isolation on one hand, and on the other hand it provides „exit points" for the impulse. P cells have a paler and more abundant cytoplasm in usual staining.

In addition to the P cells, the system also contains *transition cells* (similar in structure with the cardiac myocytes but with specifically smaller dimensions and lower conduction velocity than the cardiac contractile myocytes), as well as *Purkinje fibers* (located subendocardially).

The Purkinje fibers consist of modified muscular cells with single nuclei and large diameters of approximately 30 μm. The cells have pale, abundant cytoplasm and irregularly arranged myofibrils. On light microscopy samples they are grouped in clusters and are surrounded by satellite cells. Electron microscopy studies show that Purkinje fibers lack a transverse tubular system and have small quantities of contractile material and large quantities of intermediate filaments. They also have fewer mitochondria, a reduced enzymatic activity and large quantities of glycogen [20].

The conduction velocity is greater than that of the normal cardiac myocyte. Purkinje fibers also have an anaerobic metabolic capacity, which makes them resistant to hypoxia.

Purkinje fibers have a thin *connective tissue sheath* which gives them isolation (sheath of Curran).

Transition cells are located in the periphery of the nodes (their role is not yet clearly defined) as well as in the internodal tracts.

The excitoconductive system has the following components: *the sinoatrial node, the atrioventricular node, the bundle of His with a right bundle branch and a left bundle branch. The left bundle branch usually has three divisions. Both branches continue with the Purkinje network consisting of fibers that connect with the contractile myocytes.*

However, we should mention that although microscopy samples demonstrate the presence of extrinsic innervation in the proximity of the sinoatrial node, there is no proof of direct connections between the autonomic nervous fibers and the P cells. Furthermore, there have been no descriptions of neuromuscular junctions between the extrinsic innervation and the cardiomyocytes. The unmyelinated nerve fibers that belong to both the sympathetic and parasympathetic systems terminate in the proximity of cardiac myocytes (*Gray's anatomy*, 37th ed., page 558). See Fig. 7.7, where we have shown nerve fibers in the proximity of myocytes.

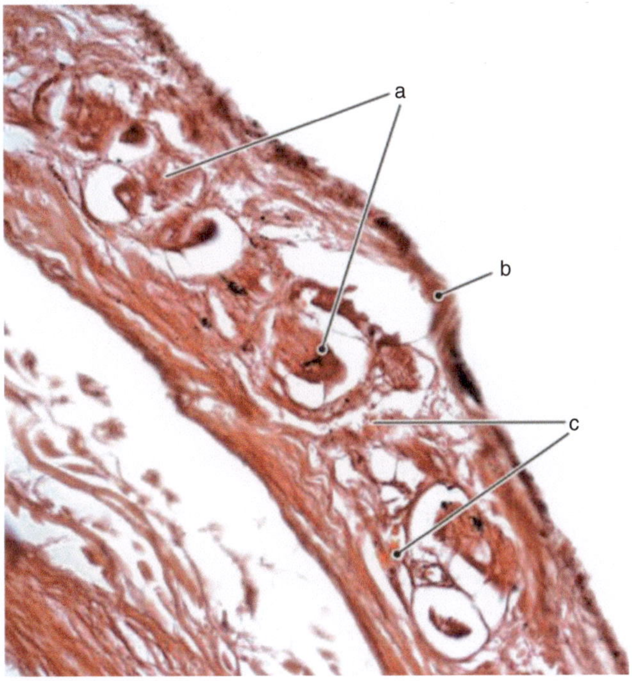

Fig. 7.83 Detail of the sinoatrial node structure highlighting some capillaries. *a* conductive myocytes, *b* connective capsule, *c* capillaries

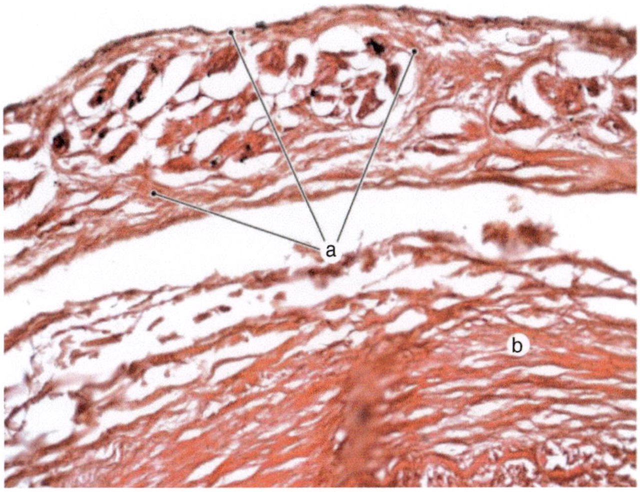

Fig. 7.84 "Nest" disposition of the conduction system cells. *a* conductive myocytes "nest", *b* artery

7.4.1 The Sinoatrial Node (Keith-Flack)

The sinoatrial node is considered to be the main cardiac pacemaker responsible for the existence of the sinus rhythm. It is located beneath the epicardium. Its subepicardial position exposes the node to various pathologies (for instance, it can be affected by pericarditis). The node is situated in front of the superior vena cava opening, at the border between the smooth part and the muscular part of the right atrium. This separation line is known as *the cavo-auricular notch* (Figs. 4.37, 7.10 and 7.11). A small atrial superior extension usually [19] covers this notch. The notch becomes visible after the epicardium is removed and the atrial extension is detached from the vena cava.

Sometimes the terminal part of the superior vena cava may consist of muscular tissue with a thickness of 1–2 cm, thereby modifying the local electrophysiology (Fig. 7.78).

The node comprises P cells and transition (intermediate) cells. *It contains an important connective tissue matrix which isolates the P cells into clusters.* Its shape varies and it has a longitudinal extension along the long axis of crista terminalis. The shape of the nodule is described in various ways in specialized literature (longitudinal, ovoid, irregular, horseshoe-shaped or bag-shaped). It is 1–2–3 cm long and 2–3 cm thick. A detailed description (Quintana) [21] describes the node as crescent-shaped and quantifying an average of ten *multidirectional extensions* into the contractile myocardium and into the intercaval region. These extensions are 1–3 mm long. The node is situated in the thickness of the hearts wall, 1–3 mm beneath the endocardium and 1–2 mm beneath the epicardium.

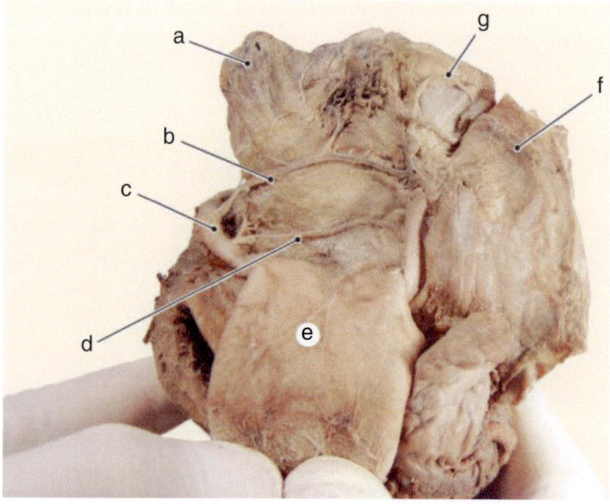

Fig. 7.85 Branches for both of the nodes originate from the right coronary artery. Anterior view of the interatrial notch with a reversed aorta. The proper artery of the sinoatrial node originates from the main trunk and courses on the right side of the superior vena cava. *a* right auricle, *b* sinoatrial node artery, *c* right coronary artery, *d* artery of the atrioventricular node, *e* aorta, *f* superior right pulmonary vein, *g* superior vena cava

The same author describes the node as being composed of a head (located superiorly), a middle part and a tail. This description must not be taken literally because the shape of the node is very irregular and extremely variable. The description (in our opinion) is rather a division into regions for didactic purposes.

The node is generally described as being unencapsulated. However, in our studies the central periarterial portion seems visibly delimited by a connective tissue capsule. (This thin capsule is mentioned in the Quintana and Anderson study, but it is paradoxically overlooked afterwards) (Figs. 7.79, 7.80, 7.81, 7.82, 7.83 and 7.84).

The node can be identified by following the point of termination of the sinoatrial node artery or, better said, the point where the artery becomes an intramural subepicardial artery. We should mention, though, that both macroscopic and histological identifications of the node are difficult.

It was not by chance that the node was the last element of the excitoconductive system to be identified. It was initially discovered by Keith and Flack [22] in *the mole. Afterwards the research was extrapolated to humans.*

7.4.1.1 The Sinoatrial Node Blood Supply

The artery of the node can be single or multiple and it usually arises from the first two centimeters of the right coronary artery or of the circumflex artery of the heart. It is classically considered that the sinoatrial node artery crosses or termi-

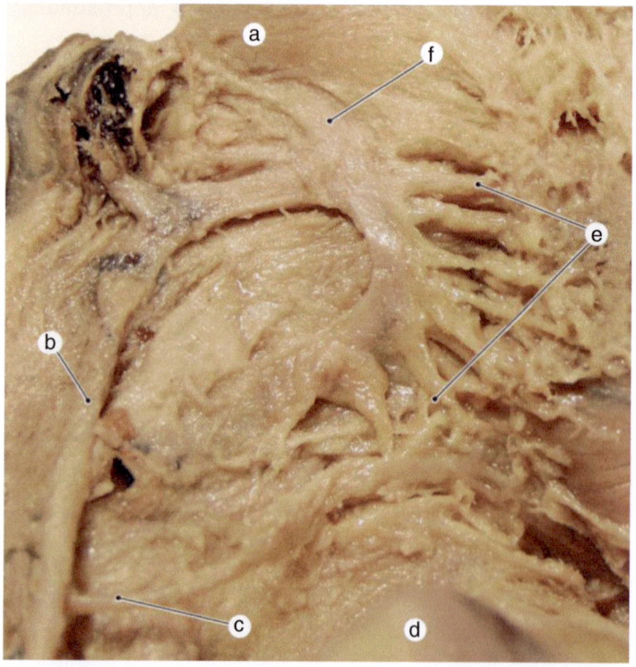

Fig. 7.86 Anterior surface of the right atrium. From the main trunk of the sinoatrial node artery emerges a "dedicated" nodal artery. The rest of the artery supplies the Bachmann fascicle. *a* superior vena cava, *b* sinoatrial nodal artery, *c* atrioventricular nodal artery, *d* aorta, *e* branches for the Bachmann fascicle, *f* nodal "dedicated" branch

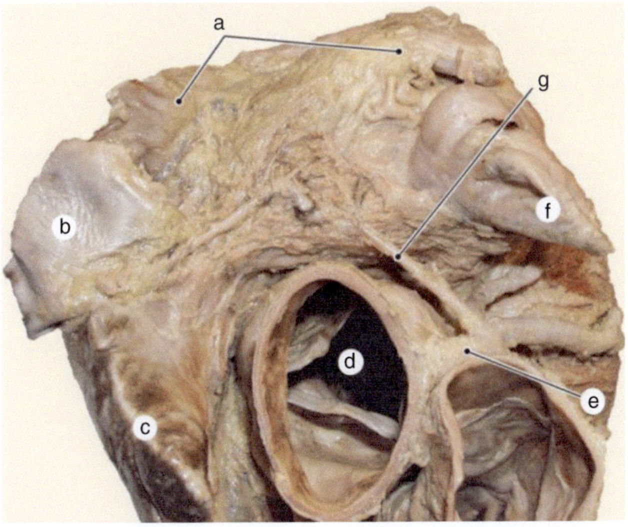

Fig. 7.87 Sinoatrial nodal artery originating from the left coronary artery. The artery courses on the anterior surface of the atria, supplies the Bachmann fascicle and ends right to the superior vena cava. *a* pulmonary veins, *b* superior vena cava, *c* right auricle, *d* aorta, *e* left coronary artery, *f* left auricle, *g* sinoatrial nodal artery

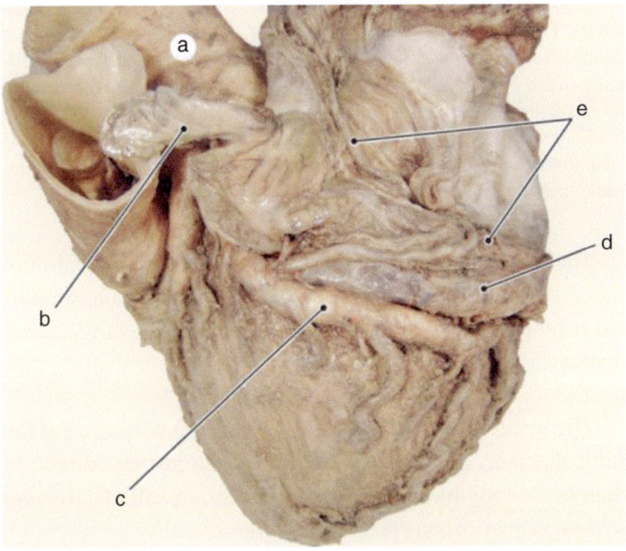

Fig. 7.88 Sinoatrial nodal artery originating from the circumflex artery with an posterior to the right auricle course. *a* aorta, *b* left auricle, *c* circumflex artery, *d* coronary sinus, *e* sinoatrial nodal artery

nates in the node. In our dissections we have observed that the artery frequently forms a loop in the proximity of the node which gives off small branches that supply the entire node surface. One of these branches is more important because it crosses the very core of the node. This is the *proper sinoatrial node artery.*

Arteries Presentation

We have found the following *variants of the sinoatrial node artery* (Figs. 7.85, 7.86, 7.87, 7.88, 7.89, 4.13, 7.10, 7.17 and 7.18):

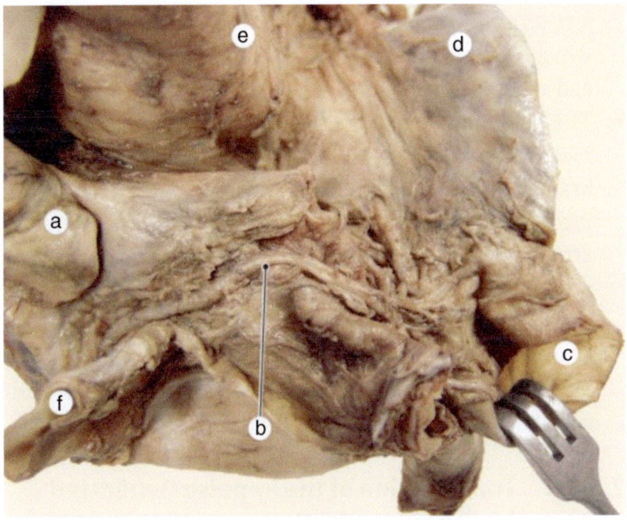

Fig. 7.89 The distal part of the artery from the previous image. Posterior view. *a* left auricle, *b* continuity of the sinoatrial nodal artery, *c* superior vena cava, *d* right auricle, *e* aorta, *f* left pulmonary veins

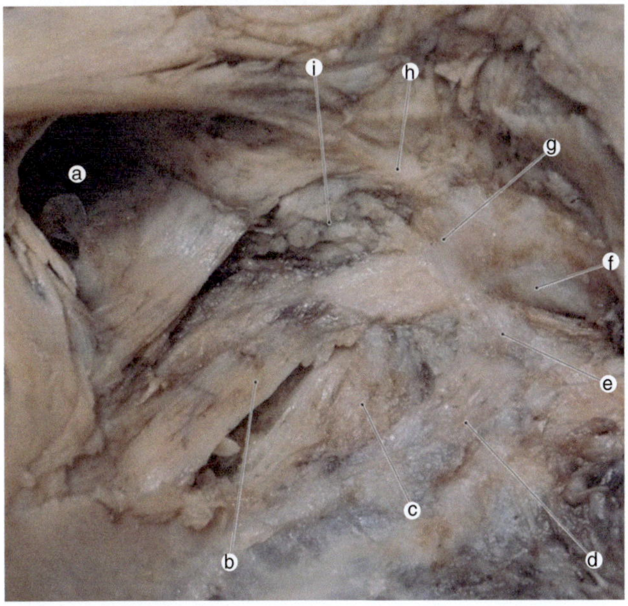

Fig. 7.90 Highlighting the subendocardial part of the atrioventricular node. A fascicle from the atrial floor (a very thin structure) that ends at the level of the atrioventricular node was kept. On both sides of this fascicle the atrial floor was resected in order to demonstrate the adipose tissue in the pyramidal space and its base (base of the right ventricle). *a* ostium of the coronary sinus, *b* atrial floor muscle fibers that end at the subendocardial part of the atrioventricular node, *c* muscle fibers from the right ventricle base, *d* septal cusp insertion, *e* extension of the septal cusp insertion, *f* atrioventricular septum, *g* tendinous center, *h* tendon of Todaro, *i* adipose septal tissue that continues into the pyramidal space

- A single sinoatrial node artery that arises from the proximal part of the right coronary artery; it then ascends subepicardially to the cavo-atrial notch, at which point it forms a loop and penetrates superficially the interatrial Bachmann bundle along which it will course toward the left atrium. The loop gives off the proper node artery which descends in the thickness of the crista terminalis and crosses the nodular area.

- The proximal part of the right coronary artery gives off two arteries which sometimes anastomose. The superior branch gives off a branch for the node and then forms a loop downward and anastomoses with the inferior artery. The inferior artery penetrates the interatrial septum and terminates in the proximity of the atrioventricular node.
- The sinoatrial node artery arises from the proximal part of the circumflex artery and passes before or behind the left auricle, and then heads toward the nodular area.

7.4.1.2 Transmission of the Impulse Generated by the Sinoatrial Node

The electric impulse generated by the sinoatrial node must activate the atrial myocytes and reach the atrioventricular node.

There are no specialized pathways for internodal or interatrial conduction (*Gray's Anatomy,* 39th ed., page 1012). The internodal pathways presented in this chapter as „the internodal conduction system" *were described rather physiologically (preferential pathways) than morphologically.*

The electric impulse generated by the main pacemaker of the heart reaches the atrioventricular node step by step, *through the atrial myocytes which it depolarizes, thus generating the atrial contraction.*

There is a time lapse between the onset of the electric impulse in the sinoatrial node and the moment it reaches and stimulates the ventricular myocytes. This time lapse explains why the atrial and ventricular contractions do not take place simultaneously but consecutively (this lapse results from the time necessary for the atrial depolarization and the time necessary for the atrioventricular activation and transmission).

The ultrastructure of the myocardium provides the reason for this delay: the conduction of the electric impulse through the myocardium is anisotropic (the myocardial conductivity varies in different directions – a higher conduction velocity in the direction parallel to the fibers and a lower velocity in the direction perpendicular to the fibers). The myocardial resistance (resistivity) is lower in the longitudinal direction than in the transverse direction.

Normally, the conduction velocity in the direction parallel to the long axis of the myocyte is approximately three times higher than the one in the transverse direction. A myocyte has approximately 11 gap junctions. Taking into consideration the spatial arrangement of these junctions, the wavefront will propagate longitudinally as well as transversely. The resistivity of the gap junction, though a few times lower than that of other types of membrane junctions, is a few times higher than the intracellular cytoplasmic resistivity [23].

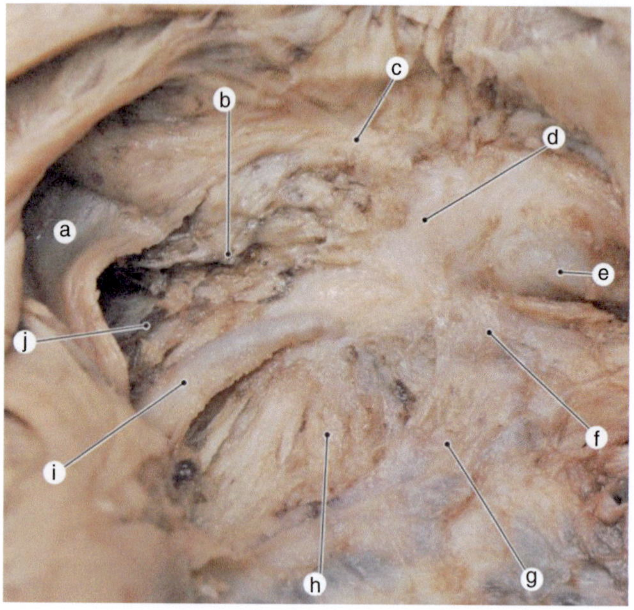

Fig. 7.91 Same heart from the previous image. The atrial floor has been resected completely. The muscle fibers of the right ventricle base are forming the base of the pyramidal space. At the apex of this space lies the deep part of the atrioventricular node, which receives the nodal artery. The insertion of the septal cusp of the tricuspid valve sends a connective extension that covers and isolates the pre-perforated segment of the Hiss bundle. *a* ostium of the coronary sinus, *b* adipose septal tissue that continues in the pyramidal space, *c* tendon of Todaro, *d* tendinous center, *e* atrioventricular septum, *f* extension of the septal cusp insertion, *g* septal cusp insertion, *h* muscle fibers of the right ventricle base, *i* atrioventricular nodal artery, *j* pyramidal space

The percentage of myocytes in the ventricular myocardium that are joined „head-to-head", thus resulting in a longitudinal arrangement, is larger than the percentage in the atrial myocardium, where head-to-head junctions are scarcer, thus resulting in a transverse arrangement.

The result is that the activating wavefront will meet, at the same distance, more gap junctions in the transverse direction than in the longitudinal direction, and as a result, *conduction will be slower transversely than longitudinally.*

Taking into consideration the fact that *the activating wavefront is more extensive transversely*, this explains the delay of the excitatory wave in the atrial area.

Although both the atrial and the ventricular myocardium have anisotropic conduction, the ventricular myocardium has a smoother depolarization wave (uniform anisotropism), whereas in the atrial myocardium the depolarization wave is segmented into smaller multiphase fragments due to the asynchronous activation of the myocytes in the transverse direction (varying anisotropism) [24].

The data suggest that there is a complex relation between electric conductivity and myocardial architecture.

Taking into consideration the lower conductivity of the fascial structures, it must be inferred that *the disposition of*

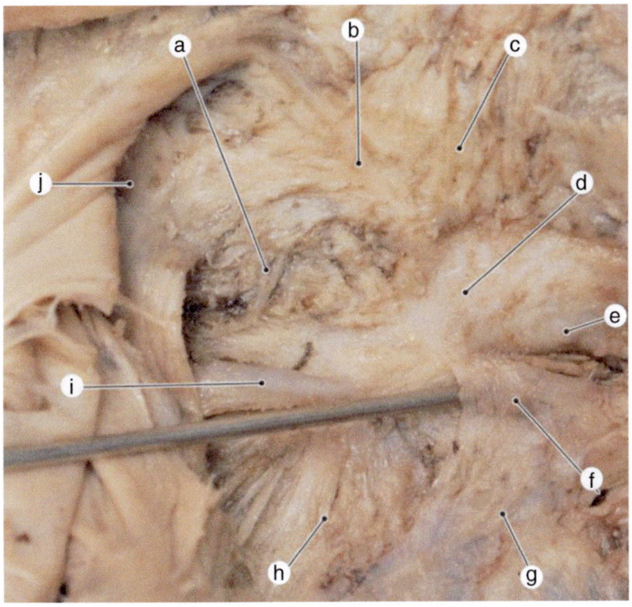

Fig. 7.92 Dissection continues. Needle elevates and individualizes the connective extension of the septal cusp insertion. *a* adipose septal tissue continues in the pyramidal space, *b* tendon of Todaro, *c* muscular fibers coming from Bachmann fascicule towards the atrioventricular node, *d* tendinous center, *e* atrioventricular septum, *f* extension of the septal cusp insertion, *g* insertion of the septal cusp, *h* muscle fibers of the right ventricle base, *i* atrioventricular nodal artery, *j* ostium of the coronary sinus

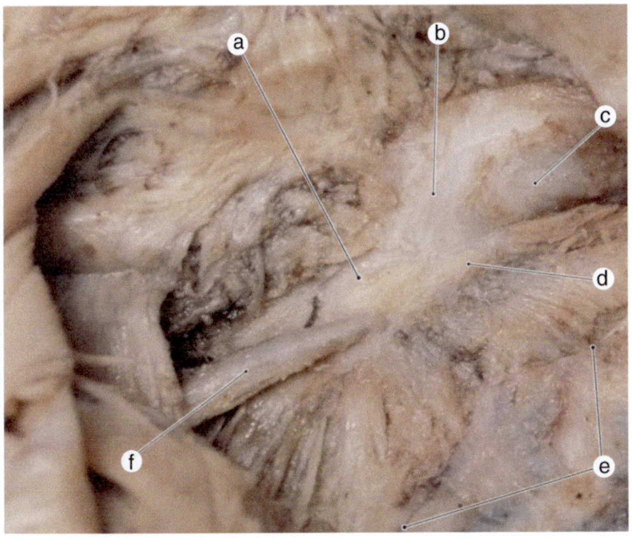

Fig. 7.93 The connective extension was resected. Preperforating part of the Hiss bundle becomes visible. *a* the compact, deep part of the atrioventricular node, *b* tendinous center, *c* atrioventricular membranous septum, *d* preperforating part of the Hiss bundle, *e* septal cusp insertion, *f* nodal artery

the perimysium can also influence the propagation direction and velocity of the excitatory wave.

As we have already mentioned, there is great architectural variability, especially with regard to the internal configuration of

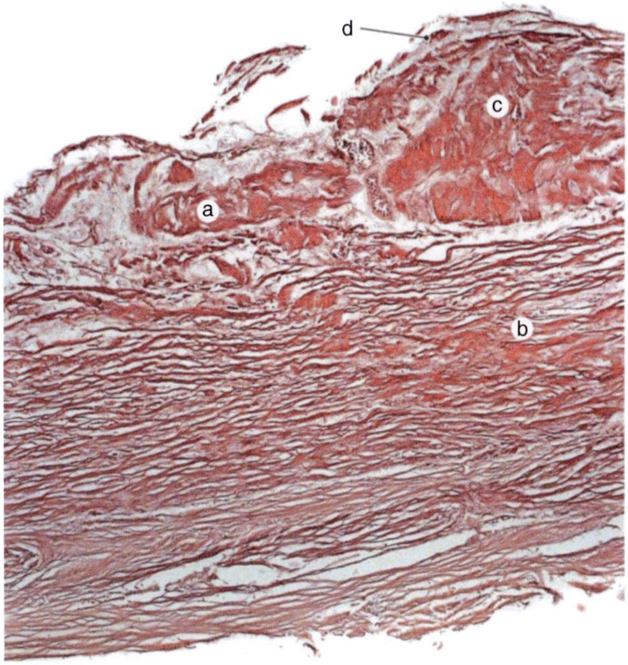

Fig. 7.94 Optical microscopic image of the atrioventricular node presented in Fig. 7.69. Note the connective capsule. Its isolation role has already been suggested. In the same way notice the presence of the connective intranodal tissue. *a* posterior extension, *b* ventricular musculature, *c* atrioventricular node, *d* capsule

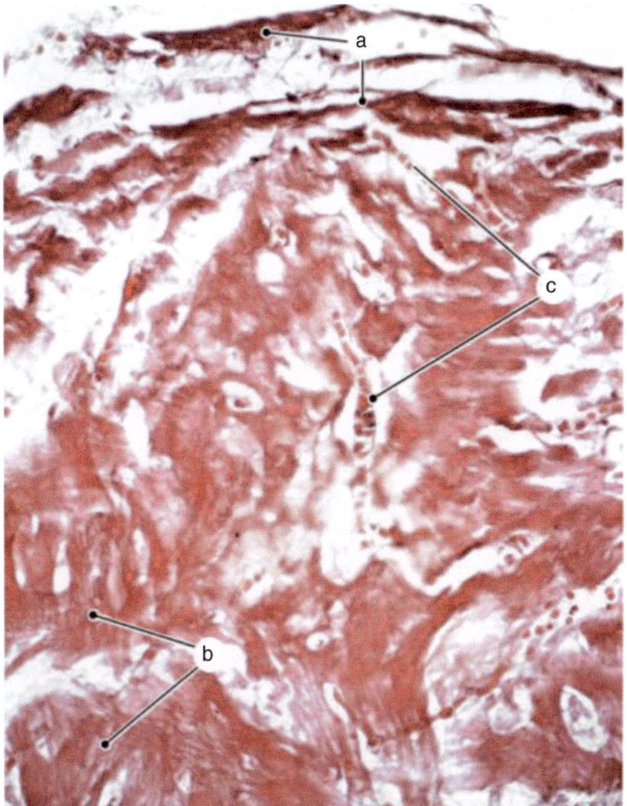

Fig. 7.95 Detail of the atrioventricular node. *a* connective capsule, *b* myocytes with irregular myofibrils, *c* capillaries

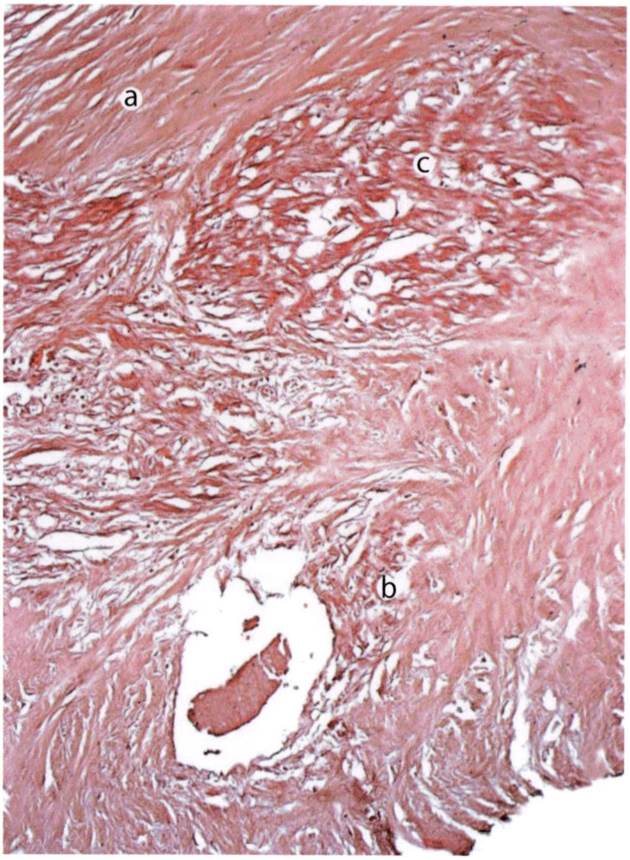

Fig. 7.96 Microscopic image of the perforating segment of the Hiss bundle. Notice the electric isolation done by the connective part of the tendinous center. A small group of conducting fibers follows the course of the atrioventricular nodal artery in its perforating course towards the interventricular septum. These fibers can be incriminated in the reentry atrioventricular node pathology. *a* fibrous connective tissue of the tendinous center, *b* perforating conducting fibers following the course of the atrioventricular nodal artery, *c* perforating part of the Hiss bundle

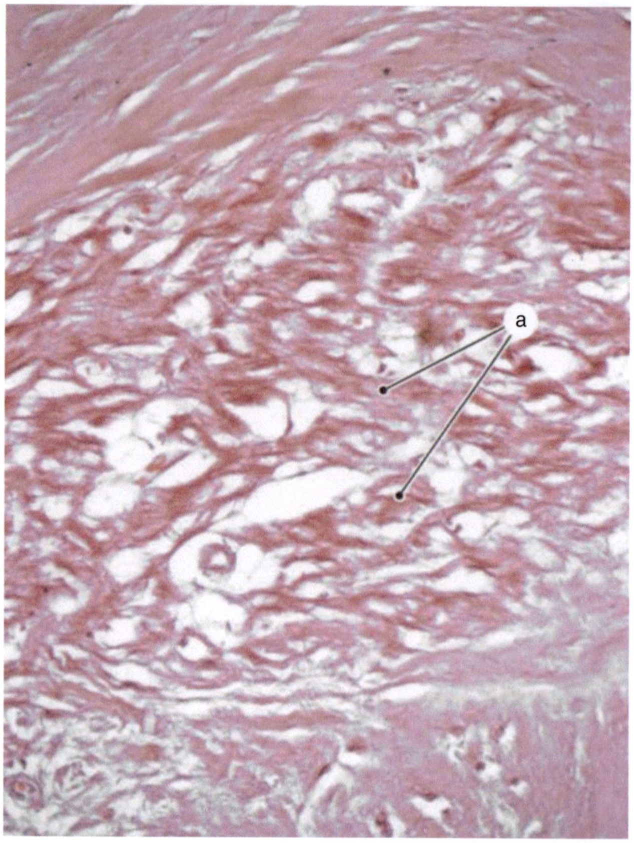

Fig. 7.97 Microscopic detail of the perforation segment of the Hiss bundle. *a* Myocytes with irregular myofibrils

the cavities. *This variability is enhanced by the microstructural transformations that take place with age* [25].

This architectural variability can influence myocardial conductivity. Areas with complex ontogenesis (the dorsosinusal space, the interatrial septum, the ligament of Marshall, the venous ostia and the periostial areas) can have varying conductivity patterns which can become pathological under certain circumstances.

The passive anisotropic electrophysiological characteristics of the myocardium – which is determined by the arrangement of the myocytes, their complex form, the spatial distribution of the intercellular junctions, and the composition of the extracellular space – play an important role in the re-entry mechanisms of atrial and ventricular arrhythmias [24].

7.4.1.3 The Atrial Conduction System

The impulse generated by the sinoatrial node reaches the atrioventricular node much faster than if it would have travelled diffusely through the entire substance of the myocardium [26]. In other words, the stimulus generated by the sinoatrial node evolves in two directions: on one hand it depolarizes the atrial myocardium, thus generating the contractions of the atria, and on the other hand it travels faster towards the atrioventricular node. There have been attempts to explain this phenomenon by demonstrating the existence of specific internodal pathways containing a mixture of Purkinje cells and cardiac myocytes.

These pathways would form the *atrial conduction system.* The system comprises *interatrial and internodal pathways.* These are represented by the Bachmann interatrial bundle, the inferior interatrial bundles and the anterior, middle and posterior internodal bundles.

!While interatrial bundles have a clear anatomic muscular substrate, the internodal bundles are more likely preferential pathways followed by the excitatory wavefront (through the myocardium), which is structurally determined to avoid or to go through elements of atrial anatomic architecture.

Interatrial Conduction Pathways

The Bachmann bundle is usually described as being a thin bundle of muscular fascicles which joins together the two atria anteriorly and superiorly (*the anterosuperior bundle*),

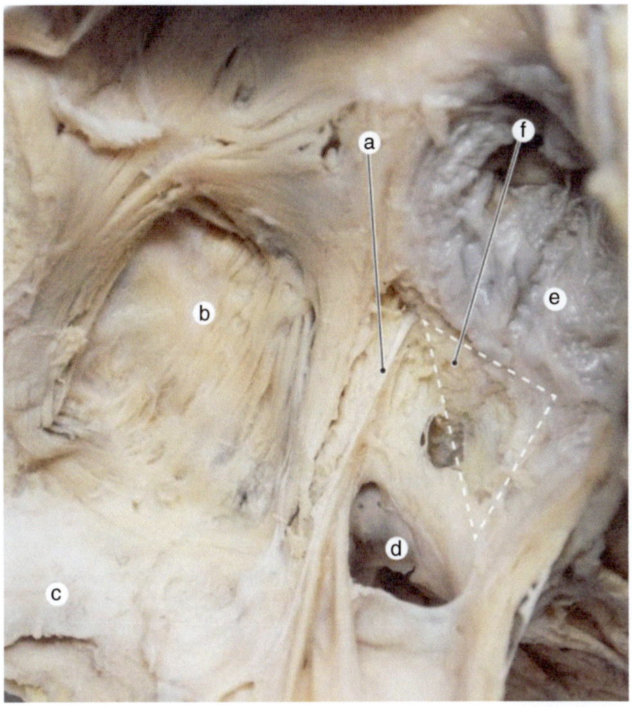

Fig. 7.98 Right atrium. View from the right side of the fossa ovalis and the atrial floor. Koch trigone is marked with a *dotted line*. Between the sinus ostium and the septal cusp, the atrium floor was dissected in order to demonstrate the pyramidal space. Tendon of Todaro is highlighted throughout its entire route. *a* tendon of Todaro, *b* fossa ovalis, *c* inferior vena cava, *d* sinus ostium, *e* septal cusp, *f* atrioventricular node at the apex of the Koch trigone

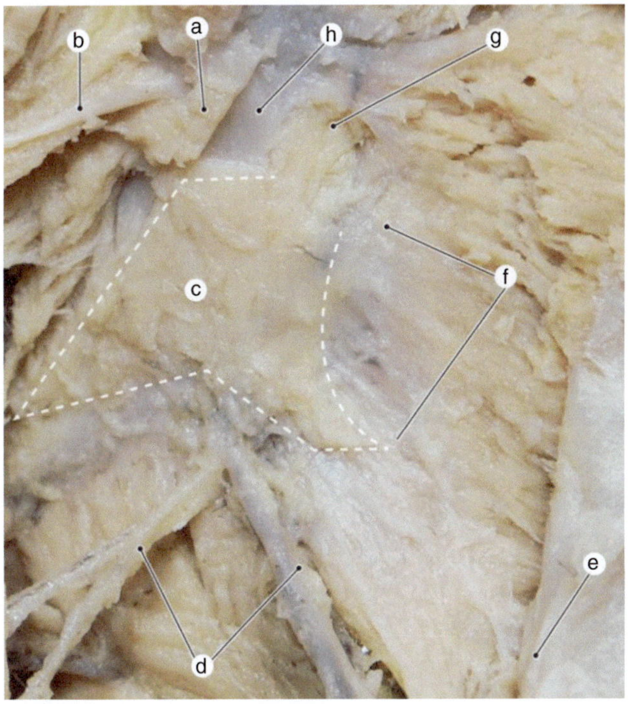

Fig. 7.99 The *dotted line* delineates the atrioventricular node and its extensions. Detail of Fig. 7.69. Notice the highlighting of the preperforating segment of Hiss bundle. *a* atrial myocardium (part of the floor), *b* tendon of Todaro, *c* atrioventricular node with two posterior extensions, *d* nodal vessels, *e* peeled ventricular endocardium, *f* fibrous insertions which secure the electrical isolation, *g* preperforating segment of the Hiss bundle, *h* tendinous centre

from the proximity of the superior vena cava ostium to the anterosuperior region of the left atrium (Figs. 7.10 and 7.17).

There are *other interatrial bundles (called inferior bundles)*. Most of them are located in the interatrial groove, above the point where the coronary sinus penetrates the wall of the right atrium (Fig. 6.36).

The atrial notch bundle has already been mentioned as a possible interatrial pathway (Fig. 7.10).

Considering the great variability of interatrial connections in all aspects (existence, position, number, thickness), one can pinpoint the reason why only some people are afflicted by interatrial conduction disorders.

The intercaval bundle and the various interatrial bundles dependant on the sinus musculature can influence or alter the interatrial conduction.

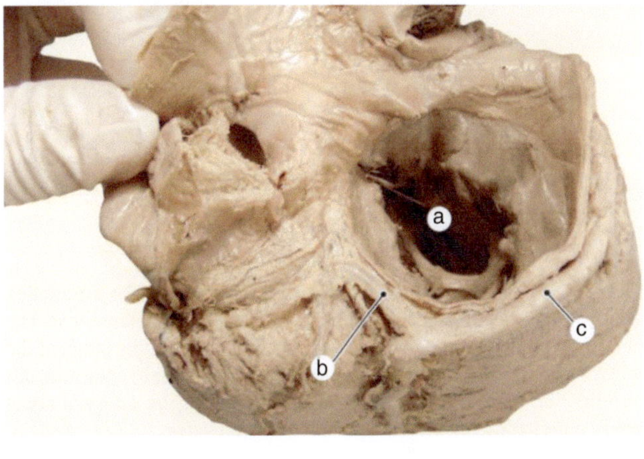

Fig. 7.100 Atrioventricular nodal artery emerges from the right coronary artery at the level of the crux cordis and passes through the pyramidal space parallel with the septal cusp insertion. *a* tricuspid valve, *b* atrioventricular nodal artery through the pyramidal space, *c* right coronary artery

The Internodal Pathways

- *The anterosuperior pathway (Bachmann)* [27] arises from the anterior extremity of the sinoatrial node, passes anteriorly to the superior vena cava opening, joins the Bachman bundle and then separates itself to descend on the atrial septum to the atrioventricular node.
- *The middle internodal pathway (Wenckebach)* arises from the inferior extremity of the sinoatrial node, passes behind the superior vena cava opening and descends on the interatrial septum (along the fossa ovalis or before it) to the atrioventricular node.
- *The inferior internodal pathway (Thorel)* arises from the inferior extremity of the node, passes through crista

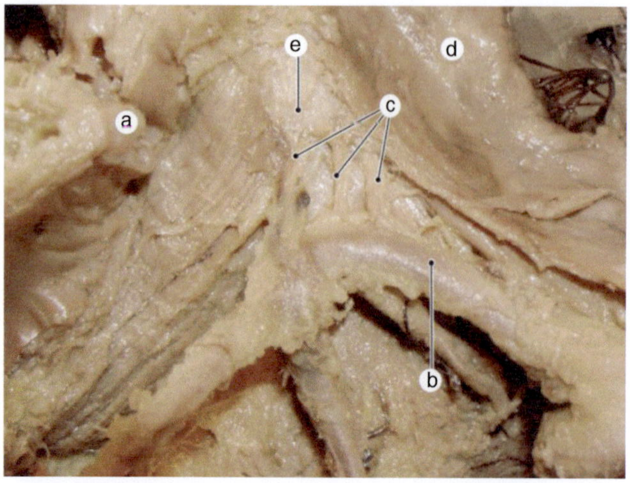

Fig. 7.101 Detail of the previous image. Near the node the artery forms a loop from which originates a group of branches in "palisade" for the node. After that the artery divides into three branches for the ventricular myocardium of the cordis. *a* left atrium, *b* nodal artery, *c* "palisade" arterial branches, *d* septal cusp, *e* atrioventricular node at the apex of the pyramidal space

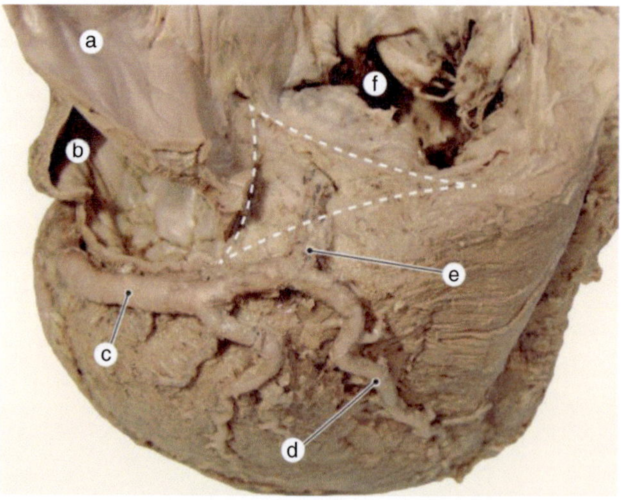

Fig. 7.102 Atrioventricular nodal artery arises from the circumflex artery at the level of the crux cordis. The right atrium was resected. The *dotted line* indicates the pyramidal space, at its apex being situated the atrioventricular node. *a* right surface of the interatrial septum, *b* left atrium, *c* circumflex artery, *d* posterior interventricular artery, *e* nodal artery entering the pyramidal space, *f* tricuspid valve

terminalis and the Eustachian margin and reaches the atrioventricular node.

– See the atrial continuum theory presented in the chapter dealing with the structure of atria!

There is room for discussion with regard to the structure, configuration and position (or even the existence) of these pathways. We should mention that although in present literature the term „bundle" is still in use, in reality they are more likely preferential pathways that were described rather electrophysiologically than morphologically.

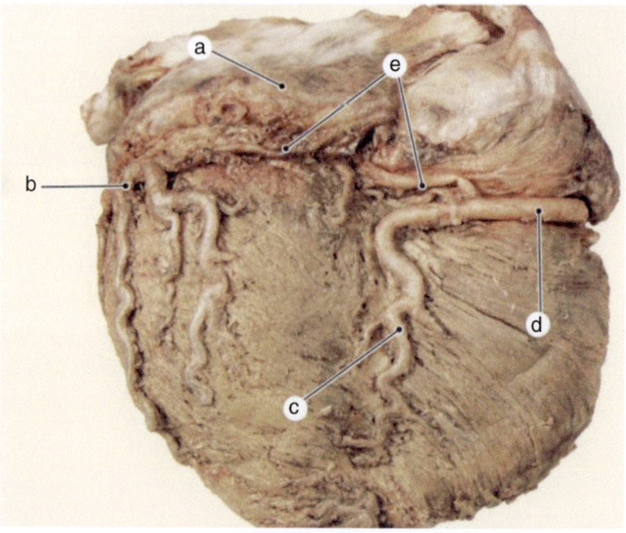

Fig. 7.103 Atrioventricular node can simultaneously receive "dedicated" vessels from both coronary arteries. *a* coronary sinus, *b* circumflex artery, *c* posterior interventricular artery, *d* right coronary artery, *e* arteries of atrioventricular node

Clinical Application

(A) Patients suffering from *re-entrant nodal tachycardia* have two distinct simultaneously functioning pathways of entry of the sinus impulse into the atrioventricular node [28] (*Pathophysiology of Heart Disease,* Leonard S. Lily. 4th ed. ISBN 0781763215):

- ***The slow pathway*** has a lower conduction velocity and a shorter refractory period. The impulse reaches the atrioventricular node through its anteroinferior *compact part*, which is located deeper. The impulse travels from the posterior area, along the base of the interatrial septum. It can involve some muscular fibers of a myocardially-transformed sinus and the dorsosinusal region in the coronary sinus ostium area. There can be two such pathways, left and right [29].
- ***The fast pathway*** has a higher conduction velocity and a longer refractory period. The impulse reaches the atrioventricular node by passing anteriorly and superiorly to the fossa ovalis and through the tip of Koch's triangle. The impulse reaches the node on the anterior side, in the common distal pathway, more precisely in the *pre-penetrating segment* of the bundle of Hiss.

The simultaneous existence of the two distinct electrophysiological pathways influences the physiology of the atrioventricular node and generates the re-entry mechanism.

(B) The cavo-tricuspid isthmus is an area specifically involved in the typical circuit of atrial flutter.

The following terminology is the one proposed by Anderson [30] for the pathways relevant to the preexcitation syndrome:

1. Atrioventricular accessory muscular fibers;
2. Nodoventricular accessory muscular fibers;

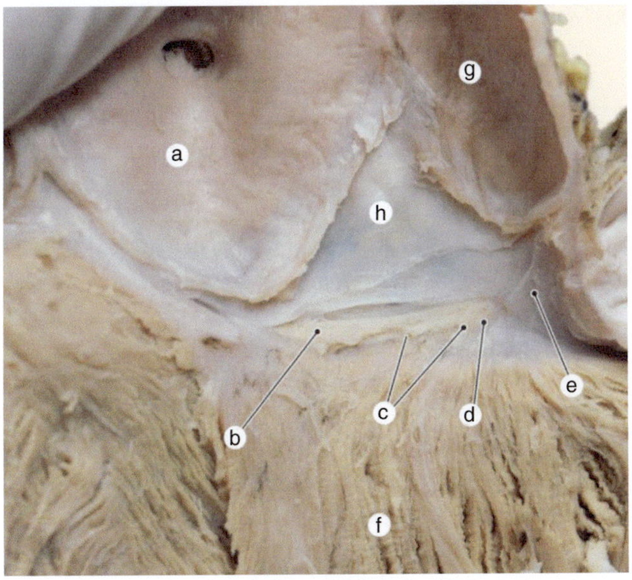

Fig. 7.104 View from the aortic vestibule (left side) of the right Henle trigone. At the base of the Henle space are visible the lines where de endocardium and the connective membrane that covered the Hiss bundle were resected. Obviously the conduction elements are passing through a "cavum" situated on the crest of the muscular interventricular septum, into the thickness of the membranous septum (see also Fig. 7.119). *a* right coronary sinus, *b* right branch inside the "cavum", *c* sectioned emergence of left branch, *d* postperforating segment of the Hiss bundle, *e* tendinous center, *f* aortic vestibule, *g* non-coronary sinus, *h* Henle trigone

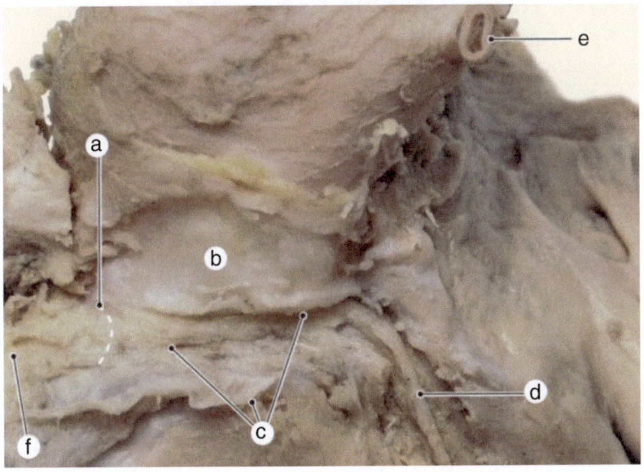

Fig. 7.105 Postperforating segment of Hiss bundle in its course through the cavum at the membranous septum base. View from the right side after removal of the right atrium and ventricle. *a* area of perforation, *b* membranous septum, *c* postperforating segment of the Hiss bundle into the cavum, *d* right branch of the Hiss Bundle, *e* right coronary artery, *f* atrioventricular node

3. Atriofascicular bypass fibers (atrial fibers which reach the pre-penetrating portion of the Hiss bundle);
4. Fasciculoventricular connection accessory fibers;
5. Intranodal bypass fibers;
6. Nodal malformations.

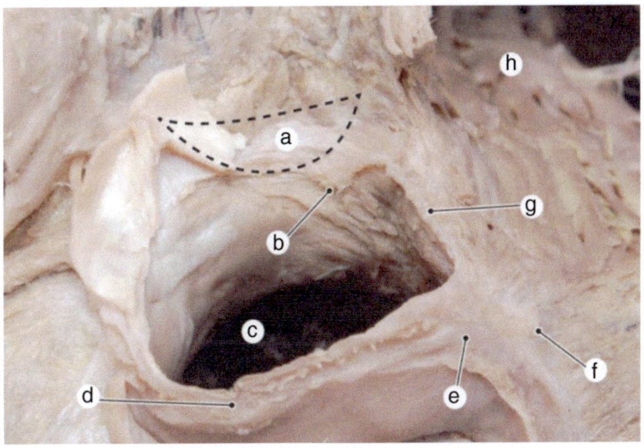

Fig. 7.106 Posterior and from the left view of the aortic root, after the removal of the atria and the mobile wall of the right ventricle. It can be observed the preperforating segment of the Hiss bundle on the tendinous center and the postperforating segment on the crest of the muscular septum. Right coronary sinus was represented with a *dotted line*. Left bundle branch emerges near the coronary sinus base. *a* right coronary sinus, *b* left branch, *c* aortic vestibule, *d* mitral- aortic continuity, *e* tendinous center, *f* preperforating segment, *g* Hiss bundle on the interventricular septum crest, *h* right ventricle

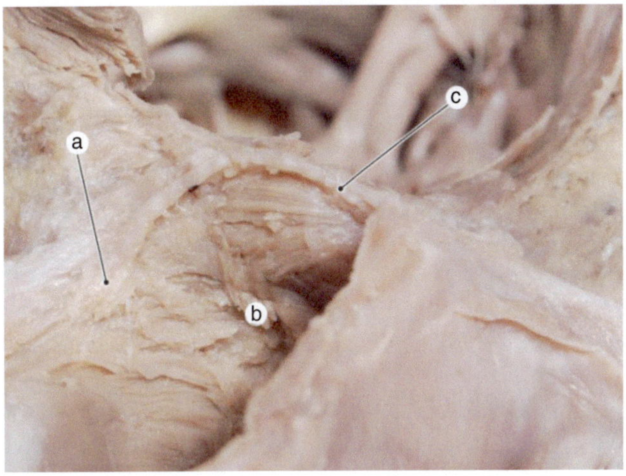

Fig. 7.107 Detail of the previous image. *a* left branch, *b* aortic vestibule, *c* Hiss bundle

The atrioventricular accessory muscular fibers are also known as *the bundle of Kent.* Such atrioventricular myocardial bridges have been reported in hearts with normal general structure as well as in hearts with congenital abnormalities. These bundles can be found almost anywhere – subepicardially, around the atrioventricular rings – but more frequently in the septal region (at the crux cordis (Fig. 6.82)) and around the tricuspid valve (in the proximity of the right subauricular vestibule). These bundles are 0.3–0.5 mm thick and under 1 cm long. Their existence is correlated to the *WPW syndrome* [31].

The atriofascicular bypass fibers are involved in the Lown-Ganong-Levine syndrome (short PR interval and normal duration of QRS).

The nodoventricular accessory fibers and the fasciculoventricular connection accessory fibers are also known in literature as *the parafascicular fibers of Mahaim.* Unlike other accessory pathways, the Mahaim fibers have *excitoconductive tissue characteristics* (they are abnormal branches of the node and of the pre-penetrating segment of the Hiss bundle) (Figs. 7.96b and 7.110).

7.4.2 The Atrioventricular Node

The atrioventricular node can be found „partially" in the right atrium, relatively beneath the endocardium, in the Koch triangle area (which is described together with the right atrium). It can be variable in shape, either ellipsoidal or with extensions. It is 0.5–1 cm long and 2–3 mm thick. Its color (on the dissection samples) is yellowish-white (Figs. 7.90, 7.91, 7.92 and 7.93).

From a histological point of view, the myocytes have irregular myofibrils and the node has a thin connective tissue capsule (Figs. 7.94, 7.95, 7.96 and 7.97).

The posterosuperior part is situated subendocardially, as a continuation of the atrial myocardial fibers on the floor of the right atrium.

The deeper, anteroinferior part, also known as the compact part, is located in the fold formed by the right atrium floor and the posterior part of the crest of the interventricular septum, in the proximity of the atrioventricular membranous septum, at the tip of the pyramidal space.

Sometimes it has a right posterior extension and a left one (horns) (Figs. 7.98 and 7.99).

In the above mentioned localization, *the compact part molds the central fibrous body of the heart. This fibrous structure provides the electric isolation paramount to the functioning of the node and of the penetrating part of the Hiss bundle.* The ventricular muscular fibers that insert on the central fibrous body around the node create the insertion through the means of a fibro-tendinous structure that *contributes to the completion of the electric isolation.*

The arterial vasculature of the atrioventricular node *originates from:*

- *The right coronary*, right after it passes the acute margin. In this case the node artery is *long* and passes in the fold between the right atrium and the base of the right ventricle, running under the atrial myocardium of the vestibular segment of the cavo-tricuspidian isthmus. Its course is relatively parallel to the tricuspid ring. Sometimes *the artery can be double.*
- *The right coronary*, in the proximity of the crux cordis. In this case the artery passes through the atrioventricular fold and has a shorter course, relatively perpendicular to the tricuspid ring.
- *The circumflex artery*. In this case, too, it can originate closer or further from the crux cordis. There can also be longer or shorter variants of the artery.
- *There can be two arteries of the node,* one originating from the right coronary and one from the circumflex artery.
- The node can also be supplied by *branches of the sinoatrial nodal artery*
- We have found a situation in which *the arteries of both nodes arose from the circumflex artery, on the diaphragmatic surface.*

The images that show the vasculature of the node are Fig. 6.40 and the images from Figs. 7.99, 7.100, 7.101, 7.102 and 7.103.

Regardless of its origin, the artery of the node is accompanied by one to two small veins. When it reaches the Koch triangle area its following course is variable:

- It either penetrates the posterior part of the nodule as a single or double branch or
- It forms a loop which gives off three to four branches that reach the node like a palisade.

The blood supply of the Hiss bundle *in the post-penetrating segment and that of its main branches is provided by* **the main septal artery** *(a branch from the anterior interventricular artery). Injury to this artery can lead to an atrioventricular block.*

7.4.3 The Hiss Bundle, Its Branches and the Purkinje Network

The atrioventricular bundle of Hiss is usually the only electric connection between the atria and the ventricles. It continues for a short distance the anteroinferior extremity of the atrioventricular node, which represents the **pre-penetrating segment** (Fig. 7.99). The bundle then penetrates the right side of the central fibrous body (representing **the penetrating segment**) and lastly penetrates (as **the post-penetrating segment**) the **septal cavum in the area of the right membranous space of Henle** (limited by the left ventricle endocardium, the interventricular membranous septum and the base of the interventricular muscular septum) (Fig. 6.142).

In this region *(cavum)* **the post-penetrating segment** of the bundle of Hiss can have two variants:

- If the segment is short it will *bifurcate immediately* after it arises from the central fibrous body. The right bundle branch descends beneath the aortic vestibule endocardium (Fig. 7.70) while the right bundle branch courses along the crest of the interventricular muscular septum to the base of the right coronary sinus and descends on the right side of the interventricular septum, in the margin of the septomarginal trabecula (Figs. 7.104, 7.105, 7.106, 7.107 and 7.108).

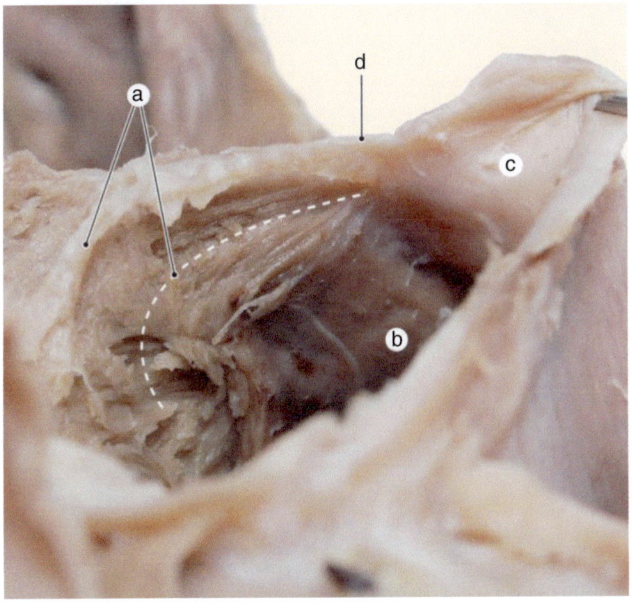

Fig. 7.108 Detail of previous image, view from the left side. *a* left branch and the initial course, *b* aortic vestibule, *c* tendinous center, *d* Hiss bundle

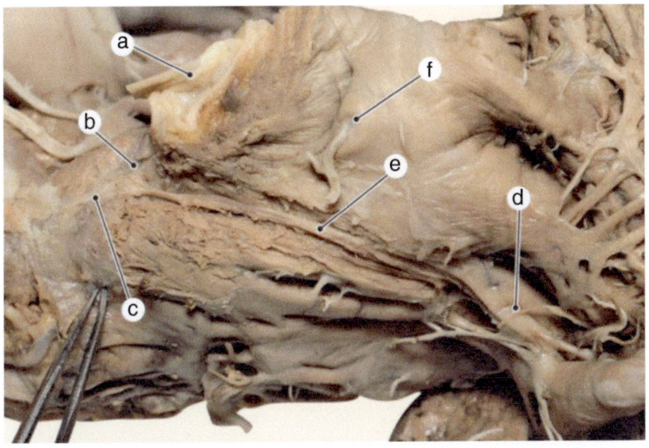

Fig. 7.109 View from the right and superior of the septal wall of the right ventricle and the crest of the interventricular muscular septum. The Hiss bundle follows the contour of the septal crest and it bifurcates at the base of the right coronary sinus. *a* right coronary sinus, *b* left branch, *c* Hiss bundle on the interventricular septum crest, *d* moderator band, *e* right branch, *f* Lancissi fascicle

- If the segment is long, the bundle will course along the crest of the interventricular muscular septum, in the base of the cavum, *to the base of the right coronary sinus where it bifurcates* (Figs. 7.109 and 7.110).

The bundle and its branches have a *fine connective tissue sheath (the sheath of Curran).*

- *Radiofrequency ablation procedures in the proximity of the Koch triangle, the fibrous central body and the base of the right coronary sinus present a high risk of injury to the normal excito-conductive tissue and to the node vasculature* [32].

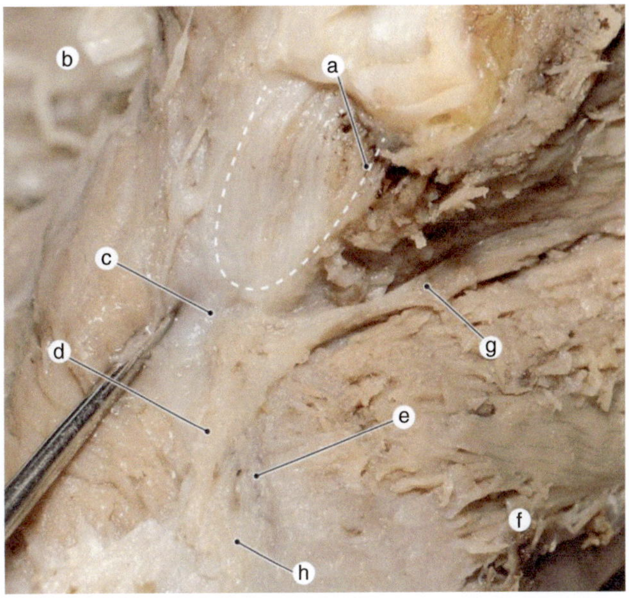

Fig. 7.110 Detail of previous image, posterior view. Besides the Hiss bundle, there is another fascicle of electrical conductive tissue with characteristics of nodal tissue (Mahaim). This originates from the node and enters the crest of the muscular interventricular septum. *a* limit of the right coronary sinus (sectioned), *b* left ventricle, *c* left branch, *d* Hiss bundle, *e* Mahaim fascicle, *f* right ventricle, *g* right branch, *h* atrioventricular node

In conclusion, the bundle of Hiss can be divided relative to the fibrous central body in *a pre-penetrating part, a penetrating part and a post-penetrating part.*

- The aortic annulus can undergo pathological transformations that can extend to the bundle of Hiss causing an atrioventricular block. Moreover, surgical procedures in the region of the aortic root may cause injury to the atrioventricular bundle or to its branches. It is for this reason that the close relations of the bundle in this area are very important.

  In this context we should mention that:
- The bundle of Hiss penetrates the central fibrous body just above the interventricular septum myocardium, to the right of the base of the non-coronary aortic sinus.
- The penetrating part is very attached to the central fibrous body, which can mean that the surgical procedures on the central fibrous body can cause injury to the atrioventricular bundle.
- The post-penetrating part perforates the cavum or the base of the membranous septum, at the junction with the muscular septum.

The left side of the bundle gives off beneath the endocardium the *left bundle branch*, a contingent of fibers molding the crest of the interventricular septum. Because

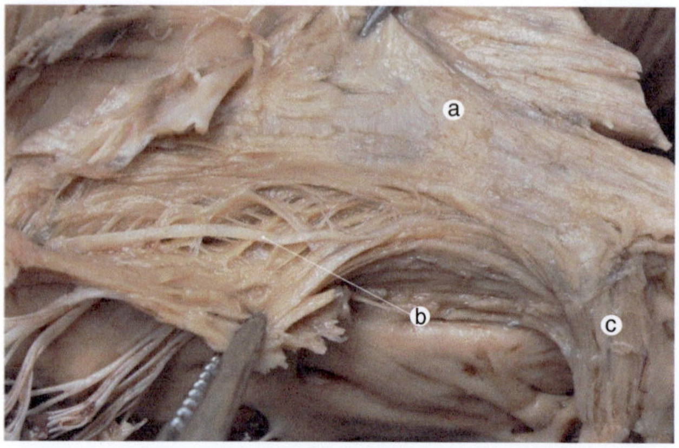

Fig. 7.111 Right branch of the Hiss bundle descends intramuscularly into the thickness of the inferior edge of septomarginal trabecula. It continues after that in the depth of the moderator band. *a* septomarginal trabecula, *b* the right branch of Hiss bundle, *c* moderator band

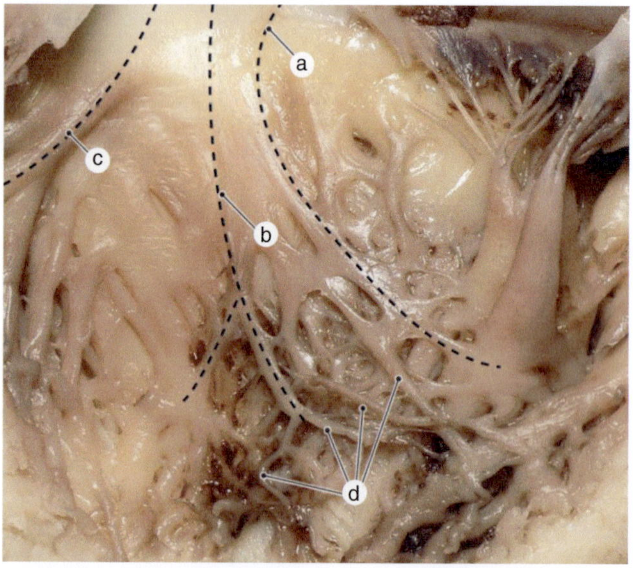

Fig. 7.112 Fetal heart. Left surface of the interventricular septum. The *dotted lines* indicate the course of the left branch elements, which continues with the Purkinje network. *a* posterior segment, *b* septal segment, *c* anterior segment, *d* Purkinje network

of its broad appearance, this contingent is also known as the widebranch.

From the point of origin of the left bundle branch the atrioventricular bundle is practically continued by the *right bundle branch.*

Again, the "cavum" varies in structure and identity. It is enclosed between the membranous septum and the ventricular endocardium of the aortic vestibule, or it can *even be found in the thickness of the base of the membranous septum.*

! The edema caused by a possible local inflammation can put pressure on the bundle in a relatively inextensible structure like the cavum. This explains the occurrence of atrioventricular blocks in local inflammatory diseases, as well as the possibility of treatment through therapeutic decompression.

The right bundle branch reaches the proximity of the base of the right coronary sinus, at which point it exits the cavum and penetrates the thin myocardium beneath the endocardium of the right ventricle.

The right bundle branch, also known as the right leg (crus dextrum) descends subendocardially covered by a thin layer of muscular fibers, on the right side of the intraventricular muscular septum, inferiorly to the small muscular prominence known as the *Lancissi bundle* (which can act as point of insertion for one tendinous chord). It courses intramyocardially after penetrating the inferior margin of the septomarginal trabecula, and then joins the *moderator band.* It then reaches the base of the anterior papillary muscle (Fig. 7.111).

In here it unfolds to form the right part of the Purkinje's network beneath the endocardium, which then reaches the cardiac myocytes. Sometimes the network forms pseudo-chordae tendinae in the ventricular cavity (Fig. 2.89). **The left bundle branch or left leg (crus sinistrum)** is also known as *the wide branch.* It descends subendocardially through the aortic vestibule, passes the left side of the muscular interventricular septum, downward and subendocardially, and forms a subendocardial network condensed into three segments:

- *The anterior segment* (anterosuperior division);
- *The septal segment*, which descends anteriorly to the apex of the heart;
- *The posterior segment* (posteroinferior division);

The anterior and posterior segments course towards the base of the homonymous papillary muscles. Some well-defined fascicles take the appearance of *pseudo-chordae tendineae* near the apex of the ventricle, and carry portions of these segments through the ventricular cavity into the myocardial substance (Figs. 7.112, 7.113, 7.114 and 7.120).

All three segments taper to the left part of the Purkinje network beneath the endocardium, which then reaches the cardiac myocytes (Figs. 7.115 and 7.116).

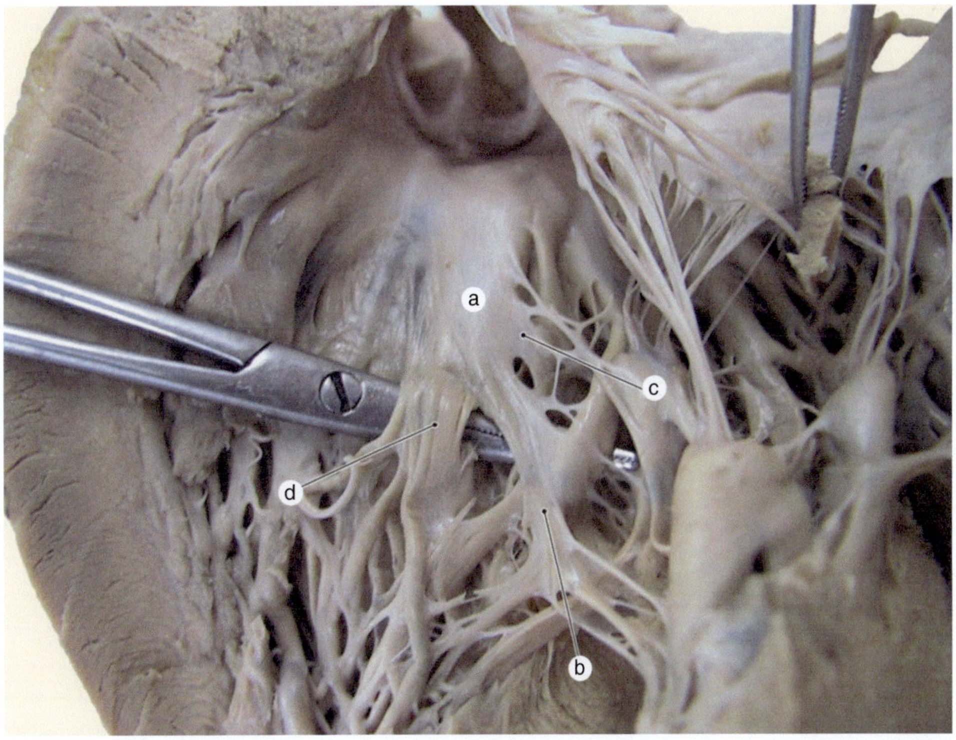

Fig. 7.113 Adult heart. Left surface of the interventricular septum. Highlighting the left branch of the Hiss bundle. *a* left branch, *b* septal segment, *c* posterior segment which continues with the Purkinje network, *d* anterior segment

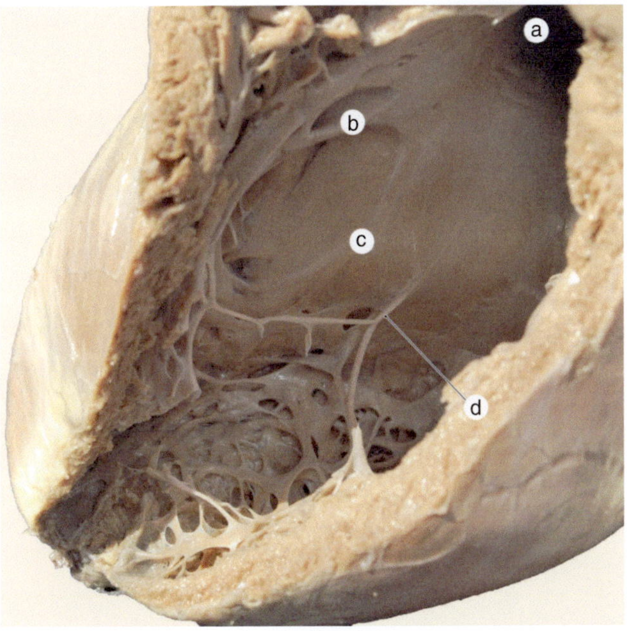

Fig. 7.114 Adult heart. Left surface of the interventricular septum. Highlighting of the left branch of the Hiss bundle and its segments. *a* aortic vestibule, *b* anterior segment (subendocardial), *c* septal segment, *d* posterior segment (intracavitary)

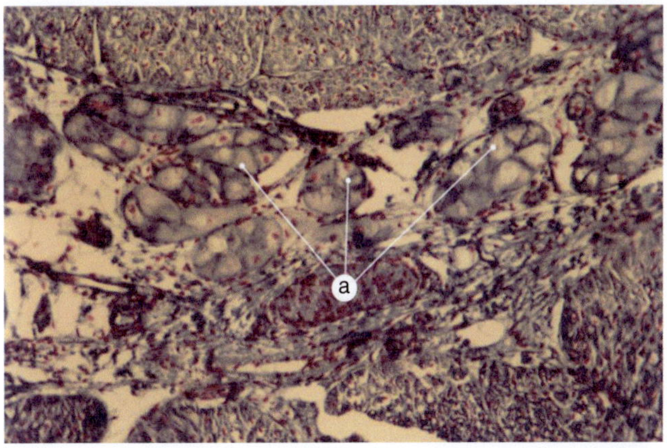

Fig. 7.115 Optical microscopy. Intramyocardial Purkinje fiber located near a vessel (Prof. Nicolae Ionescu collection) *a* Purkinje myocytes in "nests" in the structure of a Purkinje fiber

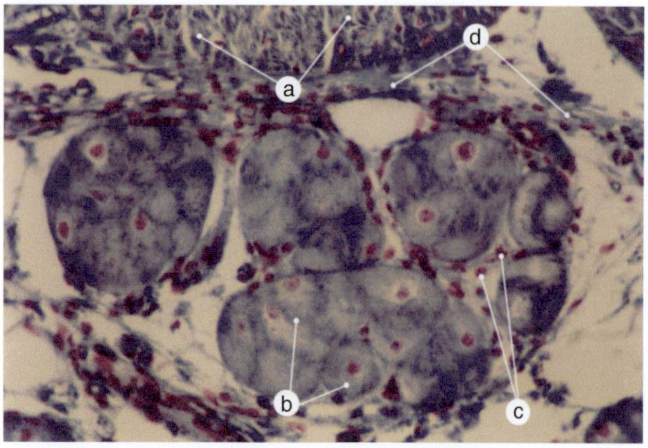

Fig. 7.116 Detail of Purkinje cells arranged in nests. Notice their large size, isolation by the connective sheath very well represented and also the multitude of satellite cells (Prof. Nicolae Ionescu collection) *a* working myocytes, *b* Purkinje cells, *c* satellite cells, *d* connective sheath

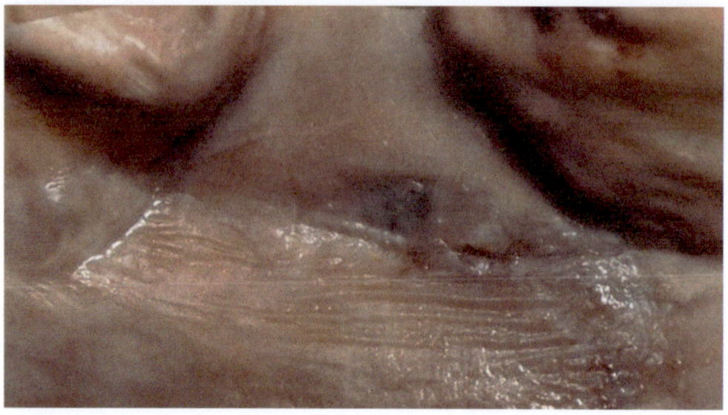

Fig. 7.117 View of the membranous septum from the aortic vestibulum

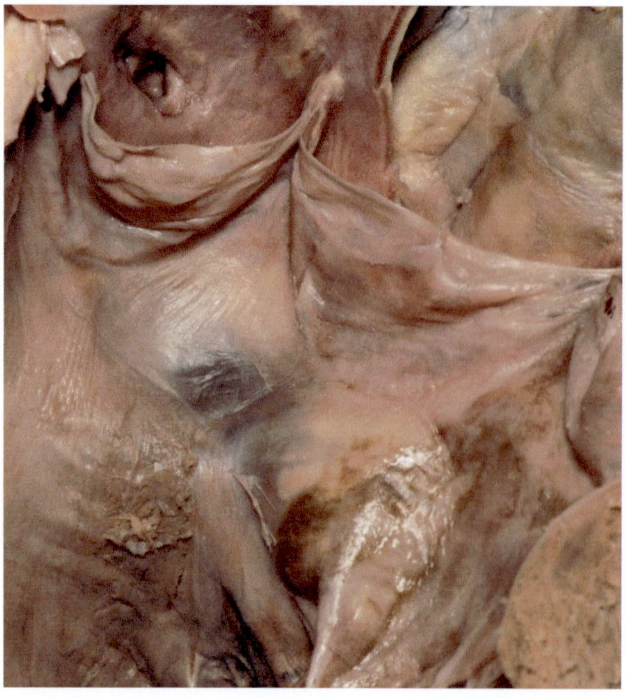

Fig. 7.118 View of the membranous septum from the aortic vestibulum

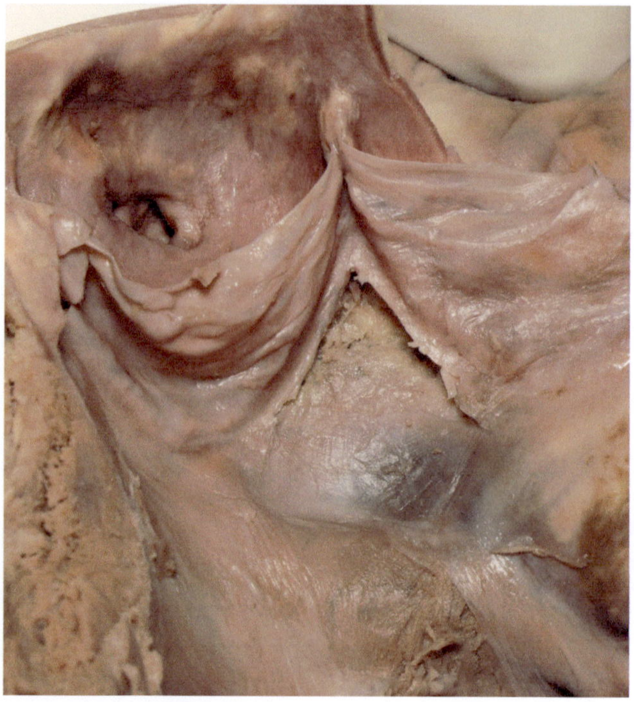

Fig. 7.119 Highlighting the septal cavum, first described by our team. View from the aortic vestibulum

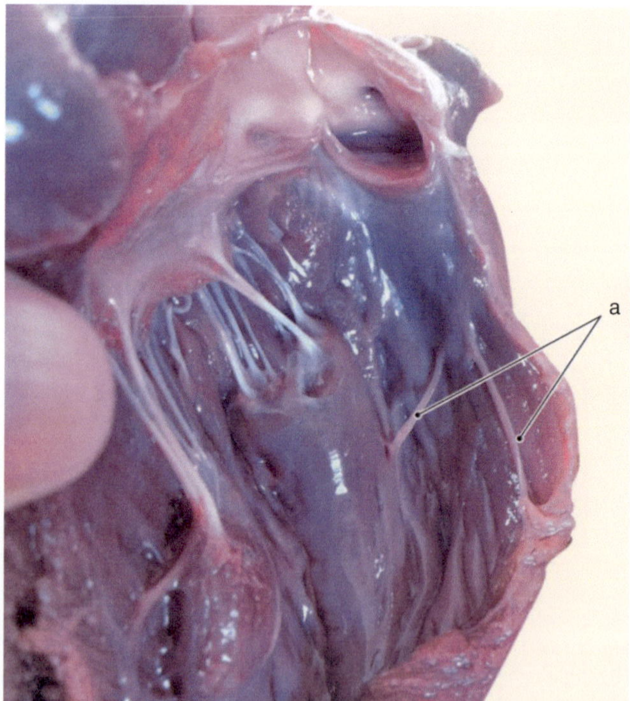

Fig. 7.120 Goat heart not preserved in formaldehyde. *a* the left branch of Hiss fascicle has an intracavitary course

References

1. Spach MS, Heidlage JF. The stochastic nature of cardiac propagation at a microscopic level – electrical description of myocardial architecture and its application to conduction. Circ Res. 1995;76:366–80.
2. Antzelevitch C, Fish J. Electrical heterogeneity within the ventricular wall. Basic Res Cardiol. 2001;96:517.
3. Weber K, Trombitas K, Granzier H. Cardiac interstitium in health and disease: the fibrillar collagen network. J Am Coll Cardiol. 1989;7:1637–52.
4. Trombitás K, Granzier H. Actin removal from cardiac myocytes shows that near Z line titin attaches to actin while under tension. Am J Physiol. 1997;273(2 Pt 1):C662–70.
5. Robison TF, et al. Structure and function of connective tissue in cardiac muscle: collagen types I and III in endomissyal struts and pericellular fibres. Scanning Microsc. 1988;2:1005–15.
6. Brown L. Cardiac extracellular matrix: a dynamic entity. Am J Physiol Heart Circ Physiol. 2005;289:H973–4.
7. Brown RD, Ambler SK, Mitchell MD, Long CS. The cardiac fibroblast: therapeutic target in myocardial remodelling and failure. Ann Rev Pharmacol Toxicol. 2005;45:657–87.
8. Brown L. Cardiac extracellular matrix: a dynamic entity. Am J Physiol Heart Circ Physiol. 2005;289(3):H973–4.
9. Cleutjens Jack PM. The role of matrix metalloproteinases in heart disease. Cardiovasc Res. 1996;32:816–21.
10. Caulfield JB, Borg TK. The collagen network of the heart. Lab Invest. 1979;40(3):364–72.
11. Sugihara N, Genda A, Shimizu M. Quantitation of myocardial fibrosis and its relation to function in essential hypertension and hypertrophic cardiomyopathy. Clin Cardiol. 1988;11:771–8.
12. Swynghedauw B. Molecular mechanisms of myocardial remodeling. Physiol Rev. 1999;79:215–62.
13. Shirwany A, Weber KT. Extracellular matrix remodeling in hypertensive heart disease. J Am Coll Cardiol. 2006;48(1):97–8.
14. Dean JW, Ho SY, Rowland E, Mann J, Anderson RH. Clinical anatomy of the atrioventricular junctions. J Am Coll Cardiol. 1994;24:1725–31.
15. Jamieson JD, Palade GE. Specific granules in atrial muscle cells. J Cell Biol. 1964;23:151–72. The Rockefeller University Press.
16. Brenner BM, Stein JH. Atrial natriuretic peptides. New York: Churchill Livingstone; 1989. p. 276.
17. Cheng A, Nguyen T, Malinowski M, Daughters GT, Miller DC, Ingels NB. Heterogeneity of left ventricular wall thickening mechanisms. Circulation. 2008;118:713–21.
18. Williams PL, Gray H. Gray's anatomy. 37th ed. Edinburgh/New York: Churchill Livingstone Inc; 1989.
19. Kwong KF, Schuessler RB, Green KG, Laing JG, Beyer EC, Boineau JP, Jeffrey E. Differential expression of gap junction proteins in the canine sinus node saffitz. Circ Res. 1998;82:604–12.
20. Virágh S, Stoeckel ME, Porte A. Light and electron microscope structure of the cardiac Purkinje fibers– review. Physiol Bohemoslov. 1987;36:233–42.
21. Sánchez-Quintana D, Cabrera JA, Farré J, Climent V, Anderson RH, Ho SY. Sinus node revisited in the era of electroanatomical mapping and catheter ablation. Heart. 2005;91(2):189–94.
22. Silverman ME, Hollman A. Discovery of the sinus node by Keith and Flack: on the centennial of their 1907 publication. Heart. 2007;93:1184–7.
23. Peters NS, Wit AL. Myocardial architecture and ventricular arrhythmogenesis. Circulation. 1998;97:1746–54.
24. Spach MS. Anisotropic structural complexities in the genesis of reentrant arrhythmias. Circulation. 1991;84:1447–50.
25. Matsuyama TA, Inoue S, Kobayashi Y, Sakai T, Saito T, Katagiri T, Ota H. Anatomical diversity and age– related histological changes in the human right atrial posterolateral wall. Europace. 2004;6(4):307–15.
26. Snell R. Clinical anatomy by regions. Philadelphia: Lippincott Williams & Wilkinson; 2008.
27. Braunwald PL. Heart disease: a textbook of cardiovascular medicine. 2007.
28. Lily LS. Pathophysiology of heart disease. 4th ed. Philadelphia: Lippincott Williams & Wilkins; 2006.
29. Asirvatham SJ. Cardiac anatomic considerations in pediatric electrophysiology. Indian Pacing Electrophysiol J. 2008;8:S75–91.
30. Anderson RH, Becker AE, Brechenmacher C, Davies MJ, Rossi L. Ventricular preexcitation. A proposed nomenclature for its substrates. Eur J Cardiol. 1975;3(1):27–36.
31. Gussak I, Antzelewitch C. Electrical disease of the heart. London: Springer; 2008.
32. El-Maasaranya SH, Elazaba EEB, Jensenb S, Henein MY. AV nodal artery anatomy and relations to the posterior septal space and its contents. Int J Cardiol. 2009;141:92–8.

8 Hearts Vessels

8.1 Arteries of the Heart

8.1.1 General Considerations

When regarding the hearts vascularization, broken rules are often the case. Here there are exceptions to almost every rule.

Perhaps more than in any other organ, individual variations of the heart's vascular supply can be the deciding factor between life and death.

We shall briefly consider some of the characteristics of the heart's vascularization, keeping in mind that these rules often have exceptions.

- At first glance, the heart seems to have **an independent vascular supply**, isolated from the other organs. In fact, there are small anastomoses in the subepicardial plexus, connecting it to small branches originating in the pericardiophrenic, esophageal, bronchial, internal thoracic and mediastinal arteries.
- Not only that, but the subepicardial space has angiogenetic properties. For instance, the greater omentum, if sutured to this plane, will develop arteriolar anastomoses with the subepicardial plexus. It is possible that other parts of the heart may have the same angiogenetic properties.
- The hearts **vascularization is terminal**. This means that there are no anastomoses between the branches of an artery supplying a certain myocardial segment and those of another artery supplying the same segment. Therefore, the obstruction of an artery must lead to the infarction of its myocardial territory. This is the rule. However, if the *arterial obstruction occurs slowly*, *gradually*, there usually is enough time for anastomoses and collateral vessels to develop ("on demand-anastomoses").
- More than that, up to the age of one, there are numerous intercoronary anastomoses. In some cases, these persist up to adulthood. These *intercoronary anastomoses* are most often to be found:
  - at the apex, between branches of the anterior interventricular, posterior interventricular, and circumflex branch;
  - around the conus, between branches from the right and left coronary arteries.
  - on the pulmonary surface, between branches of the anterior interventricular and circumflex branches
  - on the sternocostal surface of the right ventricle, between branches of the anterior interventricular branch and the right coronary artery
  - in the subendocardial plexus, especially at the base of the papillary muscles
  - in the interventricular septum
  - in the vasa vasorum of the great vessels.
- Another rule states that **arteries are continued by an arteriolar-capillary network**. However, there are arteriocavitary anastomoses (with the atrial or ventricular lumina) and even arterio-venous anastomoses, shunting the capillary bed.
- In the myocardium there are structures called *intertrabecular sinusoid spaces*, especially in the wall of the left ventricle, with a diameter of about 250 μm. Some of the arterio-cavitary anastomoses are *arterio-sinusoid anastomoses*. Specific to these vessels is that they lack the tunica media, (thus being unresponsive to vasodilatatory signals [1]).
- As a rule, **when an artery descends into the muscular layer, it does not reemerge to the surface**. This is not the case in cardiac anatomy, where myocardial bridges can cover arterial segments of various lengths. These occur most frequently over the anterior interventricular branch (Figs. 8.23 and 8.24), the obtuse marginal branch and the artery to the sinoatrial node (Fig. 7.17). Proximal, and sometimes distal to the myocardial bridge, the artery is slightly dilated.
- It is noteworthy that the coronary arteries usually have a subepicardial course. In extreme cases, the arteries may have an intracavitary course through the aortic vestibule or the pulmonary infundibulum, or, as shown in our studies, through the atrial lumen (Figs. 8.53 and 8.54). Coronary arteries with a free intrapericardial course have been described.

F.M. Filipoiu, *Atlas of Heart Anatomy and Development*,
DOI 10.1007/978-1-4471-5382-5_8, © Springer-Verlag London 2014

- As a rule, **the sympathetic and parasympathetic autonomous systems have opposite effects on arterial muscle.** *In the heart, both acetylcholine and noradrenalin are coronarodilators.*
- In **an organ consuming that much energy, one would expect a very long coronary perfusion time.** This is not the case. Coronary blood flow is mostly diastolic, *the coronary perfusion time is very short (8 s)* and gets even shorter during exercise. All this is compensated by *an immense capillary territory and a 1:1 ratio between capillaries and myocytes.* In cardiac hypertrophy, this ratio remains unchanged and an imbalance between the cardiac fibers great volume and the limited capacities of the capillary occurs.
- As there are two coronary arteries, for a long time it was thought that there is **a predefined, constant and predictable border between their vascularization-territories.** *Individual variation is the rule when concerning the heart's vascularization. Coronary* dominance *spans from moderate to extreme. It is not wrong to state that every individual has his own "coronary map".*
- In classical anatomy textbooks (*Gray's Anatomy*, ed. 39, p. 1014) **the dominant coronary artery is defined as the one supplying the posterior interventricular branch.** This is true only if this branch has the proper length and diameter, because there are cases where this branch is short and slender, and even though it is situated in the posterior interventricular sulcus, it is by far not dominant.

  We think that it is important to mention that there can be a left, a right, or a balanced dominance (a so-called co-dominance, *when branches originating in both arteries descend through the posterior interventricular sulcus).*

8.1.2 The Left Coronary Artery

The left coronary artery emerges from an ostium usually situated in the center of the left aortic sinus (Fig. 8.1). Usually, the greater part of this ostium is situated above the superior edge of the semilunar valve, but its position can vary: it can also be below this margin or completely above it (a so-called "tubular origin"). Seldom the left coronary artery can have its origin in the pulmonary trunk. Sometimes there can be two to three ostia in the left aortic sinus, the additional ones usually belonging to small branches.

The left coronary artery usually has a greater diameter than the right, of about 3–4 mm.

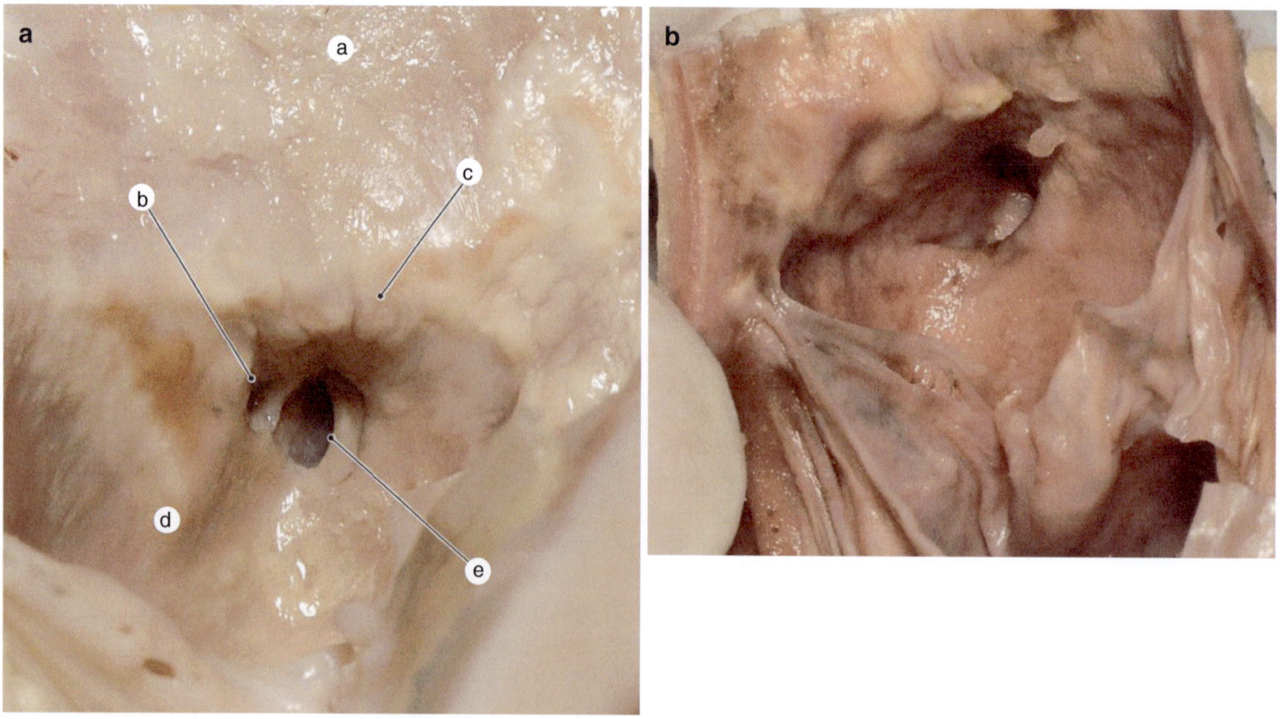

Fig. 8.1 (**a**) Left coronary sinus – detail. *a* aorta, *b* accessory coronary ostium, *c* supravalvular crest with atherosclerotic changes, *d* left coronary sinus, *e* the aortic-coronary margin at the level of the left coronary ostium. (**b**) Left coronary sinus with periostial atheromatosis – detail

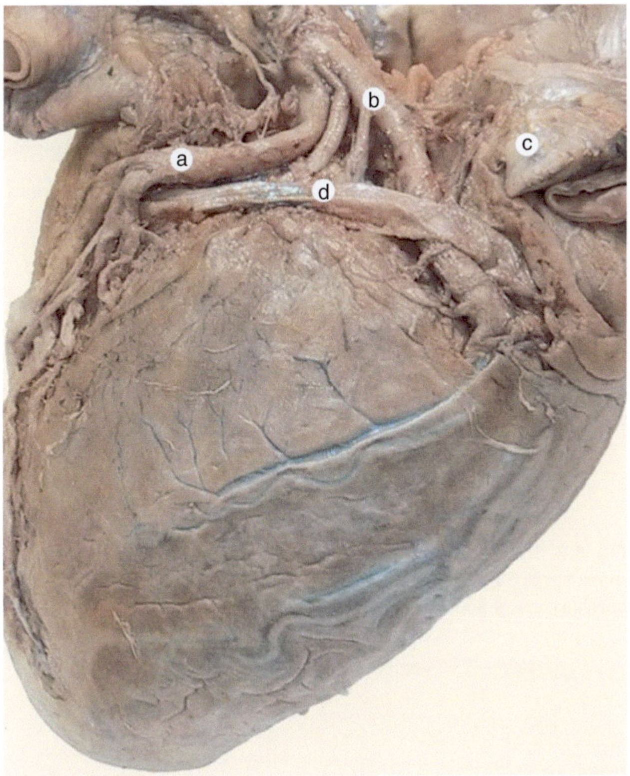

Fig. 8.2 Highlighting of the arteriovenous triangle (Brocq and Mouchet). *a* anterior interventricular artery, *b* circumflex artery, *c* left auricle, *d* great cardiac vein

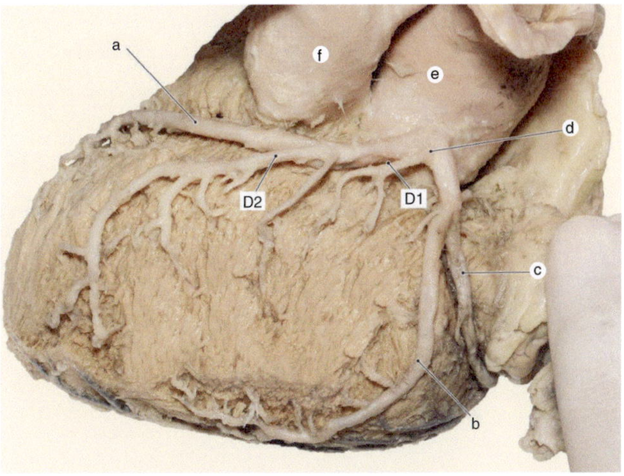

Fig. 8.3 The left coronary artery – view from the left side. *a* anterior interventriculary artery, *b* obtuse marginal artery, *c* circumflex artery, *d* left coronary artery with a short course, *e* aorta, *f* pulmonary trunk

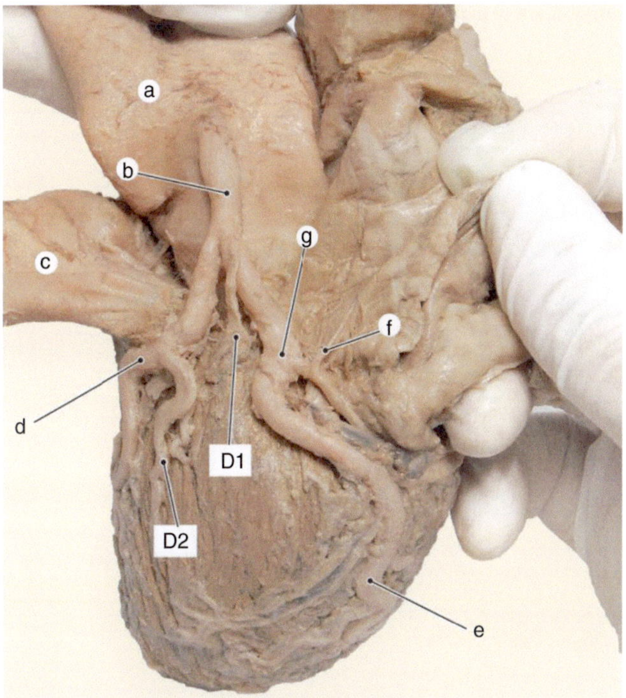

Fig. 8.4 Left coronary artery with a long course. *a* aorta, *b* left coronary artery with a long course, *c* pulmonary trunk, *d* anterior interventricular artery, *e* obtuse marginal artery, *f* an anterior atrial artery (from the circumflex artery), *g* bifurcation of the circumflex artery

The left coronary artery can create anteriorly an "aorto-coronary edge", rendering its catheterization for angiography more difficult.

The left coronary artery courses towards the left half of the coronary sulcus, being surrounded by the fatty tissue between the pulmonary trunk and the left atrial appendage (which also covers it). In this area, its bifurcation becomes a part of the arteriovenous triangle (Brocq and Mouchet): the base of the triangle is the greater cardiac vein, the two other sides are the anterior interventricular and the circumflex branches (Fig. 8.2).

The left coronary artery is considered to be *short* when its course is shorter than 0.5 cm (Figs. 8.3 and 8.6), or *long*, when over 0.5 cm; it can reach up to 2–3 cm (Fig. 8.4).

After this short course, the left coronary artery divides into two branches: *the anterior interventricular branch*, also called *left anterior descending (LAD)* by surgeons, and *the circumflex branch* (*the angle between the two branches is about 90**).

The left coronary artery can also divide into *three or four branches*.

When there are three branches, the middle can be called *the "animus intermediate" artery*, *median artery*, *left diagonal* etc (Fig. 8.5).

In the case of four branches, these are labeled, from anterior to posterior: *anterior interventricular branch*, *left ventricular diagonal artery*, *obtuse marginal artery* and *circumflex branch* (Fig. 8.6).

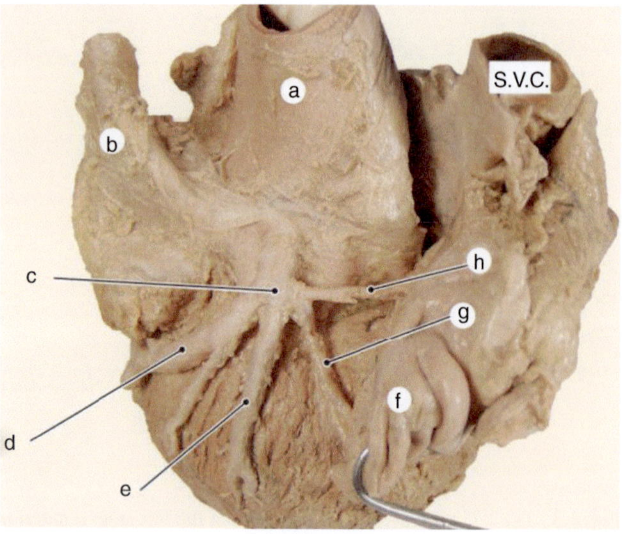

Fig. 8.5 Trifurcation of the left coronary artery. *a* aorta, *b* pulmonary trunk, *c* trifurcation of the left coronary artery, *d* anterior interventricular artery, *e* left ventricular diagonal artery, *f* left auricle, *g* circumflex artery, *h* artery to the sinoatrial node

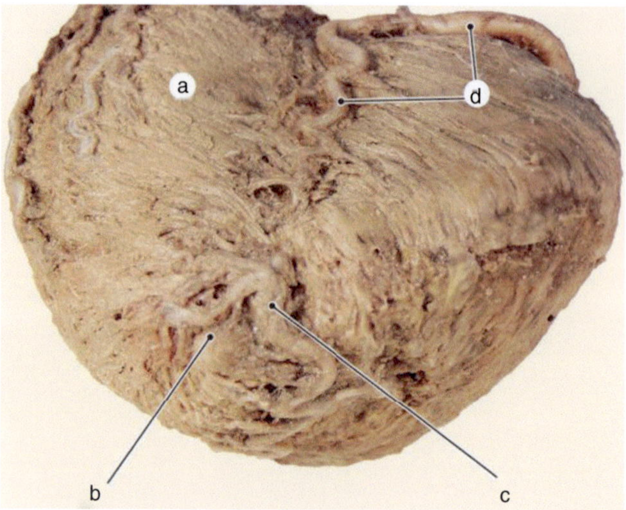

Fig. 8.7 Recurrent an posterior interventricular arteries. *a* diaphragmatic surface of the left ventricle, *b* vortex, *c* recurrent artery, *d* right coronary artery and posterior interventricular artery

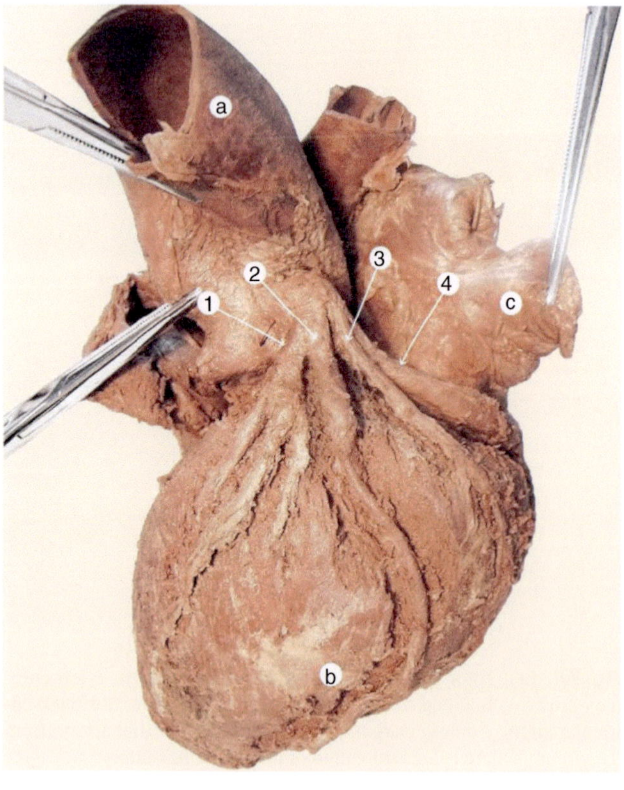

Fig. 8.6 Quadrifurcation of the left coronary artery. *1* anterior interventricular artery, *2* left ventricular diagonal artery, *3* obtuse marginal artery, *4* circumflex artery, *a* aorta, *b* obtuse margin, *c* left auricle

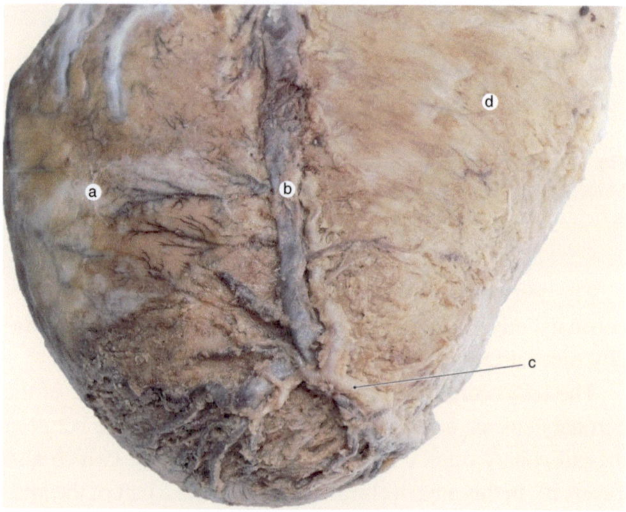

Fig. 8.8 Recurrent artery high ascending in the posterior interventricular sulcus. *a* diaphragmatic surface of the left ventricle, *b* middle cardiac vein, *c* recurrent artery, *d* diaphragmatic surface of the right ventricle

8.1.2.1 The Anterior Interventricular Branch

The anterior interventricular branch (left anterior descending) descends through the eponymous sulcus together with the greater cardiac vein. Its relation to the vein is very variable (Figs. 4.8 and 4.9). It reaches the notch at the heart's apex and then continues on the diaphragmatic surface as the *recurrent artery* (Figs. 8.7 and 8.8). It ascends 1–2 cm through the posterior interventricular sulcus and then ends by dividing into two or more branches. It can anastomose at the apex with the posterior interventricular or circumflex branch (Fig. 8.9) (*the recurrent artery rarely occupies the whole posterior interventricular sulcus*).

A special variation is the *bifurcation* of the anterior interventricular branch. We can describe a *true bifurcation* when both branches are situated in the anterior interventricular sulcus, with the shorter one also ending there (Fig. 8.11). A *pseudobifurcation* is the case when the shorter branch does not end its course in the sulcus (Fig. 8.12). These details are important in cardiac surgery.

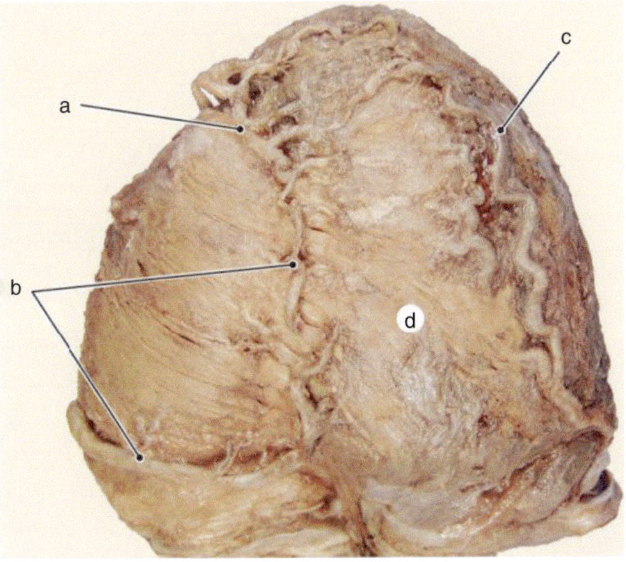

Fig. 8.9 The cardiac apex is an area where all three main coronary arteries can anastomose. *a* recurrent artery (from the anterior interventricular artery), *b* right coronary artery and posterior interventricular artery, *c* obtuse marginal artery (from the circumflex artery), *d* diaphragmatic aspect of the left ventricle

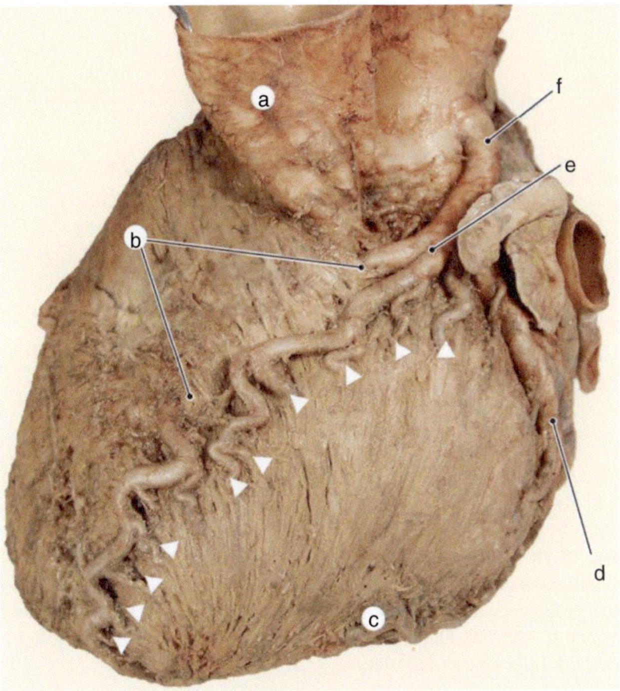

Fig. 8.11 "True" bifurcation of the anterior interventricular artery. The *arrowheads* indicate the origins of the septal arteries. *a* pulmonary trunk, *b* myocardial bridge over the anterior interventricular artery, *c* obtuse margin, *d* circumflex artery, *e* true bifurcation, *f* left coronary artery (long course)

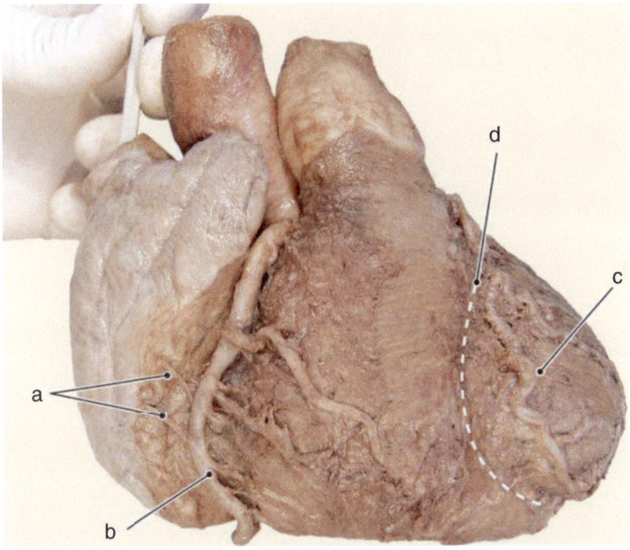

Fig. 8.10 The anterior interventricular artery actually runs left to the homonymous sulcus. *a* anterior atrial arteries, *b* right coronary artery, *c* anterior interventricular artery, *d* anterior interventricular sulcus

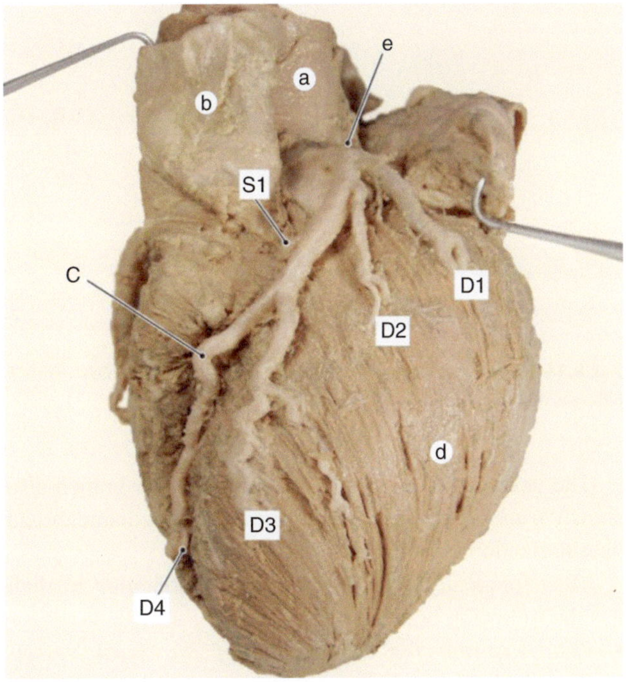

Fig. 8.12 Pseudobifurcation of the anterior descending artery – actually the emergence of D3. *a* aorta, *b* pulmonary trunk, *c* anterior interventricular artery, *d* obtuse margin, *e* left coronary artery. *S1* first septal artery, *D1–D4* diagonal arteries

In case of clinical signs of myocardial infarction around the bifurcation, it is possible that only one of the two branches is obstructed.

The angiographic visualization of the permeable branch can lead to misdiagnosing and missing the chance of performing a coronary intervention.

Clinically the anterior interventricular branch is *topographically divided* into three segments (based on angiographic criteria): *the proximal segment* (from the origin to the emergence of the main septal branch), *the middle segment* (to the origin of the second diagonal branch) and *the distal segment* (to the end of the artery) (Fig. 8.13).

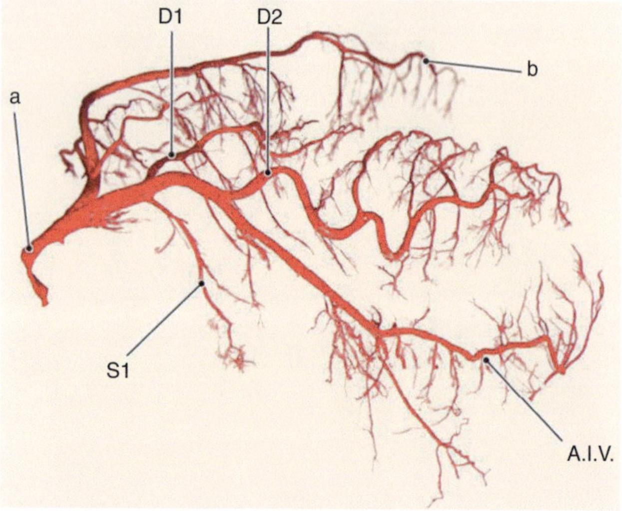

Fig. 8.13 The segments of the anterior interventricular artery (methylmetacrylate coronary mold): the proximal segment – from the emergence to S1, middle segment –between S1 and D2, distal segment – beyond D2. *a* left coronary artery, *b* circumflex artery. *A.I.V* anterior interventricular artery

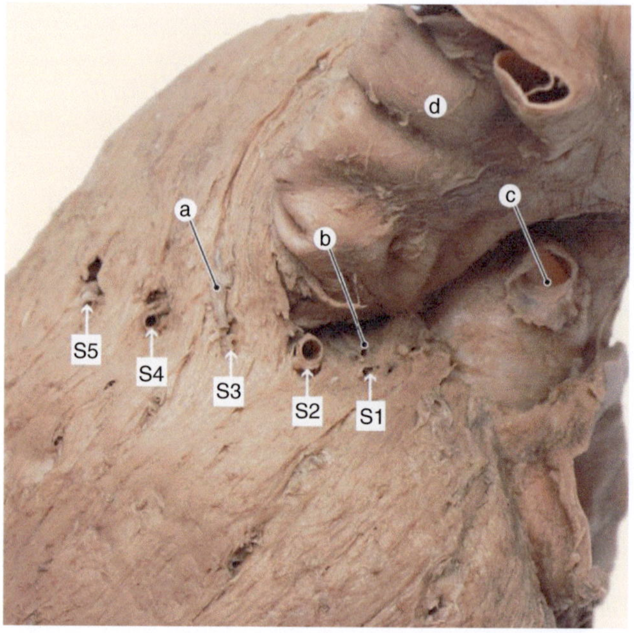

Fig. 8.15 Highlighting the septal arteries and infundibular branches. *a* preinfundibular artery, *b* retroinfundibular artery, *c* left coronary artery, *d* pulmonary trunk

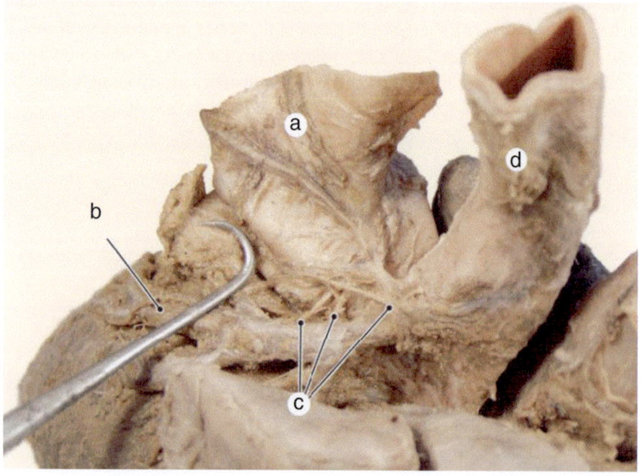

Fig. 8.14 Vasa vasorum of the aorta highlighted. *a* pulmonary trunk, *b* anterior interventricular artery, *c* vasa vasorum, *d* aorta

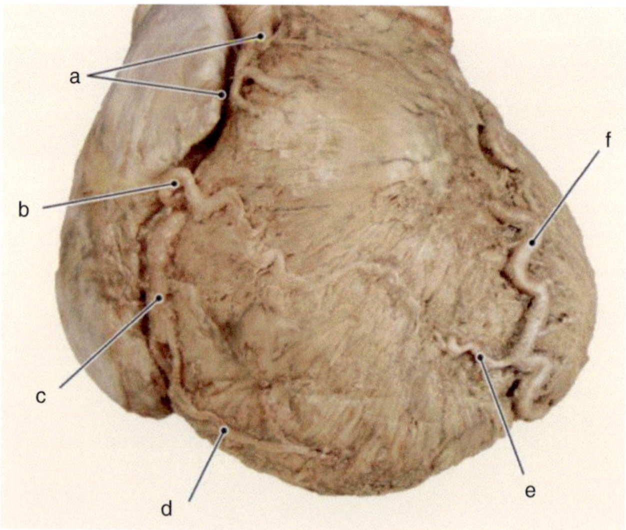

Fig. 8.16 Intercoronary anastomosis on the sternocostal aspect of the heart. *a* conal arteries, *b* right ventricular diagonal artery, *c* right coronary artery, *d* right marginal artery, *e* anterior right ventricular artery, *f* anterior interventricular artery

The branches of the anterior interventricular branch also show *variability* regarding their origin, length, diameter and vascularization territory.

Most frequently, **the anterior interventricular branch** has the following branches:

- *vasa vasorum for the origins of the great vessels* (Fig. 8.14);
- *anterior right ventricular branches*;
- *anterior left ventricular branches, also called diagonal branches* (*some of these can also be double*);
- *anterior septal branches, also called perforating branches*;
- *posterior septal branches, emerging from the recurrent artery*.

We would like to mention that the anterior ventricular branches usually have a short subepicardial course and then

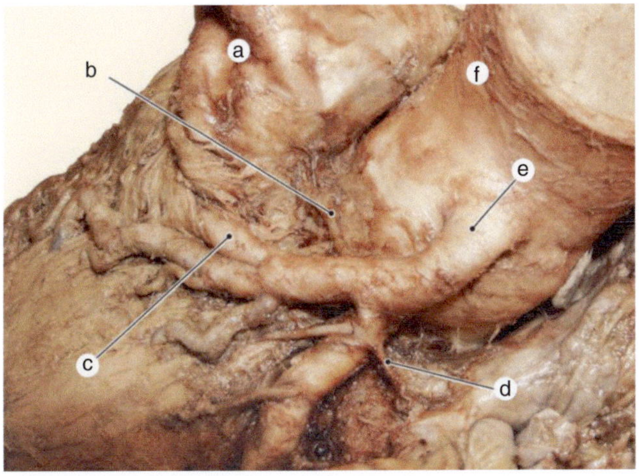

Fig. 8.17 Proximal part of the retroinfundibular artery (from the left coronary artery). *a* pulmonary trunk, *b* retroinfundibular artery, *c* anterior interventricular artery, covered by myocardial bridge, *d* anterior atrial artery, *e* left coronary artery, *f* aorta

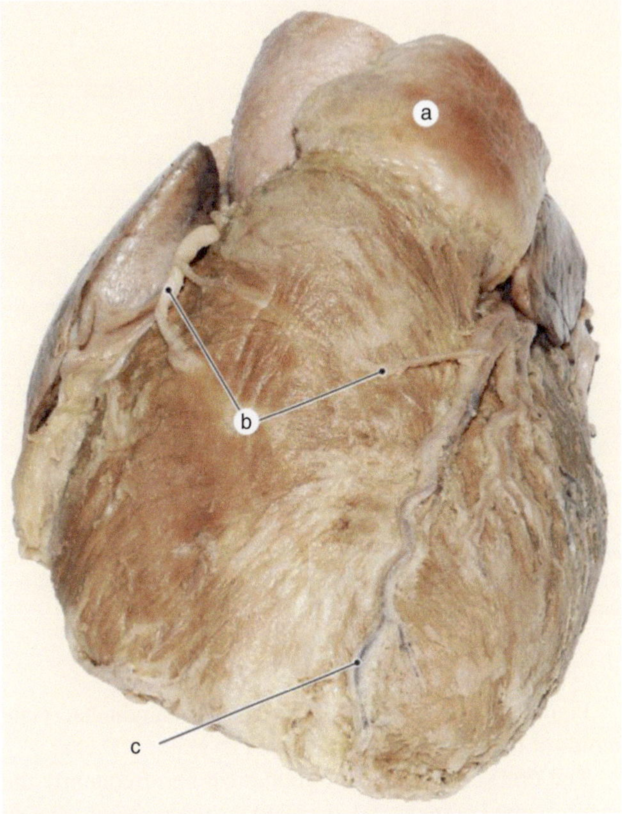

Fig. 8.18 Conal arteries. *a* pulmonary trunk (with bulbous proximal segment), *b* anterior conal arteries, *c* anterior interventricular artery

penetrate the myocardial layer. The various groups of anterior branches will now be individually described:

The anterior right ventricular branches are few and usually short. Sometimes there is a *left conal (or left periinfindibular) artery* (Figs. 8.15 and 8.19), which, together with a homonymous branch from the right coronary artery, creates "*the arterial periinfundibular ring*" (Vieussens). Sometimes there are *one to two right branches* (Fig. 4.30). One of these long subepicardial branches can anastomose with a diagonal branch of the right ventricle (Fig. 8.16).

The right-sided branches are:

- *the right conal branch* (called the "third coronary artery" when it has its own aortic ostium). It runs anteriorly to the conus (Fig. 4.35).
- the right branch running posterior to the conus is called *the right accessory conal branch* (or "the fourth coronary artery" when it has its own aortic ostium, but it can also be a branch of the former) (Figs. 8.30 and 8.43).

The left-sided branches are: *the left conal branch (left preinfundibular)* (Fig. 8.15) and a *left retroinfundibular branch* (which can emerge directly from the anterior interventricular branch or, frequently, from the first septal branch) (Figs. 8.17, 8.18, 8.19, 8.32 and 6.98).

The anterior left ventricular branches (lateral branches in N.A.I.) are more numerous (2–10) and also variable when considering their number or position. Some of these branches have a more constant course and are easier to identify, even if their origin is variable (from the left coronary artery or from the circumflex branch): *the first left ventricular diagonal branch* and *the obtuse marginal branch* (Fig. 8.3). Their names are very suggestive for their course. When describing individual branches of this type it is always important to mention their origin (e.g. the first diagonal branch of the left ventricle, a branch of the anterior interventricular branch). These arteries vascularize, completely or together with other branches, the *anterior mitral papillary group*.

All of the anterior left ventricular branches are called *diagonal* when there are more than two, when these are parallel to each other and when they course towards the acute margin and the apex (They are labeled D1, D2, etc.) (Figs. 8.12, 8.20, 8.21, 8.22, 8.23, 8.24 and 8.25).

As a general rule, when the first branches are of greater size, the others are smaller.

The anterior interventricular septal (perforating) branches emerge in a parallel pattern from the anterior interventricular branch and vascularize roughly the anterior 2/3 of the interventricular septum.

Their number varies. In clinical practice they are labeled S1, S2, S3,... (Figs. 8.26 and 8.27).

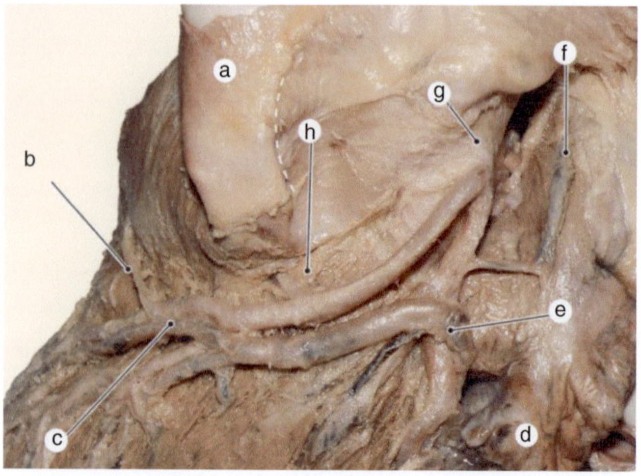

Fig. 8.19 Infundibular branches emerging from the anterior interventricular artery. *a* pulmonary trunk, *b* preinfundibular artery, *c* anterior intreventricular artery, *d* left auricle, *e* greater cardiac vein, *f* greater anastomotic artery, *g* left coronary artery, *h* retroinfundibular artery

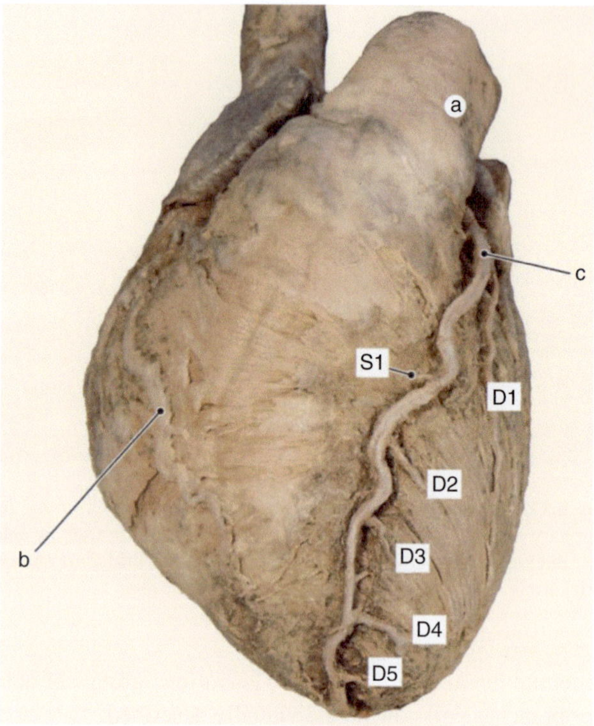

Fig. 8.20 Diagonal branches (*D1–D5*), first septal artery (*S1*), from the anterior interventricular artery. *a* pulmonary trunk, *b* right ventricular diagonal artery, *c* anterior intreventricular artery

Figures 8.13, 8.28 and 8.29 show methylmetacrylate molds of the left coronary artery and its major branches.

The first septal branch of greater caliber, frequently the second septal branch – S2, is called the *main septal branch*. It originates left of the infundibuloventricular junction, near the emergence of the first diagonal branch (Figs. 8.26 and 8.27). Angiographically, its course at a right angle to the anterior interventricular branch helps identify the latter.

It very often vascularizes the *postperforating segment of the His bundle*, thence its great clinical importance. This artery also supplies a *great part of the crista of the interventricular septum, the medial tricuspid papillary muscle*, and, together with a branch from the right coronary artery, *the anterior tricuspid papillary muscle*.

Sometimes *a big S1* has its own ostium in the left aortic sinus, and is labeled *the main septal branch*. This is Vieussens' *internal coronary artery* (Fig. 8.30).

!Regardless which is the main septal branch, a smaller branch may emerge adjacent to its ostium (Fig. 8.31).

Posterior septal branches emerge from the *recurrent artery* and supply the posterior third of the apical part of the interventricular septum (Fig. 8.29).

In some cases, especially concerning the first septal branches, two arteries may have a common emergence from the anterior interventricular branch. This can render coronary stenting very difficult or even impossible (Fig. 8.31).

Septal branches can communicate with the left ventricle, establishing arterioluminal anastomoses (Fig. 8.32).

- **The Romanian anatomist A. Crainicianu named the diagonal arteries and the myocardial bridges at the beginning of the last century** [2].

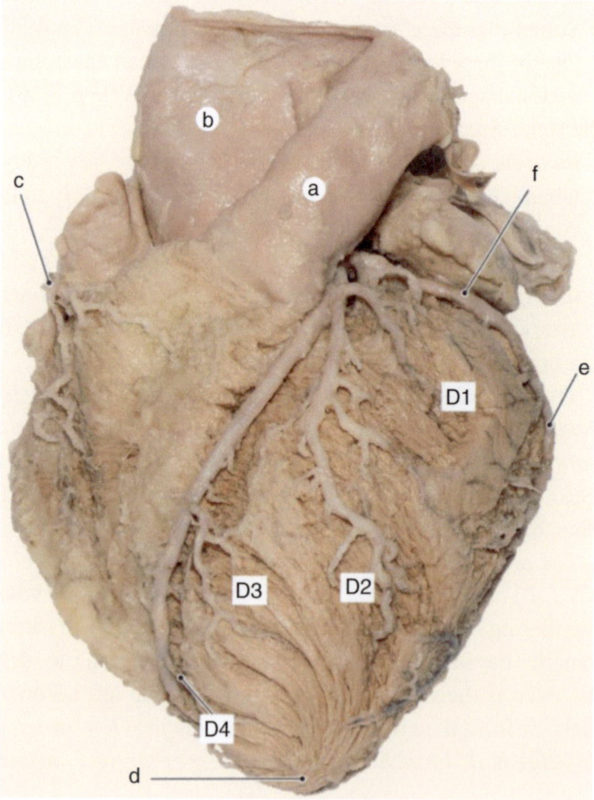

Fig. 8.21 The anterior interventricular artery and its diagonal branches (*D1–D4*). *a* pulmonary trunk, *b* aorta, *c* conal arteries, *d* vortex, *e* obtuse marginal artery, *f* circumflex artery

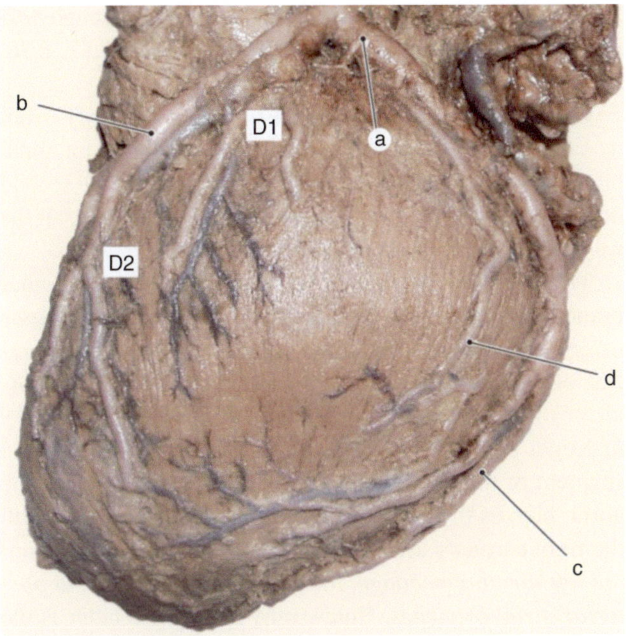

Fig. 8.22 Diagonal arteries (D1 and D2). Arterial branches for the pulmonary surface of the heart. *a* circumflex artery, *b* anterior interventricular artery, *c* obtuse marginal artery, *d* left ventricular diagonal artery, originating from the circumflex artery

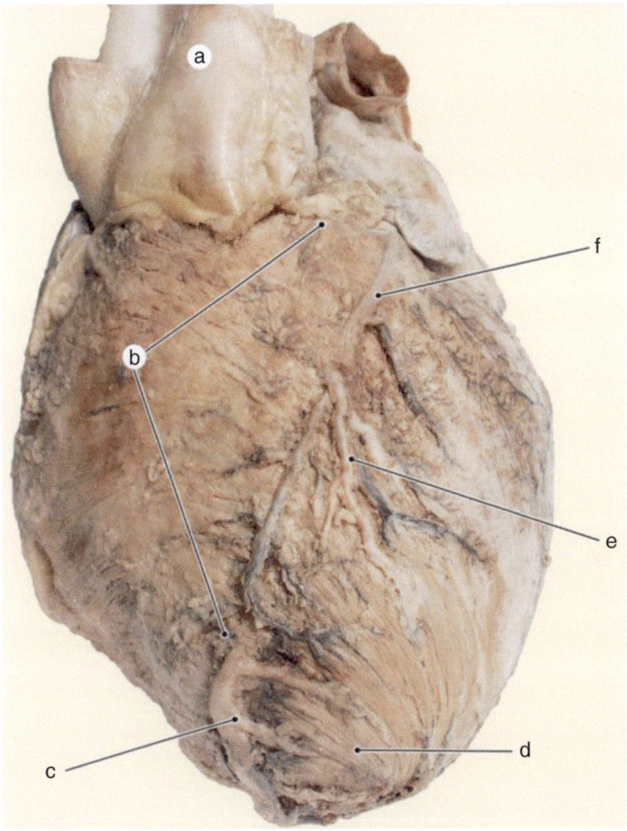

Fig. 8.23 Anterior interventricular artery, covered by a myocardial bridge throughout most of its course. *a* pulmonary trunk, *b* myocardial bridge, *c* anterior interventricular artery emerging from beneath the myocardial bridge, *d* vortex, *e* diagonal artery emerging from beneath the myocardial bridge, *f* great cardiac vein

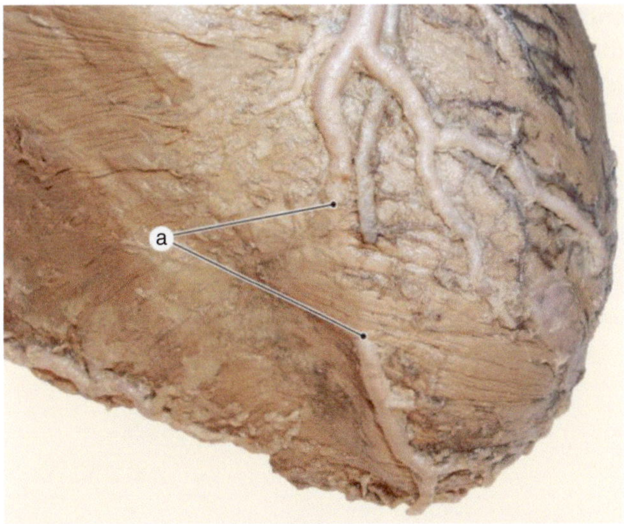

Fig. 8.24 Small myocardial bridging over the anterior interventricular artery. *a* myocardial bridge over the anterior interventricular artery

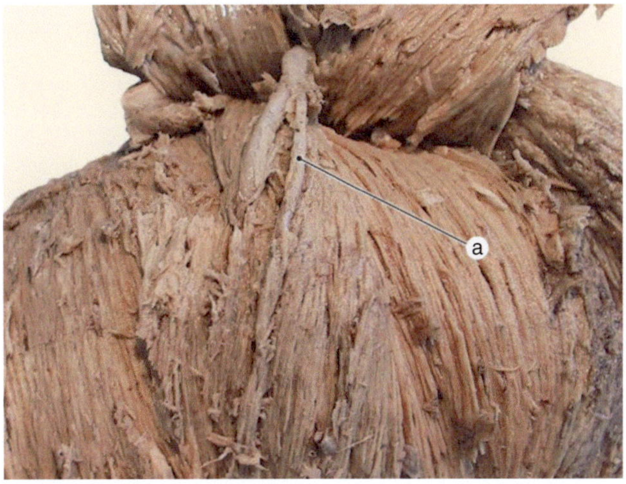

Fig. 8.25 Intramyocardial course of a diagonal artery. *a* throughout its intramyocardial course, the artery runs not perpendicular, but parallel to the myocardial fibers. Because of this, myocardial contraction does not completely block coronary arterial blood flow during systole. In the uterus, the arteries run perpendicular through the muscular layer and the uterine contraction thus perform a "biological ligature"

8.1.2.2 The Circumflex Branch

The second branch of the left coronary artery is the *circumflex branch*. In some cases it is of great size, so that clinicians say that "*the heart is vascularized by three major arteries*: the anterior interventricular branch, the circumflex branch and the right coronary artery".

The circumflex branch courses through the left half of the coronary sulcus and is initially covered by the left atrial appendage and the greater cardiac vein. At its emergence, it is situated adjacent to the greater cardiac vein (Figs. 8.2 and 8.33), and then runs together with the coronary sinus through the coronary sulcus (usually inferior to the sinus), covered by a layer of fatty tissue (Fig. 8.34). It ends left or right of the crux cordis. It often descends through the posterior interventricular sulcus as the *posterior interventricuar branch* (*posterior descending*). It can also course parallel to the sulcus which is occupied by a posterior descending branch originating in the right coronary artery. When the circumflex branch becomes a posterior interventricular branch, it also supplies

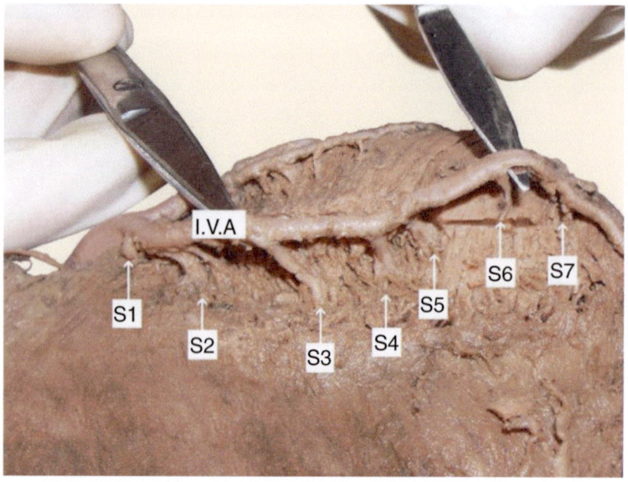

Fig. 8.26 Right view of the septal arteries (perforating) from the anterior interventricular artery (S1–S7)

the posterior part of the interventricular septum through *posterior septal branches* (Figs. 8.34, 8.35, 8.36, 8.37, 8.38, 8.39, 8.40, 8.41 and 8.42).

Clinically it has three segments: *the first segment* – from its origin to the emergence of the first major obtuse marginal branch; *the second segment* – to the emergence of the second major obtuse marginal branch, and *the third segment*, all the way to its end.

The circumflex branch has atrial and ventricular branches. *The atrial branches* are: *the sinoatrial node artery* (inconstant – see the subchapter on the vascularization of the sinoatrial node), which may run anterior or posterior to the left atrial appendage, *the anastomotic artery of* Kugel [3] (*auricularis magna* – emerges from the first segment of the circumflex branch, courses posterior to the aorta, pierces the interatrial septum and anastomoses with the right coronary artery) (Fig. 8.19), *the artery/arteries of the left atrial appendage*, *lateral atrial branches* and *posterior atrial branches*. Noteworthy among the latter is the *artery of the atrioventricular node* (inconstant – see the subchapter on the vascularization of the atrioventricular node), running profoundly in relation to the coronary sinus, in the fold between the right atrium and the crista of the interventricular septum, which it also vascularizes (Fig. 8.34).

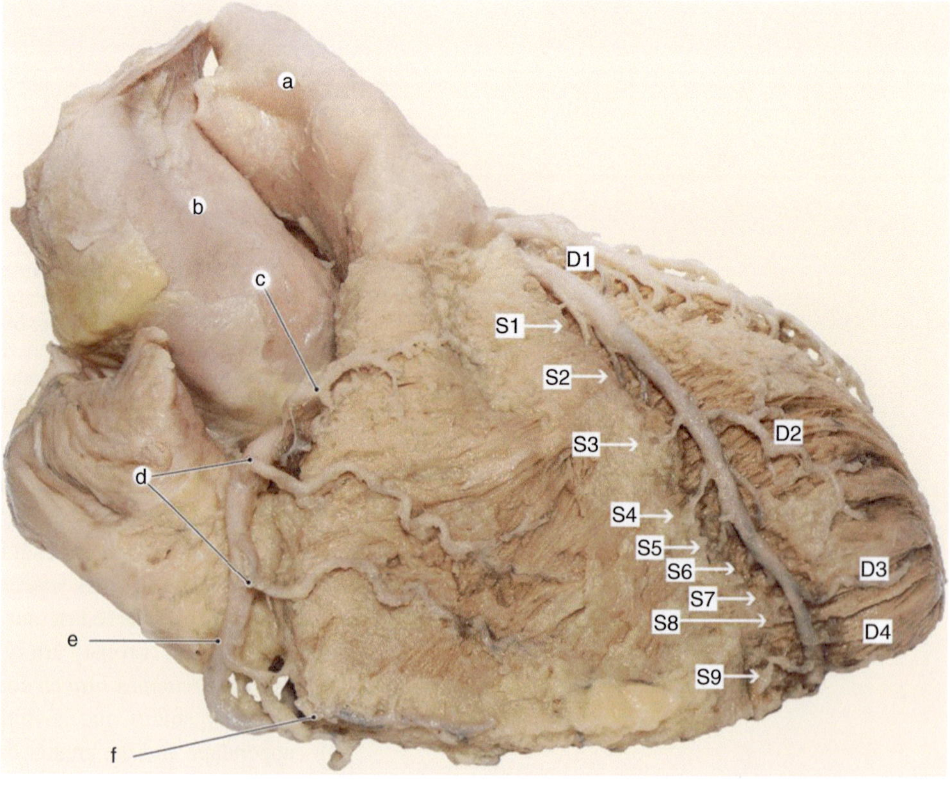

Fig. 8.27 Anterior interventricular artery and right coronary artery. *S* septal arteries, *D* left ventricular diagonal arteries. *a* pulmonary trunk, *b* aorta, *c* conal artery, *d* right ventricular diagonal arteries, *e* right coronary artery, *f* acute marginal artery

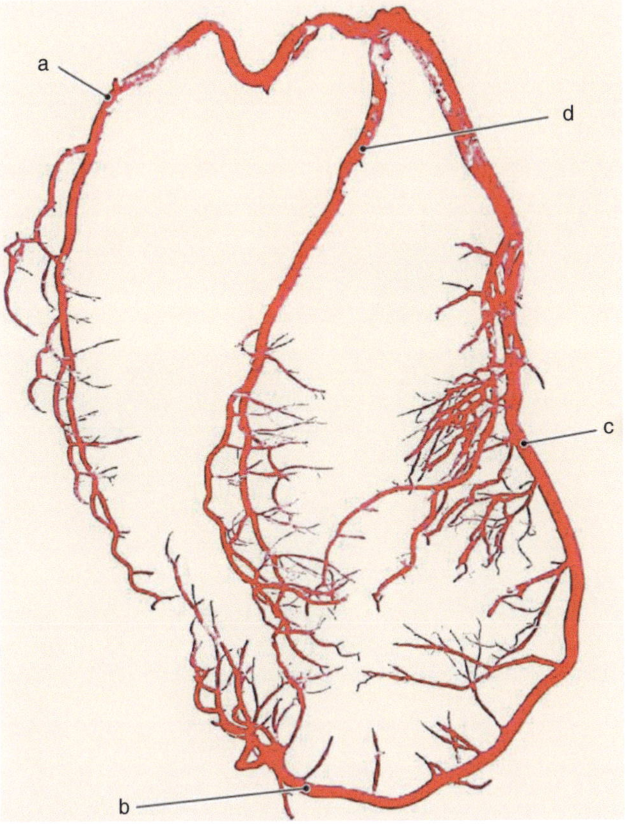

Fig. 8.28 Methylmetacrylate mold of the left coronary artery. Right view. *a* circumflex artery, *b* recurrent artery with posterior septal branches, *c* anterior interventricular artery with anterior septal branches, *d* left ventricular diagonal artery

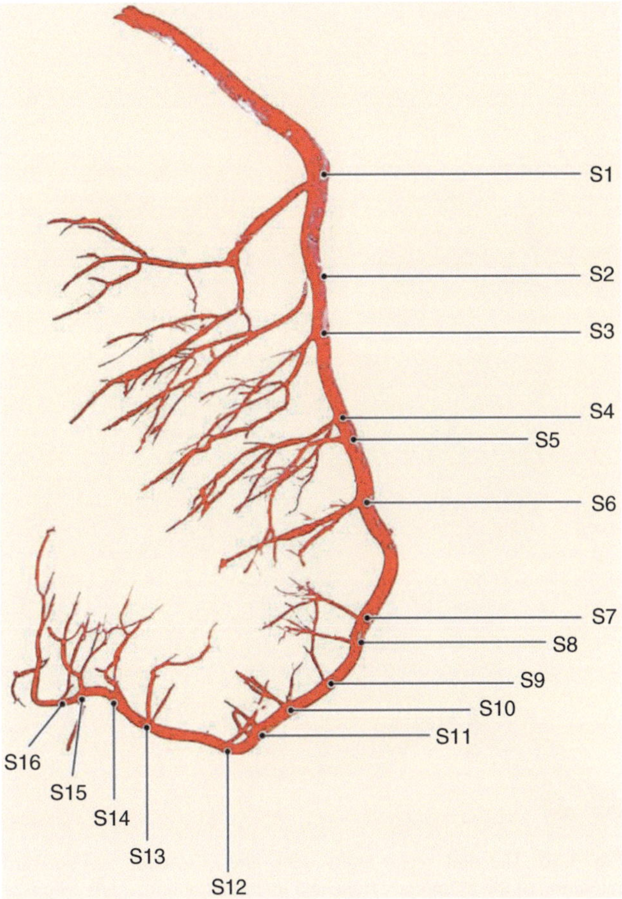

Fig. 8.29 Mold of the anterior interventricular artery. The first eight septal arteries (*S1–S8*) approach anteriorly the interventricular septum. The arteries from *S9* to *S12* approach the septum at its apex. The arteries from *S13* to *S16* are branches from the recurrent artery and approach inferiorly the interventricular septum

The ventricular branches for the sternocostal and pulmonary surface of the left ventricle can originate either in the circumflex branch, or in the anterior interventricular branch.

They are called *the left ventricular artery* and *the obtuse marginal artery*. The latter supplies *the posterior mitral papillary group*. In cases of right coronary dominance, it can be vascularized by branches from the right coronary artery.

In clinical practice the branches from the circumflex branch supplying the obtuse margin are labeled OM1, OM2, OM3, etc.

Very often the circumflex branch has *a terminal branch* of significant size, on the diaphragmatic surface of the left ventricle (*the diaphragmatic artery of the left ventricle*) and a smaller terminal branch – *the atrioventricular node artery*. The latter courses below the interatrial septum up to the triangle of Koch.

In some cases numerous ventricular branches emerge from the circumflex branch and descend for about 2–3 cm on the surface of the left ventricle. These branches do not have specific names (Fig. 8.40).

8.1.3 The Right Coronary Artery

The right coronary artery emerges from the right aortic sinus from an *ostium* situated in its greater part above the margin of the semilunar valve (Figs. 6.138, 6.139 and 8.43). Not only the position, but also the number of ostia in the right aortic sinus may vary. When there are two or three ostia, they represent the origin of the conal branches or of the artery of the sinus node.

The right coronary artery courses through the right half of the coronary sulcus, surrounded by fatty tissue (Fig. 4.11).

Initially situated between the right atrial appendage and the pulmonary trunk (Fig. 8.44), the artery passes around the acute margin of the heart to reach the diaphragmatic surface, where its later course and branching pattern are subject to great variability:

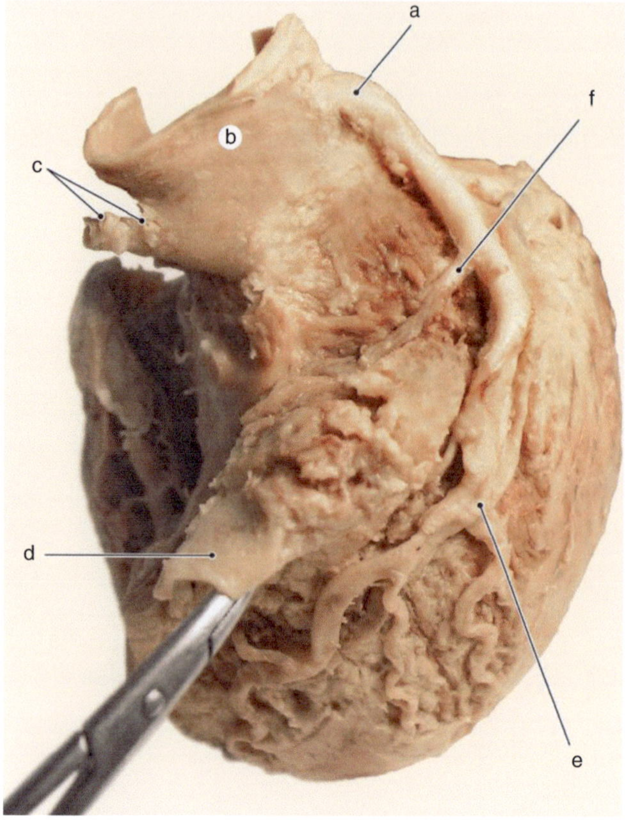

Fig. 8.30 The first septal artery, seen after dissection and forward retraction of the pulmonary trunk and its infundibulum. *a* left coronary artery, *b* aorta, *c* right coronary artery and conal branches, *d* pulmonary trunk, *e* anterior interventricular artery, *f* first septal artery

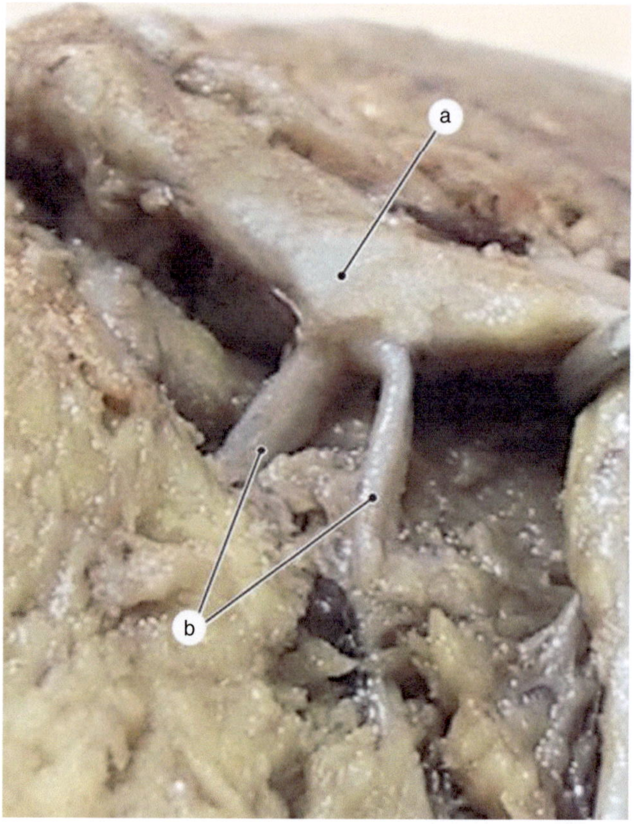

Fig. 8.31 Emergence of two septal arteries from the same segment of the anterior interventricular artery – detail. *a* anterior interventricular artery, *b* septal arteries

- Descending through the posterior interventricular sulcus as the *posterior interventricular branch* (*posterior descending*), thus supplying the posterior 1/3 of the interventricular septum through its *posterior septal branches.*
- Ending before the crux cordis, either in the coronary sulcus, or descending on the diaphragmatic surface of the left ventricle as a right ventricular diaphragmatic branch
- Ending after the crux, either in the coronary sulcus, or on the diaphragmatic surface of the left ventricle, or, in some cases, reaching the obtuse margin.

It is important to note that, because of the right coronary sulcus being in an almost frontal plane, the right coronary artery has a *vertical descending course in its proximal half*; this can clearly be seen in an angiography.

The right coronary artery is divided in a *proximal half*, from the origin to the acute margin, and a *distal half*, beyond the acute margin, on the diaphragmatic surface (Figs. 8.10, 8.16, 8.18, 8.27, 8.35, 8.45, 8.46, 8.47, 8.48, 8.49, 8.50, 8.51 and 8.52).

The right coronary artery has *anterior ventricular branches*, *posterior ventricular or diaphragmatic branches*, and *anterior, marginal and posterior atrial branches.*

The anterior ventricular branches:

- *The right conal branch* (sometimes contributing to the conal arterial ring). It is also called **the third coronary artery** when it has its separate aortic ostium. When there are two conal branches, each with its separate ostium, a **fourth coronary artery** can be described (Fig. 8.44).
- *The right ventricular diagonal branch* (inconstant) (Fig. 8.47) has a subepicardial course on the sternocostal surface and can anastomose with a branch from the anterior interventricular branch (Figs. 8.16 and 8.20).
- *The right marginal ventricular branch* (inconstant) has a long subepicardial course on the hearts (hearts) right margin. It supplies a great portion of the anterior wall of the right ventricle, but also *the posterior tricuspid papillary muscle.*
- *Small ventricular branches*, with a short subepicardial course, penetrating the myocardial mass from the coronary sulcus.

The posterior ventricular branches (2–4) usually emerge in the form of "palisade" from the convexity of the right coronary artery and have a short descending subepicardial course on the diaphragmatic surface of the right ventricle, after which they penetrate the myocardium. In this segment too there are *small ventricular branches, with a short subepicardial course.*

! Rarely there can be a long posterior ventricular branch, originating near the right margin of the heart. In case of posterior myocardial infarction it may cause confusion in

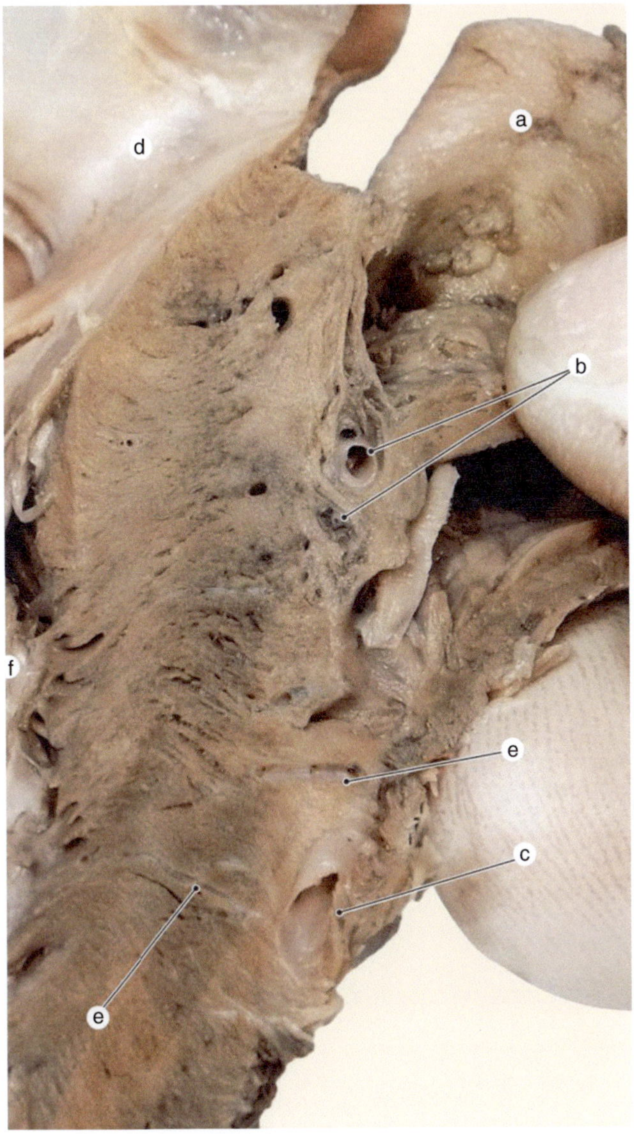

Fig. 8.32 Sagittal section through septal wall of the left ventricle. *Right view*. Small, yet macroscopically visible, septal arteries emerge from the anterior interventricular artery and open in the left ventricular cavity. *a* pulmonary trunk, *b* retroinfundibular arteries, *c* anterior interventricular artery, *d* aortic vestibule, *e* septal arteries, *f* cavity of the left ventricle

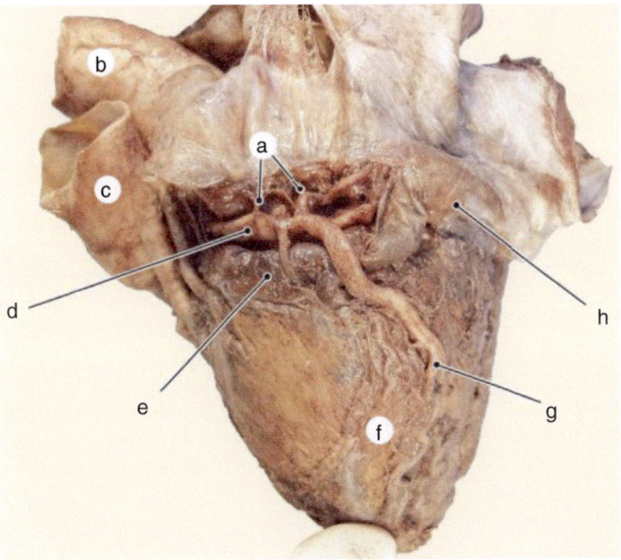

Fig. 8.33 Circumflex artery coursing superiorly to the great cardiac vein and ending as the obtuse marginal artery – *left view*. *a* atrial arteries, *b* aorta, *c* pulmonary trunk, *d* circumflex artery, *e* great cardiac vein, *f* obtuse margin, *g* obtuse marginal artery, *h* coronary sinus

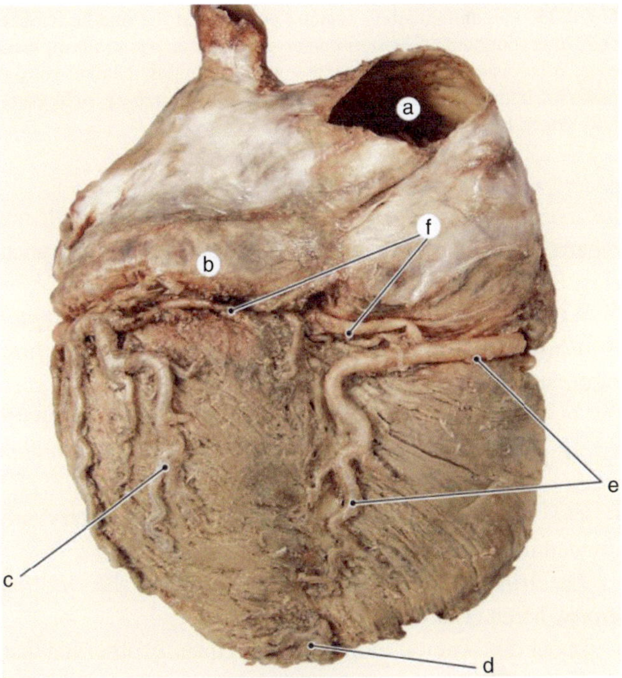

Fig. 8.34 Circumflex artery with an infravenous course, becoming a diagonal artery to the left ventricle in its distal segment. *a* inferior vena cava, *b* coronary sinus, *c* diaphragmatic artery of the left ventricle, *d* recurrent artery, *e* right coronary artery continuing as posterior interventricular artery, *f* arterial branches supplying the atrioventricular node

diagnosis. Angiographically this vessel will appear patent, thus making it possible for the angiographer to omit the obstruction of the posterior interventricular branch (whose thrombotic occlusion generated the infarction), and miss the chance of emergency recanalisation of the true posterior interventricular branch (Scandalakis).

An important ventricular branch is the *artery of the atrioventricular node* (*cf.*(*see*) *the vascularization of the atrioventricular node*), which courses below the right atrium and reaches the triangle of Koch. In our studies we have observed that in the proximity of the node, the artery makes a loop, anteriorly convex, and then courses further, sometimes to anastomose in the coronary sulcus with a branch of the circumflex branch. From the convex aspect of this loop emerge *2–3 short branches which penetrate the atrioventricular node.*

When the right coronary artery occupies the posterior interventricular sulcus it becomes *the posterior interventricular*

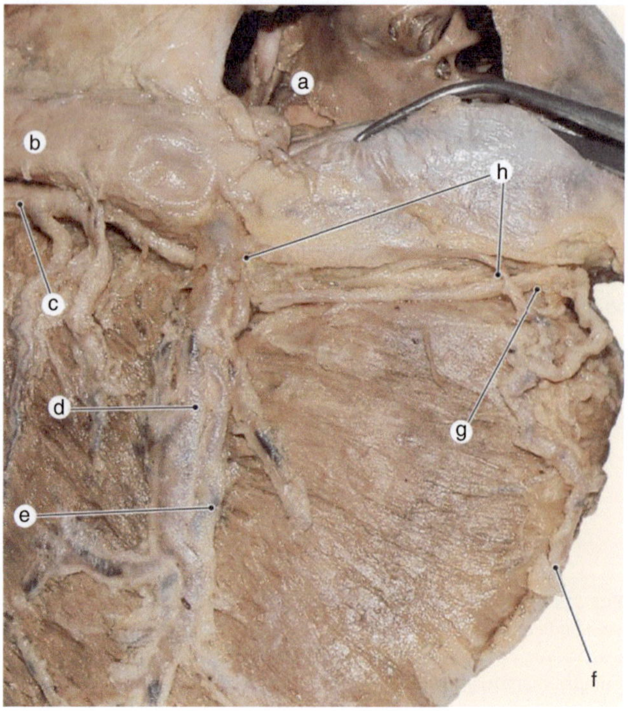

Fig. 8.35 Circumflex artery running posterior to the middle cardiac vein, then continuing as posterior interventricular artery. *a* inferior vena cava, *b* coronary sinus, *c* circumflex artery, *d* middle cardiac vein, *e* posterior interventricular artery, *f* acute marginal artery, *g* right coronary artery, *h* lesser cardiac vein

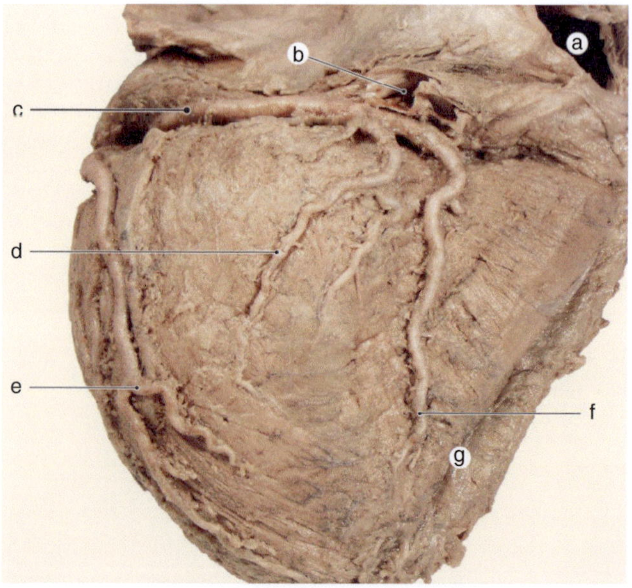

Fig. 8.36 Left dominance – posterior view of the heart. The circumflex artery has the branching, the course and the diameter necessary to sustain the left dominance, although it is not situated in the posterior interventricular sulcus. *a* inferior vena cava, *b* coronary sinus, *c* circumflex artery, *d* diaphragmatic artery of the left ventricle, *e* obtuse marginal artery, *f* diaphragmatic artery of the left ventricle, *g* posterior interventricular sulcus

(*posterior descending*) *branch*. It can anastomose with the recurrent artery and/or with branches of the circumflex branch (Fig. 8.9).

As already shown, it supplies the *posterior septal branches*. These arteries vascularize the diaphragmatic third of the septum and can anastomose with septal branches from the left coronary system. In some cases the right coronary artery ends with a *group of 2–3 posterior interventricular branches*.

The atrial branches of the right coronary artery are divided into *anterior, marginal and posterior groups*.

The artery of the sinoatrial node belongs to the *anterior group*. It can be *single or double*.

In our dissection studies we have frequently observed that the first artery emerging from the right coronary artery has a superior branch that anastomoses with the main artery of the sinoatrial node; then it descends into the interatrial septum and courses towards the atrioventricular node.

The second atrial branch is *the artery of the sinoatrial node*. It courses towards the ostium of the superior caval vein, in whose vicinity it makes a loop from which two branches emerge:

- one runs to the left of the superior caval ostium
- the second is the *true artery of the sinoatrial node*, reaches the sulcus terminalis and courses 1–3 cm through it.

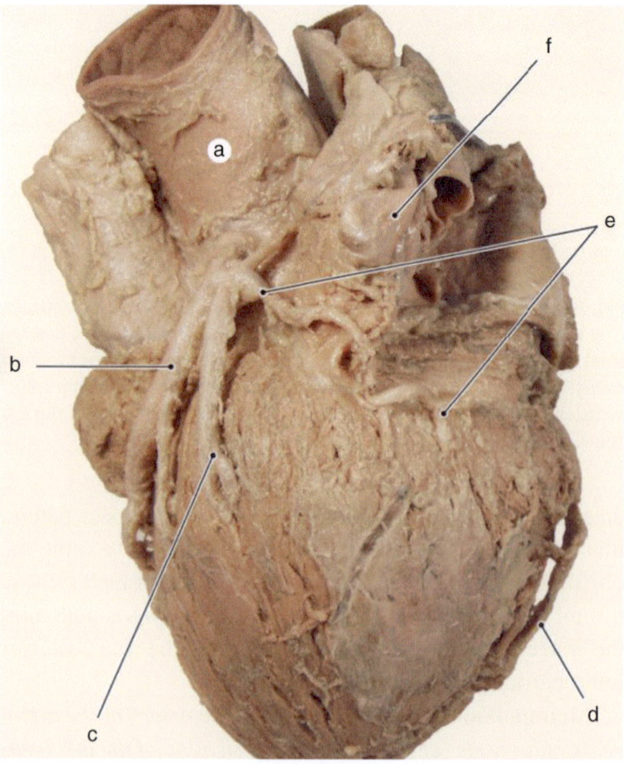

Fig. 8.37 Small circumflex artery. *a* aorta, *b* anterior interventricular artery, *c* diagonal left ventricular artery, *d* posterior interventricular artery (from the right coronary artery), *e* very small circumflex artery, *f* left auricle

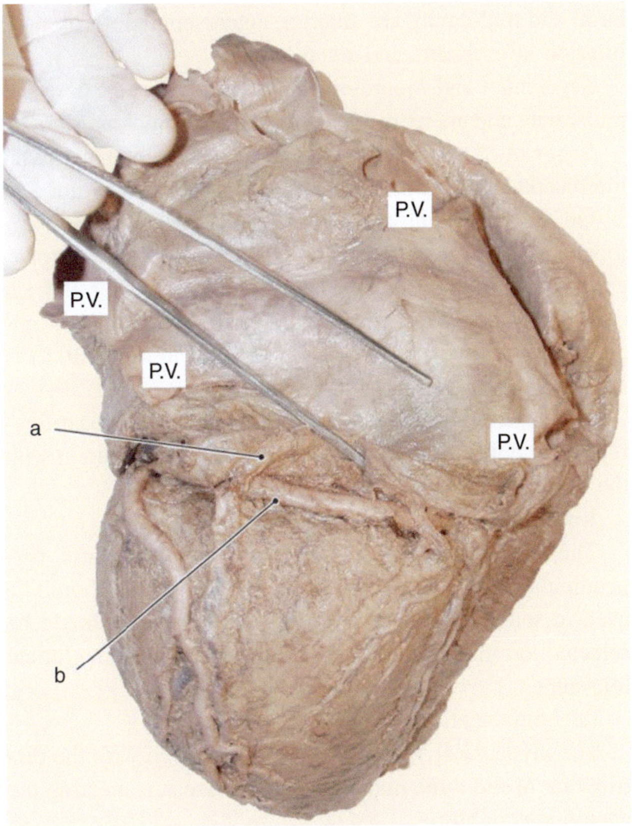

Fig. 8.38 Relation between the circumflex artery and the coronary sinus. *a* coronary sinus, *b* circumflex artery

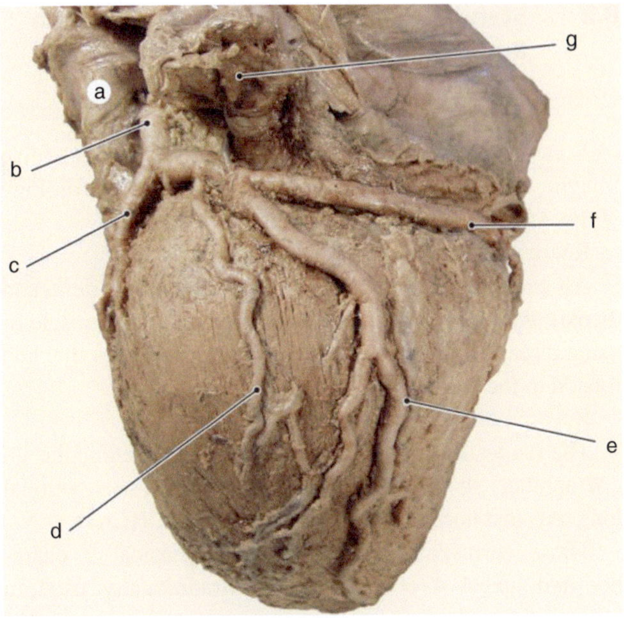

Fig. 8.39 Variant of circumflex artery with a long course, great caliber and large branches. These characteristics assure the left dominance. *a* aorta, *b* left coronary artery, *c* anterior interventricular artery, *d* obtuse marginal artery, *e* diaphragmatic left ventricular artery, *f* circumflex artery, *g* left auricle

After the emergence of these two branches, the main trunk of the artery vascularizes the Bachmann bundle.

The arteries of the right atrial appendage emerge after the artery of the sinus node.

There are few branches belonging to the *marginal and posterior groups* (*2–4*). They are small and penetrate the atrial wall after only a short course, and are somewhat difficult to dissect.

In some cases the atrial arteries can have an intracavitary course (Figs. 8.53 and 8.54).

Coronary arterial anomalies can be divided into three categories [4]:

- variations and anomalies without shunting (infra- or supernumerary coronaries, variations of the ostia, myocardial bridgings, hypoplasias, stenoses, atresias);
- anomalies with shunting (coronary fistulae and coronaries with abnormal origin in the pulmonary trunk);
- aneurysms (congenital or acquired).

8.2 Standardized Myocardial Segmentation and Nomenclature for Topographic Imaging of the Heart [5]

(A Statement for Healthcare Professionals From the Cardiac Imaging Committee of the Council on Clinical Cardiology of the American Heart Association)

Recommendation 1

All cardiac imaging modalities should define, orient, and display the heart using the long axis of the left ventricle or using three selected planes perpendicular on one another and related to the long axis.

Recommendation 2

The names of these three planes (each perpendicular on one another) should be according to the short axis, vertical long axis and horizontal long axis (SA, VLA, HLA).

These correspond to the short axis, apical 2 chamber and apical 4 chamber planes, traditionally used in echocardiography.

Recommendation 3

The heart should be divided into 17 segments for assessment of the myocardium and the left ventricular cavity.

The basal, middle (mid-cavity) and apical terms indicate the location of the segments on the long axis of the left ventricle. The circumferential locations of the segments in the basal and mid-cavity are anterior, anteroseptal, inferoseptal, inferior, inferolateral and anterolateral.

Segments 1 and 7 represent the anterior wall at the base and mid-cavity and arc named basal anterior and mid-anterior.

Segments 2 and 3 are named basal anteroseptal and basal inferoseptal and define the anterior and inferior septum.

On the same approach, segment 4 is basal inferior, segment 5 is basal inferolateral and segment 6 is basal anterolateral. The same terminology is used for segments 7 and 12. Continuing, segment 13 is apical anterior, segment 14 is apical septal, segment 15 is apical inferior and segment 16 is apical lateral. Segment 17 defines the apex.

Although the term posterior is still in use in echocardiography, for conformity it is recommended to substitute it with the term inferior.

Recommendation 4

The heart should be divided into three equal parts, perpendicular on the long axis. Anatomic landmarks should be used to select the slices, and the slice thickness should be selected on the basis of specific resolution and clinical relevance.

Recommendation 5

The myocardial segments can be correlated with the distribution of the three major coronary vessels, respecting the anatomic variability.

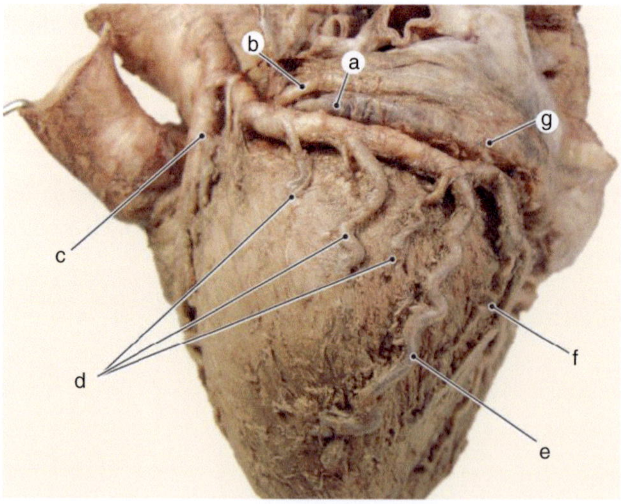

Fig. 8.40 A different branching pattern of the circumflex artery. The larger branches can be labeled OM1, OM2, OM3, etc. *a* great cardiac vein, *b* atrial artery, *c* anterior interventricular artery, *d* "raindrop-like" branches, *e* obtuse marginal artery, *f* diaphragmatic left ventricular artery, *g* coronary sinus

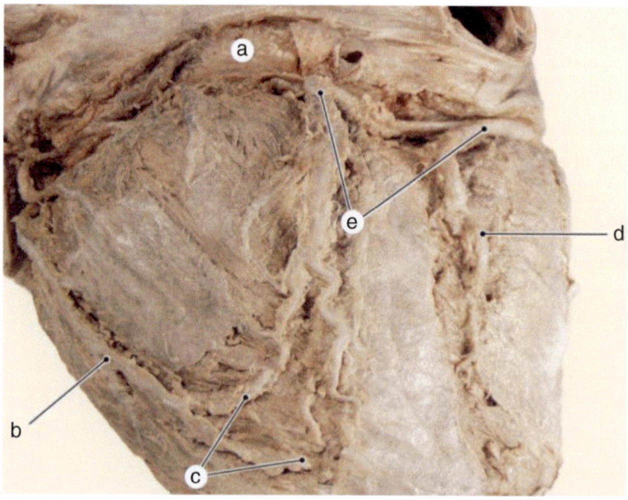

Fig. 8.41 A circumflex artery coursing up to the obtuse margin, where it anastomoses with a long, dominant right coronary artery. *a* coronary sinus, *b* circumflex artery, *c* anastomoses, *d* posterior interventricular artery, *e* the right coronary artery, reaching the obtuse margin as a diaphragmatic left ventricular artery

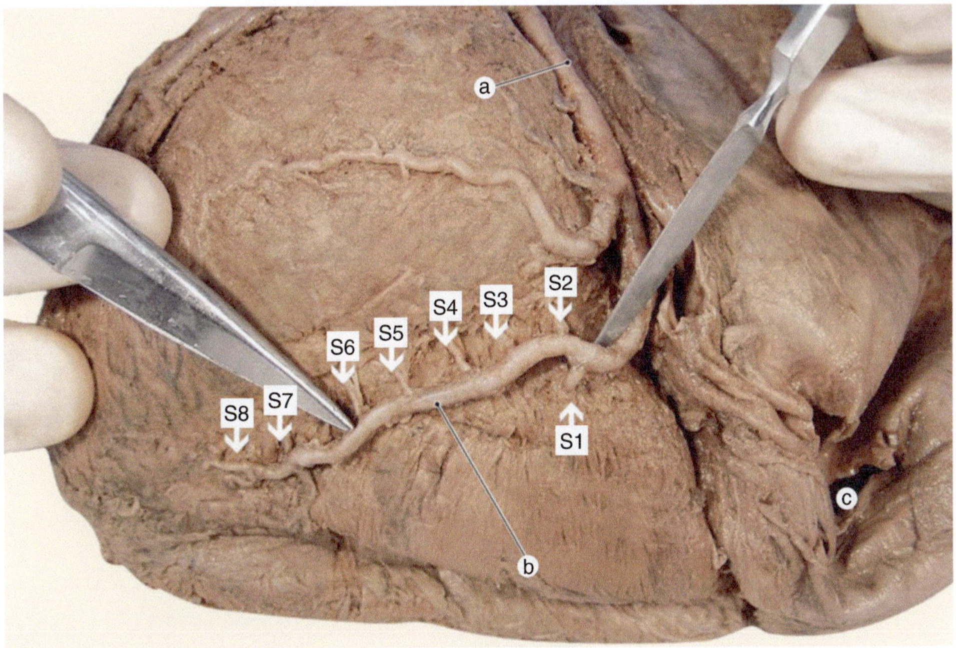

Fig. 8.42 The coronary artery reaching the posterior interventricular sulcus supplies it with septal arteries, thus becoming the dominant one. *a* circumflex artery, *b* posterior interventricular artery, *c* inferior vena cava

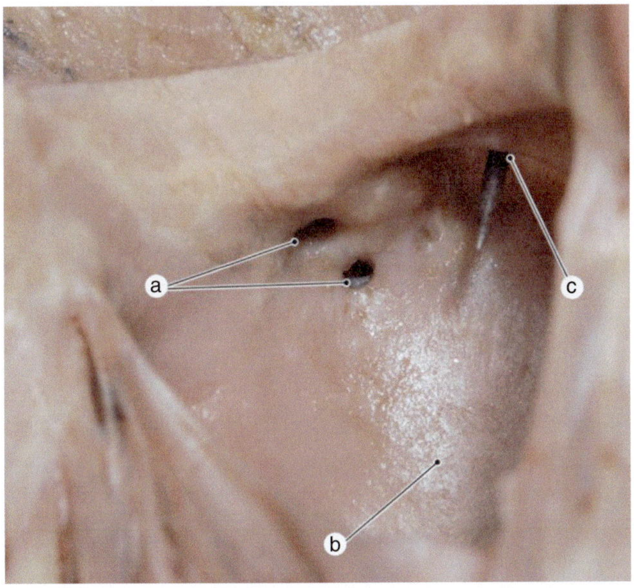

Fig. 8.43 The right coronary sinus, bounded superiorly by the supravalvular ridge. Inside the sinus a main coronary ostium and two accessory ostia are observed. *a* accessory coronary ostia, *b* right coronary sinus, *c* main coronary ostium

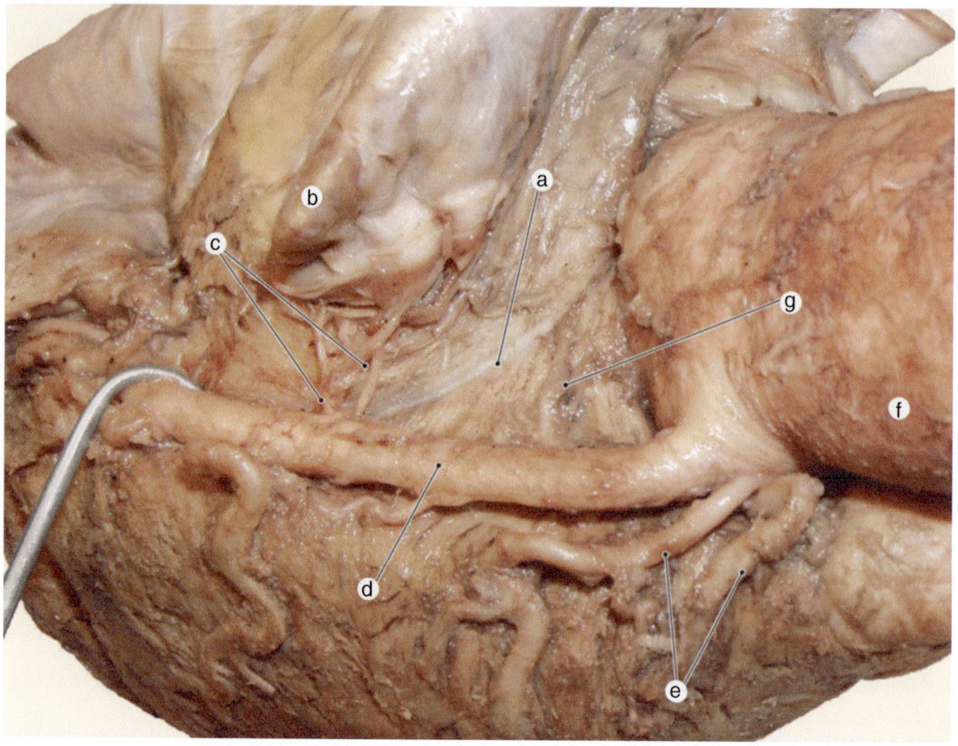

Fig. 8.44 The course, anatomical relations and branches of the right coronary artery at its origin. *a* fila coronaria, *b* auricle, *c* anterior atrial branches, *d* right coronary artery, *e* conal branches, *f* aorta, *g* atrioventricular nodal artery (variant from the origin of the right coronary artery)

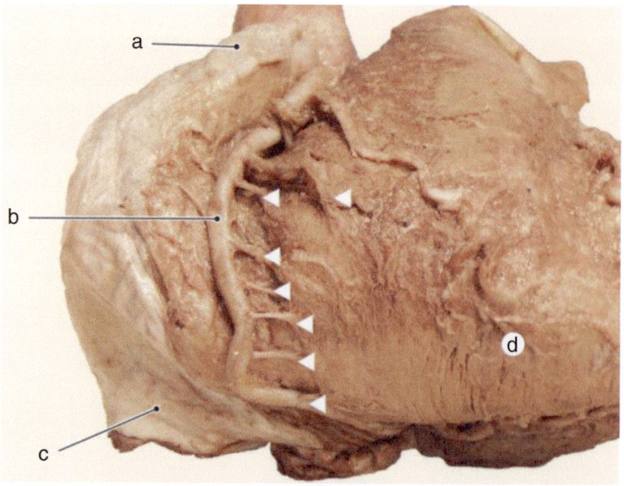

Fig. 8.45 Proximal half of the right coronary artery with "palisade" ventricular branches. *a* right auricle, *b* right coronary right, *c* inferior vena cava, *d* right margin

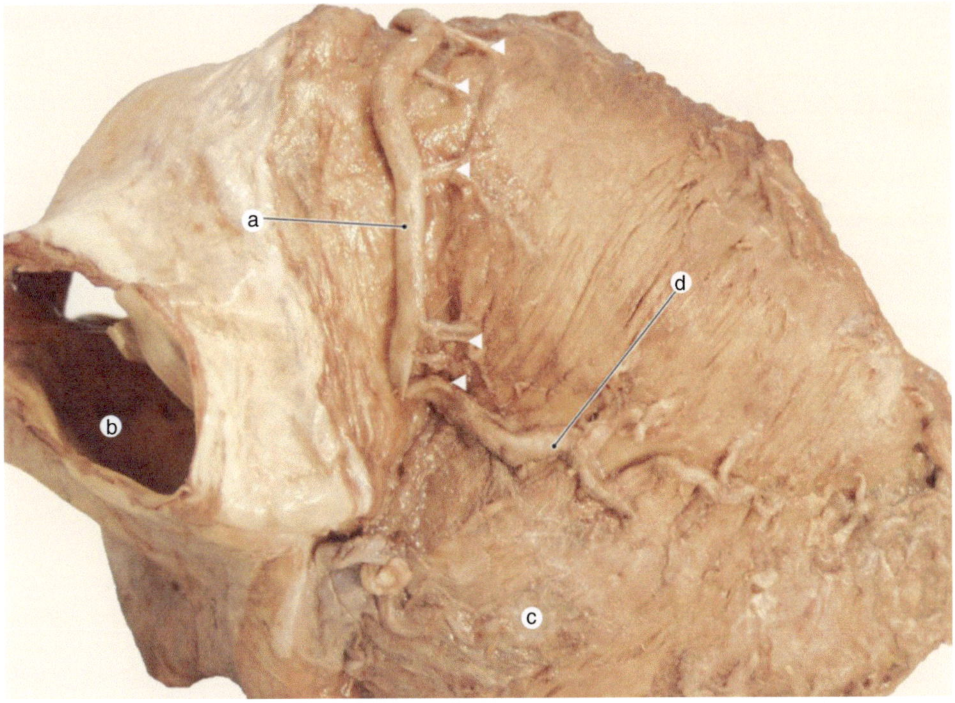

Fig. 8.46 Distal half of the right coronary artery with ventricular branches "in palisade". *a* right coronary artery, *b* inferior vena cava, *c* the diaphragmatic surface of the left ventricular, *d* posterior interventricular artery

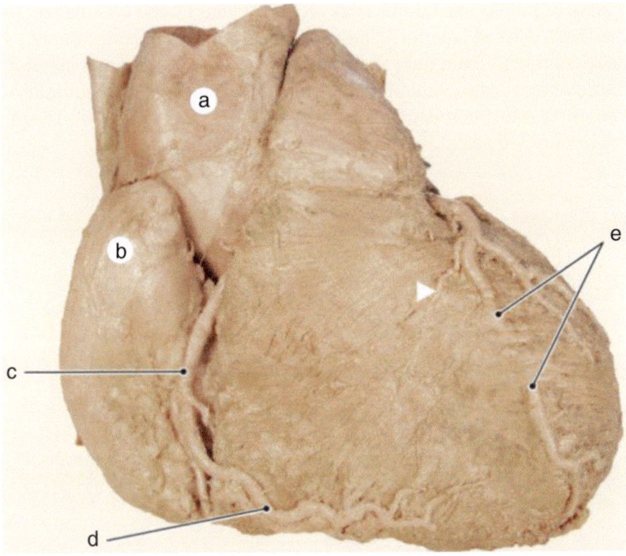

Fig 8.47 The right marginal artery reaches near the apex. The *arrow* indicates a right ventricular branch from the descending anterior artery. *a* aorta, *b* right auricle, *c* right coronary artery, *d* right marginal artery, *e* myocardial bridge over the anterior interventricular artery

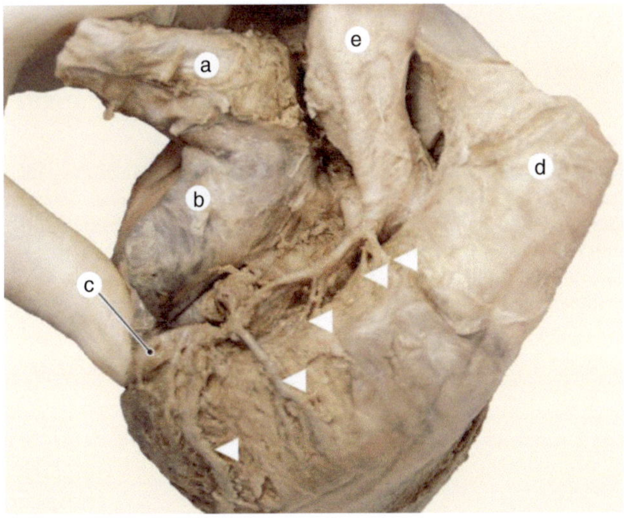

Fig. 8.48 *Arrows* indicate the sequence of conal arteries, branches of the right proximal coronary artery. *a* superior vena cava, *b* right auricle, *c* right coronary artery, *d* pulmonary trunk, *e* aorta

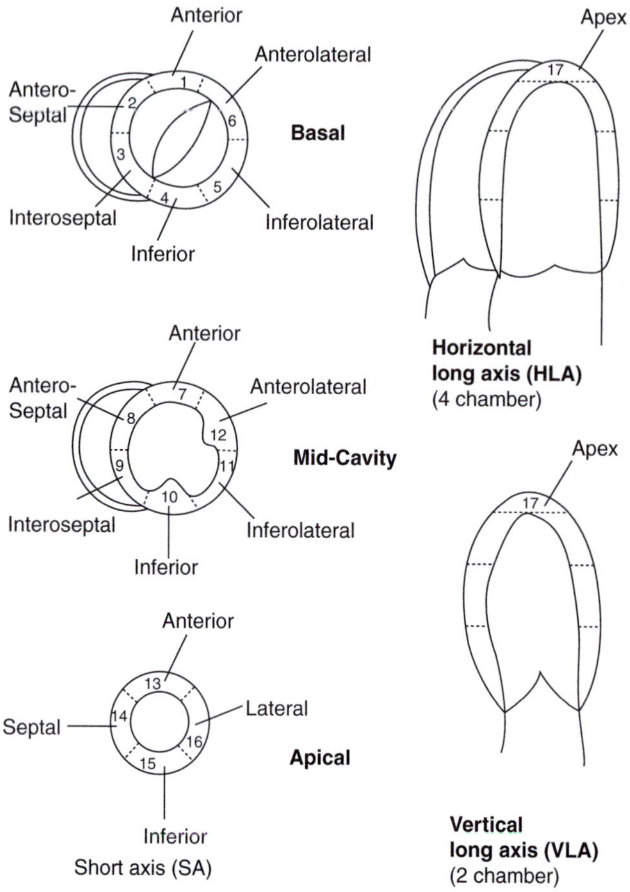

Chart 8.1 The diagram of the planes named long vertical axis, long horizontal axis and short axis. These charts indicate the names, location and anatomic landmarks of the segments in the basal (the edge of the mitral cusps), mid-cavity (papillary muscles) and apical regions (beyond the papillary muscles and before the end of the cavity). These landmarks are used in the 17 segments system

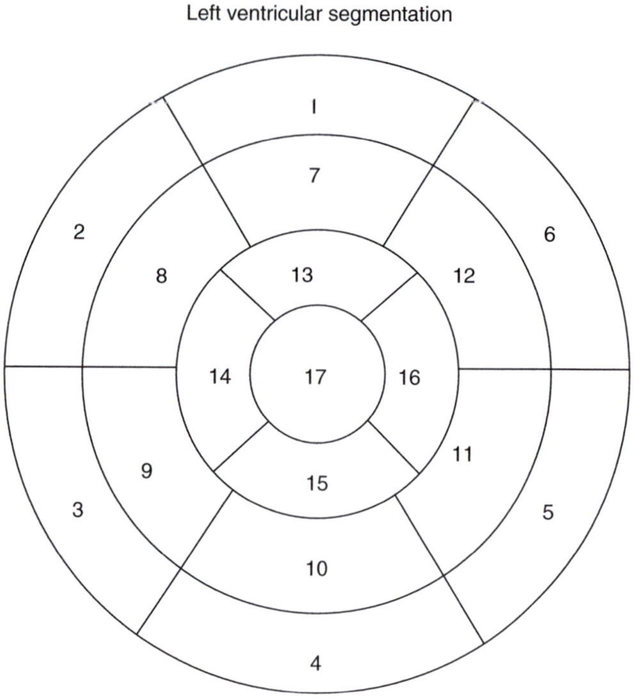

Chart 8.2 Circumferential plot (the bull's eye) displaying the 17 myocardial segments and terminology recommended for the CT imaging of the heart. *1* basal anterior, *2* basal anteroseptal, *3* basal inferoseptal, *4* basal inferior, *5* basal inferolateral, *6* basal anterolateral, *7* mid anterior, *8* mid anteroseptal, *9* mid inferoseptal, *10* mid inferior, *11* mid inferolateral, *12* mid anterolateral, *13* apical anterior, *14* apical septal, *15* apical inferior, *16* apical lateral, *17* apex

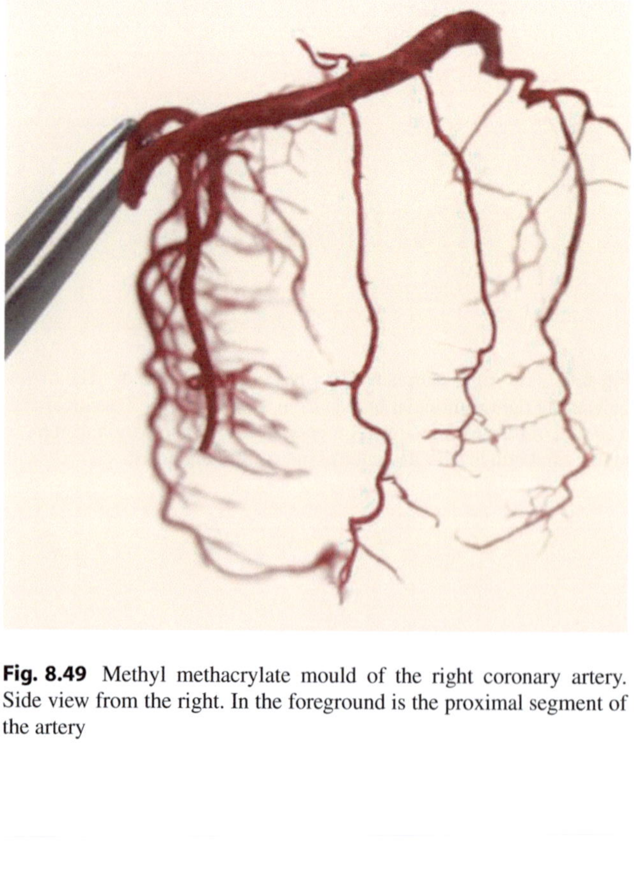

Fig. 8.49 Methyl methacrylate mould of the right coronary artery. Side view from the right. In the foreground is the proximal segment of the artery

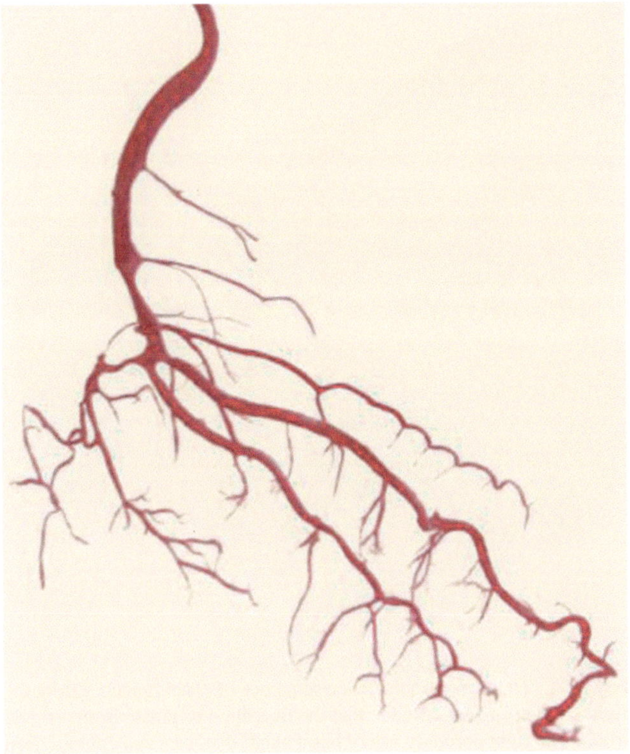

Fig. 8.50 Previous image detail with the terminal branches pattern of the posterior interventricular artery

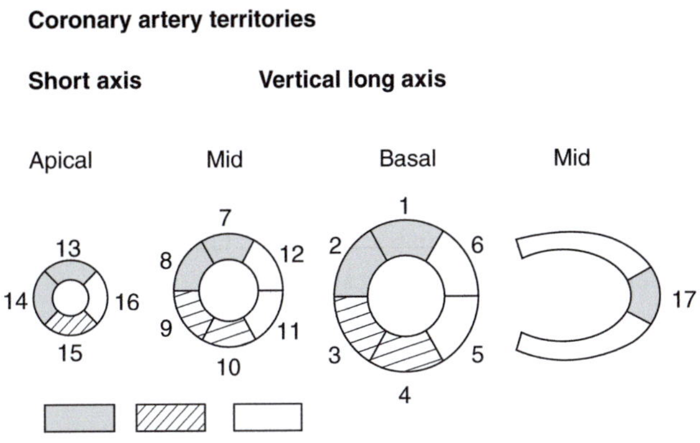

Chart 8.3 Assignment of the 17 myocardial segments to the distribution of the three major coronary vessels. Segment 17, which can be supplied by any of the three arteries, has the greatest variability of vascularization. Segments 1, 2, 7, 8, 13, 14, 17 are assigned to the anterior interventricular artery. Segments 3, 4, 9, 10, 15 are assigned to the right coronary artery when it is dominant. Segments 5, 6, 11, 12, 16 are assigned to the circumflex artery

8.3 The Cardiac Veins: General Considerations

As for the arterial territory, anatomic variability is a general rule. In the fetus heart, the intervenous anastomoses are better represented than the interarterial anastomoses.

They decrease in number after birth, but still remain better represented in the adult heart.

For the venous system there can be described anastomoses with extracardiac veins corresponding to the arteries (see) and with vasa vasorum of the large arteries.

Arteriovenous anastomoses exist and there also exist veins that open directly into cavities.

In general, collaterals of the main arteries are flanked by two veins. Usually for the large arteries there is a single corresponding vein.

The majority of the main veins have valves at their ostia.

The venous system of the heart is represented by the coronary sinus, great cardiac vein, middle cardiac vein, small cardiac vein, left marginal vein, posterior vein of the left ventricle, oblique vein of the left atrium, small cardiac veins and anterior cardiac veins.

The cardiac veins can be organized in the system of subepicardial veins and the thebessian veins.

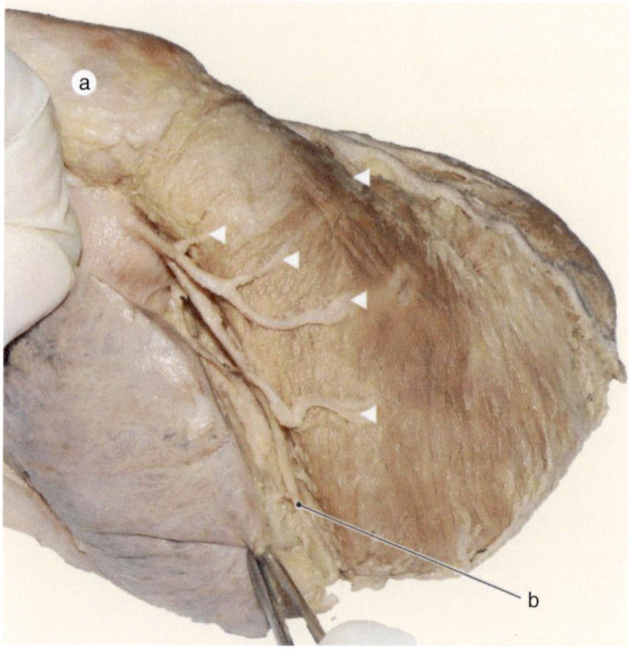

Fig. 8.51 The *arrows* indicate the sequence of conal branches from the right coronary artery . Notice that the first three originate from a single trunk. The right coronary artery has a small diameter and courses deep in the atrioventricular fold. *a* pulmonary trunk, *b* right coronary artery deep in the atrioventricular fold

8.3.1 The Coronay Sinus

The coronary sinus (see development) is the largest vein of the heart. The sinus has a variable diameter; it may be absent, unique or doubled.

The sinus wall may be covered by the myocardium in a variable degree, occasionally presenting muscular fascicles that realize electric connections between the atrial and ventricular myocardium as well as interatrial connections (see development). The fascicles are incriminated in the pathology of atrial and atrioventricular (aberrant) conduction.

The sinus is located in the left half of the coronary sulcus, subepicardial, on the diaphragmatic surface of the heart, superior to the circumflex artery which sometimes covers its branch for the atrioventricular node. In fact, the sinus begins in the lateral portion of the left coronary sulcus and ends in the right atrium. Its initial segment reaches the crux cordis, in a mass of adipose tissue. It then passes beneath the posteroinferior part of the interatrial septum, through the fold between the right atrium and the base of the right ventricle (the pyramidal space), in the depth of the dorsosinusal space (Figs. 8.56 and 8.57). In this space the sinus is accompanied by an important nervous branch from the cardiac plexus that heads to the terminal crest (see dorsosinusal space).

Finally, the sinus enters the right atrial wall and opens in its floor, at the level of the coronary sinus ostium, inferior to the

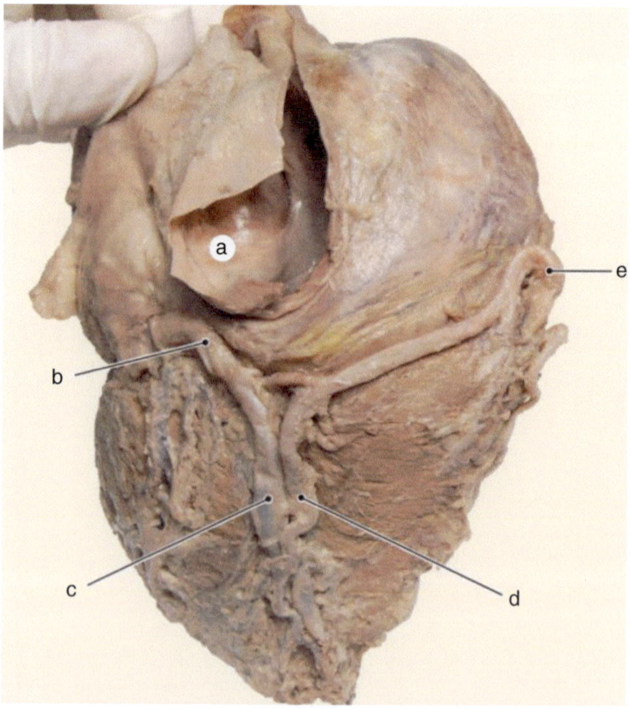

Fig. 8.52 Two posterior interventricular arteries with similar diameter, each of them giving out an artery for the atrioventricular node in the heart cross area, then descend together in the posterior interventricular sulcus. This pattern characterises the notion of codominance. *a* inferior vena cava, *b* circumflex artery, *c* posterior interventricular artery that continues the circumflex artery, *d* posterior interventricular artery that continues the right coronary artery, *e* right coronary artery

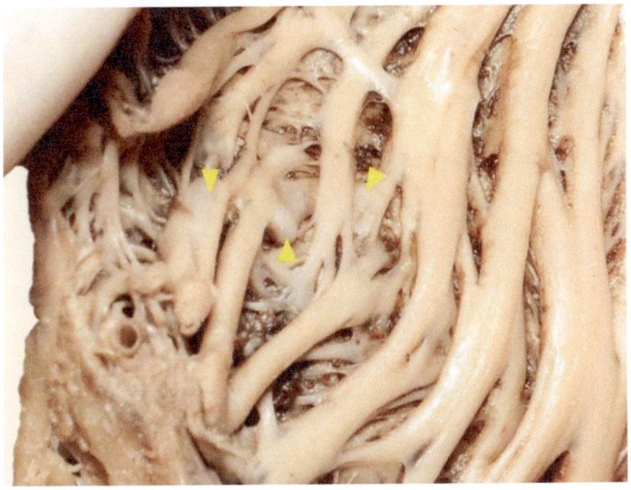

Fig. 8.53 A large caliber (*arrowheads*) artery that courses mostly intraluminal in the right atrial cavity. The artery could only be observed up to the upper part of the terminal creast. In this heart, the sinoatrial node artery could not be highlighted and we believe that the artery presented reached the node area

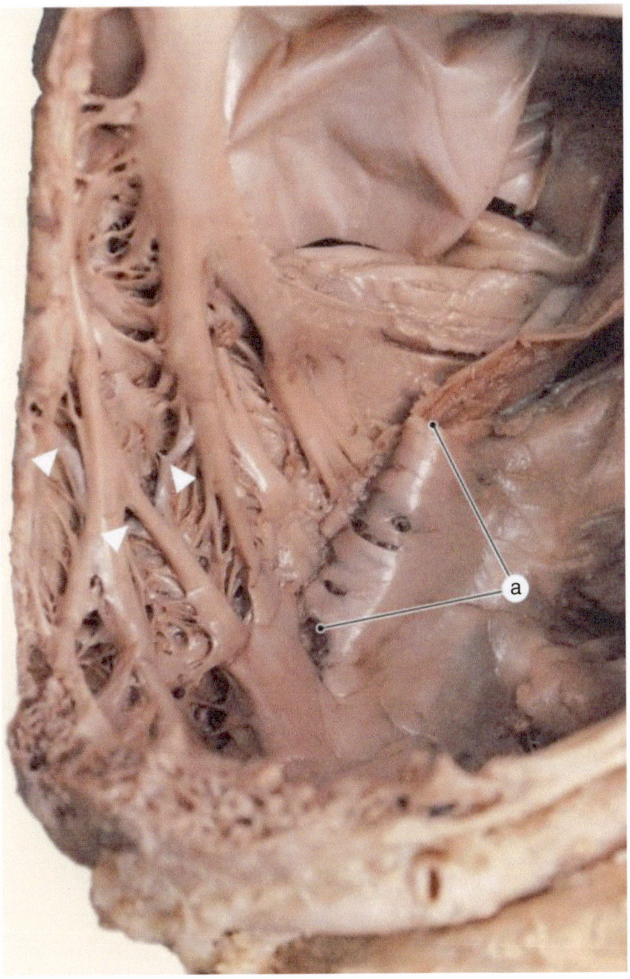

Fig. 8.54 Absolutely similar situation to the previous figure. The figure clearly shows how the artery ascends deep in the terminal creast. *a* deep venous canal in the thickness of the subauricular vestibule of the right atrium. The canal walls are fenestrated. *Arrowheads* - artery

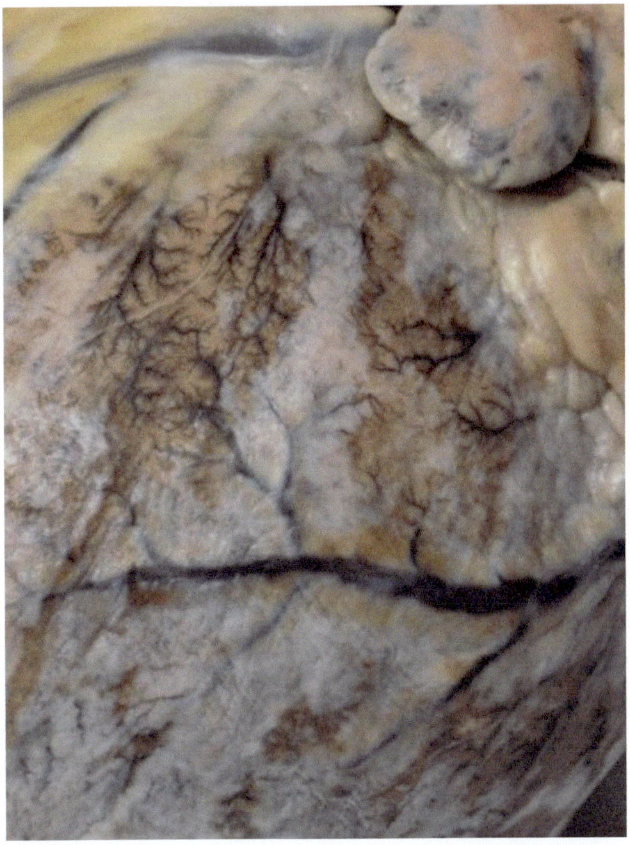

Fig. 8.55 Subepicardial intervenuous anastomosis in an adult heart, on the pulmonary surface. Detail

Eustachian ridge (Fig. 8.59). The diameter of the ostium varies widely, between 5 and 10 mm. The ostium is flanked on the right side by an incomplete semicircular valve named the valve of the coronary sinus ostium – Thebessius (see embryology). The valve may also be found on the left side of the ostium.

The characteristics of this valve became very important once catheterization of the sinus became clinical routine. In some instances, these anatomical characteristics may cause the maneuver to fail or may lead to complications.

The valve may be absent or may have a muscular or an endocardial network appearance. This endocardial network may be attached (or not) to a Chiari network and may bulge in the atrium or be retracted in the sinusal lumen.

Sometimes, the valve may have a fibromuscular aspect and/or be fenestrated. Regardless, the difference must be made between situations when the thebessian valve is an endocardial fold and the situations when this fold is absent and the ostium is limited by only a muscular flap of the atrial wall – a prolongation of the sinus septi.

Often, both structures exist and the sinus is limited by both a muscular and an endocardial flap.

The angle between the sinus ostium and the valve is important and also the degree of shielding which can vary between 0 and 90 %.

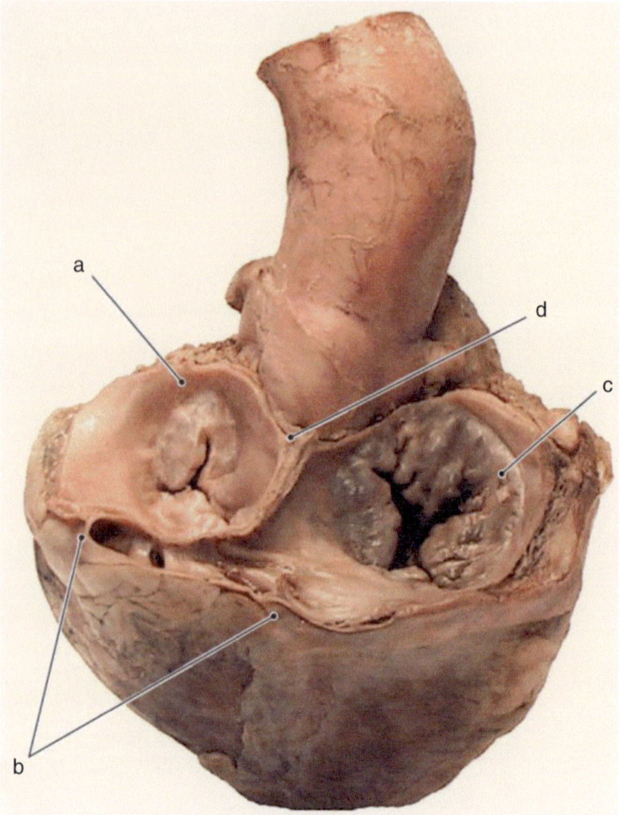

Fig. 8.56 Atria and sinus ceiling were removed. Posterior and superior view. The rear segment (lacking) of the interatrial septum overrides the coronary sinus. Sinus floor and right atrium floor mould the interventricular septum in the pyramidal area. *a* mitral valve, *b* coronary sinus (right atrium externalized), *c* tricuspid valve, *d* anterior superior part of the interatrial septum ("true" septum)

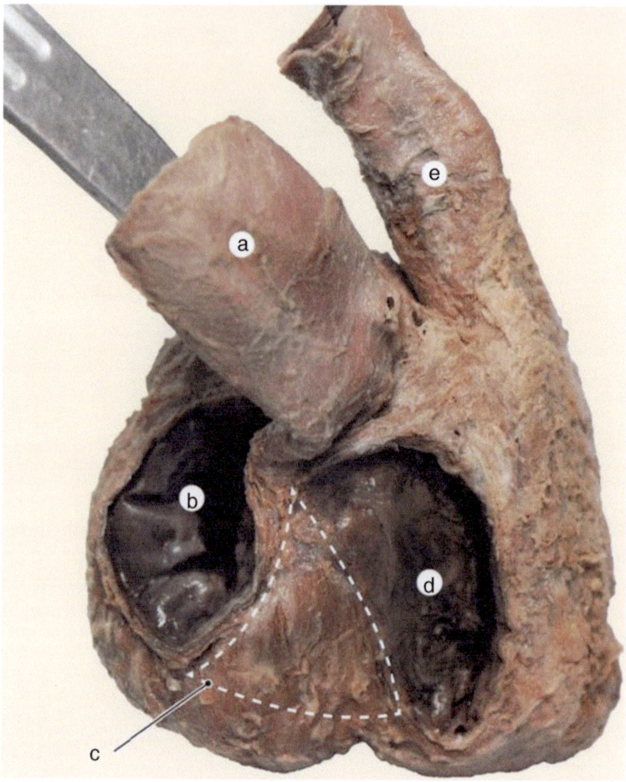

Fig. 8.57 After removing the atria and coronary sinus, the pyramidal space floor (*dotted area*) can be observed. Pyramidal space is contained in the crease of this surface – on one hand and the floor of the right atrium and coronary sinus – on the other hand. *a* aorta, *b* mitral valve, *c* pyramidal space projection, *d* tricuspid valve, *e* pulmonary trunk

- In its last part, the sinus presents all the features of the atrial wall. Adding to this its embryological development data, we understand why the sinus could be considered the "exteriorized right atrium".

  The sinus drains about two thirds of the coronary venous flow. At its origin, the sinus receives the great cardiac vein and the oblique vein of the left atrium. This last vein sometimes continues a fibrous cord named the ligament of Marshall which represents a remnant of the left superior vena cava (Fig. 8.58). The ligament of Marshall raises a pericardial fold (the triangular fold) frequently loaded with adipose tissue.
- The existence of this ligament (Marshall) is occasionally correlated with atrial electrophysiological disturbance. See figures between 2.52, 2.53, 2.54, 2.55 and 2.56.

  Practically, the opening of the oblique vein marks the origin of the coronary sinus. Usually the sinus has at its origin an incomplete valve. The middle and small cardiac veins open into the sinus at the crux cordis. In this region also, a better represented luminal valve exists (Vieussens) (Figs. 8.60 and 8.61).

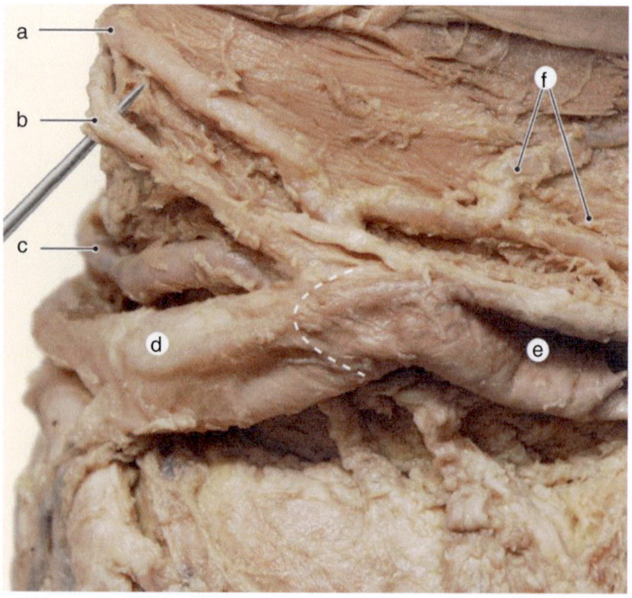

Fig. 8.58 Oblique vein of left atrium; coronary sinus limit (*dotted line*) and circumflex artery branching variant. *a* sinoatrial node artery, *b* oblique vein of left atrium, *c* circumflex artery, *d* great vein, *e* coronary sinus, *f* atrial branches

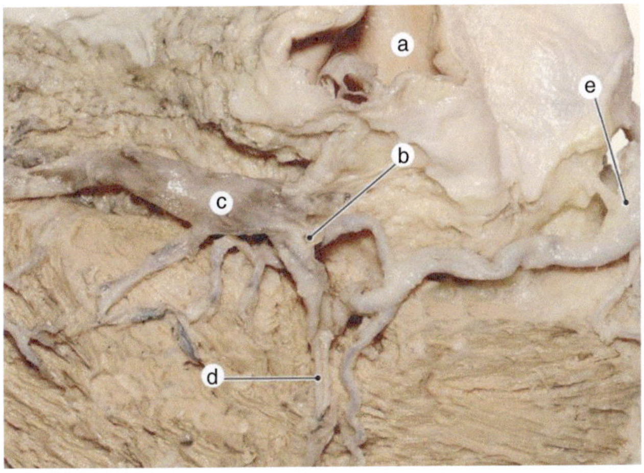

Fig. 8.59 Coronary sinus in the heart cross area and its tributaries. *a* inferior vena cava, *b* the drainage point of the lesser, *c* coronary sinus, *d* middle cardiac vein, *e* right coronary artery

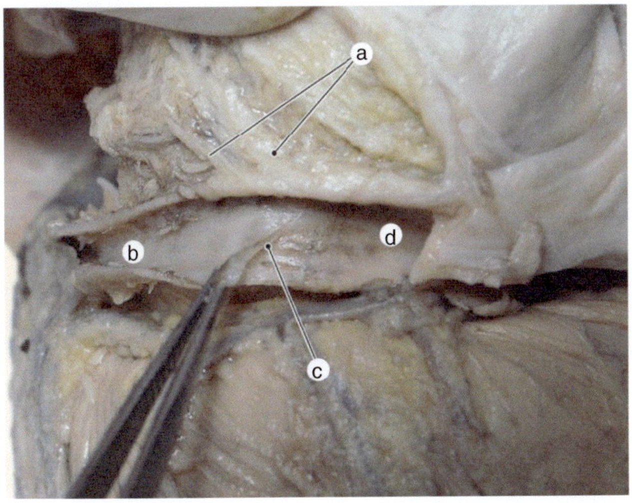

Fig. 8.60 Vieussens valvule on the lower wall and cardiac wall of the sinus. *a* sinoatrial muscle fibers, *b* great vein, *c* valve, *d* coronary sinus

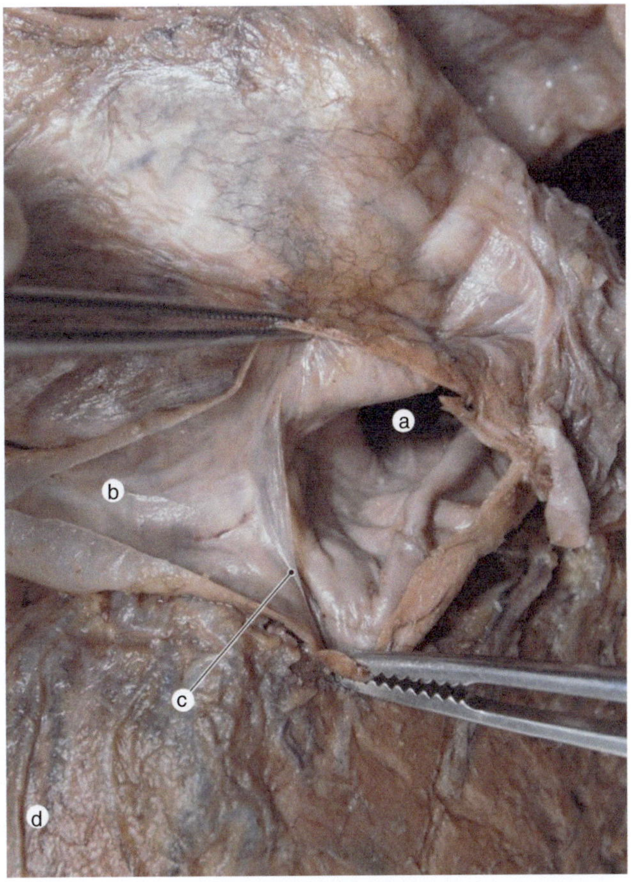

Fig. 8.61 Better represented Vieussens valve but with the same disposition as the previous. The tip of an intrasinusal catteter should follow the free wall so it would not remain trapped in the valvule. *a* ostium, *b* coronary sinus, *c* valvule, *d* diaphragmatic surface of the left ventricle

- The tip of an intrasinusal catheter may remain captive in the concavity of the valve of Vieussens.

  The posterior vein of the left ventricle ends in the middle third of the coronary sinus.

  Although traditionally, the coronary sinus is considered a simple venous conduct, recent observations of anatomy (including personal observations), embryology and electrophysiology demonstrate that in its last segment, the coronary sinus can be considered a prolongation of the right atrium. In other words, the coronary sinus is the exteriorized right atrium. And this because, just like the right atrium, the sinus has endocardium, myocardium (variable), and this myocardium, when present, has conduction proprieties (normal and abnormal) just like the myocardium of the right atrium [6].
- According to echocardiographic standards, the tributaries of the coronary sinus that drain the lateral wall are named marginal veins: anterolateral marginal vein, lateral marginal vein, inferolateral marginal vein (the term posterior is not accepted by echocardiographic standards, but this last vein may also be named the posterolateral marginal vein) [7].

8.3.2 The Tributary Veins of the Coronary Sinus

The great vein of the heart begins in the apex region, sometimes doubling the course of the recurrent artery. It ascends in the posterior interventricular sulcus, having a variable relation with the anterior descending artery (Fig. 8.62). It passes over the branches of the left coronary artery, enters the coronary sulcus in its left half and ends (possibly without an apparent limit) in the left extremity of the coronary sinus (Figs. 8.63 and 8.64).

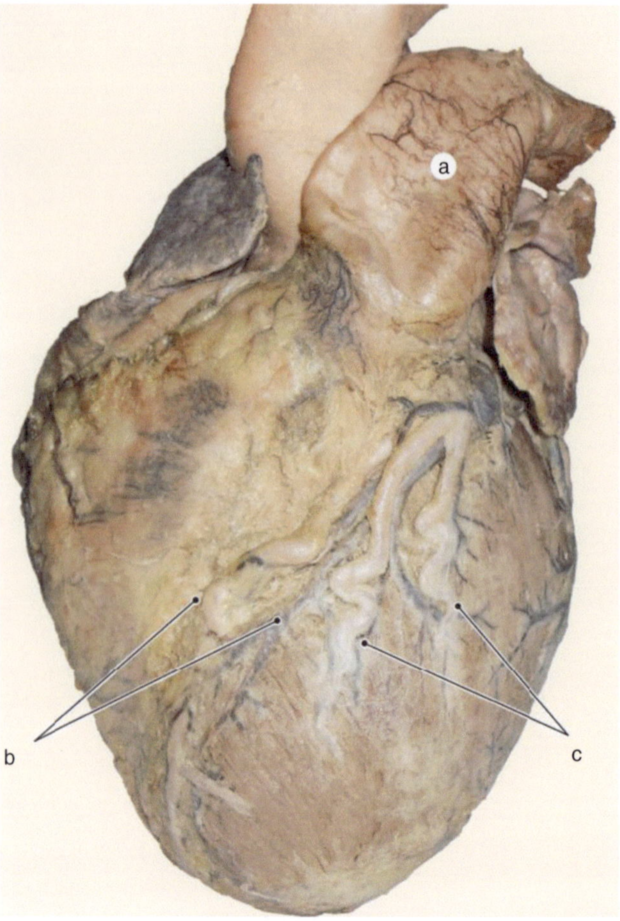

Fig. 8.62 Anatomical relations of the anterior interventricular vein. *a* pulmonary trunk, *b* interventricular anterior vein and artery, *c* diagonal arteries and veins

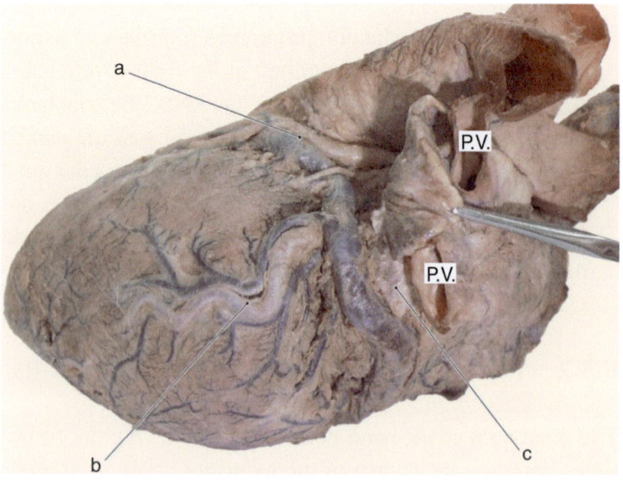

Fig. 8.63 Anatomical relations of the great vein. The left auricle is clamped. *a* great vein, *b* arteries and veins of the obtuse margin, *c* circumflex artery

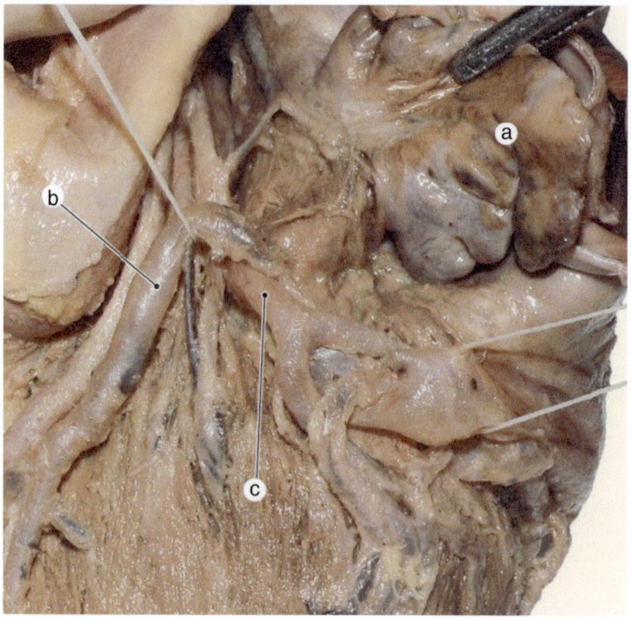

Fig. 8.64 The great vein has spiroid course (between traction wires) around the circumflex artery. In this situation it can not be catheterised. *a* left auricle, *b* great vein, *c* circumflex artery

Sometimes it receives a distinct vein of the obtuse margin (the left marginal vein). This vein occasionally ends directly in the coronary sinus. It drains the surrounding territories (Fig. 8.65).

- In imagistic studies mostly, the following terminology is used: the anterior interventricular vein continues as the great vein (the part between the anterior interventricular sulcus and the origin of the coronary sinus) [8].

The middle vein of the heart occupies the posterior interventricular sulcus. It is also called the posterior interventricular vein. An anastomosis between the middle and great veins of the heart can be found at the apex. It ends in the coronary sinus, near the crux cordis (Figs. 4.22, 4.23, 4.24 and 8.55).

The small vein of the heart (inconstant) is found in the right side of the coronary sulcus. At times, this vein continues in fact the right marginal vein that enters the right coronary sulcus on the acute margin, reaches the diaphragmatic surface of the heart and ends in the coronary sinus (Figs. 8.35 and 8.72). Obviously in this case the small vein doesn't exist in the anterior half of the coronary sulcus. This region is dominated by anterior veins.

Other times, the small vein begins in the coronary sulcus or in its proximity, near the right margin of the heart. Against expectations, it heads anteriorly, perforates the right atrial wall and ends in a deep venous canal in the subauricular vestibule structure of the right atrium. This also opens in the right atrium through an orifice surrounded by a pseudo-valve.

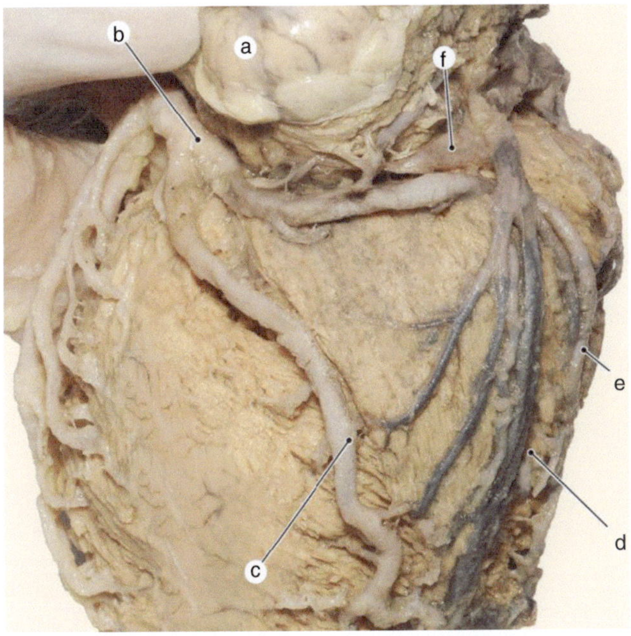

Fig 8.65 Group of veins that drain in a single trunk the diaphragmatic surface and the obtuse margin of the left ventricle. *a* left auricle, *b* circumflex artery, *c* artery of the obtuse margin, *d* veins for the diaphragmatic surface of the left ventricle, *e* diaphragmatic artery of the left ventricle, *f* venous sinus

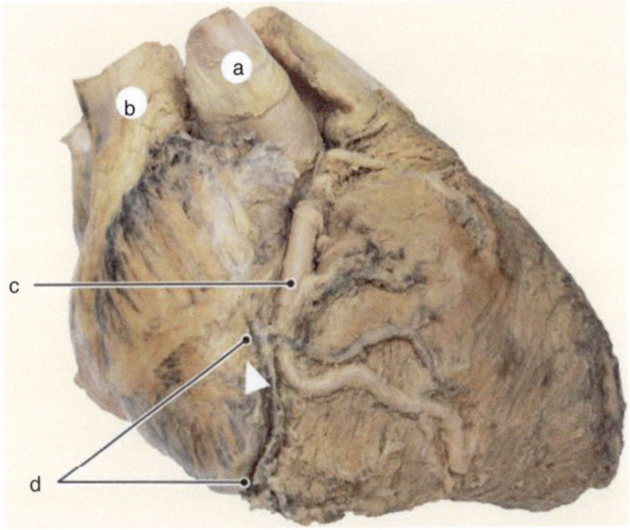

Fig. 8.66 Lesser coronary vein variant that drains the diaphragmatic surface and the right margin, receiving an anterior vein, then drains into a deep venous canal in the right atrium. The *arrow* shows the inverted drainage manner compared to the case when this vein would drain into the coronary sinus. *a* aorta, *b* superior vena cava, *c* right coronary artery, *d* lesser vein

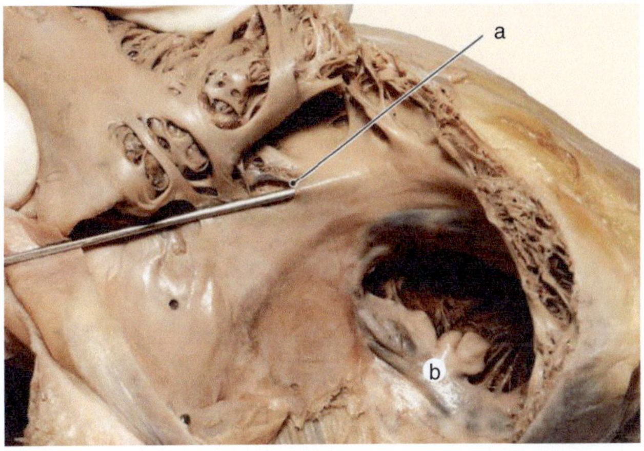

Fig. 8.67 The needle is inserted through the drainage oriffice of a deep venous canal from the subauricular vestibule of the right atrium. *a* deep venous canal ostium in the subauricular vestibule, *b* tricuspid valve

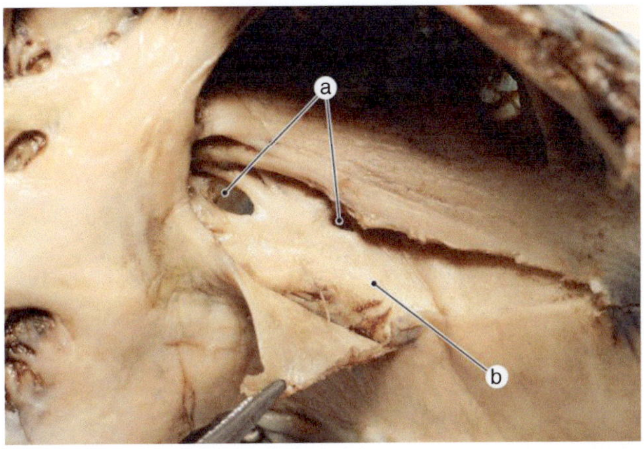

Fig. 8.68 Highlighting of the deep venous canal and anterior veins oriffices that drain into it. *a* anterior veins oriffices, *b* deep venous canal

When a venous canal like this exists (in 30–50 % of cases), it also receives the anterior veins of the heart (Figs. 8.66, 8.67 and 8.68). This deep venous canal has been described for the first time by our team.

The oblique vein of the left atrium has its origin on the posterior surface of the left atrium in the proximity of the end of the superior left pulmonary vein, where it continues inferiorly a fibrous cord called the ligament of Marshall (a remnant of the left superior vena cava). This ligament raises a pericardial fold named the left superior vena cava (triangular) fold (Marshall). The oblique vein ends in the coronary sinus (Figs. 4.17, 2.52, 2.53, 2.54, 2.55 and 2.56).

The posterior vein of the left ventricle, like the name says, is the greatest vein on the diaphragmatic surface of the left ventricle. It ends in the coronary sinus (Fig. 4.23).

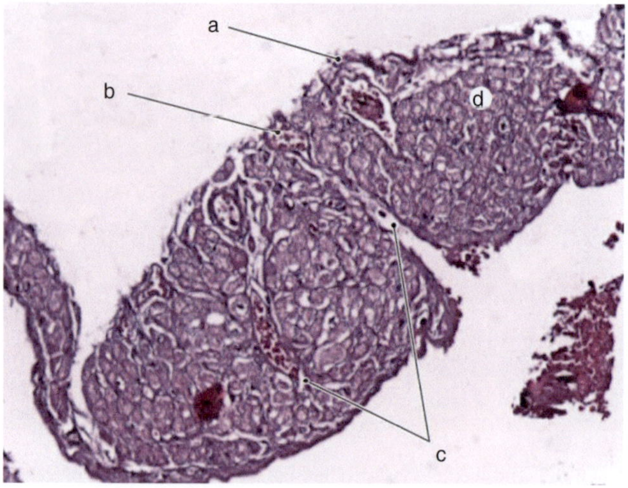

Fig. 8.69 Venous-cavitary anastomosis (thebessian vein) between a subepicardial vein and the right atrial cavity. *a* epicardium, *b* subepicardial vein, *c* Thebessian vein, *d* atrial myocardium

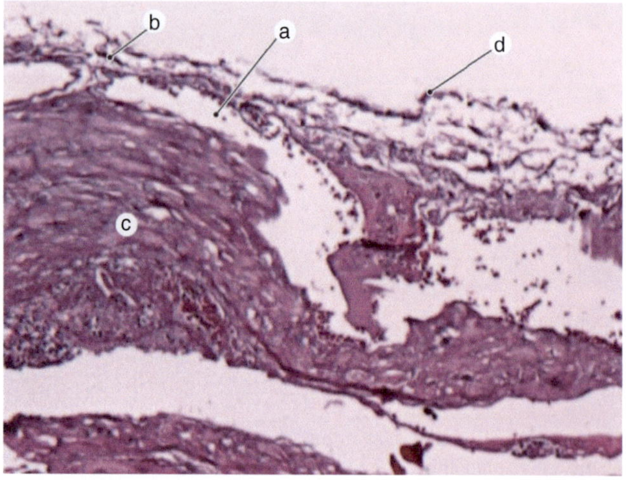

Fig. 8.70 Subepicardial vein with antireflux valvules. *a* subepicardial vein, *b* valvules, *c* atrial myocardium, *d* epicardium

8.3.3 The Veins That Don't Drain into the Coronary Sinus

There are veins that don't drain in the coronary sinus. These are the anterior and small veins.

The system of small vessels (veins), described for the first time by Viessens and Thebessius in the seventeenth century (vasa cordis minima), "the thebessian system" in clinical culture, is formed by the following types of vessels (Martin Rothman and Wearn) [6, 9, 10].

- veins that drain a network of capillaries from the ventricular wall and end directly in the ventricular lumen;
- veins that drain directly an artery and end directly in the ventricular lumen. Clearly, these veins don't drain a network of capillaries, being the equivalent of an arterioluminal anastomosis (of large caliber);

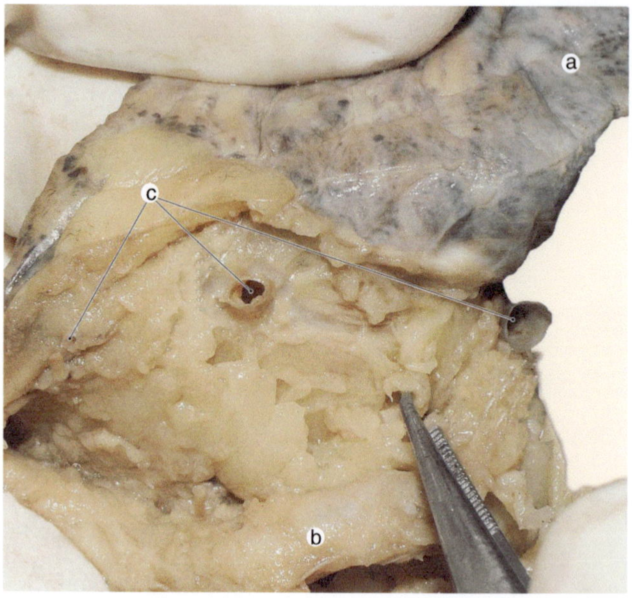

Fig. 8.71 Anterior veins that drain into the deep venous canal in the right atrium. Right coronary artery was partially removed from the coronary sulcus. Right anterior and lateral view. *a* right auricle, *b* right coronary artery, *c* ostiums of anterior veins, opening in the deep venous canal

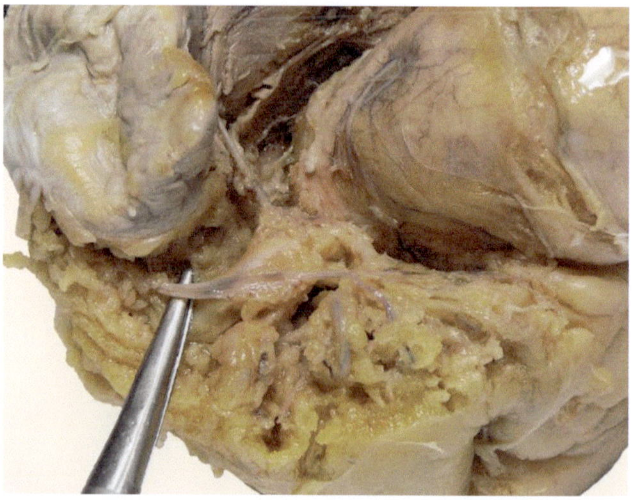

Fig. 8.72 Lesser coronary vein draining the conal territory up to the acute edge

- veins that in fact are venous shunts on the route of subepicardial veins. These veins unite a subepicardial vein with the lumen of a cavity. They practically form venoluminal anastomoses and represent the majority of the thebessians vessels (Figs. 8.69, 8.70 and 8.71).
  - The system of small veins is very compliant. Although, under normal conditions, it drains approximately 10 % of the venous return, in case of the obstruction of the subepicardial veins, it may overtake the majority of the surplus venous flow.

The anterior veins of the heart drain the venous blood of the sternocostal surface of the right ventricle and end in the small vein of the heart or (mostly) in the right atrium by larger orifices named foramina.

The largest of these veins is the right marginal vein (inconstant) that ends in the right atrium.

The opening orifices of the small veins in the cavities are named foraminules.

The distribution of the thebessian vessels ostia is remarkably varied. These are found predominantly in the ventricles rather than in the atria, the majority of them being situated around the bases of the papillary muscles and in the vicinity of the apex.

There are cases when after progressive blockage of the ostia of the two coronary arteries (syphilitic gummas) the patients survived a long period of time. In these cases, the plausible explanation consists in the existence and adaptation of the thebessian vessels by the dilation of the arterio-luminal anastomoses.

- The principle of myocardial revascularization by creating conduits in the ventricular wall using laser fascicles was truly based on the existence of the thebessian vessels. The technique wasn't successful neither in incrementing the myocardial perfusion nor in the creation of anastomoses between the ventricular cavities and the endomyocardial vessels [10].

We wish to call attention to an evocative experiment, the presence of blood flow in the coronary sinus after the simultaneous ligation of the coronary vessels [11]. The results of this experiment highlights the importance of collateral myocardial vascularization, especially during severe ischemia.

8.4 Lymphatics of the Heart

In the heart, a wide lymphatic network exists, different territories being interconnected by anastomoses. Traditionally, a subendocardial lymphatic plexus, an intramyocardial plexus and a subepicardial plexus are described. The lymphatic drainage is from the endocardium towards the epicardium.

Like with any major organ, the great veins are followed by two to three lymphatic collecting trunks. The drainage for the right heart as for the left are quite individualized. On the left side, the collecting trunks are reunited between the pulmonary trunk and left auricle and drain into an inferior tracheobronchial node.

On the right side, the collecting trunks are reunited anterior to the aorta and end in a node in the anterior mediastinum or a brachiocephalic node.

Rainer described subepicardial intermediary nodes [12], located posterior to the pulmonary trunk, anterior to the aorta and between the pulmonary veins (Fig. 8.73). We have noted the enlargement of a subepicardial node located in the left half of the coronary sulcus. We found no entries regarding this subject in specialty literature (Fig. 2.53)

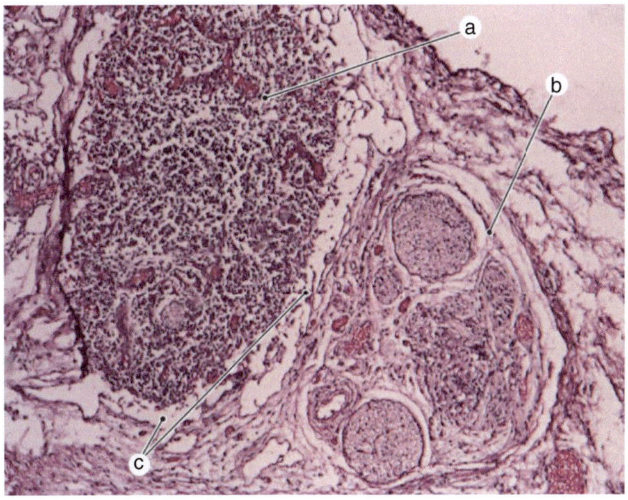

Fig. 8.73 Subepicardial lymph node surrounded by lymph vessels and in relation with a vasculonervous bundle. *a* subepicardial ganglion, *b* subepicardial vasculonervous bundle, *c* lymphatic vessels

References

1. Angelini P. Questions on coronary fistulae and microfistulae. Tex Heart Inst J. 2005;32(1):53–5.
2. Crainicianu A. Anatomische studien über die coronaraterienund experimentelle untersuchungen über die durchgängigkeit. Virchows Arch Path Anat. 1922;238:1–75.
3. Nerantzis CE, Marianou SK, Koulouris SN, Agapitos EB, Papaioannou JA, Vlahos LJ. An anatomical and angiographic study using a new technique. Tex Heart Inst J. 2004;31(3):267–70.
4. David M. Normal coronary anatomy and anatomic variations. Appl Radiol. 2007;(36 Supp 1):14–26.
5. Cerqueira MD, Weissman NJ, Dilsizian V, Jacobs AK, Kaul S, Laskey WK, Pennell DJ, Rumberger JA, Ryan T, Verani M. Standardized myocardial segmentation and nomenclature for tomographic imaging of the heart. J Nucl Cardiol. 2011;9(2):240–5.
6. Rothman MT. An alternative route of access to the myocardium: coronary venous system. J Invasive Cardiol. 2006;18(11):563–8.
7. Von Lüdinghausen M. The venous drainage of the human myocardium. Adv Anat Embryol Cell Biol. 2003;168:I–VIII, 1–104.
8. Van de Veire NR, Schuijf JD, De Sutter J, Devos D, Bleeker GB, De Roos A, Van der Wall EE, Schalij MJ, Bax JJ. Non-invasive visualization of the cardiac venous system in coronary artery disease patients using 64–slice computed tomography. J Am Coll Cardiol. 2006;48:1832–8.
9. Wearn JT. The role of the thebesian vessels in the circulation of the heart. J Exp Med. 1928;47:293–315.
10. Moosdorf R, Rybinski L, Hoffken H, Funck RC, Maisch B. Transmyocardial laser revascularization in stable and unstable angina pectoris. Herz. 1997;22:198–204.
11. Toumanidis ST, Papadopoulou S, Tsirikos N, Demestiha TD, Trika CO, Kottis G, Moulopoulos SD. Preservation of coronary sinus flow after complete ligation of all coronary arteries. Hellenic J Cardiol. 2007;48:319–24.
12. Rainer Francisc J. Le systéme lymphatique du coeur. Étude d`anatomie comparée. Ann Biol (Paris). 1911;1:60–89.

The Extrinsic Innervation of the Heart

9

9.1 Cardiac Pain: Anatomical and Clinical Considerations

Both vegetative systems, sympathetic and parasympathetic, participate in the extrinsic innervation of the heart, this being both *motor and sensitive*.

Before commencing, some comments are mandatory:

- *Low pressure baroreceptors* exist in the atrial wall. These receptors are part of a system of receptors of low pressure that can also be found in *the venous network* and are involved mainly in the *control of blood volume*. Stimulation of these receptors has both renal and vascular effects.

  If the low pressure receptors are denervated, the false impression of low blood volume is induced and the regulating mechanisms of fluid retention and rise of blood pressure are activated.
- *Receptors for pain* (*free nerve endings*) are infrequent in the working myocardium and numerous in the **endocardium**, and even more in the **epicardium**. They are also present in the **arterial and periarterial wall**. As a consequence, damage to the territories with large numbers of receptors is more painful than damage to the territories with lesser receptors.
- *Cardiac pain – referred pain*: one of the rules of development is metamerism. In principle, the development of the body is segmentary. One segment called metamer is correlated with a *viscerotome* (the viscera with origin in this metamer), a *neurotome* (the nerves of the metamer), a *myomer* (the muscles derived from that segment) and a *dermatome* (a cutaneous segment innervated by the spinal nerve of the metamer).

Without a doubt, during development *fusions occur that don't permit to follow the exact metameric origin* but as a principle, the metamer and the viscerotome derived from it have the same number and that is the number of the corresponding spinal nerve.

In the case of cardiac pain we are used to say that the pain migrates in the territories clinically known. In reality, it's about **the referred pain** *in the dermatome with the same number as the viscerotome and the respective neurotome* [1]. The viscerotomes that participate in the development of the heart are from C2 to T4.

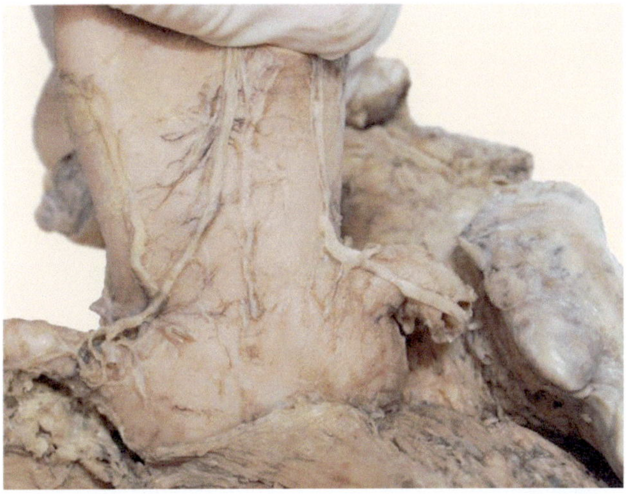

Fig. 9.1 The superficial component of the cardiac nerve plexus on the anterior aspect of the ascending aorta

The cubital side of the upper limb belongs to the C8–T1 dermatome, the anterolateral aspect of the neck belongs to the C2 dermatome and the precordial and scapular regions belong to the T1–T4 dermatomes.

We state that the vegetative sensitive fibers of cardiac origin have two ascending pathways: some are *reticulospinothalamic* and some join the *specific spinothalamic fibers* that also conduct cutaneous impulses.

This being said, *the explanations of the referred pain* are not unitary but evocative:

- *The convergence phenomenon in the spinothalamic pathway* (10/1 convergence of the peripheral fibers to a spinothalamic fibers). Following the common ascending pathway, nociceptive cardiac impulses are transmitted as belonging to a cutaneous territory.
- *Influx irradiation* from the low myelinated or non-myelinated visceral sensitive fibers into surrounding

F.M. Filipoiu, *Atlas of Heart Anatomy and Development*,
DOI 10.1007/978-1-4471-5382-5_9, © Springer-Verlag London 2014

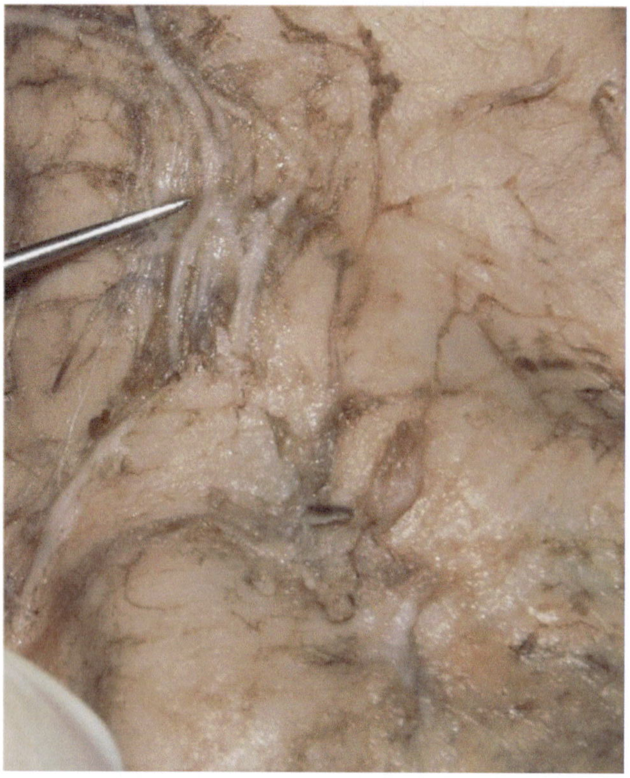

Fig. 9.2 The needle indicates a small prominance on the periaortic nervous course, which is actually a juxtavisceral nervous ganglion

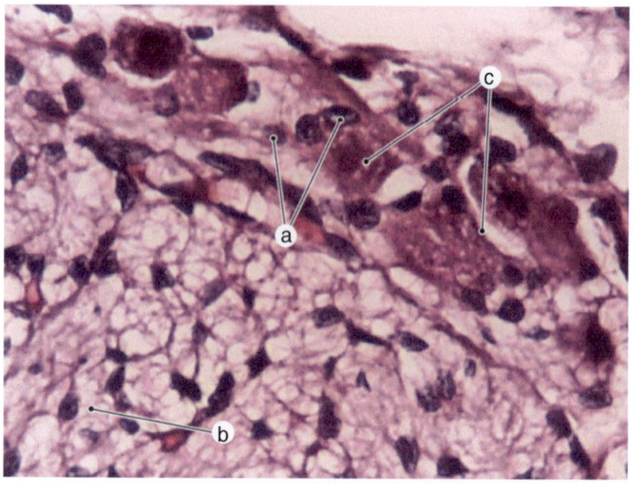

Fig. 9.3 Subepicardial ganglion in relation with the ventricular myocardium. *a* satellite cells nuclei, *b* myocardium, *c* neurons

cutaneous spinothalamic fibers. These fibers transmit the information into cerebral areas corresponding to a cutaneous territory.

- *Medullar facilitation process*: pain impulses from a suffering organ diminish the excitability threshold of the surrounding somatic neurons and the somatic sensitivity arrived at these neurons, even under the pain threshold, is transmitted to the superior centers and misinterpreted as peripheral pain.
- *Cortical facilitation process*: visceral pain projections on the cerebral cortex permit reception of cutaneous impulses under the pain threshold as false pain sensations.
  - *Visceral pain of cardiac origin has an important biological significance*. It may be accompanied by somatic and vegetative reflexes as well as relevant mood disorders. At times these may be the only signs of cardiac illness.

    We emphasize that cardiac activity is under the influence of the carotid glomus regulating reflexes (there are other glomic structures, such as those in the mediastinum and pelvis that may indirectly modify the heart function).

At the end of these comments, we stress that direct links between vegetative nerve fibers and P cells have never been reported. Furthermore, neuromuscular junctions between extrinsic innervation and "working" cardiomyocytes have never been described in literature. Amyelinic nerve fibers belonging to both sympathetic and parasympathetic end in the vicinity of the myocytes (*Gray's anatomy, ed. 37, pg. 558*).

9.2 Parasympathetic Innervation

The effector structures influenced by vegetative fibers are: the atrial and ventricular myocardium, the nodes of the conducting tissue and the coronary vessels muscles.

The cardiac nervous plexus at the base of the heart receives both sympathetic and parasympathetic fibers. The plexus lies around the great vessels and may be described in terms of a superficial component (between the aortic arch and the pulmonary trunk) (Figs. 9.1 and 9.2) and a deep component around the inferior vena cava and posterior to the ascending aorta. The plexus also contains ganglion cells generally considered *paravisceral and intramural parasympathetic ganglia.*

An intramural nervous network (that also contains subepicardial ganglion cells) exists and is organized in a subendocadial plexus, an intramyocardial plexus and a subendocardial one.

The parasympathetic innervation is realized by the cardiac cervical rami (1–2 rami) and the thoracic cardiac rami (3–4 rami) of both the vagus nerves. The right vagal rami (Fig. 5.31) reach the plexus in its superficial part and *the rami of the left vagus* reach the plexus in the deep part. *The superior cardiac cervical nerves* derive from the vagus inferior to the inferior ganglion of the vagus (Ranga, Head and Neck). *The inferior cardiac vagal rami* derive from the reccurent laryngeal nerve.

The first parasympathetic motor neuron is found in the dorsal nucleus of the vagus and in the vicinity of the ambiguus nucleus (*Gray's anatomy, ed. 39, pg. 1019*). The second parasympathetic motor neuron is found in the paravisceral and intramural ganglia (Figs. 8.76, 8.77, 8.78, 8.79, 8.80 and 8.81).

Parasympathetic action slows the heart. In literature, vagal action on the coronary arteries is in discussion. Some authors consider that the coronary arteries have no parasympathetic innervation while some consider that the vagal fibers have either a constricting or a dilating effect on the vessels (*Gray's anatomy, ed.39, pg. 1019*). We consider that there are insufficient studies on the parasympathetic innervation, and the results reflect the authors' opinions rather than scientific argumentation.

9.3 Sympathetic Innervation

The sympathetic innervation is realized by the *superior, middle and inferior cervical cardiac nerves* as well as by three to four thoracic cardiac nerves.

The cervical cardiac neurons have the first neuron in the lateral horn of the spinal cord (T1). The second neuron is in the three sympathetic cervical ganglia, the nerves being in fact formed by *postganglionic rami.*

The superior cervical cardiac nerve has its origin in the sympathetic superior cervical ganglion (C2–C4). It is the only strictly efferent cardiac nerve (*Gray's anatomy, ed. 39*). *The rest of the cardiac nerves are mixed nerves, the afferent fibers reaching the posterior and lateral horns of the spinal cord.*

The middle cervical cardiac nerve has its origin in the sympathetic middle cervical ganglion (C5–C6).

The inferior cervical cardiac nerve has its origin in the sympathetic stellate ganglion (C7–T2, T3).

The thoracic cardiac nerves have the first neuron in the lateral horn of the medullar gray matter, in the intermediolateral column (T3–T5, cardioaccelatory center) and *the second neuron* in the first four sympathetic ganglia of the thoracic paravertebral chain. These also are mixed nerves (sensitive fibers reaching the posterior medullar horns). Postganglionic nerve fibers form in fact *the so-called thoracic cardiac nerves* that reach the cardiac plexus.

From the cardiac plexus, the nerve branches form plexuses around the coronary arteries and their branches. From *the periarterial plexuses*, nerve filaments reach the atrial and ventricular myocardium and the nodes of the conducting tissue (Figs. 9.1 and 9.2).

We stress that *the arterial wall has a very dense sensitive innervation*, its injury being followed by intense pain and reflex manifestations (vomit, cold sweat, cardiac rhythm disturbances, anxiety).

9.4 The Adrenergic and Cholinergic Receptors in the Myocardium [2, 5]

9.4.1 The Sympathetic Component

The sympathetic innervation reaches the conducting system and the cardiomyocytes. *The neurotransmitter involved is norepinephrine.* Its binding with the receptor activates a chain of reactions whose finality is the modification of cardiac function.

Besides norepinephrine, the main neurotransmitter of the sympathetic system, in the heart *co-neurotransmitters can be found.* Among these are:

- *Adenosine* acts as a norepinephrine inhibitor, slows the heart rate, and has vasodilator and antiarrhythmic effects.
- *Neuropeptide Y* is the most abundant peptide in the heart. It inhibits catecholamine release and modulates the vasoconstrictor effect of norepinephrine. It has a vasoconstrictor effect on the coronary vessels. It may inhibit the response of the sinus and atrioventricular nodes to vagal stimulation.

Sympathetic activation produces a short and reduced coronary vasoconstriction, mediated by the *alfa 1 adrenoreceptors*. This is followed by production of mediators that cause vasodilation due to the activation of *beta 1 receptors*. The global effect is coronary vasodilation, elevation in heart rate and contractility, in spite of the short period of vasoconstriction. *This phenomenon is called functional sympatholysis.*

Adrenergic receptors are in fact activated by two agonists: the classic neurotransmitter of the sympathetic system – *norepinephrine*, and the circulating hormone – *epinephrine* (produced by the adrenal medulla).

Alfa and beta adrenergic receptors are found in the heart.

The most important is the *beta 1 receptor*, which if activated by agonists, produces a rise in heart rate (chronotropic effect), in the speed of conduction (dromotrope effect) and in the myocyte relaxation rate (lusitrope effect).

Activation of the *beta 2 receptors* by agonists has similar effects with beta 1 receptors activation, and their activation becomes significant in heart failure.

Stimulation of alfa 1 receptors by the two sympathetic agonists produces a light inotropic effect.

9.4.2 The Parasympathetic Component

The parasympathetic innervation reaches the conducting system and the atrial myocardium. The neurotransmitter involved is acetylcholine, which is an agonist for muscarinic receptors.

Acetylcholine is the main parasympathetic neurotransmitter. There are *two types of cholinergic receptors*:

- *Muscarinic* – is the main type, and can be found at the level of cardiac effector cells;
- *Nicotinic* – can be found in the postganglionic neurons.

Cholinergic co-neurotransmitters exist:

- *Intestinal vasoactive peptide* – elevates the heart rate efficiently;
- *Somatostatin* – slows the heart rate;
- *Substance P* – a vasodilator.
- *Nitric oxide* – a coronary dilator.

Parasympathetic stimulation of the heart has a low coronary dilation effect, slows the heart rate and lowers contractility. As a consequence, if the effect lasts, the reduction in oxygen demand will lead eventually, through metabolic mechanisms, to vasoconstriction.

Binding of choline with the muscarinic receptor M2 (myocardial specific receptor) has negative dromotrope, chronotrope, lusitrope and inotrope effects in the atria (these effects are scarce in the ventricles.

The vegetative nervous pathways also have pre-junctional receptors. Thus, the prejunctional alfa 2 receptor inhibits the norepinephrine release and the prejunctional beta 2 receptor facilitates norepinephrine release. The prejunctional M2 receptor inhibits acetylcholine release.

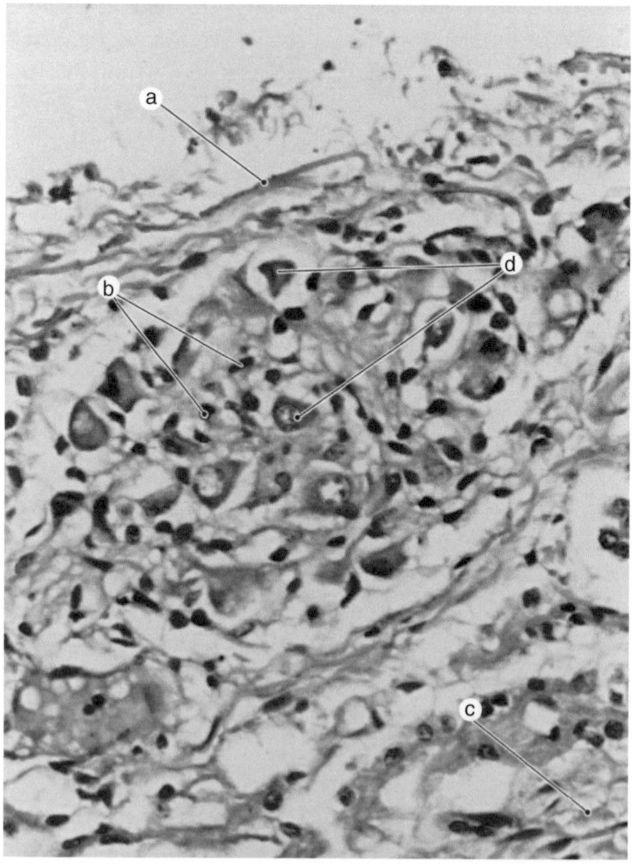

Fig. 9.4 Subepicardial ganglion, in relation with the atrial myocardium. Notice the abundant periganglionic connective fibers. Consequencial, superficial acute inflammations and subepicardial fibrosis will legitimately affect the activity of these nerve structures with logical effects on cardiac function. *a* epicardium, *b* satellite cells nuclei, *c* myocardium, *d* neurons

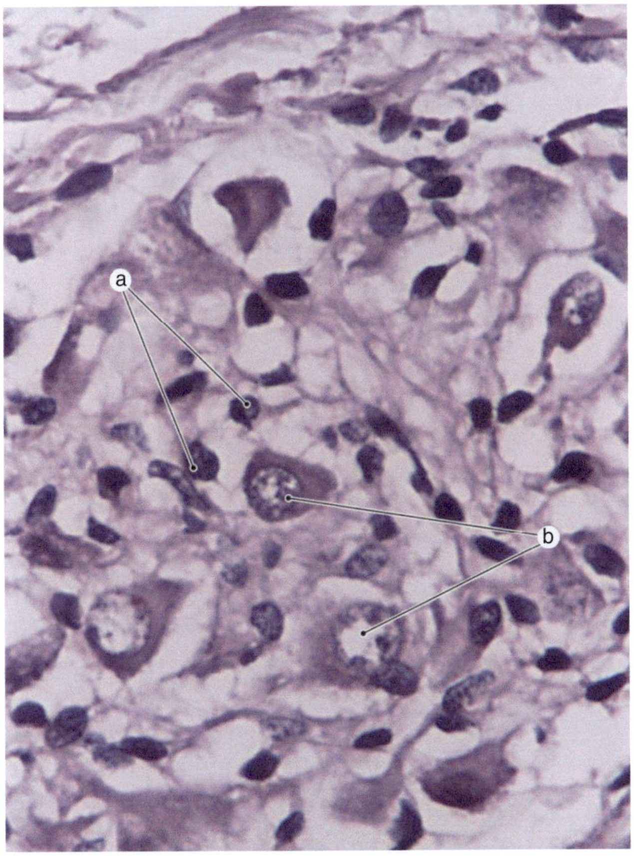

Fig. 9.5 Previous image detail indicating the presence of many satellite intraganglionar cells. Their function is unknown. *a* satellite cells nuclei, *b* neurons

9.5 Adrenergic and Cholinergic Receptors at the Level of the Coronary Arteries

9.5.1 The Sympathetic Component [3]

The coronary vessels have both alpha and beta adrenergic receptors. Coronary flow adaptation results from the interaction of the activation of these two subtypes of receptors.

Stimulation of the coronary alpha receptors produces vasoconstriction. There are two subtypes of alpha adrenergic receptors: alpha 1 and alpha 2. These receptors are localized at the level of the smooth muscle fibers of the vessels. Alpha 1receptors are found mostly in larger caliber vessels while alpha 2 receptors are found in the arterioles. Alpha 2 receptors are also found at the level of the endothelial cells, where their activation leads to nitric oxide production and subsequent vasodilation (indirect effect of alpha 2 stimulation).

Stimulation of coronary beta receptors produces vasodilation. There are three subtypes of receptors: beta 1, beta 2 and beta 3. Large caliber vessels have fewer beta receptors while at the levels of the arterioles, beta receptors are much more numerous.

9.5.2 The Parasympathetic Component [4, 5]

Parasympathetic stimulation leads to the release of acetylcholine which activates the muscarinic receptors M3 at the level of the coronary endothelium (smooth muscle fiber of vessel wall specific receptors). Activation of this receptor in the case of normal endothelium leads to nitric oxide production and subsequent vasodilation. The nitric oxide mediated vasodilation effect is in part counteracted by a direct effect of

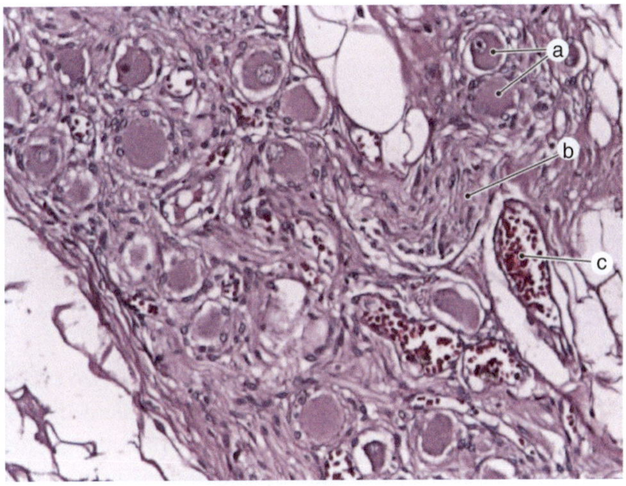

Fig. 9.6 Subepicardial nervous ganglion located at the top of the terminal sulcus. Notice the large number of intraganglionar neurons. *a* neurons, *b* bundle of nerve fibers, *c* venule

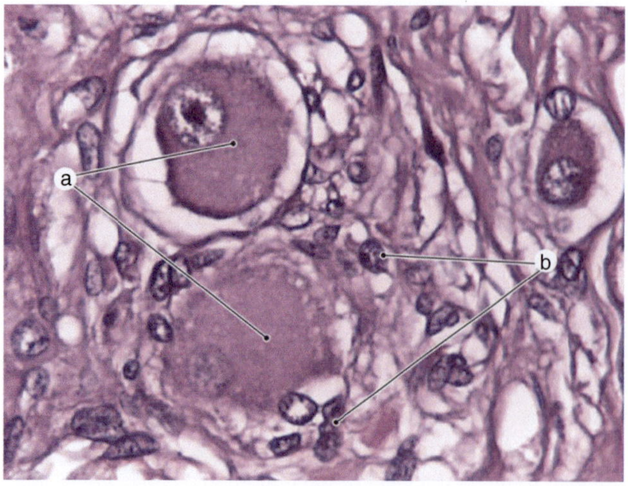

Fig. 9.7 Detail of several intraganglionar neurons. Notice the large number of satellite cells. *a* neurons, *b* satellite cells nuclei

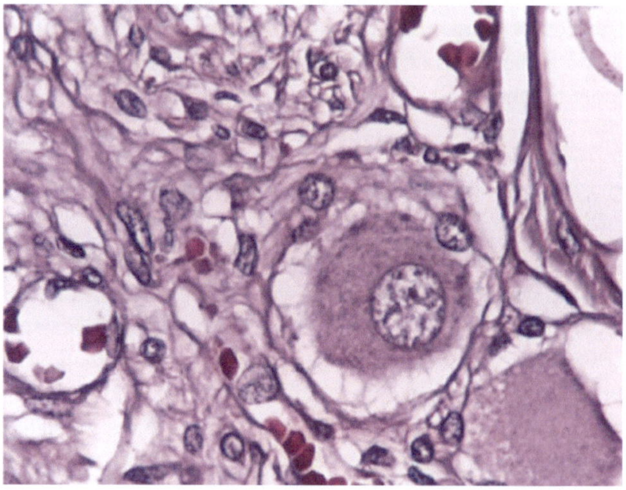

Fig. 9.8 Detail of an intraganglionar neuron. Such large neurons, spherical, located near the sinoatrial node, suggest an important involvement of the extrinsic innervation in the nodal activity

M3 activation at the level of the smooth coronary muscle that leads to vasoconstriction.

The direct effect of vasoconstriction is dominant in the presence of endothelial dysfunction.

In the heart, numerous *non-adrenergic*, *non-cholinergic transmitters* have been found: opioids, neurotensin, and a peptide called histidine-isoleucine. Their actions haven't been sufficiently defined.

The myocardium also produces *endocrine factors* that regularize the activity of the cardiac nervous system. These are: the atrial natriuretic peptide and the brain natriuretic peptide. They also have natriuretic and diuretic effects and inhibit the renin angiotensin aldosterone system.

References

1. Andronescu A. Anatomia funcţională a SNC, Ed. Didactică şi Pedagogică, Bucuresti; 1979.
2. Mohrman DE, Heller LJ. Cardiovascular physiology, 7th edn. McGraw–Hill Prof Med /Tech; New York 2010.
3. Barbato E. Role of adrenergic receptors in human coronary vasomotion. Heart. 2008;95:603–8.
4. Lanzer P, Topol EJ. Pan vascular medicine: integrated clinical management. Heidelberg: Springer; 2002.
5. Klabunde RE. Cardiovascular physiology concepts. Philadelphia: Lippincott Williams & Wilkins; 2005.

Projection of the Heart, Pericardium and the Cardiac Auscultation Sites

10

10.1 The Projection of the Pericardium

The projection of the pericardium has a rectangular shape with convex borders, obtained by uniting four points:

- The right superior point is on the superior margin of the second right rib, two centimeters from the sternum.
- The right inferior point is on the superior margin of the seventh rib, two centimeters from the sternum.
- The left superior point is marked by the first left chondrosternal joint.
- The left inferior point is found in the fifth left intercostal space on the midclavicular line.

Some *comments* are required: the pericardium ascends on the superior vena cava up to the opening of the arch of the azygos vein.

The pericardium ascends on the pulmonary artery following an oblique line that passes under the bifurcation of the pulmonary trunk. This oblique line then reaches the aorta up close to the origin of the brachiocephalic artery.

10.2 The Projection of the Pleural Recesses

The projection of the costomediastinal pleural recesses partially covers the anterior pericardium and projects on the anterior thoracic wall forming two triangles (Fig. 5.7):

- *The superior triangle called the "thymic triangle"* points downward towards the sternal angle and has its base upwards at the jugular notch.
- *The inferior triangle called "pericardial"* points upwards towards the fourth chondrosternal joints and has its base downwards at the xiphoid process. The lateral borders are formed by the margins of the costomediastinal pleural recesses. In the area of this triangle, the pericardium has direct, unmediated contact with the sternocostal wall.

This pericardial triangle has a "*costal*" part, where the pericardium is not covered by the sternum. The medial margin of this part is the left margin of the sternum, between the fourth and sixth left sternocostal joints. The lateral margin is the border of the left costomediastinal recess, which in the fifth left intercostal space is 1 cm lateral to the sternum and in the sixth left intercostal space is 2 cm lateral to the sternum. This pericardial "costal" trigon can be used for cardiac puncture, in the fourth or fifth left intercostal space, entering perpendicularly and grazing the sternum (in order to avoid injury to the internal thoracic artery, which passes 1 cm lateral to the sternum).

The pericardial puncture is made in the space between the xiphoid process and the left costal margin, with the needle oriented obliquely and upwards.

Due to the interposing costomediastinal pleural recesses, the projection of the heart obtained by percussion is enclosed in the so-called *relative cardiac dullness area*.

This area has a smaller surface than the pericardial projection and is formed by uniting four points:

- *the superior right point* is marked by the third right chondrosternal joint (the third right rib 2 cm lateral to the sternum)
- *the inferior right point* is marked by the sixth right chondrosternal joint (the sixth right rib lateral to the sternum)
- *the superior left point* is in the second left intercostal space, 2 cm lateral to the sternum.
- *the inferior left point* is in the fifth intercostal space on the midclavicular line.

The absolute cardiac dullness area is contained by the relative dullness area. Here the heart comes into direct contact with the thoracic wall. This area also has a triangular shape and can be obtained by uniting three points. *The vertex* of this triangular area corresponds to the fourth left sternocostal joint, the inferior right point corresponds to the sixth right sternocostal joint and the inferior left point corresponds to the fifth left intercostal space, 2–3 cm lateral to the sternum (Fig. 10.1).

F.M. Filipoiu, *Atlas of Heart Anatomy and Development*,
DOI 10.1007/978-1-4471-5382-5_10, © Springer-Verlag London 2014

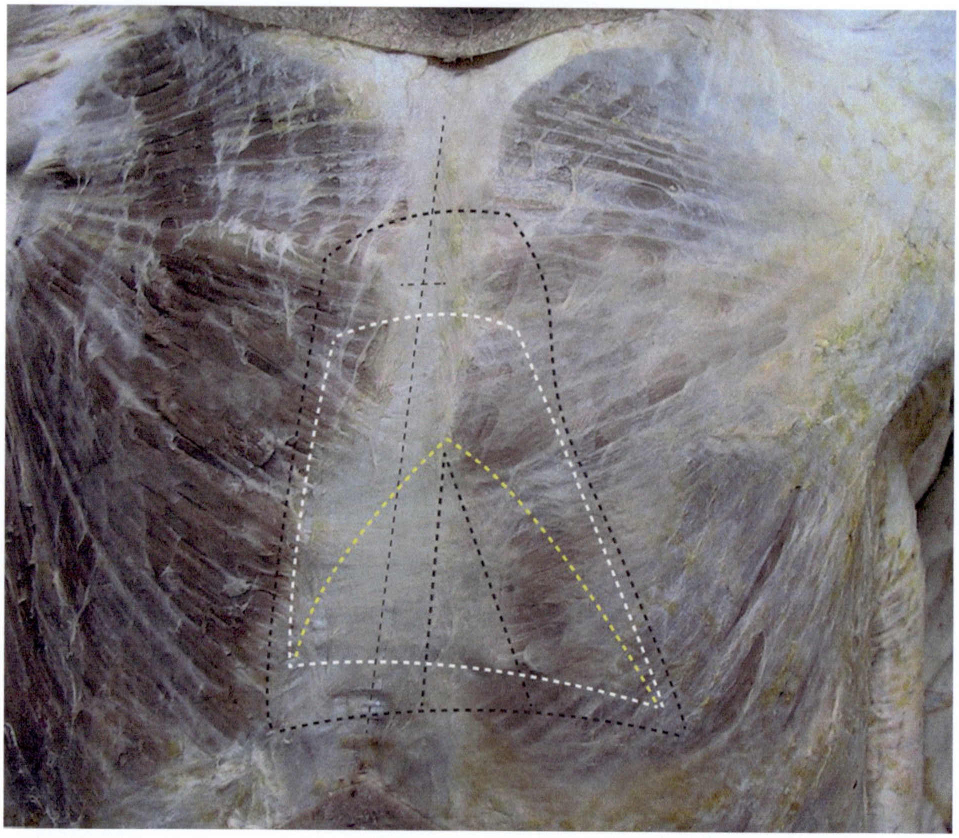

Fig. 10.1 The largest area represents the pericardial projection. The *dotted white line* delineates the relative dullness of the heart. The *yellow dotted line* delineates the absolute dullness cardiac area. The *inner triangle* represents the "pericardial costal triangle" useful during pericardial puncture

10.3 The Projection of the Heart Orifices and Auscultation Sites

The projection of the cardiac orifices is relative. With consideration to anatomic tradition, we reproduce the projections:

- *the mitral orifice* is projected on the left margin of the sternum, in the third intercostal space. Its axis is on the line that unites the extremity of the third intercostal space with the extremity of the fourth right intercostal space.
- *the tricuspid orifice* is projected on the inferior half of the line that unites the extremity of the fourth left intercostal space with the extremity of the sixth right intercostal space.
- *the aortic orifice* is projected on a transversal line that passes through the extremity of the third left intercostal space. Only a third of the long axis of this orifice extends to the left of the sternal margin.
- *the pulmonary orifice* is projected on a transverse line that passes through the third left sternocostal joint. Only a half of the long axis of this orifice extends to the left of the sternal margin.

The auscultation sites are regions where through auscultation we have the best perception of cardiac sounds. These sites don't correspond with the projection of the respective orifices due to the physical characteristics of sound transmission.

The projection of the auscultation sites is:

- *the mitral focus* is in the fifth left intercostal space on the midclavicular line;
- *the tricuspid focus* at the apex of the sternum, right on the sternum:
- *the pulmonary focus* is in the second left intercostal space, lateral to the sternum.
- *the aortic focus* is in the second right intercostal space, lateral to the sternum.

On the vertebral column, the heart corresponds to T6–T8.

Index

F.M. Filipoiu, *Atlas of Heart Anatomy and Development*,
DOI 10.1007/978-1-4471-5382-5, © Springer-Verlag London 2014

D

E

MIX
Papier aus verantwortungsvollen Quellen
Paper from responsible sources
FSC® C105338

If you have any concerns about our products,
you can contact us on
ProductSafety@springernature.com

In case Publisher is established outside the EU,
the EU authorized representative is:
Springer Nature Customer Service Center GmbH
Europaplatz 3, 69115 Heidelberg, Germany

Printed by Libri Plureos GmbH
in Hamburg, Germany